THE DIRECTORY OF

Ethnic Minority Professionals in Psychology

FOURTH EDITION

Compiled and Edited by
The Office of Ethnic Minority Affairs
Sherry T. Wynn
Bertha G. Holliday, PhD

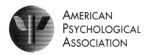

AMERICAN
PSYCHOLOGICAL
ASSOCIATION

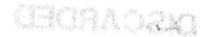

ISBN: 1-55798-824-2

Copies may be ordered from:
APA Order Department
P.O. Box 92984
Washington, DC 20090-2984

Printed in the United States of America

In Memory Of

DALMAS A. TAYLOR, PhD
September 9, 1933–January 26, 1998
Scholar, Activist, and Founding Director
of the APA Minority Fellowship Program

and

LOGAN WRIGHT, PhD
December 6, 1933–December 18, 1999
Psychologist, Osage Indian, and
Former President of the
American Psychological Association

"Always mindful of the shoulders on which we stand..."

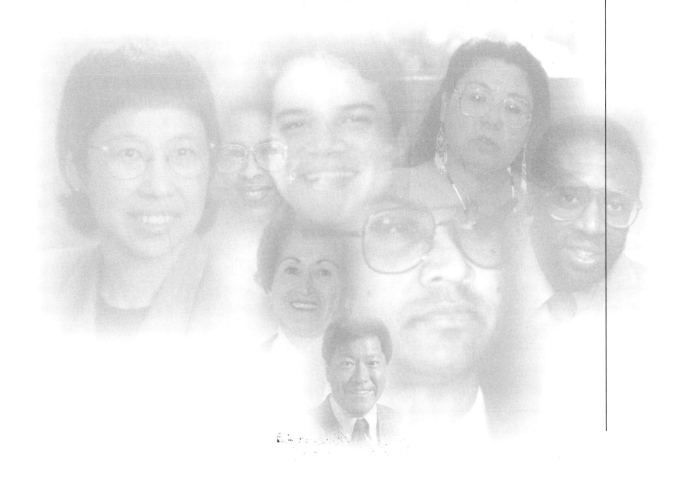

Table 1

Geographical Distribution of Ethnic Minority Professionals in Psychology In The Year 2000

STATE	ETHNIC GROUP						TOTAL	PERCENT
	African American/Black	American Indian/ Alaska Native	Asian American/ Pacific Islander	Hispanic/Latino(a)	Multi-Ethnic	Unknown[a]		
Alabama	8	0	4	5	1	0	18	0.75%
Alaska	1	2	0	1	0	0	4	0.17%
Arizona	4	0	8	15	0	0	27	1.12%
Arkansas	1	0	0	1	0	0	2	0.08%
California	120	12	167	176	13	0	488	20.28%
Colorado	7	3	16	22	2	0	50	2.08%
Connecticut	10	0	7	6	1	0	24	1.00%
Delaware	4	0	1	1	0	0	6	0.25%
District of Columbia	44	1	7	8	1	0	61	2.54%
Florida	24	2	9	90	1	0	126	5.24%
Georgia	42	2	7	10	1	0	62	2.58%
Hawaii	1	1	43	3	0	0	48	2.00%
Idaho	0	0	0	0	0	0	0	0.00%
Illinois	34	3	24	25	1	0	87	3.62%
Indiana	14	0	7	5	1	0	27	1.12%
Iowa	3	1	4	3	0	0	11	0.46%
Kansas	1	0	2	0	0	0	3	0.12%
Kentucky	2	1	3	2	0	0	8	0.33%
Louisiana	9	3	5	1	0	0	18	0.75%
Maine	1	0	0	1	0	0	2	0.08%
Maryland	49	5	18	18	2	0	92	3.82%
Massachusetts	32	2	20	30	4	0	88	3.66%
Michigan	45	3	15	13	0	0	76	3.16%
Minnesota	8	2	12	3	1	0	26	1.08%
Mississippi	0	0	1	1	1	0	3	0.12%
Missouri	11	3	5	4	1	0	24	1.00%
Montana	0	3	1	1	0	0	5	0.21%
Nebraska	1	1	1	2	0	0	5	0.21%

Table 1 Continued

STATE	ETHNIC GROUP						TOTAL	PERCENT
	African American/Black	American Indian/ Alaska Native	Asian American/ Pacific Islander	Hispanic/Latino(a)	Multi-Ethnic	Unknown[a]		
Nevada	0	4	2	4	0	0	10	0.42%
New Hampshire	0	1	2	1	0	0	4	0.17%
New Jersey	40	1	15	26	1	0	83	3.45%
New Mexico	2	0	3	11	2	0	18	0.75%
New York	86	3	38	70	5	0	202	8.40%
North Carolina	19	1	4	6	1	0	31	1.29%
North Dakota	0	0	1	0	0	0	1	0.04%
Ohio	27	3	19	9	0	0	58	2.41%
Oklahoma	0	9	0	2	0	0	11	0.46%
Oregon	2	1	7	4	0	0	14	0.58%
Pennsylvania	33	2	17	24	1	0	77	3.20%
Puerto Rico	0	0	0	55	1	0	56	2.33%
Rhode Island	5	1	2	3	1	0	12	0.50%
South Carolina	9	1	2	0	0	0	12	0.50%
South Dakota	0	1	0	0	0	0	1	0.04%
Tennessee	17	1	4	6	1	0	29	1.21%
Texas	26	9	25	57	1	0	118	4.90%
Utah	0	1	3	6	0	0	10	0.42%
Vermont	1	0	1	0	1	0	3	0.12%
Virgin Islands	2	0	0	2	1	0	5	0.21%
Virginia	33	4	14	11	2	0	64	2.66%
Washington	5	8	28	10	2	0	53	2.20%
West Virginia	2	1	2	1	0	0	6	0.25%
Wisconsin	7	3	5	10	1	0	26	1.08%
Wyoming	0	0	0	2	0	0	2	0.08%
Foreign Country	7	2	77	22	1	0	109	4.53%
No Information	0	0	0		0	0		0.00%
TOTALS	799	107	658	789	53	0	2406	100.00%
PERCENT	33.21%	4.45%	27.35%	32.79%	2.20%	0.00%	100.00	

a - "Unknown" indicates persons who did not identify an ethnic group.

TABLE OF CONTENTS

LIST OF TABLES

FOREWORD

In this Year 2001, we stand on the precipice of wonder. And from this vantage point we can only vaguely comprehend the forthcoming radical transformations in our understanding of human behavior and its potential, the breadth of its diversity, and its remarkable adaptability and resilience. Such new knowledge of human behavior will be engendered not only by the new technology epitomized by computers and biotechnology, but even more profoundly by the global mobility of racial/ethnic groups, the increasing multiple and uncontrolled intersections of cultures and their knowledges, and the concomitant de-hegemonization of "whiteness" as a racial/social/political concept. Thus the ensuing transformations of our behavioral knowledge are inevitable outcomes of the de-colonization and liberation movements of the twentieth century.

In the face of such transformations, notions such as "normative patterns of development and behavior", "standardized tests of achievement", "acculturation", and "mental health" are undergoing rapid erosion of their core meanings. Concerns for norms and standards increasingly are rivaled by demands for behavioral and intellectual flexibility and breadth. Fundamental questions related to the integrity of the assumed behavioral boundaries of humans and their institutions are emerging. Confronted with the prospect of truly free and open intellectual, cultural, political and economic marketplaces, we increasingly recognize that things must be re-thought.

Wonder is not readily understood. On topics of human behavior, psychologists are recognized experts. Thus, hopefully, psychologists will seek to be at the center of research and innovations related to both transforming our understanding of human behavior, and more effectively promoting human potential. Changing the face of psychology, through the inclusion of a large cadre of culturally diverse psychologists and psychologists skilled in understanding, interacting, and conducting research with culturally diverse individuals and communities, will be critical to the success of such efforts.

From this perspective, the ethnic minority members of the American Psychological Association (APA) comprise a major national treasure. In 1999, 4,471 APA members self-identified as ethnic minorities (i.e., as African-American/Black, American Indian/Alaska Native, Asian American/Pacific Islander, Hispanic/Latino[a]). This represented 5.3% of all APA members, as well as a 19% increase since 1993 in the number of ethnic minority members of APA. These 4,471 persons constitute the largest organized group of behavioral scientists of color in the world and represent a critical link in shaping a more global perspective of human behavior.

This *Fourth Edition of the Directory of Ethnic Minority Professionals in Psychology* will hopefully serve as a major guide for identifying the nation's ethnic minority psychologists. This *Fourth Edition...* includes updated and expanded information on **2406 psychologists of color who are members of APA.** Thus, 53.7% of all self-identified ethnic minority members of APA provided information for inclusion in this Directory. Significant efforts were made to ensure the Directory's comprehensiveness and accuracy. In April 1998, a special computerized database matching routine was conducted between persons who self-identified as ethnic minority on the APA membership database and all persons with current addresses (i.e., postmaster had not returned mail) on the database maintained by APA's Office of Ethnic Minority Affairs(OEMA). These two databases also were matched on a computerized address search-and-comparison routine for those persons whose addresses were known to not be current in the OEMA database. When updated addresses were present in the APA membership database, these were entered into the OEMA database. A month later, in May 1998, all ethnic minority persons on the APA membership database who were <u>not</u> listed on the OEMA database were forwarded a letter describing the uses of the OEMA database, and requesting completion and return of the recipient's vita along with an attached "Biosketch" form, which is used for obtaining permission and data for entry into the OEMA database. A total of 2,092 such letters were mailed. Later, individual printouts of all "Biosketch" information in the OEMA database were prepared for review and update by each person with a current or updated address in the OEMA database. A total of over 2,500 of these printouts were mailed in September 1998 along with a request for an updated vita.

Throughout the latter half of 1998 and all of 1999, notices were repeatedly placed in the APA's monthly newspaper, *The Monitor,* and in the semi-annual OEMA newsjournal, *The Communique,* announcing the preparation of the *Fourth Edition...* and encouraging persons to request, update or complete, and return "Biosketch" forms. Data entry proceeded throughout 1999. To minimize variability in systematic error in data entry, all returned "Biosketches" were entered into the OEMA database by a single technician.

During the first quarter of the year 2000, the OEMA database was subjected to extensive and repeated manual and electronic proofing and text editing. Systematic glitches in the database and its Directory format were identified and corrected by staff of APA's Management Information Systems Office. In March, APA's Public Communication's Office was asked to initiate cover and book design efforts. In May 2000, the Directory text was downloaded into Page Maker format as requested by the publisher. This involved additional proofing and text editing. In February 2001, a camera ready and electronic copy of the Directory were submitted to APA Books for publication.

Thus the *Fourth Edition...* consists of all known ethnic minority APA members who submitted a "Biosketch" since May, 1998, or who submitted revisions to a printout of their OEMA database information as of September, 1999, or who were listed in the OEMA database as of September 1998 with a current address. Despite the great care that was taken in preparing the *Fourth Edition...*, we are certain that errors are present. OEMA updates its database continuously. So, in the event you note such errors, or wish to update information, or desire to be included in the Directory's next edition, please contact APA's Office of Ethnic Minority Affairs (email: oema@apa.org). A copy of the "Biosketch" form is available on the web for downloading: Go to OEMA's homepage (www.apa.org/pi/oema) and click on "Publications".

In terms of the real work of compiling this *Fourth Edition...* all accolades and all glory should be give to OEMA's Program Associate, Ms. Sherry T. Wynn. Ms. Wynn is the keeper of OEMA's database: She does all the data entry, produces all of its reports and tables; she keeps the database clean and identifies any glitches in its programming. She identifies needed revisions to the "Biosketch" form and coordinates any required database matching routines. She orchestrated the printout of individual database information, coordinated the various mailings required to ensure a comprehensive update of database information, and single-handedly addressed the tedious work of repeated manual and electronic proofing and text editing of the Directory's text. She did all this with great professionalism and high competence, while maintaining a full load of other job responsibilities. Consequently, Ms. Wynn is the designated first editor of the *Fourth Edition...*

OEMA is committed to providing high quality services and products. We welcome your suggestions for improving the Directory's utility and design.

Bertha G. Holliday, PhD
Director
Office of Ethnic Minority Affairs
American Psychological Association
Washington, DC
February 1, 2001

DIRECTORY USER'S GUIDE

The *Fourth Edition of the Directory of Ethnic Minority Professionals in Psychology* is designed as a user-friendly reference -- with special attention accorded the networking and information needs of APA Divisions (representing various sub-disciplines and special interests), State Psychological Associations, and the nation's four major communities of color (i.e., African American/Black, American Indian/Alaska Native, Asian American/Asian/Pacific Islander, and Hispanic/Latino[a]). In addition, the Directory may be used as an employment recruitment tool, for identifying consultants and speakers, and for research and marketing purposes. (Please note: those interested in extensive employment recruitment searches and access to mailing labels should consider use of OEMA's Job Bank Search service.)

The Directory is divided into the following six (6) major sections.

1. **MASTER ALPHABETICAL LISTING:** This section is the **comprehensive listing of information for each person** listed in the directory, with entries alphabetically arranged by last name. Whenever sufficient data were provided, each listing includes the following information.

    - *Name*
    - *Address* (street, city, state, country)
    - *Telephone and facsimile numbers*
    - *E-mail address*
    - *Ethnicity*
    - *Language capabilities*
    - *Type and year of highest graduate or professional degree(s)*
    - *Major field*
    - *Specialty areas*

2. **ETHNIC GROUP LISTING: Names** of psychologists are listed by **ethnic group** membership. Four major ethnic groups are identified: (a)African American/Black, (b) American Indian/Alaska Native, (c) Asian American /Asian/Pacific Islander, and (d) Hispanic/Latino (who may be of any race). The names of persons who identified themselves as a member of two ethnic/racial groups are listed under a fifth category ("Multi-Ethnic"), with a notation of the ethnic/racial groups in which membership is claimed. Information in this section is ordered as follows.

    - *Ethnic Group* (and under each:)
        Names (alphabetized)

3. **GEOGRAPHICAL LISTING:** In this section, the **names** of psychologists of color are listed by **foreign country of domicile** or **U.S. State or Possession of residence**, and within these categories, by **ethnic group**. Information in this section is ordered as follows.

- *Foreign Countries* (alphabetized and under each:)
    Ethnic Group (and under each:)
        Names (alphabetized)

- *U.S. States* (alphabetized and under each:)
    Ethnic Group (and under each:)
        Names (alphabetized)

4. **DIVISION LISTING:** APA members may voluntarily affiliate with one or more of APA's 53 Divisions (representing subdisciplines, specialty areas, or special interests). In this section, the **names** of those psychologists of color who are affiliated with one or more divisions are listed by **division** and by **ethnic group**. Individuals claiming membership in more than one division and/or ethnic group are listed under <u>all</u> membership categories claimed. Information in this section is ordered as follows:

- *Divisions* (numerically ordered and under each:)
    Ethnic Group (and under each:)
        Names (alphabetized)

5. **DIVISION FELLOW LISTING:** This is a new section for the *Directory*. Qualified APA members may, on nomination by an APA division and election by the APA Council of Representatives, become Fellows of the APA. Fellows must "...present evidence of unusual or outstanding contribution or performance in the field of psychology". In this section, the **names** of those psychologists of color who have reported "fellow" status with one or more divisions are listed by **division** and by **ethnic group**. Information in this section is ordered as follows:

- *Divisions* (numerically ordered and under each:)
    Ethnic Group (and under each:)
        Names (alphabetized)

6.   **MAJOR FIELD AND PROFESSIONAL ROLE LISTING:** For survey purposes, APA recognizes 21 major fields. In addition, the OEMA "Biosketch" form asks persons to identify their major professional roles -- that is, academician, administrator, consultant, practitioner, researcher or "other". In this section, **names** are listed by **major field** and **major professional role**, and this information is ordered as follows.

   - *Major Fields* (alphabetized and under each:)
     Professional Roles (Primary and Secondary and under each:)
     Names (alphabetized)

7.   **LANGUAGE (Non-English) LISTING:** This new section in the *Directory* was developed in response to numerous inquiries to OEMA for names of psychologists in specific geographical locations with specific linguistic capabilities. The "Biosketch" form requests respondents to identify whether they have "Non-English language fluency " in 14 major categories of language and related dialects (i.e., American Sign Language, Arabic, Chinese, Filipino, French, German, Hindi, Italian, Japanese, Korean, Portuguese, Spanish, Urdu, and "Other"). In this section, **names** are listed by **language** and **state of residency,** and this information is order as follows.

   - *Language Categories* (alphabetized and under each:)
     State of Residency (alphabetized and under each:)
     Names

8.   **STATISTICAL PROFILE:** This section consists of narrative highlights and associated statistical tables. These constitute a statistical profile of those psychologists of color listed in the *Fourth Edition.*

Master Alphabetical Listing

CODES USED IN THIS SECTION

B Business Phone Number

H Home Phone Number

F Facsimile (fax) Number

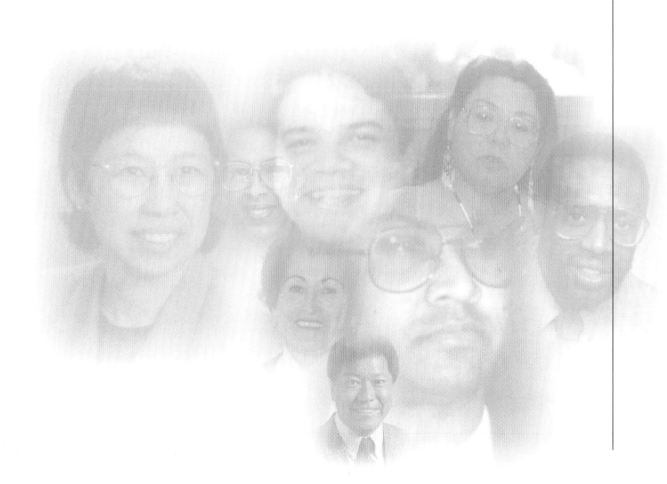

MASTER ALPHABETICAL LISTING

ABELLO, Ana L.
3128 Lakeshore Drive
Deerfield Beach, FL 33442-7977
(305) 537-1194-**B**, (305) 570-7153-**H**
Ethnicity: Hispanic/Latino
Languages: Spanish
Degree and Year: PhD 1989
Major Field: Clinical Psychology
Specialty: Assessment/Diagnosis/Evaluation;Eating Disorders;Stress

ABERCOMBIE, Delrita
137 Garfield Place
Brooklyn, NY 11215
(718) 240-6415-**B**, (718) 260-8921-**H**, (718) 788-0663-**F**
Ethnicity: African-American/Black
Languages: French, Spanish
Degree and Year: PhD 1975
Major Field: Clinical Psychology
Specialty: Assessment/Diagnosis/Evaluation;Clinical
Neuropsychology;School Psychology;Depression;Learning
Disabilities

ABERCROMBIE, Maria M.
9502 Cotesworth Lane
Knoxville, TN 37922-3429
SAME-**B**, (615) 691-2205-**H**
Ethnicity: Hispanic/Latino
Degree and Year: PhD 1983
Major Field: Clinical Psychology
Specialty: Alcoholism & Alcohol Abuse;Adolescent Therapy;Family
Therapy;Marriage & Family;Drug Abuse

ABERNETHY, Alexis D.
Fuller Theological Seminary
Graduate School of Psychology
180 North Oakland Avenue
Pasadena, CA 91101
(626) 584-5359-**B**, (626) 398-9630-**H**, (626) 584-9630-**F**
aabernet@fuller. edu
Ethnicity: African-American/Black
Degree and Year: PhD 1985
Major Field: Clinical Psychology
Specialty: Ethnic Minorities;Stress;Group Psychotherapy

ABORDO, Enrique J.
Porterville Development Center
PO Box 2000
Porterville, CA 93258-2000
(209) 781-0284-**B**
Ethnicity: Hispanic/Latino
Degree and Year: PhD 1971
Major Field: unknown
Specialty: Behavior Therapy;Mental Health Services;Applied Behavior
Analysis;Mentally Retarded

ABRAIDO-LANZA, Ana F
Columbia University
School of Public Health
Division of Sociaomedical Sciences
600 West 168th Street, 7th Floor
New York, NY 10032
(212) 305-1859-**B**, (516) 775-4014-**H**, (212) 305-0315-**F**
afl7@columbia.edu
Ethnicity: Hispanic/Latino
Languages: Spanish
Degree and Year: PhD 1994 MA 1991
Major Field: Health Psychology
Specialty: Health Psychology;Ethnic Minorities;Stress;Pain & Pain
Management;Cultural & Social Processes;Social Psychology

ABSTON, JR., Nathaniel
4811 Henry Road
Eightmile, AL 36613
(205) 415-3940-**B**
Ethnicity: African-American/Black
Degree and Year: PhD 1984
Major Field: Clinical Psychology
Specialty: Clinical Psychology;Alcoholism & Alcohol
Abuse;Gerontology/Geropsychology;Health
Psychology;Ethnic Minorities

ABUDABBEH, Nuha
3000 Connecticut Avenue, NW
Suite #135
Washington, DC 20008
(202) 462-5715-**B**, (202) 234-1765-**H**, (202) 462-7794-**F**
Ethnicity: Asian-American/Asian/Pacific Islander
Languages: Arabic, Turkish
Degree and Year: PhD 1974
Major Field: Counseling Psychology
Specialty: Cross Cultural Processes;Forensic
Psychology;Psychopathology;Psychotherapy

ACKA-POPE, Zeynep K
3413 Grand Forest Drive Apt. C
St. Louis, MO 63033
314/340-3354-**B**, 314/533-4821-**H**
Ethnicity: Asian-American/Asian/Pacific Islander
Languages: German, Turkish
Degree and Year: PhD 1986
Major Field: Counseling Psychology
Specialty: Counseling Psychology;Mental Disorders;Chronically
Mentally Ill;Crisis Intervention & Therapy;Mental Health
Services;Mental Disorders

ACOSTA, Frank X.
USC Department of Psychiatry
1934 Hospital Place
Los Angeles, CA 90033-1071
(213) 226-5350-**B**

Ethnicity: Hispanic/Latino
Degree and Year: PhD 1974
Major Field: Clinical Psychology
Specialty: Clinical Psychology;Community Psychology

ADAMS, JR., Clarence L.
200 W 90th Street
Apartment #12G
New York, NY 10024
(212) 724-6650-**H**
Ethnicity: African-American/Black
Degree and Year: EdD 1972
Major Field: Clinical Psychology

ADAMS-ESQUIVEL, Henry
1643 Sixth Avenue
San Diego, CA 92101-2706
619 232-5628-**B**, (619) 232-0373-**F**
Ethnicity: Hispanic/Latino
Languages: French, Italian, Portuguese, Spanish
Degree and Year: PhD 1979
Major Field: Physiological Psychology
Specialty: Consumer Psychology;Psycholinguistic;Market
   Analysis;Mass Media Communication;Cross Cultural
   Processes

ADAMS, Afesa M.
University of North Florida
Department of Psychology
4567 St. Johns Bluff Road
Jacksonville, FL 32224-2645
(904) 646-2807-**B**, (904) 642-7972-**H**, (904) 642-6891-**F**
Ethnicity: African-American/Black
Degree and Year: PhD 1975
Major Field: Social Psychology
Specialty: Ethnic Minorities;Community Psychology;Cultural & Social
   Processes;Interpersonal Processes & Relations;Family
   Processes

ADAMS, C. Jama
P.O. Box 499
New York, NY 10037
(212) 283-3100-**B**, (212) 947-7111-**H**, (212) 281-7377-**F**
Ethnicity: African-American/Black
Degree and Year: PhD 1986
Major Field: Clinical Psychology
Specialty: Cultural & Social Processes;Child Therapy;Parent
   Education;Assessment/Diagnosis/Evaluation;Adolescent
   Therapy

ADLER, Peter J.
10410 Amestoy Avenue
Granada Hills, CA 91344
(310) 284-4893-**B**, (818) 368-5510-**H**
Ethnicity: Hispanic/Latino
Languages: Spanish, Hungarian
Degree and Year: EdD 1981
Major Field: Educational Psychology
Specialty: Clinical Psychology;Hypnosis/Hypnotherapy;Mentally
   Retarded;Parent Education;Stress

ADVANI, Nisha
Advani Associates
12750 Lika Court
Saratoga, CA 95070-3805

(408) 741-1749-**B**, (408) 741-1450-**H**
nadvani@pacbell.net
Ethnicity: Asian-American/Asian/Pacific Islander
Degree and Year: PhD 1991
Major Field: Social Psychology

AGUILAR, Martha C.
1757 South Pearl
Denver, CO 80210
(303) 765-1248-**B**, (303) 765-1250-**F**
Ethnicity: Hispanic/Latino
Languages: Spanish
Degree and Year: PsyD 1990
Major Field: Clinical Psychology
Specialty: Clinical Psychology;Cross Cultural Processes

AGUILERA, David M.
900 Lafayette Street
Suite #605
Santa Clara, CA 95050-4967
(408) 244-9552-**B**, (408) 244-9552-**F**
Ethnicity: Hispanic/Latino
Degree and Year: PhD 1980 BS 1976
Major Field: Clinical Psychology
Specialty: Clinical Psychology;Clinical Child Psychology;Assessment/
   Diagnosis/Evaluation;Community Mental Health;Crisis
   Intervention & Therapy;Psychotherapy

AGUIRRE-DEANDREIS, Ana I.
6325 Executive Building
Rockville, MD 20852
(301) 571-2324-**B**, (301) 571-1985-**H**, (3010 770-0276-**F**
Ethnicity: Hispanic/Latino
Languages: Spanish
Degree and Year: PhD 1991
Major Field: Clinical Psychology
Specialty: Clinical Psychology;Cross Cultural Processes;Attention
   Deficit Disorders;Assessment/Diagnosis/Evaluation;Parent-
   Child Interaction;Learning Disabilities

AHANA, Ellen
14042 NE 8th Street
Bellevue, WA 98007
(206) 746-3782-**B**, (206) 643-0543-**F**
Ethnicity: Asian-American/Asian/Pacific Islander
Languages: Chinese, Hawaiian
Degree and Year: PhD 1965
Major Field: Clinical Psychology
Specialty: Clinical Psychology;Depression;Health
   Psychology;Psychosomatic Disorders;Psychotherapy

AHMED, Mohiuddin
57 Puddingstone Lane
Bellingham, MA 02019
(401) 766-3330-**B**, (508) 966-1342-**H**
Ethnicity: Asian-American/Asian/Pacific Islander
Languages: Hindi, Bengali
Degree and Year: PhD 1969
Major Field: Clinical Psychology
Specialty: Assessment/Diagnosis/Evaluation;Group
   Psychotherapy;Mental Health Services;Mentally Retarded

AHSEN, Akhter
22 Edgecliff Terrace
Yonkers, NY 10705-1606
(914) 423-5291-**B**

Ethnicity: Asian-American/Asian/Pacific Islander
Degree and Year: PhD 1973
Major Field: Clinical Psychology

AHUJA, Harmeen
3309 North Lakewood
Chicago, IL 60657
(773) 445-1616-B
Ethnicity: Asian-American/Asian/Pacific Islander
Languages: Hindi, Punjabi
Degree and Year: PhD 1994
Major Field: Clinical Psychology
Specialty: Adolescent Development;Clinical Psychology;Adolescent Therapy;Psychotherapy

AI, Amy L.
University of Michigan
1080 South University
Ann Arbor, MI 48109
(734) 786-8472-B, (736) 936-1961-F
Ethnicity: Asian-American/Asian/Pacific Islander
Degree and Year: PhD 1996
Major Field: Gerontology

AINSLIE, Ricardo C.
University of Texas @ Austin
Department of Educational Psychology
Suite EDB-504
Austin, TX 78712
(512) 471-4409-B, (512) 473-2214-H, (512) 471-4607-F
Ethnicity: Hispanic/Latino
Languages: Spanish
Degree and Year: PhD 1979
Major Field: Clinical Psychology
Specialty: Psychoanalysis;Projective Techniques;Counseling Psychology;Individual Psychotherapy;Emotional Development

AKAMATSU, T. John
Kent State University
Department of Psychology
Kent, OH 44242
(330) 672-2048-B, (330) 673-2522-H, (330) 672-3786-F
Ethnicity: Asian-American/Asian/Pacific Islander
Degree and Year: PhD 1972
Major Field: Clinical Psychology
Specialty: Assessment/Diagnosis/Evaluation;Family Therapy;Professional Issues in Psychology;Psychotherapy

AKCA, Zeynep K.
Harris-Stowe State College
Comprehensive Mental Health Center
East St. Louis, IL 62105
(314) 340-3354-B, (314) 533-4821-H, (314) 340-3692-F
akca@email.hssc.edu
Ethnicity: Asian-American/Asian/Pacific Islander, European/White
Languages: German, Turkish
Degree and Year: PhD 1986 MA 1979
Major Field: Counseling Psychology
Specialty: Counseling Psychology;Drug Abuse;Mental Health Services;Mental Disorders;Crisis Intervention & Therapy;Mental Disorders

AKIMOTO, Sharon A
Carleton College
Department of Psychology
Northfield, MN 55057
(507) 646-4503-B, (612) 435-1612-H, (507) 646-7005-F
sakimoto@carleton.edu
Ethnicity: Asian-American/Asian/Pacific Islander
Languages: Japanese
Degree and Year: PhD 1993 MA 1989
Major Field: Social Psychology
Specialty: Ethnic Minorities;Social Cognition

AKIYAMA, M. Michael
University of Michigan-Dearborn
4260 Washtenaw
Ann Arbor, MI 48108-1009
(313) 593-5520-B
Ethnicity: Asian-American/Asian/Pacific Islander
Degree and Year: PhD 1977
Major Field: Developmental Psychology
Specialty: Thought Processes

AKUTAGAWA, Donald
10845 Main Street
Bellevue, WA 98004
(206) 454-8461-B, (206) 747-0472-H
Ethnicity: Asian-American/Asian/Pacific Islander
Languages: Italian
Degree and Year: PhD 1956
Major Field: Clinical Psychology
Specialty: Cognitive Behavioral Therapy;Crisis Intervention & Therapy

AKUTSU, Phillip D.
Pacific Graduate School of Psychology
940 East Meadow Drive
Palo Alto, CA 94303-4233
(650) 843-3541-B, (510) 528-2715-H, (650) 856-6734-F
itj6pda@cmsa.berkeley.edu
Ethnicity: Asian-American/Asian/Pacific Islander
Degree and Year: PhD 1993
Major Field: Clinical Psychology
Specialty: Ethnic Minorities;Community Psychology;Family Processes;Social Problems;Program Evaluation;Mental Health Services

AL-TAI, Nazar M.
4301 Linton Ave, Apt 7
Montreal, PQ H3S1T-5
CANADA
(514) 398-4240-B, (514) 735-7252-H, (514) 398-6968-F
Ethnicity: Asian-American/Asian/Pacific Islander
Languages: Arabic, French
Degree and Year: PhD 1976
Major Field: Educational Psychology
Specialty: Vocational Psychology;Personality Measurement;Industrial/Organizational Psychology;Clinical Psychology;Religious Psychology

ALBERT, Rosita D.
41 Line Street
Apartment #1
Cambridge, MA 02138
(-B, 617/492-6813-H
Ethnicity: Hispanic/Latino
Degree and Year: PhD 1972
Major Field: Social Psychology
Specialty: Communication; Cross Cultural Processes

5

ALDABA-LIM, Estefania
10-C Legaspi Towers 300
Roxas Boulevard
Manila,
PHILIPPINES
(632) 523-1797-**B**, (632) 523-1702-**H**, (632) 522-1246-**F**
nlyuson@globe.com.ph
Ethnicity: Asian-American/Asian/Pacific Islander
Degree and Year: PhD 1942
Major Field: Clinical Psychology

ALDRICH, John W.
Aldrich Associates
265 East Village Road
Shelton, CT 06486
(203) 929-6234-**B**, (203) 929-8035-**H**, (203) 925-0800-**F**
jwaldrich@prodigy.net
Ethnicity: African-American/Black
Degree and Year: MS 1974
Major Field: Industrial/Organizational Psy.
Specialty: Cross Cultural Processes;Industrial/Organizational
Psychology;Management & Organization;Organizational
Development;Training & Development

ALEXANDER, Allen T.
24 Pennington Way
Spring Valley, NY 10977
(212) 873-4867-**B**, (914) 354-2549-**H**
Ethnicity: African-American/Black
Degree and Year: PhD 1976
Major Field: School Psychology
Specialty: Individual Psychotherapy;Assessment/Diagnosis/
Evaluation;Clinical Psychology;Counseling Psychology;School
Psychology

ALEXANDER, Charlene M.
Ball State University
Department of Counseling and
Guidance Service - Room 607
Muncie, IN 47306
(765) 285-8040-**B**, (765) 281-6968-**H**, *765) 285-2067-**F**
cmalexander@bsuvc.bsu.edu
Ethnicity: African-American/Black
Degree and Year: PhD 1992
Major Field: Counseling Psychology
Specialty: Counseling Psychology;Cross Cultural Processes;School
Counseling

ALFARO-GARCIA, Rafael A.
PO Box 3535
Carolina, PR 00984-3535
(787) 768-3368-**B**, (787) 768-3368-**F**
Ethnicity: Hispanic/Latino
Languages: Spanish
Degree and Year: PhD 1983
Major Field: Industrial/Organizational Psy.
Specialty: Industrial/Organizational Psychology;Ethnic
Minorities;Mass Media Communication;Organizational
Development;Leadership

ALLEN-CLAIBORNE, Joyce G.
Dougherty County School, System Psychological
Services/Exceptional Student Program
400 South Monroe Street
PO Box 1470

Albany, GA 31703
(912) 431-3455-**B**
allenclai@aol.com
Ethnicity: African-American/Black
Degree and Year: PhD 1975
Major Field: Clinical Psychology
Specialty: Assessment/Diagnosis/Evaluation;Clinical Psychology;School
Psychology;Child Therapy;Individual Psychotherapy

ALLEN, Christeen
1209 Lark Lane
Fort Washington, MD 20744-6850
(301) 567-0373-**B**, 301 567-7583-**H**, 301 203-0962-**F**
Ethnicity: African-American/Black
Degree and Year: PsyD 1987
Major Field: Clinical Psychology
Specialty: Assessment/Diagnosis/Evaluation;Clinical Child
Neuropsychology;Clinical Neuropsychology;Learning
Disabilities;School Psychology

ALLEN, Jane E.
Cellulan One
250 Australian Avenue, South
West Palm Beach, FL 33401-5087
Ethnicity: African-American/Black
Degree and Year: PhD 1985
Major Field: unknown
Specialty: Human Resources;Industrial/Organizational
Psychology;Management & Organization;Organizational
Development;Training & Development

ALLEN, Winnie M.
2354 Fletcher Drive
Suite #223
Los Angeles, CA 90039-4032
(213) 564-7911-**B**
Ethnicity: African-American/Black
Degree and Year: PhD 1978
Major Field: Clinical Psychology
Specialty: Psychotherapy

ALLEN, Wise E.
1020 Sierra Street
Berkeley, CA 94707
(510) 466-7311-**B**, (510) 527-7177-**H**, (510) 835-4078-**F**
Ethnicity: African-American/Black
Degree and Year: PhD 1976
Major Field: Social Psychology
Specialty: Clinical Psychology

ALLGOOD-HILL, Barbara A.
Community Services
The Kennedy Institute
2911 East Biddle Street
Baltimore, MD 21213-3939
(410) 550-9700-**B**, (410) 768-4106-**H**
Ethnicity: African-American/Black
Degree and Year: PhD 1987
Major Field: Clinical Psychology
Specialty: Mentally Retarded

ALLSOPP, Ralph N
5590 Long Island Drive NW
Atlanta, GA 30327-3928
404 434-0677-**B**, 404 843-3089-**H**, 404 256-9121-**F**
Ethnicity: African-American/Black

Degree and Year: PhD 1982 MA 1977
Major Field: Clinical Psychology
Specialty: Crime & Criminal Behavior;Psychology & Law

ALONSO, Mario
  1727 Jonathan Street
  Allentown, PA 18104
  (215) 437-2277-**B**, (215) 542-79766-**H**
Ethnicity: Hispanic/Latino
Languages: Spanish
Degree and Year: PhD 1979
Major Field: Clinical Psychology
Specialty: Employee Assistance Programs;Managed Care;Industrial/
    Organizational Psychology;Management &
    Organization;Clinical Psychology

ALONSO, Martha R.
  8550 W Flagler Street
  Suite #118
  Miami, FL 33144
  (305) 223-8225-**B**
Ethnicity: Hispanic/Latino
Languages: Spanish
Degree and Year: PhD 1973
Major Field: Clinical Psychology
Specialty: Developmental Psychology;Personality
    Measurement;Psychometrics;Projective Techniques;Individual
    Psychotherapy

ALSTON, Denise A.
  619 10th St NE
  Washington, DC 20002-5315
  (202) 822-7734-**B**
Ethnicity: African-American/Black
Degree and Year: PhD 1985
Major Field: Social Psychology

ALTARRIBA, Jeanette
  State University of New York
  @ Albany
  Department of Psychology
  Social Science 112
  Albany, NY 12222
  (518) 442-5004-**B**, (518) 464-1567-**H**, (518) 442-4867-**F**
  ja087@csc.albany.edu
Ethnicity: Hispanic/Latino
Languages: French, Spanish
Degree and Year: PhD 1990
Major Field: Cognitive Psychology
Specialty: Cognitive Psychology;Language Process;Psycholinguistic

ALVAREZ, Blanca M. De
  Apartado 69
  Chihuahua,
  MEXICO
  12-97-08-**B**
Ethnicity: Hispanic/Latino
Degree and Year: PhD 1967
Major Field: Educational Psychology

ALVAREZ, Carlos M.
  7420 Sunset Drive
  Miami, FL 33143
  (305) 348-3472-**B**, (305) 667-4291-**H**, (305) 348-1515-**F**
Ethnicity: Hispanic/Latino
Languages: Spanish

Degree and Year: PhD 1974
Major Field: Clinical Psychology
Specialty: Clinical Psychology;Consulting Psychology;Cross Cultural
    Processes;Ethnic Minorities;Group Processes

ALVAREZ, Gary L.
  St. Catherine Hospital of Ancilla Systems
  4321 First Street
  East Chicago, IN 46312
  219/398-0905-**H**
Ethnicity: Hispanic/Latino
Degree and Year: PsyD 1993
Major Field: Clinical Psychology
Specialty: Clinical Psychology;Community Mental Health;Ethnic
    Minorities;Hospital Care;Administration;Program Evaluation

ALVAREZ, Manuel E.
  782 Northwest 42nd Avenue
  Suite 633
  Miami, FL 33126-5547
  (305) 443-8841-**B**, (305) 279-4346-**H**, (305) 443-8628-**F**
Ethnicity: Hispanic/Latino
Languages: Spanish
Degree and Year: PhD 1981
Major Field: Clinical Psychology
Specialty: Cognitive Behavioral Therapy;Forensic Psychology;Health
    Psychology;Managed Care;Pain & Pain Management

ALVAREZ, Maria D.
  1706 NW 26th Way
  Gainesville, FL 32605
  (352) 955-7612-**B**, (352) 374-4149-**H**, (352) 374-4020-**F**
Ethnicity: Hispanic/Latino
Languages: French, Spanish, Haitian Creole
Degree and Year: PhD 1983
Major Field: School Psychology
Specialty: Assessment/Diagnosis/Evaluation;Special Education;Cultural
    & Social Processes;Ethnic Minorities;Learning Disabilities

ALVAREZ, Mauricia
  Boston International Psychotherapy
  52 Moore Road
  Wayland, MA 01778
  (617) 236-7719-**B**, (808) 358-7606-**H**, (617) 236-7729-**F**
Ethnicity: Hispanic/Latino
Languages: Spanish
Degree and Year: PsyD 1985
Major Field: Clinical Psychology

ALVAREZ, Mildred M.
  Cornell University
  Psychology Department
  San Jose State University
  San Jose, CA 95192-0001
  (408) 924-5604-**B**
Ethnicity: Hispanic/Latino
Degree and Year: PhD 1985
Major Field: Developmental Psychology
Specialty: Emotional Development

ALVAREZ, Paul A.
  3910 Five Mile Drive
  Stockton, CA 95219-3258
  (209) 949-6393-**B**, (209) 948-0868-**F**
Ethnicity: Hispanic/Latino
Languages: Spanish

Degree and Year: EdD 1983
Major Field: Counseling Psychology
Languages: Thai, Loa
Degree and Year: PhD 1985
Specialty: Correctional Psychology;Juvenile
Delinquency;Psychotherapy;Suicide;Drug Abuse;Humanistic
Psychology

ALVAREZ, Roland
1209 Ferdinand Street
Coral Gables, FL 33134-2138
(305) 558-2480-**B**, (305) 552-0936-**H**
Ethnicity: Hispanic/Latino
Degree and Year: PhD 1987
Major Field: Counseling Psychology
Specialty: Psychotherapy

ALVAREZ, Rosaligia
PO Box 11964
San Juan, PR 00922-1964
(787) 782-2117-**H**
rosaligiaa@hot
Ethnicity: Hispanic/Latino
Languages: Spanish
Degree and Year: PhD 1995
Major Field: Clinical Psychology
Specialty: Drug Abuse;HIV/AIDS;Psychotherapy;Ethnic
Minorities;Psychology & Law

ALVAREZ, Vivian
12304 Santa Monica Boulevard
Apartment 210
Los Angeles, CA 90025
(310) 473-1210-**B**, (310) 477-5668-**H**
Ethnicity: Hispanic/Latino
Languages: Spanish
Degree and Year: PhD 1987
Major Field: Clinical Psychology
Specialty: Clinical Child Psychology;Assessment/Diagnosis/
Evaluation;Community Mental Health;Affective
Disorders;Ethnic Minorities

AMARO, Hortensia
Boston University
BUSPH
715 Albany Street, TW2
Boston, MA 02118-2340
(617) 638-5146-**B**, (617) 638-4483-**F**
hamaro@bu.edu
Ethnicity: Hispanic/Latino
Languages: Spanish
Degree and Year: PhD 1982
Major Field: Developmental Psychology
Specialty: Psychology of Women;Drug Abuse;Social Change;Health
Psychology;HIV/AIDS

AMAWATTANA, Tipawadee
Thammasat University
Deptartment of Psychology
Fac. Liberal Arts
Bangkok 10200,
THAILAND
221-6111-2609-**B**, 66-2-413-4158-**H**, 66-2-224-8099-**F**
csgpsy@alpha.tu.ac.th
Ethnicity: Asian-American/Asian/Pacific Islander

Major Field: Counseling Psychology
Specialty: Counseling Psychology;Drug Abuse;Family Therapy;HIV
AIDS;Behavior Therapy

AMBADY, Nalina
Harvard University
33 Kirkland Street
Cambridge, MA 02138
(617) 495-3898-**B**
na@wjn.harvard.edu
Ethnicity: Asian-American/Asian/Pacific Islander
Languages: Hindi
Degree and Year: PhD 1991
Major Field: Social Psychology
Specialty: Nonverbal Communication;Cultural & Social
Processes;Statistics;Social Cognition;Social
Psychology;Personality Psychology

AMEZAGA, JR., Alfredo M.
PO Box 8069
University Station
Reno, NV 89507-8069
(775) 746-8993-**B**, (775) 746-8993-**F**
amezaga_am@attglobal.net
Ethnicity: Hispanic/Latino
Languages: Spanish
Degree and Year: PhD 1996
Major Field: Clinical Psychology
Specialty: Alcoholism & Alcohol Abuse;Case Management;Program
Evaluation;Assessment/Diagnosis/Evaluation;Ethnic
Minorities;Labor & Management Relations

AMEZCUA, Charlie A.
8348 Fable Avenue
West Hills, CA 91304
(213) 265-8744-**B**, (818) 340-5587-**H**
Ethnicity: Hispanic/Latino
Languages: Spanish
Degree and Year: MS 1960
Major Field: Counseling Psychology
Specialty: Counseling Psychology;Rehabilitation;School
Counseling;Educational Psychology;Physically Handicapped

AMIN, Kiran
Samaritan Rehabilitation Institute
1012 E Willetta
Phoenix, AZ 85006-2749
(602) 285-3688-**B**
Ethnicity: Asian-American/Asian/Pacific Islander
Degree and Year: PhD 1987
Major Field: Clinical Psychology
Specialty: Rehabilitation;Clinical Neuropsychology

ANAND, Shashi
2543-B W. Howard Street
Chicago, IL 60645
(219) 888-3950-**B**, (773) 465-1576-**H**
anad@mailhostchi.ameritech.net
Ethnicity: Asian-American/Asian/Pacific Islander
Languages: Hindi, Urdu
Degree and Year: PhD 1988

Major Field: Counseling Psychology
Specialty: Clinical Child Neuropsychology;Cultural & Social
  Processes;Depression;Assessment/Diagnosis/
  Evaluation;Conduct Disorders;Child Therapy

ANDERSON, Claudia J.
  4747 Belllaire Blvd, Ste 342
  Bellaire, TX 77401-4519
  (713) 661-1515-**B**, (713) 660-8768-**H**
Ethnicity: Hispanic/Latino
Degree and Year: PhD 1987
Major Field: Clinical Psychology
Specialty: Assessment/Diagnosis/Evaluation;Child
  Therapy;Communication;Family Therapy;Child Development

ANDERSON, Linda
  412 Sixth Avenue
  Suite #702
  New York, NY 10012
  (212) 243-0202-**B**, (718) 499-2925-**H**
Ethnicity: African-American/Black
Languages: Spanish
Degree and Year: PhD 1983
Major Field: Clinical Psychology

ANDERSON, Louis P.
  Georgia State University
  Department of Psychology
  University Plaza
  Georgia State University
  Atlanta, GA 30303-
  (404) 651-1615-**B**, (404) 593-0284-**H**
Ethnicity: African-American/Black
Degree and Year: PhD 1982
Major Field: Clinical Psychology
Specialty: Cultural & Social Processes;Ethnic
  Minorities;Stress;Personality Measurement;Professional
  Issues in Psychology

ANDERSON, Norman B.
  Office of Behavioral & Social Sciences Reser
    Research - Building 1, Room 326
  National Institutes of Health
  One Center Drive
  Bethesda, MD 20892-0001
  (301) 402-1146-**B**, (301) 402-1150-**F**
  norman_anderson@nih.gov
Ethnicity: African-American/Black
Degree and Year: PhD 1983
Major Field: Clinical Psychology

ANDERSON, Shirley G.
  Johnson C. Smith University
  100 Beatties Ford Road
  Charlotte, NC 28216
  (704) 378-1055-**B**, (704) 568-1992-**H**, (704) 378-3556-**F**
  sanderson@jcsu.edu
Ethnicity: African-American/Black
Degree and Year: PhD 1972
Major Field: School Psychology
Specialty: Educational Psychology

ANDERSON, William H.
  109 Quince Lane
  Charlottesville, VA 22902
  (804) 924-3751-**B**, (804) 971-7931-**H**, (804) 924-6476-**F**

Ethnicity: African-American/Black
Languages: French, Spanish
Degree and Year: PhD 1974
Major Field: Clinical Psychology
Specialty: Behavior Therapy;Cognitive Behavioral Therapy;Lesbian &
  Gay Issuues;Psychopathology;Values & Moral
  Behavior;Clinical Child Psychology

ANDRIEU, Brenda J.
  21 Elm St #2
  Middlebury, VT 05753-1127
  (802) 388-3711-**B**, (802) 388-0362-**H**, (802) 388-6436-**F**
Ethnicity: African-American/Black, American Indian/Alaska Native
Degree and Year: PhD 1975
Major Field: Counseling Psychology
Specialty: Assessment/Diagnosis/Evaluation;Cross Cultural
  Processes;Ingestive Behavior & Nutrition;Learning
  Disabilities;Psychotherapy

ANDUJAR, Carlos A.
  University of Puerto Rico
  Avenue Ponce De Leon
  Rio Piedras, PR 00931
  (787) 273-0643-**B**, (787) 273-0643-**H**, (787) 273-0643-**F**
Ethnicity: Hispanic/Latino
Languages: Spanish
Degree and Year: PhD 1994
Major Field: Industrial/Organizational Psy.
Specialty: Management & Organization;Organizational
  Development;Quantitative/Mathematical,
  Psychometrics;Measurement;Training &
  Development;Psychometrics

ANSELMO, Fe
  Lansing Community College
  1024 N Magnolia Ave
  Lansing, MI 48912-3235
  (517) 484-3764-**B**, (517) 484-3764-**H**
Ethnicity: Asian-American/Asian/Pacific Islander
Degree and Year: PhD 1967
Major Field: Developmental Psychology
Specialty: Adolescent Development

ANTHONY, Bobbie M.
  Chicago State University
  PO Box 19104
  Chicago, IL 60619
  (773) 783-5712-**B**, (773) 783-4424-**H**, (312) 995-3767-**F**
Ethnicity: African-American/Black
Degree and Year: PhD 1967 MSEd 1959
Major Field: Quan/Math & Psychometrics/Stat
Specialty: Counseling Psychology;Curriculum Development/
  Evaluation;Cross Cultural Processes;Educational
  Psychology;Ethnic Minorities

ANTOKOLETZ, Juana C.
  2802 Horseshoe Bend Cove
  Austin, TX 78704
  (512) 343-2823-**B**, (512) 441-7520-**H**
Ethnicity: Hispanic/Latino
Languages: Spanish
Degree and Year: PhD 1970
Major Field: Educational Psychology
Specialty: Clinical Psychology;Child Abuse;Clinical Child
  Psychology;Ethnic Minorities

ANTONUCCIO, David
V.A. Medical Center (116B2)
1000 Locust Street
Reno, NV 89520
(702) 328-1490-**B**, (702) 746-0930-**H**, (702) 328-1464-**F**
oliver2@aol.com
Ethnicity: Hispanic/Latino
Languages: Spanish
Degree and Year: PhD 1980
Major Field: Clinical Psychology
Specialty: Behavior Therapy;Depression;Sexual
Dysfunction;Smoking;Psychotherapy

ANTON, William D.
University of So. Florida
Counseling Center
SVC 2124
Tampa, FL 33620
(813) 961-7544-**B**, (813) 920-3778-**H**, (813) 974-3089-**F**
Ethnicity: Hispanic/Latino
Languages: Spanish
Degree and Year: PhD 1975
Major Field: Clinical Psychology
Specialty: Psychotherapy;Neuroses;Personality
Measurement;Administration;Counseling Psychology

ANZAI, Yuichiro
Keio University
Dept. of Information & Computer Science
Faculty of Science and Engineering
3-14-1 Hiyoshi
Yokohama, 223 JAPAN
anzai@aa.cs.keio.ac.jp
Ethnicity: Asian-American/Asian/Pacific Islander
Degree and Year: PhD
Major Field: Experimental Psychology
Specialty: Thought Processes;Memory

AOKI, Bart K.
2477 Washington Street
San Francisco, CA 94115
(415) 541-9285-**B**, (415) 441-1233-**H**, (415) 541-9986-**F**
Ethnicity: Asian-American/Asian/Pacific Islander
Degree and Year: PhD 1980
Major Field: Clinical Psychology
Specialty: Clinical Psychology;Psychotherapy;Drug Abuse;HIV/AIDS;Mental
Health Services

AOKI, Melanie F.
Northwestern Memorial
Healthsouth Back and Neck Institute
680 North Lakeshore Drive #1316
Chicago, IL 60611
(312) 926-6219-**B**
maoki@nmh.org
Ethnicity: Asian-American/Asian/Pacific Islander
Languages: Japanese
Degree and Year: PhD 1993
Major Field: Health Psychology

AOKI, Wayne T.
Fuller Theological Seminary
Graduate School of Psychology
180 North Oakland Avenue
Pasadena, CA 91101
(818) 584-5531-**B**, (818) 794-8406-**H**, (818) 584-9630-**F**
aoki@fuller.edu
Ethnicity: Asian-American/Asian/Pacific Islander
Degree and Year: PhD 1980
Major Field: Clinical Psychology
Specialty: Adolescent Therapy;Assessment/Diagnosis/Evaluation;Clinical
Child Psychology;Depression;Family Therapy

APENAHIER, Leonard
P.O. Box 5434
Takoma Park, MD 20912
(202) 362-0691-**B**, (202) 832-0619-**H**, (202) 362-1675-**F**
Ethnicity: African-American/Black
Degree and Year: PhD 1993
Major Field: Educational Psychology
Specialty: Research Design & Methodology;Statistics

APONTE, Evelyn I.
3636 Greystone Avenue
Suite #1J
Bronx, NY 10463-2022
(914) 576-4360-**B**, (718) 543-7911-**H**
Ethnicity: Hispanic/Latino
Languages: Spanish
Degree and Year: PhD 1991
Major Field: School Psychology
Specialty: Clinical Child Psychology;Counseling Psychology;Special Education

APONTE, Joseph F.
University of Louisville
Department of Psychology
Louisville, KY 40292
(502) 588-6782-**B**, (502) 426-9418-**H**
Ethnicity: Hispanic/Latino
Degree and Year: PhD 1970
Major Field: Clinical Psychology
Specialty: Community Mental Health;Ethnic
Minorities;Psychotherapy;Counseling Psychology

ARADOM, Tesfay A
Roxbury Community College
Social Sciences
53 Bristol Road
Medford, MA 02155
617 427-0060-**B**, 617 625-4316-**H**
Ethnicity: African-American/Black
Languages: Italian, Tigrigna Amharic
Degree and Year: PhD
Major Field: General Psy./Methods & Systems

ARANA, Olga R.
Center for Psychiatric Medicine
7800 Fannin S-400
Houston, TX 77054
(713) 795-5999-**B**, (713) 771-2246-**H**, (713) 795-5261-**F**
Ethnicity: Asian-American/Asian/Pacific Islander
Languages: Filipino
Degree and Year: EdD 1980
Major Field: Clinical Psychology
Specialty: Clinical Psychology;Individual Psychotherapy;Mental Health
Services;Pain & Pain Management;Projective Techniques

ARAOZ, Daniel L.
66 Gates Avenue
Malverne, NY 11565-1912

(516) 599-5905-**B**, (516) 599-5905-**F**
taoist23@argentinamail.com
Ethnicity: Hispanic/Latino
Languages: French, German, Spanish
Degree and Year: EdD 1969
Major Field: Counseling Psychology
Specialty: Hypnosis/Hypnotherapy;Family Processes;Sex/Marital
    Therapy;Management & Organization;Counseling Psychology

ARBOLEDA, Catalina
    328 Broadway
    Cambridge, MA 02139
    (617) 876-6535-**B**, (978) 443-3689-**H**, (978) 443-4694-**F**
    catarbol@aol.com
Ethnicity: Hispanic/Latino
Languages: Spanish
Degree and Year: PhD 1982
Major Field: Developmental Psychology
Specialty: Individual Psychotherapy

ARBONA, Consuelo
    University of Houston
    Educational Psychology, Dept. FH491
    4800 Calhoun Rd
    Houston, TX 77004-2610
    (713) 743-9814-**B**, (713) 485-8486-**H**
    anzai@aa.cs.keio.ac.jp
Ethnicity: Hispanic/Latino
Languages: Spanish
Degree and Year: PhD 1986
Major Field: Counseling Psychology
Specialty: Cultural & Social Processes;Vocational Psychology;Research
    & Training

ARCAYA, Jose M.
    141 Parkway Road
    Suite #9
    Bronxville, NY 10708
    (914) 779-5034-**B**, (914) 478-7607-**H**
Ethnicity: Hispanic/Latino
Languages: French, Spanish
Degree and Year: PhD 1984
Major Field: Clinical Psychology
Specialty: Philosophy of Science;Memory;Clinical Psychology;Ethnic
    Minorities;Projective Techniques

ARCHIBALD, Eloise M.
    400 Central Park, West
    Suite #16M
    New York, NY 10025
    (212) 316-4380-**H**
Ethnicity: African-American/Black
Degree and Year: PhD 1979
Major Field: Clinical Psychology
Specialty: Assessment/Diagnosis/Evaluation;Individual
    Psychotherapy;Employee Assistance Programs;Selection &
    Placement

ARDILA, Ruben
    Carribean Center - Advance Studies
    Old San Juan Station
    San Juan, PR 00902-3711
    (571) 256-7527-**H**

carbon@bayou.uh.edu
Ethnicity: Hispanic/Latino
Languages: French, Spanish
Degree and Year: PhD 1970
Major Field: Experimental Psychology
Specialty: Experimental Analysis of Behavior;Experimental
    Psychology;Health Psychology;Learning/Learning
    Theory;Social Psychology

ARELLANO-LOPEZ, Juan
    A&A Psychotherapy Associates, PC
    PO Box 564
    Okemos, MI 48805-0564
    (517) 349-4111-**B**, (517) 347-6999-**F**
Ethnicity: Hispanic/Latino
Languages: Spanish
Degree and Year: MSW 1979
Major Field: Clinical Psychology
Specialty: Psychotherapy;Hypnosis/Hypnotherapy;Pain & Pain
    Management;Cognitive Behavioral Therapy;Marriage &
    Family;Sports Psychology

ARELLANO, Charleanea
    Tri-Ethnic Center for Prevention Research
    Department of Psychology, C-78
    Andrew G. Clark Building,
    Colorado State University
    Fort Collins, CO 80523-1879
    (970) 491-663-**B**, (303) 254-9707-**H**, (970) 491-0527-**F**
    carellan@lamar.colostate.edu
Ethnicity: Hispanic/Latino
Degree and Year: PhD 1993
Major Field: Clinical Child Psychology
Specialty: Clinical Child Psychology;Family Processes

ARENAS, JR., Silverio
    P.O. Box 306
    Mount Vernon, WA 98273
    (206) 428-9233-**B**, (206) 428-8851-**H**
Ethnicity: Hispanic/Latino
Languages: Spanish
Degree and Year: PhD 1983
Major Field: Clinical Psychology
Specialty: Health Psychology;Cognitive Behavioral Therapy;Cross
    Cultural Processes;Neuropsychology;Pain & Pain Management

AREVALO, Luis E.
    2712 E 5th Street
    La Verne, CA 91750
    (714) 838-4193-**B**, (909) 596-7118-**H**, (714) 838-4194-**F**
Ethnicity: Hispanic/Latino
Languages: Spanish
Degree and Year: PhD 1987
Major Field: Clinical Psychology
Specialty: Clinical Psychology;Cross Cultural Processes;Alcoholism &
    Alcohol Abuse;Affective Disorders

ARIZA-MENEDEZ, Maria
    300 NW Le Jeune Road
    Apartment #409
    Miami, FL 33126
    (305) 995-7544-**B**, (305) 443-0329-**H**, (305) 995-7571-**F**
Ethnicity: Hispanic/Latino
Languages: French, Italian, Spanish
Degree and Year: PhD 1982

Major Field: Social Psychology
Specialty: Program Evaluation;Educational Research;Research Design & Methodology;Quantitative/Mathematical, Psychometrics;Psycholinguistic

ARIZMEUDI, Thomas
5060 Lexington Circle
Loomis, CA 95650
(916) 444-6408-**B**
Ethnicity: Hispanic/Latino
Degree and Year: PhD 1983
Major Field: Clinical Psychology
Specialty: Psychotherapy;Adolescent Therapy

ARMENGOL, Carmen G.
Northeastern University
203 lake Hall
360 Huntington Avenue
Boston, MA 02115
617/373-5917-**B**, 617/522-7061-**H**, 617/524-0606-**F**
carmengo@lynx.neu.edu
Ethnicity: Hispanic/Latino
Languages: French, Spanish
Degree and Year: PhD 1985
Major Field: Clinical Psychology
Specialty: Neuropsychology;Attention Deficit Disorders;Eating Disorders;Learning Disabilities;Rehabilitation

ARMILLA, Jose
1347 Stokley Way
Vienna, VA 22182-1666
Ethnicity: Asian-American/Asian/Pacific Islander
Degree and Year: PhD 1961
Major Field: Social Psychology
Specialty: Mass Media Communication

ARNAU-GRAS, Jamie
Rambla Del Poblenou
32, 4,1
Barcelona, SPAIN
08005 398, 0733093326-**B**
Ethnicity: Hispanic/Latino
Degree and Year: PhD 1973
Major Field: Experimental Psychology
Specialty: Thought Processes

ARNOLD, John F.
Spokane Valley Family Medicine
13102 East Mission
Spokane, WA 99216
(509) 747-7754-**B**, (509) 927-9348-**H**, (509) 928-0300-**F**
Ethnicity: American Indian/Alaska Native
Degree and Year: PhD 1994
Major Field: Clinical Psychology
Specialty: Cross Cultural Processes;Community Mental Health;Mental Health Services;Psychotherapy

ARREDONDO, Patricia
Empowerment Workshops, Inc.
251 Newbury St.
Boston, MA 02116
(617) 266-9100-**B**, (617) 926-0168-**H**, (617) 266-7370-**F**
empow@aol.com
Ethnicity: Hispanic/Latino
Languages: Spanish
Degree and Year: EdD 1978

Major Field: Counseling Psychology
Specialty: Adult Development;Counseling Psychology;Cultural & Social Processes;Feminist Therapy;Organizational Development

ARREOLA-ROCKWELL, Fran Pepitone
The Fielding Institute
2112 Santa Barbara Street
Santa Barbara, CA 93105
(805) 898-2923-**B**, (805) 966-5556-**H**, (805) 687-4590-**F**
frock@fielding.edu
Ethnicity: Hispanic/Latino
Degree and Year: PhD 1984
Major Field: Clinical Psychology
Specialty: Gender Issues;Ethnic Minorities;Psychology of Women;Suicide;Medical Psychology;Health Psychology

ARRISO, Roberta H
99-16 67 Road
Apartment 2L
Forest Hills, NY 11375
718 993-5765-**B**, 718 896-8992-**H**
Ethnicity: Hispanic/Latino
Languages: Spanish
Degree and Year: PhD 1989
Major Field: Developmental Psychology
Specialty: Developmental Psychology;Special Education;Cognitive Behavioral Therapy;Rational-Emotive Therapy;Cross Cultural Processes

ARROYO, Judith A.
University of New Mexico
Department of Psychology
Albuquerque, NM 87131
(505) 277-8947-**B**, (505) 277-1394-**F**
jarroyo@unm.edu
Ethnicity: Hispanic/Latino
Languages: Spanish
Degree and Year: PhD 1989
Major Field: Clinical Psychology
Specialty: Alcoholism & Alcohol Abuse;Community Psychology;Cross Cultural Processes;Domestic Violence;Ethnic Minorities

ARROYO, Patricia M.
7 Ropeferry Rd
Dartmouth Col
Hanover, NH 03755-1404
(603) 650-1442-**B**, (603) 795-3120-**H**
Ethnicity: Hispanic/Latino
Degree and Year: PhD 1990
Major Field: Clinical Child Psychology
Specialty: Clinical Child Psychology;Ethnic Minorities

ARSUAGA, Enrique N.
PO Box 9021616
Old San Juan Station
San Juan, PR 00902-1616
(809) 736-8921-**B**, (809) 731-2464-**H**
Ethnicity: Hispanic/Latino
Languages: Spanish
Degree and Year: PhD 1988
Major Field: Clinical Psychology
Specialty: Individual Psychotherapy;Clinical Psychology;Assessment/ Diagnosis/Evaluation

ARTILES, Alfredo J.
UCLA
405 Hilgard Avenue
3335 Moore Hall
Los Angeles, CA 90095
(310) 206-2111-**B**, (310) 206-6293-**F**
aartiles@ucla.edu
Ethnicity: Hispanic/Latino
Languages: Spanish
Degree and Year: PhD 1992
Major Field: Educational Psychology
Specialty: Educational Psychology;Ethnic Minorities;Special
Education;Educational Research;Learning Disabilities;Thought
Processes

ARTILES, Laura M.
10300 SW 72 Street, #280
Miami, FL 33173
(305) 270-3737-**B**, (305) 270-3014-**H**, (305) 270-3736-**F**
Ethnicity: Hispanic/Latino
Languages: Spanish
Degree and Year: PhD 1990
Major Field: Clinical Psychology
Specialty: Assessment/Diagnosis/Evaluation;Giftedness;Attention
Deficit Disorders;Clinical Psychology;School
Psychology;Learning Disabilities

ARTIOLA, Lydia
6147 E Grant Rd
Tucson, AZ 85712-5829
(520) 290-1700-**B**, (520) 749-5829-**H**, (602) 290-1102-**F**
Ethnicity: Hispanic/Latino
Languages: French, Italian, Portuguese, Spanish, Catalan
Degree and Year: PhD 1977
Major Field: Physiological Psychology
Specialty: Neuropsychology;Neurological Disorders

ARTIS, Daphne J.
2290 North State College Boulevard
Fullerton, CA 92831
(714) 680-5132-**B**, (714) 537-2158-**H**, (714) 537-2345-**F**
Ethnicity: African-American/Black
Degree and Year: PsyD 1982
Major Field: Clinical Psychology
Specialty: Affective Disorders;Cognitive Behavioral Therapy;Ethnic
Minorities;Individual Psychotherapy

ARVELO, Luis E.
1913 East 17th Street #202
Santa Ana, CA 92705-8627
(714) 569-0067-**B**, (909) 596-7118-**H**
mtona@aol.com
Ethnicity: Hispanic/Latino
Degree and Year: PhD 1987
Major Field: Clinical Psychology

ASAMEN, Joy K.
Pepperdine University
Graduate School
400 Corporate Pointe
Culver City, CA 90230
(310) 568-5654-**B**, (310) 568-5755-**F**
jasamen@pepperdine.edu
Ethnicity: Asian-American/Asian/Pacific Islander

Degree and Year: PhD 1983 MA 1977
Major Field: Educational Psychology
Specialty: Counseling Psychology;Ethnic Minorities

ASBURY, Charles A.
School of Education
Howard University
Washington, DC 20059
(202) 806-7350-**B**, (301) 439-6875-**H**
Ethnicity: African-American/Black
Degree and Year: PhD 1969
Major Field: Educational Psychology

ASBURY, Jo-Ellen
Department of Psychology
Bethany College
Bethany, WV 26032
(304) 829-7431-**B**, (304) 829-4487-**H**
j.asbury@mail.bethanywv.edu
Ethnicity: African-American/Black
Degree and Year: PhD 1985
Major Field: Social Psychology
Specialty: Gender Issues;Ethnic Minorities;History & Systems of
Psychology;Program Evaluation;Social
Psychology;Psychology of Women

ASCANO, Ricardo
Ascano & Associates
PO Box 325
Breckenridge, MN 56520-0325
(218) 643-3867-**B**, (218) 643-1630-**F**
Ethnicity: Asian-American/Asian/Pacific Islander
Languages: Filipino
Degree and Year: PsyD 1979
Major Field: Clinical Psychology
Specialty: Forensic Psychology;Child Abuse

ASCENCAO, Erlete M.
Tennessee State University
3500 John A. Merritt Boulevard
Nashville, TN 37206
(615) 963-2177-**B**, (615) 650-2697-**H**
Ethnicity: Hispanic/Latino
Languages: Portuguese, Spanish
Degree and Year: PhD 1995 PhD 1986
Major Field: Clinical Psychology
Specialty: Clinical Psychology;Personality Disorders;Interpersonal
Processes & Relations;Individual Psychotherapy;Health
Psychology;Group Processes

ASGHAR, Anila
4943 Keota Run, NE
Roswell, GA 30075-1660
(770) 517-6133-**H**, (770) 425-7175-**F**
anilaa@aol.com
Ethnicity: Asian-American/Asian/Pacific Islander
Languages: Hindi, Urdu, Pujabi
Degree and Year: PhD 1997
Major Field: Counseling Psychology
Specialty: Assessment/Diagnosis/Evaluation;Counseling
Psychology;Forensic Psychology;Cognitive Behavioral
Therapy;Crisis Intervention & Therapy;Drug Abuse

ASHIDA, Sachio
SUNY College at Brockport
53 Sweden Hill Road

Brockport, NY 14420-2543
(716) 395-2685-**B**, (716) 637-3036-**H**, (716) 395-2116-**F**
sashida@pobrockport.edu
Ethnicity: Asian-American/Asian/Pacific Islander
Languages: Japanese
Degree and Year: PhD 1963
Major Field: Experimental Psychology
Specialty: Experimental Psychology;Computer Applications and
        Programming;Creativity;Memory;Research Design &
        Methodology

ASHMORE-HUDSON, Anne
2200 20th Street , NW
Washington, DC 20009-5004
(202) 234-0432-**B**, (202) 234-0432-**H**, (202) 234-0433-**F**
AnnMachele@aol.com
Ethnicity: African-American/Black
Degree and Year: PhD 1979
Major Field: Clinical Psychology
Specialty: Cognitive Psychology;Psychotherapy;Training &
        Development;Motivation;Human Resources

ATILANO, Raymond B.
7800 Charter Oak Court
Ft. Worth, TX 76179-2702
(817) 429-2288-**B**, (817) 236-2532-**H**
Ethnicity: Hispanic/Latino
Degree and Year: PhD 1982
Major Field: unknown

ATKINSON, Michael B.
744 Castle Kirk Drive
Baton Rouge, LA 70808
(504) 388-8774-**B**, (504) 769-4365-**H**, (504) 388-5655-**F**
Ethnicity: American Indian/Alaska Native
Degree and Year: PhD 1976
Major Field: Clinical Psychology
Specialty: Behavior Therapy;Group Psychotherapy

ATTORE, Lois
1328 N Saratoga
Orange, CA 92669-1446
(714) 895-8740-**B**, (714) 639-6260-**H**
Ethnicity: Asian-American/Asian/Pacific Islander
Degree and Year: PhD 1984
Major Field: Counseling Psychology

ATWAL, Baljit K,
Department of California Youth Authority
7650 South Newcastle
O.H. Close School, Humboldt Hall
Stockton, CA 95213
(209) 944-6323-**B**, (916) 684-2237-**H**, (209) 944-6361-**F**
baljit@midtown.net
Ethnicity: Asian-American/Asian/Pacific Islander
Languages: Hindi, Punjabi
Degree and Year: PhD 1993
Major Field: Clinical Psychology
Specialty: Correctional Psychology;Cross Cultural Processes;Crime &
        Criminal Behavior;Juvenile Delinquency;Forensic
        Psychology;Conduct Disorders

ATWELL, Robert L.
1723 S Logan
Denver, CO 80210-3123
(303) 440-7225-**B**

Ethnicity: African-American/Black
Degree and Year: PsyD 1982
Major Field: Clinical Psychology

AUSTRIA, Asuncion M.
Cardinal Stritch University
Department of Psychology
Milwaukee, WI 53217-3985
(414) 410-4471-**B**, (414) 352-6281-**H**, (414) 247-1703-**F**
aaustria@acs.stricth.edu
Ethnicity: Asian-American/Asian/Pacific Islander
Languages: Filipino
Degree and Year: PhD 1970
Major Field: Clinical Psychology
Specialty: Ethnic Minorities;Psychology of Women;Pain & Pain
        Management;Medical Psychology;Psychotherapy

AUUILAS-GAXIOLA, Sergio A.
728 E Wood Duck Circle
Fresno, CA 93720
(209) 278-2822-**B**, (209) 434-2704-**H**
Ethnicity: Hispanic/Latino
Languages: Spanish
Degree and Year: PhD 1986
Major Field: Clinical Psychology
Specialty: Depression;Cognitive Behavioral Therapy;Family
        Therapy;Clinical Psychology;Clinical Research

AVIERA, Arlene T.
435 N Bedford Drive #408
Suite #408
Beverly Hills, CA 90210
(310) 247-1808-**B**
Ethnicity: Hispanic/Latino
Languages: Spanish
Degree and Year: PhD 1984
Major Field: Clinical Psychology
Specialty: Child Abuse;Parent Education;Affective
        Disorders;Personality Disorders;Psychoanalysis

AVILES, Alice A.
10 Valley Lane East
North Woodmere, NY 11581-3629
(516) 791-8326-**B**, (516) 791-8326-**H**
Ethnicity: Hispanic/Latino
Languages: Spanish
Degree and Year: PhD 1984
Major Field: Clinical Psychology
Specialty: Affective Disorders;Individual Psychotherapy;Personality
        Disorders;Psychoanalysis;Psychotherapy

AYLLON, Teodoro
Georgia State University
University Park
Atlanta, GA 30303-3044
(404) 325-7479-**B**
Ethnicity: Hispanic/Latino
Degree and Year: PhD 1959
Major Field: Clinical Psychology

AYOUB, Catherine C.
8 Sheffield Circle
Andover, MA 01810
617-495-3614-**B**, 508-470-0906-**H**, 617-495-3626-**F**

Ethnicity: Hispanic/Latino
Languages: Spanish
Degree and Year: EdD 1990
Major Field: Counseling Psychology
Specialty: Child Abuse;Child Development;Forensic
Psychology;Prevention;Psychology & Law

AZARET, Marisa
7800 SW 87th Avenue
Suite #B-250
Miami, FL 33173
(305) 595-0918-**B**, (305) 271-0532-**H**, (305) 595-0581-**F**
Ethnicity: Hispanic/Latino
Languages: Spanish
Degree and Year: PsyD 1986
Major Field: Clinical Child Psychology
Specialty: Adolescent Therapy;Child Therapy;Autism;Learning
Disabilities;Clinical Child Psychology

AZCARATE, Eduardo M.
6201 Leesburg Pike
Suite #216
Falls Church, VA 22044
(703) 237-0725-**B**, (703) 379-0424-**H**
eazcarate@aol.com
Ethnicity: Hispanic/Latino
Languages: Spanish
Degree and Year: PhD 1969
Major Field: Clinical Psychology
Specialty: Clinical Psychology;Adolescent Therapy;Child Therapy

AZEVEDO, Don Fernando
1150 SE Maynard Road
Suite 140
Cary, NC 27511-4164
919 469-0864-**B**, 919 387-3475-**H**
Ethnicity: Hispanic/Latino
Languages: Portuguese
Degree and Year: PhD 1988
Major Field: Clinical Psychology
Specialty: Individual Psychotherapy;Marriage & Family;Family
Therapy;Parent-Child Interaction;Parent Education

AZMITIA, Margarita
University of Santa Cruz
Department of Psychology
Santa Cruz, CA 95064
(408) 459-3146-**B**, (408) 459-8996-**H**, (408) 459-3519-**F**
Ethnicity: Hispanic/Latino
Languages: Spanish
Degree and Year: PhD 1986
Major Field: Developmental Psychology
Specialty: Cultural & Social Processes;Adolescent
Development;Cognitive Development;Ethnic
Minorities;Developmental Psychology

BABA, Masao
3-20-14 Nishioizumi
Nerima-Ku,JAPAN
039223561-**B**
Ethnicity: Asian-American/Asian/Pacific Islander
Degree and Year: MA 1960
Major Field: Industrial/Organizational Psy.

BABA, Vishwanath V.
Concordia University
Department of Managment
1455 de Massonneuve Blvd., West
Montreal
Quebec H3G 1M8,
CANADA
(514) 848-2933-**B**, (450) 672-6448-**H**, (514) 848-4292-**F**
baba@vax2.concordia.ca
Ethnicity: Asian-American/Asian/Pacific Islander
Languages: Tamil
Degree and Year: PhD 1979
Major Field: Industrial/Organizational Psy.
Specialty: Industrial/Organizational Psychology;Cross Cultural
Processes;Job Satisfaction;Stress;Work
Performance;Management & Organization

BABB, Harold
Binghamton University
SUNY
Department of Psychology
PO Box 6000
Binghamton, NY 13902-6000
(607) 777-4862-**B**, (717) 553-4268-**H**, (607) 777-4890-**F**
hbabb@binghamton.edu
Ethnicity: American Indian/Alaska Native
Degree and Year: PhD 1953
Major Field: General Psy./Methods & Systems
Specialty: Learning/Learning Theory;Motivation;General
Psychology;Experimental Psychology;Emotion

BACAL, Sergio
10 Heaton Street
Downsville, ONTARIO,CANADA   M3H 4Y6
(416) 630-2104-**B**, (416) 630-5665-**H**, (416) 244-1761-**F**
Ethnicity: Hispanic/Latino
Languages: French, Portuguese, Spanish
Degree and Year: PhD 1982
Major Field: Clinical Psychology
Specialty: Rehabilitation;Health Psychology;Biofeedback;Ethnic
Minorities;Vocational Psychology

BACA, Sandra G.
25410 Longfellow Pl
Stevenson Ranch, CA 91381-1508
(213) 384-7084-**B**, (805) 255-6454-**H**, (805) 255-2709-**F**
dbaca31483@aol.com
Ethnicity: Hispanic/Latino
Languages: Spanish
Degree and Year: PhD 1993
Major Field: General Psy./Methods & Systems
Specialty: Domestic Violence;Feminist Therapy;Child Abuse;Family
Therapy;Ethnic Minorities

BACIGALUPE, Gonzalo M.
University of Massachusetts, Boston
Graduate College of Education
Boston, MA 02125-3393
(617) 287-7631-**B**, (617) 630-9153-**H**, (617) 630-9153-**F**
bacigalupe@umbsky.cc.umb.edu
Ethnicity: Hispanic/Latino
Languages: Spanish
Degree and Year: EdD 1995

Major Field: Counseling Psychology
Specialty: Domestic Violence;Child Abuse;Family Therapy;Ethnic Minorities;Cross Cultural Processes;Policy Analysis

BADILLO, Diana
115 Old Ridge Road
New Milford, CT 06776
(203) 775-5183-**B**, (203) 355-4975-**H**, (203) 775-8453-**F**
Ethnicity: Hispanic/Latino
Languages: Spanish
Degree and Year: PhD 1984
Major Field: Neurosciences
Specialty: Clinical Neuropsychology;Pain & Pain Management;Assessment/Diagnosis/Evaluation;Cognitive Behavioral Therapy;Neurological Disorders

BAEZ, Luis
The Joshua Group
333 West Wacker
Suite #700
Chicago, IL 60606
(312) 444-2072-**B**, (708) 789-3992-**H**
Ethnicity: Hispanic/Latino
Languages: Spanish
Degree and Year: PhD 1973
Major Field: Physiological Psychology
Specialty: Industrial/Organizational Psychology;Consulting Psychology;Human Resources;Leadership;Management & Organization

BAILEY, Joan W.
600 First St, #5
Hoboken, NJ 07030-6502
(201) 200-3064-**B**, (201) 653-6741-**H**
Ethnicity: African-American/Black
Degree and Year: PhD 1988
Major Field: Social Psychology
Specialty: Attribution Theory;Interpersonal Processes & Relations;Social Cognition;Social Psychology;Personality

BAINUM, Charlene K.
1155 Las Posadas Road
Angwin, CA 94508
(707) 965-2571-**H**
cbainum@puc.edu
Ethnicity: Asian-American/Asian/Pacific Islander
Languages: French
Degree and Year: PhD 1979
Major Field: Developmental Psychology
Specialty: Child Development;Gerontology/Geropsychology

BAKER, III, Carl E.
3030 Bogle Road
Bensalem, PA 19020-1722
(215) 757-0289-**H**
Ethnicity: African-American/Black
Languages: German, Spanish
Degree and Year: MA 1985
Major Field: Educational Psychology
Specialty: Human Relations

BAKER, Christine
West Essex Associates
99 Northfield Avenue
West Orange, NJ 07050
(201) 731-2331-**B**, (201) 763-0363-**H**

Ethnicity: African-American/Black
Degree and Year: PhD 1990
Major Field: Clinical Child Psychology
Specialty: School Psychology;Clinical Child Psychology

BAKER, Octave V.
1250 Oakmead Parkway
Suite #210
Sunnyvale, CA 94086-4027
Ethnicity: African-American/Black
Degree and Year: PhD 1977
Major Field: Industrial/Organizational Psy.
Specialty: Human Relations;Organizational Development;Community Psychology

BALBONA, Manuel
106 Woodland Drive
Lewisville, KY 75067
(214) 317-2883-**B**, (214) 317-6270-**H**
Ethnicity: Hispanic/Latino
Languages: Spanish
Degree and Year: PhD 1965
Major Field: Clinical Psychology
Specialty: Adolescent Therapy;Clinical Psychology;Computer Applications and Programming;Correctional Psychology;Cross Cultural Processes

BALCAZAR, Fabricio E.
University of Illinois at Chicago
1640 Roosevelt Road
Chicago, IL 60608
(312) 413-1646-**B**, (847) 673-3-**H**, (312) 996-4744-**F**
fabricio@uic..edu
Ethnicity: Hispanic/Latino
Languages: Spanish
Degree and Year: PhD 1987
Major Field: Developmental Psychology
Specialty: Applied Behavior Analysis;Community Psychology;Rehabilitation

BALDERRAMA, Sylvia R.
Vassar College
PO Box 706
124 Raymond Avenue
Poughkeepsie, NY 12604
(914) 437-5700-**B**, (914) 437-5715-**F**
sybalderrama@vassar.eou
Ethnicity: Hispanic/Latino
Languages: Spanish
Degree and Year: EdD 1990
Major Field: Counseling Psychology
Specialty: Adolescent Development;Crisis Intervention & Therapy;Cross Cultural Processes;Eating Disorders;Individual Psychotherapy

BALLERING, Lawrence R.
17803 Cypress Spring
Spring, TX 77388-4984
Ethnicity: American Indian/Alaska Native
Degree and Year: PhD 1979
Major Field: unknown
Specialty: Clinical Psychology;Developmental Psychology

BALY, Iris E.
Kaiser Permanente Medical Center
1761 Broadway

Suite 100
Vallejo, CA 94589-2227
(707) 645-2700-**B**, (707) 65-2181-**F**
irisbaly@ncalkaiperm.org
Ethnicity: African-American/Black
Degree and Year: PhD 1984
Major Field: Counseling Psychology
Specialty: Family Therapy;Clinical Psychology;Cognitive Behavioral
      Therapy;Individual Psychotherapy

BAMGBOSE, Olujiimi O.
PO Box 91426-1595
Encino, CA 91426-1595
(818) 788-6463-**B**, (818) 780-9588-**H**
Ethnicity: African-American/Black
Languages: Yoruba
Degree and Year: PhD 1977
Major Field: Clinical Psychology
Specialty: Assessment/Diagnosis/Evaluation;Consulting
      Psychology;Forensic Psychology;Hospital Care

BANAJI, Mahzarin R.
Yale University
Department of Psychology
PO Box 208205
New Haven, CT 06520-8205
(203) 432-4547-**B**, (203) 432-7172-**F**
mahzarin.banaji@yale.edu
Ethnicity: Asian-American/Asian/Pacific Islander
Languages: Hindi
Degree and Year: PhD 1986
Major Field: Social Psychology
Specialty: Attitudes & Opinions;Child & Pediatric Psychology;Social
      Cognition;Social Psychology;Memory;Thought Processes

BANIK, Sambhu N.
President's Commission
On Mental Retardation
8606 Bradmoor Drive
Bethesda, MD 20817-3633
Ethnicity: Asian-American/Asian/Pacific Islander
Degree and Year: PhD 1964
Major Field: Clinical Psychology
Specialty: Clinical Psychology

BANKS, Hobart M.
2 Amber Drive
San Francisco, CA 94131-1648
(415) 557-3575-**B**
Ethnicity: African-American/Black
Degree and Year: PhD 1982
Major Field: Clinical Psychology
Specialty: Psychotherapy

BANKS, Karel L.
128 Forest Street
Stanford, CT 06901
(914) 934-8797-**B**, (203) 323-3073-**H**
Ethnicity: African-American/Black
Languages: French
Degree and Year: PhD 1988
Major Field: Clinical Psychology
Specialty: Individual Psychotherapy;Affective
      Disorders;Psychotherapy;Ethnic Minorities;Death & Dying

BANKS, Martha E.
ABackans Diversified Computer
Research & Development Division
PO Box 1017
Uniontown, OH 44685-1017
(330) 699-0606-**B**, (330) 836-7261-**H**, (330) 699-0606-**F**
abackan.@en.com
Ethnicity: African-American/Black
Languages: French
Degree and Year: PhD 1980
Major Field: Neurosciences
Specialty: Neuropsychology;Computer Applications and
      Programming;Assessment/Diagnosis/Evaluation;Gerontology/
      Geropsychology;Rehabilitation;Psychology of Women

BARATTA, Frank S.
Director of District Research
Contra Costa CC Dist
500 Court Street
Martinez, CA 94553-1203
(415) 229-1000-**B**
Ethnicity: Hispanic/Latino
Degree and Year: PhD 1976
Major Field: Social Psychology
Specialty: Social Change;Program Evaluation

BARBARIN, Oscar A.
1943 Ivywood Drive
Ann Arbor, MI 48103
(313) 763-7778-**B**, (313) 995-1500-**H**, (313) 763-7864-**F**
Ethnicity: African-American/Black
Degree and Year: PhD 1975
Major Field: Clinical Psychology
Specialty: Administration;Child & Pediatric Psychology;Clinical Child
      Psychology;Clinical Research;Family Processes

BARBER, Kevin V.
18401 Midway Road
Southfield, MI 48075
(313) 271-0499-**B**, (313) 646-1131-**H**
Ethnicity: African-American/Black
Degree and Year: PhD 1990
Major Field: Clinical Psychology
Specialty: Clinical Child Psychology;Clinical Child
      Neuropsychology;Managed Care;School Psychology;Sports
      Psychology

BARDENSTEIN, Karen K.
21961 Rye Road
Shaker Heights, OH 44122-3033
Ethnicity: Hispanic/Latino
Degree and Year: PhD 1985
Major Field: Clinical Psychology
Specialty: Psychotherapy

BARKER-HACKETT, Lori
Behavioral Science Department
California State Polytechnic Univeristy Pomona
3801 West Temple Avenue
Pomona, CA 91768
(909) 869-3904-**B**, (909) 393-1901-**H**, (909) 869-4930-**F**
labarker@csupomona.edu
Ethnicity: African-American/Black
Degree and Year: PhD
Major Field: unknown

BARNER, II, Pearl
1928 Rome Avenue
St. Paul, MN 55116-2031
(612) 624-1444-**B**, (612) 291-2668-**H**
Ethnicity: African-American/Black
Degree and Year: PhD 1983
Major Field: Counseling Psychology
Specialty: Psychotherapy;Assessment/Diagnosis/Evaluation;Ethnic
    Minorities;Disadvantaged;Cognitive Behavioral Therapy

BARNES, Charles A.
2909 Ellesmere Avenue
Costa Mesa, CA 92626-3608
(714) 546-6713-**H**
Ethnicity: Hispanic/Latino
Languages: Spanish
Degree and Year: PhD 1949
Major Field: Clinical Psychology
Specialty: Measurement;Social Psychology;Client-Centered
    Therapy;Clinical Psychology;Assessment/Diagnosis/
    Evaluation;Brain Damage

BARNES, Denise R.
510 Holloway Street
Durham, NC 27701-3458
Ethnicity: African-American/Black
Degree and Year: PhD 1980
Major Field: Clinical Psychology
Specialty: Depression

BARNES, Michael J.
996 Baldwin Court
Uniondale, NY 11553-1102
(516) 997-6878-**B**
Ethnicity: African-American/Black
Degree and Year: PhD 1981
Major Field: School Psychology

BARONA, Andres
Arizona State University
Division of Psychology in Education
Box 0611
Tempe, AZ 85283-0211
(602) 965-2920-**B**, (602) 965-0300-**F**
Ethnicity: Hispanic/Latino
Languages: Spanish
Degree and Year: PhD 1982
Major Field: School Psychology
Specialty: Ethnic Minorities;Psychometrics;Educational
    Research;Research & Training;Counseling Psychology

BARON, Augustine
University of Texas at Austin
Counseling and Mental Health Center
100A West Dean Keeton Street
Austin, TX 7812-1001
(512) 475-6990-**B**, (512) 447-2048-**H**, (512) 471-8875-**F**
shrinkrap@mail.utexas.edu
Ethnicity: Hispanic/Latino
Languages: Spanish
Degree and Year: PsyD 1977
Major Field: Clinical Psychology
Specialty: Cultural & Social Processes;Lesbian & Gay
    Issuues;Management & Organization;Organizational
    Development;Training & Development

BARRERA, JR., Manuel
Arizona State University
Psychology Department
Tempe, AZ 85287-1104
(602) 965-3826-**B**, (602) 831-2615-**H**, (602) 965-8544-**F**
Ethnicity: Hispanic/Latino
Degree and Year: PhD 1977
Major Field: Clinical Psychology
Specialty: Clinical Psychology;Community Psychology;Ethnic
    Minorities

BARRERA, Francisco J.
SRC
Rural Route 1
Blenheim, ONTARIO, N0P-1A0 CANADA
(519) 676-5431-**B**, (519) 676-2389-**H**, (519) 676-5836-**F**
barrerdr@epo.gov.on.ca
Ethnicity: Hispanic/Latino
Languages: Spanish
Degree and Year: PhD 1974
Major Field: Experimental Psychology
Specialty: Applied Behavior Analysis;Mentally
    Retarded;Psychopathology;Clinical
    Research;Psychopharmacology

BARRIOS, Francisco X.
University of Northern Iowa
Department of Psychology
Cedar Falls, IA 50614
(319) 273-2419-**B**
Ethnicity: Hispanic/Latino
Degree and Year: PhD 1977
Major Field: Clinical Psychology
Specialty: Cognitive Behavioral Therapy;Pain & Pain Management

BARRY, Martha J.
P.O. Box 10593
Portland, ME 04104
(207) 774-6065-**B**, (207) 767-2112-**H**, (207) 772-2670-**F**
mbarry@usm.maine.edu
Ethnicity: Hispanic/Latino
Languages: Spanish
Degree and Year: PhD 1987
Major Field: Counseling Psychology
Specialty: Psychotherapy;Psychology of Women;Gender
    Issues;Feminist Therapy;Cross Cultural Processes

BARTEE, Robert L.
University of California at Santa Cruz
Counseling and Psychological Services
Santa Cruz, CA 95064
(831) 459-2377-**B**
rlbartee@cats.ucsc.edu
Ethnicity: African-American/Black
Degree and Year: PhD 1993
Major Field: Clinical Psychology
Specialty: Community Psychology;Crisis Intervention &
    Therapy;Ethnic Minorities;Depression

BARTHOLOMEW, Charles
1345 Druid Park Avenue
Augusta, GA 30904
(706) 738-5057-**B**, (706) 868-0460-**H**, (706) 738-4124-**F**
Ethnicity: African-American/Black

Degree and Year: PhD 1987
Major Field: School Psychology
Specialty: Juvenile Delinquency;Mental Health
  Services;Prevention;Conduct Disorders;Ethnic
  Minorities;Cognitive Behavioral Therapy

BASCO, Monica A.
  2930 Central Drive
  Bedford, TX 76021
  (817) 355-9479-**B**, (817) 239-1289-**H**, (817) 239-1289-**F**
  mbasco@msn.com
Ethnicity: Hispanic/Latino
Languages: Spanish
Degree and Year: PhD 1987
Major Field: Clinical Psychology
Specialty: Affective Disorders;Chronically Mentally Ill;Assessment/
  Diagnosis/Evaluation;Cognitive Behavioral
  Therapy;Interpersonal Processes & Relations

BASCUAS, Joseph W.
  Dean, Georgia School
  Georgia School Professional Psychology
  990 Hammond Dr
  Atlanta, GA 30328-5529
  (770) 671-1200-**B**, (404) 671-0476-**F**
Ethnicity: Hispanic/Latino
Languages: Spanish
Degree and Year: PhD 1981
Major Field: Clinical Psychology
Specialty: Administration;Adolescent Therapy;Child Therapy;Family
  Therapy;Individual Psychotherapy

BASTIEN, IV, Samuel A.
  St. Lawrence Psychiatric Center
  1 Chimney Point Drive
  Ogdensburg, NY 13669
  (315) 393-3000-**B**, (315) 379-0805-**H**, (315) 393-4496-**F**
Ethnicity: Hispanic/Latino
Languages: Spanish
Degree and Year: PhD 1986
Major Field: Clinical Psychology
Specialty: Sexual Dysfunction;Behavior Therapy;Clinical
  Psychology;Forensic Psychology;Hypnosis/Hypnotherapy

BASTIEN, Rochelle T.
  2988 Jamacha Road
  El Cajon, CA 92019
  (619) 670-5190-**B**, (619) 670-3667-**H**, (619) 670-0280-**F**
Ethnicity: African-American/Black
Degree and Year: PhD 1982
Major Field: Clinical Psychology
Specialty: Psychotherapy;Family Therapy;Gender Issues;Social
  Change;Problem Solving

BATTIEST, William V.
  1201 East Drachman Street
  #104
  Tuscon, AZ 85719
Ethnicity: African-American/Black
Languages: Spanish
Degree and Year: PhD 1986
Major Field: Counseling Psychology
Specialty: Marriage & Family;Pastoral Psychology

BAUERMEISTEN, Jose J.
  177 Las Caobas
  San Juan, PR 00927
  (809) 763-1946-**H**
Ethnicity: Hispanic/Latino
Languages: Spanish
Degree and Year: PhD 1970
Major Field: Clinical Child Psychology
Specialty: Assessment/Diagnosis/Evaluation;Attention Deficit
  Disorders;Learning Disabilities;Child Therapy;Behavior
  Therapy

BAVON, Moises
  637 Third Avenue
  Suite #F
  Chila Vista, CA 91910
  (619) 498-0904-**B**, (619) 484-7120-**H**
Ethnicity: Hispanic/Latino
Languages: Spanish
Degree and Year: PhD 1986
Major Field: Clinical Psychology
Specialty: Psychotherapy;Crisis Intervention & Therapy;Ethnic
  Minorities;Marriage & Family;Affective Disorders

BAXLEY, Gladys B.
  1329 Emerald Street, NE
  Washington, DC 20002-5431
  (202) 396-2150-**B**, (202) 397-7071-**H**, (202) 396-2150-**F**
Ethnicity: African-American/Black
Degree and Year: PhD 1973
Major Field: Developmental Psychology
Specialty: Program Evaluation;Prevention

BAXTER-BOEHM, Alva
  22 Glendale Road
  Ossining, NY 10562-1608
  (718) 262-2317-**B**
Ethnicity: Hispanic/Latino
Degree and Year: MA, 1974
Major Field: unknown

BAXTER, Anthony G.
  University of Massachusetts at Boston
  100 Morrissey Boulevard
  Boston, MA 02125
  (617) 287-7653-**B**, (781) 596-2317-**H**, (617) 287-7664'-**F**
  baxter@umbsky.cc.umb.edu
Ethnicity: African-American/Black
Degree and Year: PhD 1989
Major Field: Educational Psychology
Specialty: Statistics;Educational Research;Program
  Evaluation;Quantitative/Mathematical,
  Psychometrics;Psychometrics;Measurement

BAXTER, Bernice K.
  110 West End Avenue
  Apartment #4A
  New York, NY 10023-6348
Ethnicity: African-American/Black
Degree and Year: PhD 1963
Major Field: Social Psychology

BAYON, E. Paul
  2022 Cirone Way
  San Jose, CA 95124-1402
  (510) 795-3877-**B**, (510) 795-3551-**F**

epbayon@stanfordalumni.org
Ethnicity: Hispanic/Latino
Degree and Year: PsyD 1993 BAS 1985
Major Field: Clinical Psychology
Specialty: Cognitive Behavioral Therapy;Professional Issues in Psychology;Eating Disorders;Affective Disorders;Clinical Psychology;Psychotherapy

BEAM, Micheline
PO Box 6272
Oakland, CA 94603-0272
(510) 638-0617-**B**, (510) 521-3678-**H**, (510) 521-3678-**F**
Ethnicity: African-American/Black
Degree and Year: PhD 1980
Major Field: Clinical Child Psychology
Specialty: Assessment/Diagnosis/Evaluation;Parent-Child Interaction;Preschool & Day Care Issues;Emotional Development;Training & Development;Child Therapy

BEATO-SMITH, Vera
440 West End Avenue
Apartment 16E
New York, NY 10024-5358
(212) 787-4582-**B**, (212) 595-8098-**H**
Ethnicity: Hispanic/Latino
Languages: Portuguese, Spanish
Degree and Year: PhD 1992
Major Field: Clinical Psychology
Specialty: Psychotherapy;Assessment/Diagnosis/Evaluation;Cross Cultural Processes;Cultural & Social Processes

BEATTIE, Muriel Y.
12 Gault Avenue
Oneonta, NY 13820
(607) 436-3212-**B**, (607) 432-7085-**H**
Ethnicity: Asian-American/Asian/Pacific Islander
Degree and Year: PhD 1971
Major Field: Social Psychology
Specialty: Environmental Psychology;Gender Issues;Health Psychology

BEATTY, Lula A.
9007 Wallace Road
Lanham, MD 20706
(301) 443-0441-**B**, (301) 577-5779-**H**, (301) 443-9127-**F**
Ethnicity: African-American/Black
Degree and Year: PhD 1989
Major Field: Developmental Psychology
Specialty: Ethnic Minorities;Drug Abuse;Prevention

BECKLES, Nicola
148 Greenwich Street
Suite #103
Hempstead, NY 11550-5625
(516) 691-7900-**B**
Ethnicity: African-American/Black
Degree and Year: PhD 1988
Major Field: School Psychology
Specialty: Cognitive Behavioral Therapy

BELEN, Ines I.
Calle 1 Bloque A-14
Parque San Miguel
Bayamon, PR 00959
(809) 250-1912-**B**, (809) 251-7583-**H**
Ethnicity: Hispanic/Latino
Languages: Spanish

Degree and Year: PhD 1977
Major Field: Clinical Psychology
Specialty: Adult Development;Clinical Psychology;Counseling Psychology;Decision & Choice Behavior;Personality

BELGRAVE, Faye Z.
George Washington University
2125 G Street, NW
Washington, DC 20052
202 994-6314-**B**, 301 839-6198-**H**, 202 994-1602-**F**
belgrave@gwuvm
Ethnicity: African-American/Black
Degree and Year: PhD
Major Field: Social Psychology
Specialty: Cultural & Social Processes;Social Psychology;Ethnic Minorities;Rehabilitation;Drug Abuse

BELGRAVE, Jeffrey
49 Willow Avenue
Rockaway, NJ 07866
(201) 579-8675-**B**, (201) 586-9872-**H**
Ethnicity: African-American/Black
Degree and Year: PhD 1983
Major Field: Clinical Psychology
Specialty: Alcoholism & Alcohol Abuse;Drug Abuse;Marriage & Family;Cross Cultural Processes;HIV/AIDS

BELIZ, JR., Efrain A.
16055 Ventura Blvd.
Suite #545
Encino, CA 91346
(888) 857-2772-**B**, (818) 204-8139-**H**, (818) 990-6773-**F**
Ethnicity: Hispanic/Latino
Languages: Spanish
Degree and Year: PhD 1984
Major Field: Clinical Psychology
Specialty: Administration;Assessment/Diagnosis/Evaluation;Attention Deficit Disorders;Chronically Mentally Ill;Consulting Psychology

BELL, Anita G.
6800 S Tenton Ave
Philadelphia, PA 19150-
(215) 849-9088-**B**, (215) 844-2941-**H**
Ethnicity: African-American/Black
Degree and Year: PsyD 1980
Major Field: Clinical Psychology
Specialty: Adolescent Therapy;Affective Disorders;Child Therapy;Clinical Psychology;Family Therapy

BELL, K. Pat
Bureau of Prisons
FCI Tallahassee
501 Capital Circle, NE
Tallahassee, FL 32301
(850) 878-2173-**B**, (850) 893-5175-**H**
Ethnicity: African-American/Black
Degree and Year: PhD 1982
Major Field: Clinical Psychology
Specialty: Assessment/Diagnosis/Evaluation;Correctional Psychology;Employee Assistance Programs;Ethnic Minorities

BELTON, Monique
35 Dix Hills Road
Huntington, NY 11743
(516) 549-7314-**B**, (516) 549-7314-**H**

Ethnicity: African-American/Black
Degree and Year: PhD 1983
Major Field: Clinical Psychology
Specialty: Adolescent Therapy;Affective Disorders;Clinical
Psychology;Client-Centered Therapy;Ethnic Minorities

BELTRAN, Joe
1855 W Brownstone Court
Decatur, AL 35603
(205) 351-1424-**B**, (205) 350-5606-**H**
Ethnicity: Hispanic/Latino
Languages: Spanish
Degree and Year: PsyD 1990
Major Field: Clinical Psychology
Specialty: Affective Disorders;Depression;Drug Abuse;Individual
Psychotherapy;Group Psychotherapy

BELZUNCE, Philip R.
22380 Berry Road
Rocky River, OH 44116-2016
(216) 327-8140-**B**
Ethnicity: Asian-American/Asian/Pacific Islander
Degree and Year: PhD 1980
Major Field: Counseling Psychology
Specialty: Psychotherapy

BENAMU, Icem
ICD International Center for the Disabled
340 East 24th Street
New York, NY 10010
(212) 585-6017-**B**, (718) 382-7587-**H**
urpi@aol.com
Ethnicity: Hispanic/Latino
Languages: Spanish, Hebrew
Degree and Year: MA 1993
Major Field: Cognitive Psychology
Specialty: Assessment/Diagnosis/Evaluation;Learning
Disabilities;Psychometrics;Developmental
Psychology;Mentally Retarded;Rehabilitation

BENAVIDES, JR., Robert
Z455 Bennett Valley Road # Z10C
Santa Rosa, CA 95404
(707) 542-2081'-**B**, (707) 546-4206-**H**, (707) 542-2082-**F**
rbjpsy@aol.com
Ethnicity: Hispanic/Latino
Languages: Spanish
Degree and Year: EdD 1986
Major Field: Clinical Psychology
Specialty: Adolescent Therapy;Alcoholism & Alcohol Abuse;Behavior
Therapy;Family Therapy;Assessment/Diagnosis/
Evaluation;Individual Psychotherapy

BENCOMO, Armando A.
14827 S 44th Place
Phoenix, AZ 85044-6828
(602) 266-0700-**B**, 602 266-1263-**H**, (602) 266-1263-**F**
Ethnicity: Hispanic/Latino
Languages: Italian, Spanish
Degree and Year: PhD 1973
Major Field: Clinical Psychology
Specialty: Assessment/Diagnosis/Evaluation;Child Abuse;Forensic
Psychology;Rehabilitation;Learning Disabilities

BENET-MARTINEZ, Veronica
University of Michigan
525 East University Street
Department of Psychology
Ann Arbor, MI 48129
(313) 647-6706-**B**
veronica@umich.edu
Ethnicity: Hispanic/Latino
Languages: Spanish, Catalan
Degree and Year: PhD 1995
Major Field: Personality Psychology
Specialty: Cultural & Social Processes;Cross Cultural Processes

BENITEZ, John C.
405 N. Wabash
Suite #1815
Chicago, IL 60611
(312) 245-5269-**B**, (312) 226-3499-**H**, (312) 527-0849-**F**
jcbenitez@msn.com
Ethnicity: Hispanic/Latino
Languages: Arabic, Spanish
Degree and Year: PhD 1982
Major Field: Clinical Psychology
Specialty: Psychotherapy;Lesbian & Gay Issuues;Ethnic
Minorities;Psychoanalysis

BENNASAR, Mari C.
Boston Medical Center
Harrison Avenue Campus
Dowling 7 North
One Boston Medical Center Place
Boston, MA 02118
(617) 414-4646-**B**, (508) 303-6722-**H**, (508) 303-6726-**F**
maridan@erols.com
Ethnicity: Hispanic/Latino
Languages: Spanish
Degree and Year: PsyD 1993 MS 1990
Major Field: Clinical Psychology
Specialty: Cognitive Behavioral Therapy;Cross Cultural Processes;Drug
Abuse;Child Abuse;Health Psychology

BENNETT, Maisha H.
222 N La Salle St, Suite
Chicago, IL 60601-1005
(312) 946-8000-**B**, (312) 288-0702-**H**, (312) 946-0254-**F**
Ethnicity: African-American/Black
Languages: French
Degree and Year: PhD 1973
Major Field: Clinical Psychology
Specialty: Ethnic Minorities;Health Psychology;Marriage &
Family;Gerontology/Geropsychology;Drug Abuse

BENZAQUEN, Isaac
143 Maple Ave
Cedarhurst, NY 11516-2225
(516) 295-4104-**B**, (516) 764-2243-**H**, (516) 764-2243-**F**
Ethnicity: Hispanic/Latino
Languages: Spanish, Hebrew
Degree and Year: PhD 1983
Major Field: Clinical Psychology
Specialty: Forensic Psychology;Assessment/Diagnosis/Evaluation;Child
& Pediatric Psychology;Family Therapy;Drug Abuse

BERNAL, Alberto J.
4541 SW 132nd Avenue
Miami, FL 33175-4500
(303) 551-0149-**B**
Ethnicity: Hispanic/Latino
Degree and Year: PhD 1962
Major Field: Clinical Psychology
Specialty: Psychotherapy

BERNAL, Guillermo A.
Medical College of Ohio
Department of Psychiatry
3129 Glendale Avenue
Toledo, OH 43614-5811
(419) 381-5695-**B**, (419) 874-0619-**H**
gargnretabernal@mco.edu
Ethnicity: Hispanic/Latino
Languages: Spanish
Degree and Year: PhD 1978
Major Field: Clinical Psychology
Specialty: Health Psychology;Hypnosis/
   Hypnotherapy;Biofeedback;Individual Psychotherapy;Stress

BERNAL, Guillermo
University of Puerto Rico Station
P.O. Box 23174
Rio Piedras, PR 00931
(787) 763-3965-**B**, (787) 760-1047-**H**, (787) 758-4213-**F**
gbernal@upracd.upr.clu.edu
Ethnicity: Hispanic/Latino
Languages: Spanish
Degree and Year: PhD 1978
Major Field: Clinical Psychology

BERNAL, Martha E
PO Box 1091
Black Canyon City, AZ 85324
602 965-7606-**B**, 602 374-9662-**H**, 602 374-9662-**F**
atmeb@imap1.asu.edu
Ethnicity: Hispanic/Latino
Languages: Spanish
Degree and Year: PhD 1962 MA 1957
Major Field: Clinical Psychology
Specialty: Clinical Child Psychology;Conduct Disorders;Ethnic
   Minorities;Behavior Therapy

BERNAT, Gloria S.
1200 N El Dorado Place
Suite #F640
Tucson, AZ 85715
(602) 298-9746-**B**, (602) 299-0138-**H**, (602) 886-0162-**F**
gbernat@primenet.com
Ethnicity: Hispanic/Latino
Languages: Spanish
Degree and Year: PhD 1978
Major Field: Clinical Psychology
Specialty: Group Psychotherapy;Hypnosis/Hypnotherapy;Individual
   Psychotherapy;Psychosomatic Disorders;Stress

BERRILL, Naftali G.
The New York Center for Neuropsychology
   and Forensic Behavioral Science, P.C.
26 Court Sstreet

Suite #900
Brooklyn Heights, NY 11242
(718) 237-2127-**H**, (718) 237-0831-**F**
Ethnicity: Hispanic/Latino
Languages: Spanish
Degree and Year: PhD 1986
Major Field: Clinical Psychology
Specialty: Forensic Psychology

BERRIOS, Zaida R.
982 Gutenberg
Jardines Metropolitanos
Rio Piedras, PR 0092
(809) 764-0973-**B**, (809) 765-5941-**H**, (809) 764-0973-**F**   **Ethnicity:**
Hispanic/Latino
Languages: Spanish
Degree and Year: PhD 1985
Major Field: Clinical Psychology
Specialty: Child & Pediatric Psychology;Neuropsychology;Mentally
Retarded;Infancy;Learning Disabilities

BERRY, Joyce Hamilton
6357 Windharp Way
Columbia, MD 21045
(202) 544-0072-**B**, (301) 596-2438-**H**, (202) 544-0357-**F**
Ethnicity: African-American/Black
Degree and Year: PhD 1970
Major Field: Clinical Psychology
Specialty: Adolescent Therapy;Affective Disorders;Cognitive
Behavioral Therapy;Assessment/Diagnosis/Evaluation;Individual
Psychotherapy

BERSING, Doris S.
CENTERPOINT
240 Lombard Street #336
San Francisco, CA 94901
(415) 956-1757-**B**, (415) 459-2395-**H**, (415) 459-1292-**F**
Ethnicity: Hispanic/Latino
Languages: French, Spanish
Degree and Year: PhD 1998
Major Field: unknown
Specialty: Individual Psychotherapy;Alcoholism & Alcohol
Abuse;Psychotherapy;Clinical Psychology;Medical Psychology

BETANCOURT, Hector
Loma Linda University
Department of Psychology
11130 Anderson Street
Loma Linda, CA 92350
909558-8577-**B**, (909) 783-1544-**H**, (909) 824-4171-**F**
hbetancourt@ccmail.llu.ed
Ethnicity: Hispanic/Latino
Languages: Spanish
Degree and Year: PhD 1983
Major Field: Social Psychology
Specialty: Attribution Theory;Cultural & Social
Processes;Aggression;Ethnic Minorities;Political Psychology

BHANTHUMNAVIN, Duangduen
Graduate School of Social Development
National Institute of Dev. Admin.

Sukapiban Rd 2
Bangkok   10240, THAILAND
662 377 6764-**B**, 662 719 0207-**H**, 662 319 6875-**F**
vutthi@mort.inet.co.th
Ethnicity: Asian-American/Asian/Pacific Islander
Languages: Thai
Degree and Year: PhD 1972
Major Field: Social Psychology
Specialty: Values & Moral Behavior;Research & Training;Human Development & Family Studies;Work Performance;Training & Development;Social Development

BHATIA, Kiran
20222 Laverton
Katy, TX 77450
(809) 764-0973-**B**, (809) 765-5941-**H**, (809) 764-0973-**F**
Ethnicity: Hispanic/Latino
Languages: Spanish
Degree and Year: PhD 1985
Major Field: Clinical Psychology
Specialty: Child & Pediatric Psychology;Neuropsychology;Mentally Retarded;Infancy;Learning Disabilities

BIGGS, Bradley
142 North Allen Street
Albany, NY 12203
(518) 482-8363-**B**, (518) 452-1745-**H**
Ethnicity: African-American/Black
Degree and Year: PhD 1984
Major Field: Counseling Psychology
Specialty: Affective Disorders;Ethnic Minorities;Family Therapy;Neurological Disorders;Psychotherapy

BILD-LIBBIN, Raguel
1111 Kane Concourse
Suite #302
Bay Harbor Island, FL 33154
(305) 865-7551-**B**, (305) 864-4703-**H**, (305) 864-0919-**F**
Ethnicity: Hispanic/Latino
Languages: Spanish
Degree and Year: PhD 1976
Major Field: Counseling Psychology
Specialty: Assessment/Diagnosis/Evaluation;Clinical Child Psychology;Depression;Child Abuse;Family Therapy

BINGHAM, Rosie P.
University of Memphis
205 Scates Hall
Memphis, TN 38152
(901) 678-5426-**B**, (901) 386-2124-**H**, (901) 678-5425-**F**
rbingham@latte.memphis.edu
Ethnicity: African-American/Black
Degree and Year: PhD 1977
Major Field: Counseling Psychology

BINION, Victoria J.
18620 Muirland
Detroit, MI 48221
(993) 993-3497-**B**, (313) 861-5183-**H**, (313) 993-3421-**F**
vbinion@wayne.edu
Ethnicity: African-American/Black
Degree and Year: PhD 1981
Major Field: Clinical Psychology

Specialty: Ethnic Minorities;Psychology of Women;Community Psychology;Mental Health Services;Mental Disorders;Research & Training

BINNS, Derrick
PO Box 315
Devonshire 059,
BERMUDA
(441) 292-3049-**B**, (441) 236-9209-**H**, (809) 234-3075-**F**
Ethnicity: African-American/Black
Degree and Year: PhD 1986
Major Field: Clinical Psychology
Specialty: Individual Psychotherapy;Correctional Psychology;Group Psychotherapy

BIRKY, Ian
Lehigh University
6311 Domarray St
Coopersburg, PA 18036-8939
(610) 758-3880-**B**, (610) 282-4807-**H**, (215) 758-6207-**F**
itb0@lehigh.edu
Ethnicity: Asian-American/Asian/Pacific Islander
Degree and Year: PhD 1982
Major Field: Clinical Psychology
Specialty: Crisis Intervention & Therapy;Family Therapy;Group Psychotherapy;Sports Psychology;Psychotherapy

BLACKBURN, Winona K.
3523 Porter St Nw
Washington, DC 20016-3177
(202) 244-4917-**H**
Ethnicity: Asian-American/Asian/Pacific Islander
Degree and Year: PhD 1983
Major Field: General Psy./Methods & Systems
Specialty: Sensory & Perceptual Processes;Psycholinguistic;Training & Development;Nonverbal Communication;Moral Development

BLACKETT-SULLIVAN, Gwendolyn A.
New York City Board of Education
CES 55 Bronx
450 St. Paul Place
New York, NY 10456
(718) 681-6227-**B**, (914) 788-0941-**H**, (718) 681-6247-**F**
Ethnicity: African-American/Black
Degree and Year: MA 1988
Major Field: Clinical Psychology
Specialty: Forensic Psychology;Crisis Intervention & Therapy;Chronically Mentally Ill;Emotional Development;Special Education;Drug Abuse

BLAIR, Deborah G.
9900 Shelbyville Road
Suite 11-B
Louisville, KY 40223
(502) 426-4153-**B**, (502) 245-2254-**H**
Ethnicity: American Indian/Alaska Native
Languages: Spanish
Degree and Year: PsyD 1988
Major Field: Clinical Psychology
Specialty: Clinical Psychology;Adolescent Development;Clinical Child Psychology;Family Therapy;Attention Deficit Disorders

BLANCO-BELEDO, Ricardo
Centro de Investigaciones Interdisciplinarias
Cerro de la Estrella 291-2
Mexico City, DF 04200 MEXICO

905 698-2816-**B**, 905 689-3770-**H**, 905 568-0392-**F**
beledo@servidor.unam.mx
Ethnicity: Hispanic/Latino
Languages: French, Italian, Spanish
Degree and Year: PhD 1986
Major Field: Counseling Psychology
Specialty: Psychotherapy;Psychoanalysis;Clinical Psychology;Pastoral Psychology

BLANDING, Benjamin
Crossing Apartments
Apartment C-223
515 Mullica Hill Road
Glassboro, NJ 08028-1061
(609) 256-4500-**B**, (601) 881-1025-**H**, (609) 256-4892-**F**
blandingz@sbs.rowan.edu
Ethnicity: African-American/Black
Degree and Year: PsyD 1984
Major Field: Clinical Psychology
Specialty: Clinical Psychology;Hypnosis/Hypnotherapy;Alcoholism & Alcohol Abuse;Affective Disorders;Smoking

BLANDINO, Ramon A.
233-40 56th Road
Bayside, NY 11364
(212) 219-1618-**B**, (718) 631-2944-**H**, (212) 219-2087-**F**
Ethnicity: Hispanic/Latino
Languages: Spanish
Degree and Year: MA 1990
Major Field: Community Psychology
Specialty: Chronically Mentally Ill;Clinical Psychology;Community Psychology;Ethnic Minorities;HIV/AIDS

BLOCK, Carolyn B.
1947 Divisadero Street
Suite 2
San Francisco, CA 94115
(415) 922-9013-**B**, (415) 239-4744-**H**, (415) 333-1833-**F**
Ethnicity: African-American/Black
Degree and Year: PhD 1972
Major Field: Clinical Psychology
Specialty: Clinical Psychology;Cross Cultural Processes;Ethnic Minorities;Clinical Child Psychology;Individual Psychotherapy;Forensic Psychology

BLUBAUGH, Victoria G.
Lakes Region Community Services Council
PO Box 509
Laconia, NH 03247
(603) 524-5373-**B**, (603) 528-8017-**H**
Ethnicity: American Indian/Alaska Native
Degree and Year: PhD 1987
Major Field: Developmental Psychology
Specialty: Developmental Psychology;Forensic Psychology;Sexual Behavior;Deviant Behavior;Mentally Retarded

BLUE, Arthur W.
PO Box 1020
Carberry, MB, R0K0H-0
CANADA

(204) 834-3331-**H**
ablue@mail.techplus.com
Ethnicity: American Indian/Alaska Native
Degree and Year: PhD 1969
Major Field: Developmental Psychology

BOGGS, Minnie
1102 19th Avenue
Honolulu, HI 96816
(808) 739-5300-**B**, (808) 737-6342-**H**
Ethnicity: Asian-American/Asian/Pacific Islander
Degree and Year: PhD 1974
Major Field: Educational Psychology
Specialty: Psychotherapy;Marriage & Family

BOLDEN, Wiley S.
975 Veltre Circle SW
Atlanta, GA 30311
(404) 755-6135-**H**
Ethnicity: African-American/Black
Degree and Year: EdD 1957
Major Field: Clinical Psychology
Specialty: Developmental Psychology;Program Evaluation

BONAL, Kathleen A.
Institute of Living
Harvard Hospital's Mental Health Network
400 Washington Street
Hartford, CT 06106
(860) 545-7167-**B**
Ethnicity: Asian-American/Asian/Pacific Islander, European/White
Degree and Year: PhD 1990
Major Field: Clinical Psychology
Specialty: Psychotherapy;Assessment/Diagnosis/Evaluation;Group Psychotherapy;Projective Techniques

BOODOO, Gwyneth M.
Educational Testing Service
Mail Stop 03-T
Princeton, NJ 08541-0001
(609) 734-5982-**B**, (609) 890-6110-**H**, (609) 734-5420-**F**
gboodoo@ets.org
Ethnicity: Asian-American/Asian/Pacific Islander
Degree and Year: PhD 1978
Major Field: Quan/Math & Psychometrics/Stat
Specialty: Psychometrics;Quantitative/Mathematical, Psychometrics;Research Design & Methodology;Statistics;Educational Research

BOONE, Martin
West Virginia University
School of Medicine
Department of Behavioral Medicine/Psychiatry
Morgantown, WV 26505
(304) 293-2411-**B**, (304) 598-3611-**H**

mboone2@wvu.edu
Ethnicity: Hispanic/Latino
Degree and Year: PhD 1993
Major Field: Clinical Psychology
Specialty: Neuropsychology

BORGATTA, Edgar F.
98 Union Street
Suite #608
Seattle, WA 98101-2068
(206) 622-9158-**H**, (206) 344-6302-**F**
borgatta@u.washington.edu
Ethnicity: Hispanic/Latino
Languages: Italian, Spanish
Degree and Year: PhD 1952
Major Field: Social Psychology
Specialty: Quantitative/Mathematical,
Psychometrics;Measurement;Statistics;Social
Psychology;Social Problems

BORREGO, Richard L.
Borrego and Associates, Inc.
7790 East Arapahoe Roade
Suite 200
Englewood, CO 80112-1274
(303) 850-7510-**B**, (303) 791-8251-**H**, (303) 779-3035-**F**
Ethnicity: Hispanic/Latino
Degree and Year: PhD 1980
Major Field: Clinical Psychology
Specialty: Adolescent Therapy;Clinical Neuropsychology;Crisis
Intervention & Therapy;Assessment/Diagnosis/
Evaluation;Clinical Psychology;Stress

BORRERO-HERNANDEZ, Alejo
U.S. Public Health Service
U.S. Department of Justice-FCI Talladega
565 East Renfroe Road
Talladega, AL 35160-2380
(265) 3125-4454-**F**
alejobh@aol.com
Ethnicity: Hispanic/Latino
Degree and Year: PhD 1979 MAe 1974
Major Field: Counseling Psychology
Specialty: Psychotherapy;Drug Abuse;Mental Health
Services;Correctional Psychology;Industrial/
Organizational Psychology

BOSCH, Isora
513 70th Street
Guttenburg, NJ 07093
(201) 868-5454-**B**, (201) 868-5454-**H**, (201) 868-2886-**F**
Ethnicity: Hispanic/Latino
Languages: Spanish
Degree and Year: EdD 1987
Major Field: Industrial/Organizational Psy.
Specialty: HIV/AIDS;Organizational
Development;Stress;Training & Development;Job
Satisfaction

BOSTICK, Rosie M.
Dept. VAMC
2002 Holcombe Boulevard (116B)
Houston, TX 77030
(713) 794-7044-**B**, (713) 794-7835-**F**
Ethnicity: African-American/Black
Degree and Year: PhD 1977
Major Field: Clinical Psychology
Specialty: Clinical Psychology;Rehabilitation;Sexual Dysfunction

BOSTWICK, Allen D.
S 1403 Grand Blvd.
Suite #202-N
Spokane, WA 99203
(509) 747-7700-**B**, (509) 535-2241-**H**
Ethnicity: American Indian/Alaska Native
Degree and Year: PhD 1980
Major Field: Clinical Psychology
Specialty: Brain Damage;Clinical Psychology;Medical
Psychology;Neuropsychology;Psychotherapy

BOUFFARD, R. Gerard
International Institute for Non-Violence
527 Cherrier
C.P. 414
Montreal, Quebec, H3B3J7
CANADA
(514) 272-2710-**B**, (514) 289-1913-**H**, (514) 272-6377-**F**
iintotal.net
Ethnicity: American Indian/Alaska Native
Languages: French
Degree and Year: PhD 1978
Major Field: Developmental Psychology
Specialty: Clinical Psychology;Assessment/Diagnosis/
Evaluation;Developmental Psychology;School
Psychology;Training & Development

BOULETTE, Tersea R.
PO Box 4789
Santa Barbara, CA 93103
(805) 681-5229-**B**, (805) 965-8429-**H**, (805) 681-5262-**F**
Ethnicity: Hispanic/Latino
Languages: Spanish
Degree and Year: PhD 1972
Major Field: Clinical Psychology
Specialty: Clinical Psychology;Health Psychology;Cognitive
Psychology;Community Psychology

BOULON-DIAZ, Frances E.
Alturas de Borinquen Gardens
LL-12 Rose Street
San Juan, PR 00926
(787) 289-4645-**B**, (787) 731-6897-**H**, (787) 289-4640-**F**
americo@caribe.net
Ethnicity: Hispanic/Latino
Languages: Spanish
Degree and Year: Phd 1992 MA 1972
Major Field: School Psychology
Specialty: Industrial/Organizational
Psychology;Administration;Employee Assistance
Programs;Human Resources;Training & Development;School
Psychology

BOWEN, Peggy C.
Rte 3, Box 5600
Bartlesville, OK 74003-9570
(918) 336-2272-**B**, (918) 336-4530-**H**
Ethnicity: American Indian/Alaska Native
Degree and Year: PhD 1979
Major Field: Social Psychology
Specialty: Attitudes & Opinions;Correctional Psychology;Crime & Criminal Behavior;Research Design & Methodology;Child Abuse

BOWEN, Tanya U.
Oswego State University
Counseling Center
Walker Health Center
Oswego, NY 13126
(315) 341-4416-**B**, (315) 699-9921-**H**
tbowen@oswego.edu
Ethnicity: African-American/Black
Degree and Year: PhD 1995
Major Field: Clinical Psychology
Specialty: Clinical Psychology;Lesbian & Gay Issuues;Training & Development;Cross Cultural Processes;Feminist Therapy;Marriage & Family

BOWMAN, Sharon L.
Ball State University
Department of Counseling and
 Guidance Services
Muncie, IN 47306-1099
(317) 285-8040-**B**, (317) 282-1385-**H**
Ethnicity: African-American/Black
Degree and Year: PhD 1989
Major Field: Counseling Psychology
Specialty: Cross Cultural Processes;Lesbian & Gay Issuues;Counseling Psychology;Vocational Psychology

BOXLEY, Russell L.
1518 Cheviotdale Drive
Pasadena, CA 91105
(213) 724-3388-**B**, (213) 259-1192-**H**, (213) 258-1192-**F**
Ethnicity: African-American/Black
Degree and Year: PhD 1973
Major Field: Clinical Psychology
Specialty: Psychotherapy;Ethnic Minorities;Homicide;Affective Disorders

BOYD, Naughne L.
846 Stevens Drive
Richland, WA 99352
(509) 946-9613-**B**, (509) 375-1360-**H**, (509) 946-6814-**F**
Ethnicity: African-American/Black
Degree and Year: PhD 1974
Major Field: Clinical Psychology
Specialty: Clinical Child Psychology;Psychotherapy;Marriage & Family;Assessment/Diagnosis/Evaluation;Child Abuse

BOYD, Vivian S.
University of Maryland
Counseling Center
Shoemaker Hall
College Park, MD 20742-0001
(301) 314-7675-**B**, (301) 384-8514-**H**, (301) 314-9206-**F**
vboyd@umdacc.umd.edu

Ethnicity: African-American/Black
Degree and Year: PhD 1975
Major Field: Counseling Psychology
Specialty: Psychotherapy;Community Mental Health

BOYER, Michele C.
Indiana State University
Department of Counseling SE
Room #1507
Terre Haute, IN 97803
(812) 237-7602-**B**, (812) 877-9662-**H**, (812) 237-4348-**F**
egboyer@befac.indstate.edu
Ethnicity: African-American/Black
Degree and Year: PhD 1984
Major Field: Counseling Psychology
Specialty: Training & Development;Feminist Therapy;Assessment/Diagnosis/Evaluation;Cross Cultural Processes

BRACERO, William
Sunset Park Mental Health Center
 of Lutheran Medical Center
514 49th Street
Brooklyn, NY 11220
(718) 437-5217-**B**, (212) 725-5297-**H**
Ethnicity: Hispanic/Latino
Languages: Spanish
Degree and Year: PhD 1990
Major Field: Clinical Psychology
Specialty: Ethnic Minorities;Cultural & Social Processes;Group Processes;Cross Cultural Processes;Gender Issues;Group Psychotherapy

BRADMAN, Leo H.
7777 Davie Road
Extension #100-A
Hollywood, FL 33204-2513
(954) 704-8686-**B**, (-**F**
Ethnicity: Hispanic/Latino
Languages: Spanish
Degree and Year: PsyD 1982
Major Field: Clinical Psychology
Specialty: Managed Care

BRADSHAW, Carla K.
22015 NE 183rd Place
Woodinville, WA 98072
(206) 441-5749-**B**
Ethnicity: Asian-American/Asian/Pacific Islander
Degree and Year: PhD 1987
Major Field: Clinical Psychology

BRANCHE, Leota Susan
1623 3rd Avenue
Apartment #22C, West
New York, NY 10128
(212) 722-1044-**B**
Ethnicity: African-American/Black, American Indian/Alaska Native
Languages: Italian, Portuguese, Spanish
Degree and Year: PhD 1988
Major Field: Clinical Psychology
Specialty: Clinical Child Psychology;Behavior Therapy;Assessment/Diagnosis/Evaluation;Pastoral Psychology;Family Therapy

BRANDENBURG, Carlos E.
7390 Pinehurst
Reno, NV 99502

(702) 688-1900-**B**, (702) 857-3422-**H**, (702) 699-1909-**F**
Ethnicity: Hispanic/Latino
Languages: Spanish
Degree and Year: PhD 1978
Major Field: Clinical Psychology
Specialty: Assessment/Diagnosis/Evaluation;Chronically Mentally Ill;Correctional Psychology;Cross Cultural Processes;Forensic Psychology

BRANNON, Lorraine
4527 Georgia Avenue, NW
Washington, DC 20011
(202) 882-2663-**B**, (202) 882-5905-**F**
Ethnicity: African-American/Black
Degree and Year: PhD 1975
Major Field: Clinical Psychology
Specialty: Child Therapy;Marriage & Family

BRATTESAMI, Karen A.
336 NW 50th Street
Seattle, WA 98107-3521
Ethnicity: Hispanic/Latino
Degree and Year: PhD 1984
Major Field: Social Psychology
Specialty: Consumer Psychology

BRICE, Janet R.
81 Drake Road
Somerset, NJ 08873-2366
(908) 937-9454-**B**
Ethnicity: African-American/Black
Degree and Year: PhD 1985
Major Field: Clinical Psychology

BRIGGS, Felicia H.
Bay Counseling Services
Frank Gibson, Jr. , PhD, PA & Associates
3727 Nortonia Road
Baltimore, MD 21716
(410) 501-6172-**B**, (410) 566-7138-**H**
Ethnicity: African-American/Black
Degree and Year: PhD 1994
Major Field: Clinical Psychology
Specialty: Clinical Psychology;Rehabilitation;Health Psychology;Gerontology/Geropsychology;Clinical Neuropsychology

BRINSON, Les
4617 Limerick Drive
Raleigh, NC 27604-3525
Ethnicity: African-American/Black
Degree and Year: PhD 1970
Major Field: Counseling Psychology

BROADFIELD, Charles S.
5750 Chesapeake Blvd.
P.O. Box 10083
Norfolk, VA 23513-0083
(804) 853-1409-**B**, (804) 853-4437-**H**, (804) 853-4437-**F**
Ethnicity: African-American/Black
Languages: German
Degree and Year: PhD 1988
Major Field: School Psychology
Specialty: Alcoholism & Alcohol Abuse;Child Abuse;Drug Abuse;Projective Techniques;Family Therapy;Forensic Psychology

BRODIE, Debra A.
559 Fisher Building
3011 W Grand Boulevard
Detroit, MI 48202-3012
(313) 875-4240-**B**
Ethnicity: African-American/Black
Degree and Year: PhD 1984
Major Field: unknown
Specialty: Physiological Psychology;Motor Performance

BROOKINS, Geraldine K
W.K. Kellogg Foundation
One Michigan Avenue East
Ford Hall
Battle Creek, MI 49017
(616) 969-2093-**B**, (616) 353-5826-**H**, (616) 969-2188-**F**
gkb@wkkf.org
Ethnicity: African-American/Black
Degree and Year: PhD 1977
Major Field: Developmental Psychology
Specialty: Adolescent Development;Family Processes;Child Development;Psychology of Women;Developmental Psychology

BROOKS, JR., Glenwood C.
3213 Pinkney Road
Baltimore, MD 21215-3710
Ethnicity: American Indian/Alaska Native
Degree and Year: PhD 1972
Major Field: Counseling Psychology
Specialty: Counseling Psychology

BROOKS, Juanita O.
Independent Practice
2210 S Front Street Street
Suite #204
Melbourne, FL 32901
(407) 951-0400-**B**, (407) 723-4320-**H**, (407) 951-0672-**F**
jbrooks@myshoes.com
Ethnicity: African-American/Black, American Indian/Alaska Native
Degree and Year: PhD 1982
Major Field: Clinical Psychology
Specialty: Psychotherapy;Marriage & Family;Depression;Humanistic Psychology;Neuroses

BROOKS, Lewis A.
9 Cobb Lane
Apartment F
Middletown, NY 10940-7008
(914) 434-7100-**B**, (914) 434-0331-**F**
Ethnicity: African-American/Black
Languages: Spanish, Hungarian
Degree and Year: PhD 1992
Major Field: Educational Psychology
Specialty: Mental Disorders;Cognitive Development;Developmental Psychology;Mentally Retarded

BROWN, Anita B.
259 Woodland Road
Hampton, VA 23669
202 336-5878-**B**, 301 460-2554-**H**
Ethnicity: African-American/Black
Degree and Year: PhD 1979
Major Field: Clinical Psychology
Specialty: Psychotherapy

BROWN, Barbara J.
Barbara J. Brown, PhD, F.A.C.T.S.,P.L.L.C.
650 Pennsylvania Avenue, SE
Suite 440
Washington, DC 20003
(202) 544-5440-**B**, (202) 901-8142-**H**, (202) 544-3004-**F**
bbrown2778@aol.com
Ethnicity: African-American/Black
Degree and Year: PhD 1985
Major Field: Clinical Psychology
Specialty: Adolescent Therapy;Child Abuse;Domestic
        Violence;Affective Disorders;Child Therapy;Family Therapy

BROWNE, Ronald H.
Browne Psychological Services
526 East Chapel
Suite A
Santa Maria, CA 93458
(805) 347-7411-**B**, (805) 473-8030-**H**, (805) 347-1306-**F**
psychor@msn.com
Ethnicity: African-American/Black
Degree and Year: PhD 1993
Major Field: Clinical Psychology
Specialty: Crisis Intervention & Therapy;Family
        Therapy;Psychopathology;Forensic Psychology;Attention
        Deficit Disorders

BROWN, John R.
6950 E Exposition Avenue
Denver, CO 80224-1512
(303) 355-2147-**B**
Ethnicity: African-American/Black
Degree and Year: PhD 1975
Major Field: Developmental Psychology

BROWN, Marilyn F.
California School of
Professional Psychology
1000 South Fremont Avenue
Alhambra, CA 91803
(213) 939-3323-**H**
Ethnicity: African-American/Black
Degree and Year:
Major Field: Clinical Psychology

BROWN, Michael T.
University of California, Santa Barbara
Graduate School of Education
1330 Phelps Hall
Santa Barbara, CA 93106-2003
(805) 893-3375-**B**
mbrown@education.ucsb.edu
Ethnicity: African-American/Black
Degree and Year: PhD 1985
Major Field: Counseling Psychology

BROWN, Pamela
1518 Walnut Street
Suite #907
Philildelphia, PA 19102
(215) 985-1213-**B**, (215) 247-6374-**H**
Ethnicity: African-American/Black
Degree and Year: PsyD 1986

Major Field: Clinical Psychology
Specialty: Clinical Psychology;Ethnic Minorities;Feminist
        Therapy;Psychotherapy;Depression

BRUGUERA, Mark R.
2810 Belmont Canyon Road
Belmont, CA 94002-1231
(408) 299-8757-**B**
Ethnicity: Hispanic/Latino
Languages: Spanish
Degree and Year: PhD 1984
Major Field: Counseling Psychology
Specialty: Adolescent Therapy;Ethnic Minorities;Group
        Psychotherapy;Clinical Neuropsychology;Chronically
        Mentally Ill

BRYANT-TUCKETT, Rose M.
23 Old Snake Hill Road
Pound Ridge, NY 10576
(914) 764-4413-**B**, (914) 764-5081-**H**
Ethnicity: African-American/Black
Degree and Year: PhD 1980
Major Field: Clinical Psychology
Specialty: Conduct Disorders;Clinical Child Psychology;Clinical
        Psychology;Adolescent Therapy;Assessment/Diagnosis/
        Evaluation

BRYANT, Gerard W.
Federal Bureau of Prisons
U.S. Custom House, 7th Floor
2nd and Chestnut Streets
Philadelphia, PA 19106
(215) 597-6391-**B**, (212) 595-9801-**H**, (215) 597-6392-**F**
Ethnicity: African-American/Black
Languages: French
Degree and Year: PhD 1989
Major Field: School Psychology
Specialty: Correctional Psychology;Industrial/Organizational
        Psychology;Clinical Child Psychology;School
        Psychology;Ethnic Minorities

BUENO, Luis F.
1401 Lancaster Drive
Memphis, TN 38120
(901) 683-4870-**H**
Ethnicity: Hispanic/Latino
Languages: Spanish
Degree and Year: PhD 1955
Major Field: Clinical Psychology
Specialty: Child & Pediatric Psychology;Child Therapy;Clinical
        Psychology;Cognitive Behavioral Therapy;Hypnosis/
        Hypnotherapy

BUFFIN, Janice E.
96 Fifth Avenue
Suite #1-C
New York, NY 10011-7605
(212) 924-4709-**B**, (212) 932-9770-**H**, (212) 924-4709-**F**
Ethnicity: African-American/Black
Degree and Year: PhD 1985
Major Field: Clinical Psychology
Specialty: Adult Development;Clinical Psychology;Group
        Psychotherapy;Individual Psychotherapy;Management &
        Organization

BUKI, Lydia P.
Georgetown University
2901 Connecticut Avenue, NW
Apartment 107
Washington, DC 20008
(202) 687-1403-**B**, (202) 518-8434-**H**
bukil@gunet.georgetown.edu
Ethnicity: Hispanic/Latino
Languages: Spanish
Degree and Year: PhD 1995
Major Field: Counseling Psychology
Specialty: Cross Cultural Processes;Gerontology/
Geropsychology;Health Psychology

BURCHELL, Charles R.
1581 Carol Sue Avenue
Suite 211
Grenta, LA 70056-5100
(504) 392-3498-**H**
Ethnicity: African-American/Black
Degree and Year: PhD 1980
Major Field: Clinical Psychology
Specialty: Clinical Psychology;Community Psychology

BURCIAGA, Lawrence E.
1600 Medical Center Street
Suite #203
ElL Paso, TX 79902-5008
(915) 542-0153-**B**
Ethnicity: Hispanic/Latino
Degree and Year: PhD 1976
Major Field: unknown
Specialty: Neuropsychology

BURKS, Eura O.
6639 Trigate
Missouri City, TX 77489-3513
(713) 772-8518-**H**
Ethnicity: African-American/Black
Degree and Year: EdD 1971
Major Field: Counseling Psychology

BURNETT YOUNG, Myra N.
415 Stone Arbor Court SW
Atlanta, GA 30331-7387
(404) 223-7568-**B**, (404) 344-3580-**H**
mburnett@spelman.edu
Ethnicity: African-American/Black
Degree and Year: PhD 1987
Major Field: Clinical Psychology

BURNETT, John H.
John H. Burnett & Associates, Inc.
70 West Madison
Suite 1400
Chicago, IL 60602
(312) 781-9616-**B**
Ethnicity: African-American/Black
Degree and Year: PhD 1977
Major Field: Social Psychology
Specialty: Human Resources;Performance
Evaluation;Psychometrics;Industrial/Organizational
Psychology;Computer Applications and Programming

BURNETT, Judith A.
1269 Massman Drive
Nashville, TN 37217
(615) 860-7300-**B**, (615) 860-7313-**F**
Ethnicity: African-American/Black
Degree and Year: PhD 1991
Major Field: Clinical Psychology
Specialty: Mental Health Services;Community Mental
Health;Individual Psychotherapy;Cross Cultural
Processes;Managed Care

BURNHAM, Lem
340 South Almonesson Road
Deptford, NJ 08096-3758
(609) 227-5629-**B**
Ethnicity: African-American/Black
Degree and Year: PhD 1984
Major Field: unknown
Specialty: Sports Psychology;Employee Assistance Programs

BURR, Sharon S.
1222 Ottawa Circle
Richardson, TX 75080-3925
(972) 251-3687-**B**
Ethnicity: African-American/Black
Degree and Year: PhD 1981
Major Field: Clinical Psychology
Specialty: Psychotherapy;Assessment/Diagnosis/
Evaluation;Psychology of Women;Managed Care;Ethnic
Minorities

BURSZTYN, Alberto M.
Brooklyn College - CUNY
2900 Bedford Avenue
Brooklyn, NY 11210
(718) 951-5214-**B**, (718) 768-2813-**H**, (718) 95104816-**F**
aburstyn@brooklyn.cuny.edu
Ethnicity: Hispanic/Latino
Languages: Spanish
Degree and Year: PhD 1992
Major Field: Counseling Psychology
Specialty: Counseling Psychology;Cross Cultural Processes;Special
Education;School Psychology;Ethnic Minorities;Program
Evaluation

BURTON, Roger V.
211 Lebrun Road
Eggertsville, NY 14226
(716) 645-3650-**B**, (716) 835-5062-**H**, (716) 645-3801-**F**
psyburt@acsu.buffalo.edu
Ethnicity: Hispanic/Latino, European/White
Languages: French, Spanish
Degree and Year: PhD 1959
Major Field: Developmental Psychology
Specialty: Moral Development;Parent-Child Interaction;Cross Cultural
Processes;Child Development;Social Development

BUSTAMANTE, Eduardo M.
48 N Pleasant Street
Suite #205
Amherst, MA 01002
(413) 256-1869-**B**, (413) 256-1869-**H**, (413) 253-4089-**F**
drb@javanet.com
Ethnicity: Hispanic/Latino
Languages: Spanish

Degree and Year: PhD 1983
Major Field: Clinical Psychology
Specialty: Attention Deficit Disorders;Conduct Disorders;Cognitive
    Behavioral Therapy;Clinical Child Psychology;Clinical Child
    Neuropsychology

BUTLER, B. LaConyea
    Spelman College
    350 Spelman Lane, S.W.
    Box 372
    Atlanta, GA 30314-4399
    (404) 223-7564-**B**, (404) 792-2747-**H**, (404) 215-7863-**F**
    (404) 223-7564
Ethnicity: African-American/Black
Degree and Year: PhD 1972
Major Field: Counseling Psychology

BYNUM, Edward B.
    University of Massachusetts
    Health Services
    127 Hills North
    Amherst, MA 01003
    (413) 545-2337-**B**, (413) 253-3901-**H**
Ethnicity: African-American/Black
Degree and Year: PhD 1977
Major Field: Clinical Psychology
Specialty: Biofeedback;Ethnic Minorities;Family Processes;Family
    Therapy;Psychotherapy

BYRD, Robert D.
    St. Johns Health Center
    1333 20th Street
    Santa Monica, CA 90404
    (310) 829-8535-**B**, (2130 933-9594-**H**, (310) 829-8455-**F**
Ethnicity: American Indian/Alaska Native
Languages: American Sign Language
Degree and Year: PsyD 1994
Major Field: Clinical Child Psychology
Specialty: Forensic Psychology;Neuropsychology;Community
    Psychology;Clinical Psychology

CABERTO, Steven C.
    12th MOOS/SGOH
    1985 First Street, West
    Suite #1
    Randolph AFB, TX 78150-4311
    (210) 652-2448-**B**, (210) 497-4633-**H**, (210) 652-3173-**F**
Ethnicity: Asian-American/Asian/Pacific Islander
Degree and Year: PhD 1989
Major Field: Clinical Psychology
Specialty: Mental Health Services;Military Psychology;Sports
    Psychology;Human Factors;Selection & Placement;Work
    Performance

CADE, Bonita G.
    BG Cade, PhD, JD
    63 Ash Street
    New Bedford, MA 02740
    (508) 990-1077-**B**, (508) 990-1077-**H**, (508) 990-1077-**F**
Ethnicity: African-American/Black
Degree and Year: PhD 1981
Major Field: Clinical Psychology
Specialty: Forensic Psychology;Cross Cultural Processes;Personality
    Measurement;Counseling Psychology;Individual
    Psychotherapy;Assessment/Diagnosis/Evaluation

CAESAR, Robert
    313 Shillingford Road
    Irmo, SC 29063-2331
    (803) 734-7419-**B**, (803) 781-8738-**H**
Ethnicity: African-American/Black
Degree and Year: PhD 1985
Major Field: Clinical Psychology
Specialty: Clinical Neuropsychology

CAETANO, Elizabeth
    5632 Hazel Avenue
    Richmond, CA 94805-1904
Ethnicity: Hispanic/Latino
Degree and Year: PhD 1987
Major Field: Clinical Psychology

CALDERA, Yvonne M.
    Texas Technical University
    Department of Human Development
        and Family Studies
    Box 91162
    Lubbock, TX 79409
    (806) 742-3000-**B**, (8060 767-0756-**H**, (806) 742-0285-**F**
    q2yvo@ttacs.ttu.edu
Ethnicity: Hispanic/Latino
Languages: Spanish
Degree and Year: PhD 1990
Major Field: Developmental Psychology
Specialty: Cross Cultural Processes;Human Development & Family
    Studies;Parent-Child Interaction;Ethnic
    Minorities;Infancy;Developmental Psychology

CALDERON, Vivian
    866 Noe St
    San Francisco, CA 94114-2926
    (415) 239-3473-**B**, (510) 376-5448-**H**
Ethnicity: Hispanic/Latino
Degree and Year: PhD 1984
Major Field: Social Psychology
Specialty: Educational Research

CALDWELL-COLBERT, A. Toy
    University of Illinois
    378 Henry Administration Building
    506 South Wright Street
    Urbana, IL 61801
    (217) 333-3079-**B**, (217) 355-3500-**H**, (217) 244-5763-**F**
    toycc@uillinois.edu
Ethnicity: African-American/Black
Degree and Year: PhD 1977
Major Field: Clinical Psychology
Specialty: Administration;Behavior Therapy;Cognitive Behavioral
    Therapy;Psychology of Women;Ethnic Minorities;Social Skills

CALDWELL, Barrett S.
    University of Wisconsin, Madison
    1513 University Avenue
    Room 393
    Madison, WI 53706
    (608) 262-2414-**B**, (608) 251-7583-**H**, (608) 262-8454-**F**
    caldwell@engr.wisc.edu
Ethnicity: African-American/Black
Degree and Year: PhD 1990

Major Field: Industrial/Organizational Psy.
Specialty: Engineering Psychology;Industrial/Organizational
    Psychology;Human Factors;Systems Analysis

CALLAHAN, Michelle R.
  Yale University
  135 College Street
  Suite 323
  New Haven, CT 06510
  (203) 785-3441-**B**, (203) 787-5740-**H**, (203) 764-4837-**F**
  michelle.callahan@yale.edu
Ethnicity: African-American/Black
Degree and Year: PhD 1998 MA 1995
Major Field: Developmental Psychology
Specialty: Adolescent Development;Gender Issues;HIV/AIDS;Ethnic
    Minorities;Domestic Violence;Industrial/Organizational
    Psychology

CAMARGO, Robert J.
  679 Davis Drive
  Suite #308
  Newmarket, Ontario, L3Y 5G8
  CANADA
  (416) 895-7442-**B**, (416) 895-5757-**H**, (905) 727-4214-**F**
Ethnicity: Hispanic/Latino
Languages: Spanish
Degree and Year: PhD 1978
Major Field: Clinical Psychology
Specialty: Community Mental Health;Clinical
    Neuropsychology;Epidemiology & Biometry;Attention Deficit
    Disorders;Gender Issues

CAMARILLO, Max
  186 E Seacliff Drive
  Aptos, CA 95003
  (408) 459-2628-**B**, (408) 688-6870-**H**
Ethnicity: Hispanic/Latino
Languages: Spanish
Degree and Year: PhD 1985
Major Field: Clinical Psychology
Specialty: Clinical Psychology;Stress;Biofeedback;Managed Care

CAMERON, Linda S.
  100 Northfield Avenue
  West Orange, NJ 07052
  (973) 325-2006-**B**, (973) 761-5796-**H**, (973) 325-2006-**F**
Ethnicity: African-American/Black
Degree and Year: PhD 1982
Major Field: Clinical Psychology
Specialty: Ethnic Minorities;Depression;Group
    Psychotherapy;Community Psychology;Psychology of
    Women;HIV/AIDS

CAMPBELL-FLINT, Maxine E
  Felician Forensic Facility
  PO Box 888
  Jackson, LA 70748
  505 634-0118-**B**, 504 634-9914-**H**, 504 634-7302-**F**
Ethnicity: African-American/Black
Degree and Year: PhD 1994
Major Field: unknown

Specialty: Forensic Psychology;Clinical Psychology;Deviant
Behavior;Crime & Criminal Behavior;Community
Psychology;Correctional Psychology

CAMPBELL, Barbara L.
  242 Myrtle Street
  San Francisco, CA 94109
  (415) 775-1400-**B**, (415) 239-6254-**H**
Ethnicity: African-American/Black
Degree and Year: PhD 1978
Major Field: unknown
Specialty: Child Abuse;Child Development;Child Therapy;Clinical
    Psychology;Family Therapy

CAMPBELL, Kamal E.
  Bradley Center of St. Francis
  PO Box 7000
  Columbus, GA 31908-7000
  (706) 320-3700-**B**, (706) 660-8537-**H**, (706) 320-3704-**F**
Ethnicity: Asian-American/Asian/Pacific Islander
Languages: Hindi, Gujerati
Degree and Year: PhD 1980
Major Field: Clinical Psychology
Specialty: Individual Psychotherapy;Group Psychotherapy;Projective
    Techniques;Psychopathology;Administration

CAMPBELL, Stephen N.
  11894 SW 12th Place
  Davie, FL 33325-3880
  (305) 967-7251-**B**, (305) 792-8422-**H**
Ethnicity: African-American/Black
Degree and Year: PhD 1978
Major Field: Clinical Psychology
Specialty: Administration;Alcoholism & Alcohol Abuse;Child
    Development;Clinical Psychology;Schizophrenia

CAMPOS, Joseph J.
  University of California @ Berkeley
  Department of Psychology
  Berkeley, CA 94720
  (510) 643-9975-**B**, (510) 649-8860-**H**, (510) 649-9765-**F**
  jcampos@socrates.berkeley.edu
Ethnicity: Asian-American/Asian/Pacific Islander
Languages: Spanish
Degree and Year: PhD 1966
Major Field: Developmental Psychology
Specialty: Infancy;Emotional Development;Emotion

CAMPOS, Leonard P.
  1606 Oakview Drive
  Roseville, CA 95661
  (916) 786-2290-**B**, (916) 786-7976-**H**
  lcampos@vlink.net
Ethnicity: Hispanic/Latino
Languages: Spanish
Degree and Year: PhD 1963
Major Field: Clinical Psychology

CAMPOS, Peter E.
  Emory University
  School of Medicine
  Grady Infectious Disease Prog.
  341 Ponce de Leon Avenue
  Atlanta, GA 30329
  (404) 616-9710-**B**, 404 321-1027-**H**

pcampos@emory.edu
Ethnicity: American Indian/Alaska Native
Degree and Year: PhD 1989
Major Field: Clinical Psychology
Specialty: HIV/AIDS;Lesbian & Gay Issuues;Health
      Psychology;Behavior Therapy

CANEDO, Angelo R.
  Bayside
  38-11 Corporal Stone Street
  New York, NY 11361
  (718) 262-6595-**B**, (718) 428-1742-**H**, (718) 262-6599-**F**
Ethnicity: Hispanic/Latino
Languages: Spanish
Degree and Year: PhD 1980
Major Field: Clinical Psychology
Specialty: Neuropsychology;Rehabilitation;Child & Pediatric
      Psychology;Clinical Psychology;Counseling Psychology

CANOVAS WELLES, Nydia L.
  5225 Old Orchard Road
  Suite 45
  Skokie, IL 60077
  (847) 676-3440-**B**, (847) 256-2200-**H**, (847) 676-3486-**F**
  nlwelles@aol.com
Ethnicity: Hispanic/Latino
Languages: Spanish
Degree and Year: PhD 1986
Major Field: Counseling Psychology

CAPP, Larry D.
  20622 NW 33 Court
  Miami, FL 33056-1348
  305 442-8800-**B**, 305 836-8459-**H**
Ethnicity: African-American/Black
Degree and Year: PhD 1980
Major Field: Clinical Psychology

CAPPON, Jorge
  Sierra Gudarrama 50-501
  Los de Chapultepec
  Mexico D.F. 11000,
  MEXICO
  52-5-520-9124-**B**, 52-5-540-3678-**F**
  cappon@servidor.unam.mx
Ethnicity: Hispanic/Latino
Languages: Spanish
Degree and Year: PhD 1979
Major Field: Clinical Psychology
Specialty: Psychoanalysis;Group Psychotherapy;Nonverbal
      Communication;Organizational Development;Clinical
      Psychology

CARAVEO, Libardo E.
  5585 E Paseo Cimarron
  Tucson, AZ 85715
  (602) 881-5118-**B**, (602) 577-7690-**H**
Ethnicity: Hispanic/Latino
Languages: Spanish
Degree and Year: PhD 1986
Major Field: School Psychology
Specialty: Assessment/Diagnosis/Evaluation;Child & Pediatric
      Psychology;Forensic Psychology;Family Therapy;Learning
      Disabilities

CARBALLO-DIEGUEZ, Alex
  HIV Center
   for Clinical and Behavioral Studies
  722 West 168th Street
  New York, NY 10032
  (212) 543-5261-**B**, (212) 666-6686-**H**, (212) 543-6003-**F**
  ac72@columbia.edu
Ethnicity: Hispanic/Latino
Languages: French, Spanish
Degree and Year: PhD 1986
Major Field: Clinical Psychology
Specialty: HIV/AIDS;Sexual Behavior;Lesbian & Gay Issuues

CARCAS, Marilyn B.
  11588 SW 91st Terrace
  Miami, FL 33176-1046
  (305) 551-0072-**B**
Ethnicity: Hispanic/Latino
Degree and Year: MA 1980
Major Field: Clinical Psychology

CARDALDA, Elsa B.
  Caribbean Center for Advance Studies
  Box 9023711 Old San Juan
  San Juan, PR 00902-3711
  (787) 725-6500-**B**
Ethnicity: Hispanic/Latino
Languages: Spanish
Degree and Year: PhD 1995
Major Field: Social Psychology
Specialty: Child Development;Psychoanalysis;Social
      Psychology;Ethnic Minorities;School Psychology;Systems,
      Methods & Issues

CARDENA, Etzel A.
  USUHS
  Department of Psychiatry
  4301 Jones Bridge Road
  Building B
  Bethesda, MD 20814
  (202) 782-5098-**B**, (301) 963-2561-**H**, (202) 782-7003-**F**
  ecardena@usuhs.mil
Ethnicity: Hispanic/Latino
Languages: French, Spanish
Degree and Year: PhD 1988
Major Field: Clinical Psychology
Specialty: Psychosomatic Disorders;Psychopathology

CARDONA, Gilbert
  1014 South Gramercy Drive
  Los Angeles, CA 90019
  (213) 487-6808-**B**, (213) 734-5507-**H**
Ethnicity: Hispanic/Latino
Languages: Spanish
Degree and Year: PhD. 1976
Major Field: Clinical Psychology
Specialty: Cognitive Behavioral Therapy;Community Mental
      Health;Consulting Psychology;Depression;Family Therapy

CARDOZA, Desdemona
  California State University, Los Angeles
  5151 State University Drive
  Los Angeles, CA 90032
  (626) 574-8586-**H**, (3230 343-6469-**F**

dcardoz@calstatela.edu
Ethnicity: Hispanic/Latino
Degree and Year: PhD 1982
Major Field: Social Psychology
Specialty: Educational Research;Psychology of Women

CAREY, Patricia M.
New York University
82 Washington Square East #32
New York, NY 10003
(212) 998-5025-**B**, (212) 534-8834-**H**, (212) 995-4353-**F**
patricia.carey@nyu.edu
Ethnicity: African-American/Black
Degree and Year: PhD 1982
Major Field: Educational Psychology
Specialty: Developmental Psychology;Psychology of Women;Gender
Issues;Counseling Psychology;Administration;Educational
Psychology

CARO, Yvette
34-22 81st Street
Suite #31
Jackson Heights, NY 11372
(212) 267-4800-**B**, (718) 397-9193-**H**
Ethnicity: Hispanic/Latino
Languages: Spanish
Degree and Year: PhD 1987
Major Field: Clinical Psychology
Specialty: Chronically Mentally Ill;Homelessness & Homeless
Populations;Cross Cultural Processes

CARPENTER, Gerald A.
1655 Winona Court
Denver, CO 80204-1144
(303) 436-6393-**B**
Ethnicity: Hispanic/Latino
Degree and Year: PhD 1982
Major Field: Clinical Psychology
Specialty: Medical Psychology;Cognitive Behavioral Therapy;Clinical
Neuropsychology;Rehabilitation;Health Psychology

CARR-CASANOVA, Rosario
711 D Street
Suite #208
San Rafael, CA 94901
(415) 899-9919-**B**, (415) 899-9749-**H**, (415) 899-9769-**F**
Ethnicity: Hispanic/Latino
Languages: Spanish
Degree and Year: PhD 1983
Major Field: Clinical Psychology
Specialty: Cross Cultural Processes;Psychology of
Women;Psychotherapy;Sex/Marital Therapy;Language Process

CARRA, Sylvia F.
2715 West Sligh Avenue
Tampa, FL 33614
(813) 932-3469-**B**, (8130 289-8194-**H**, (813) 933-8214-**F**
sfcarra@aol.com
Ethnicity: Hispanic/Latino
Degree and Year: PhD 1973
Major Field: Clinical Psychology
Specialty: Learning Disabilities;Psychometrics;Parent-Child
Interaction;Neuropsychology;Family Therapy

CARRINGTON, Christine H.
6269 Gay Topaz
Columbia, MD 21045-4509
(301) 596-2558-**B**, (202) 285-6611-**H**
Ethnicity: African-American/Black
Degree and Year: PhD 1979
Major Field: Counseling Psychology
Specialty: Cognitive Behavioral Therapy;Depression

CARR, Paquita R.
2405 49th Street, NW
Washington, DC 20007
(202) 338-4788-**B**, (202) 338-4788-**H**
Ethnicity: Hispanic/Latino
Languages: Spanish
Degree and Year: PhD 1946
Major Field: Clinical Psychology
Specialty: Clinical Psychology;Clinical Child Psychology;Client-
Centered Therapy;Child Therapy;Group Psychotherapy

CARTER, Allen C.
600 West Peachtree Street
One Georgia Center
Suite #1570
Atlanta, GA 30308
(404) 874-9207-**B**, (404) 987-3521-**H**, (404) 876-4262-**F**
Ethnicity: African-American/Black
Degree and Year: PhD 1973
Major Field: Clinical Psychology

CARTER, Charles A.
238 57th Place, NE
Washington, DC 20019-6865
(202) 727-1323-**B**
Ethnicity: African-American/Black
Degree and Year: PhD 1974
Major Field: unknown
Specialty: Mentally Retarded

CARTER, Lamore J.
PO Box 1087
Marshall, TX 75671-1087
(318) 274-3717-**B**, (318) 247-6286-**H**, (318) 274-3230-**F**
Ethnicity: African-American/Black
Languages: Spanish
Degree and Year: PhD 1958
Major Field: Educational Psychology
Specialty: Administration;Curriculum Development/
Evaluation;Educational Psychology;Management &
Organization;School Psychology

CARTER, Lonnie T.
1840 N Farwell Avenue
Suite #300
Milwaukee, WI 53202
(414) 276-8381-**B**
Ethnicity: African-American/Black
Degree and Year: PhD 1973
Major Field: Counseling Psychology
Specialty: Psychometrics;Counseling Psychology;Marriage &
Family;Group Psychotherapy;School Psychology

CARTER, Robert T.
Columbia University - Teachers College
525 W 120th Street
New York, NY 10027-6625

(212) 678-3346-**B**
Ethnicity: African-American/Black
Degree and Year: PhD 1987
Major Field: Counseling Psychology

CARTER, William J.
Texas Tech University
3405 68th Drive
Lubbock, TX 79413
(806) 742-3671-**B**, (806) 797-8735-**H**
Ethnicity: American Indian/Alaska Native
Degree and Year: PhD 1972
Major Field: Counseling Psychology
Specialty: Counseling Psychology;Consulting
Psychology;Statistics;Educational Psychology;Educational
Research;Neuropsychology

CASAS, Eduardo F.
Center for Psychological Services
275 Nicholas Street
Ottawa, ON K1N6N5
CANADA
Ethnicity: Hispanic/Latino
Degree and Year: PhD 1958
Major Field: Clinical Psychology

CASCALLAR, Eduardo C.
ETS Mail Rte. 10-P
5505 Seminary Rd
Unit #1305-N
Falls Church, VA 22041-3500
(212) 794-5438-**B**, (703) 820-6727-**H**
Ethnicity: Hispanic/Latino
Degree and Year: PhD 1985
Major Field: Cognitive Psychology
Specialty: Memory;Psycholinguistic

CASON, Valerie K.
2758 Thornbrook Road
Ellicott City, MD 21042
(410) 653-0454-**B**, (410) 750-7827-**H**
Ethnicity: African-American/Black
Degree and Year: PhD 1989
Major Field: Clinical Psychology
Specialty: Child Abuse;Cognitive Behavioral Therapy;Consulting
Psychology;Cross Cultural Processes;Group Psychotherapy

CASTILLO, Diane T.
ALB, VAMC
Psychology Service (116B)
2100 Ridgecrest Drive, SE
Albuquerque, NM 87108
(505) 265-1711-**B**, (505) 266-1308-**H**, (505) 256-2819-**F**
castillo.diane@albuquerque.va.
Ethnicity: Hispanic/Latino
Languages: Spanish
Degree and Year: PhD 1985
Major Field: Counseling Psychology
Specialty: Stress;Psychotherapy;Cognitive Behavioral Therapy;Cross
Cultural Processes;Emotion

CASTRO-BLANCO, David R.
Phildelphia College of Osteo Medicine
Department of Psycyology

4190 City Avenue
Philadelphia, PA 19131-1626
(215) 871-6495-**B**, (215) 635-7473-**H**
davidcb@pcom.edu
Ethnicity: Hispanic/Latino
Degree and Year: PhD 1990
Major Field: Clinical Psychology
Specialty: Mentally Retarded

CATARINA, Mathilda B.
821 Summit Avenue
River Edge, NJ 07661
(718) 951-5262-**B**, (201) 262-0952-**H**
Ethnicity: Asian-American/Asian/Pacific Islander
Degree and Year: PhD 1990
Major Field: School Psychology
Specialty: Administration;Cross Cultural Processes;Family
Therapy;Gender Issues;Preschool & Day Care Issues;School
Psychology

CATHCART, Conrad W.
327 Fourth Street
Apartment 4C
Brooklyn, NY 11215-7414
(212) 864-7879-**B**, (718) 965-0331-**H**, (718) 965-0331-**F**
Ethnicity: African-American/Black
Degree and Year: PhD 1984
Major Field: Clinical Psychology
Specialty: Psychotherapy;Psychopathology;Alcoholism & Alcohol
Abuse;Eating Disorders;Clinical Psychology

CEBOLLERO, Ana Margarita
23 Flint Road
Watertown, MA 02472
(617) 735-6706-**B**, (617) 731-8934-**H**, (617) 730-0457-**F**
Ethnicity: Hispanic/Latino
Languages: Spanish
Degree and Year: PhD 1989
Major Field: Clinical Psychology
Specialty: Child & Pediatric Psychology;Clinical
Research;Psychotherapy;Domestic Violence;Ethnic
Minorities;Ethnic Minorities

CEPEDA-BENITO, Antonio
Texas A&M University
Department of Psychology
College Station, TX 77843-4235
(409) 845-8038-**B**, (409) 696-1369-**H**, (409) 845-4727-**F**
acb@tamu.edu
Ethnicity: Hispanic/Latino
Languages: Spanish
Degree and Year: PhD 1994
Major Field: Clinical Psychology
Specialty: Psychopharmacology;Clinical Psychology;Ethnic Minorities

CEREIJIDO, Margarita
1913 S Street, NW
Washington, DC 20009-1106
(202) 373-6563-**B**
Ethnicity: Hispanic/Latino
Degree and Year: PhD 1989
Major Field: Clinical Psychology

CERVANTES, Joseph M.
California State University
School of Human Development and
  Community Service
Department of Counseling
Fullerton, CA 92831
(714) 744-9754-**B**, (714) 637-2695-**H**, (714) 744-1830-**F**
Ethnicity: Hispanic/Latino
Languages: Spanish
Degree and Year: PhD 1977
Major Field: Clinical Psychology
Specialty: Clinical Child Psychology;Cross Cultural Processes;Ethnic
    Minorities;Family Therapy;Community Psychology;Health
    Psychology

CHAN, Adrian
Professor/Director
University of Wisconsin System
University of Wisconsin - Milwaukee
Institute on Race and Ethnicity
Milwaukee, WI 53201
(414) 229-6701-**B**, (414) 962-2271-**H**, (414) 229-4581-**F**
achan@uwm.edu
Ethnicity: Asian-American/Asian/Pacific Islander
Languages: Chinese
Degree and Year: PhD 1968
Major Field: Counseling Psychology
Specialty: Cross Cultural Processes;Educational Psychology;Ethnic
    Minorities

CHAN, Connie S.
University of Massachusetts
@ Boston
91 Beals Street #2
Brookline, MA 02146-3010
(617) 287-7231-**B**, (617) 739-1222-**H**, (617) 287-7099-**F**
chanc@umbsky.cc.umb.edu
Ethnicity: Asian-American/Asian/Pacific Islander
Languages: Chinese
Degree and Year: PhD 1981
Major Field: Clinical Psychology
Specialty: Ethnic Minorities;Sports Psychology;Psychology of
    Women;Lesbian & Gay Issuues

CHAN, Daniel S.
11107 McVine Ave
Sunland, CA 91040-2121
(714) 957-5075-**B**, (818) 352-6262-**H**, (626) 284-3926-**F**
Ethnicity: Asian-American/Asian/Pacific Islander
Languages: Chinese
Degree and Year: PhD 1984
Major Field: Clinical Psychology
Specialty: Psychotherapy

CHAN, Darrow A.
Northwest Psychological Services
1104 Market Street
Kirkland, WA 98033-5441
(206) 827-3019-**B**, (206) 324-6769-**H**
dartchan@aol.com
Ethnicity: Asian-American/Asian/Pacific Islander
Degree and Year: PhD 1985
Major Field: Clinical Child Psychology
Specialty: Cognitive Behavioral Therapy;Conduct Disorders;Mentally
    Retarded;Parent-Child Interaction;Attention Deficit Disorders

CHAN, David C.
1116 - 750 W Broadway
Vancouver, BC V5Z1J1
CANADA
Ethnicity: Asian-American/Asian/Pacific Islander
Degree and Year: EdD 1971
Major Field: unknown
Specialty: Clinical Neuropsychology;Rehabilitation

CHANG, Alice F.
P.O. Box 31837
Tucson, AZ 85751-1837
(602) 621-7136-**B**
afchang@azstarnet.com
Ethnicity: Asian-American/Asian/Pacific Islander
Degree and Year: PhD 1973
Major Field: Clinical Psychology
Specialty: Clinical Psychology;Clinical Research;Ethnic
    Minorities;Individual Psychotherapy;Stress

CHANG, Barbara
157 West 57th Street
Room #1103
New York City, NY 10019
(212) 757-6620-**B**, (212) 741-0897-**H**
Ethnicity: Asian-American/Asian/Pacific Islander
Languages: Chinese
Degree and Year: PhD 1975
Major Field: Clinical Psychology
Specialty: Assessment/Diagnosis/Evaluation;Eating Disorders;Individual
    Psychotherapy;Attention Deficit Disorders;Parent-Child
    Interaction

CHANG, Bradford W.
6139 147th Pl Se
Bellevue, WA 98006-4601
(206) 361-3468-**B**, (425) 957-9912-**H**
Ethnicity: Asian-American/Asian/Pacific Islander
Degree and Year: PhD 1989
Major Field: Clinical Psychology
Specialty: Family Therapy;Child Therapy;Clinical Child
    Psychology;Adolescent Therapy;Clinical Neuropsychology

CHANG, Theodore C. H.
105 N Park Lane Drive
Knoxville, IA 50138
(515) 842-6351-**H**
Ethnicity: Asian-American/Asian/Pacific Islander
Languages: Chinese
Degree and Year: PhD 1957
Major Field: Clinical Psychology
Specialty: Clinical Psychology;Experimental Psychology;Educational
    Psychology;Comparative Psychology;School Psychology

CHANG, Thomas M.C.
1493 Akeakamai Street
Honolulu, HI 96816
(808) 737-6496-**H**
Ethnicity: Asian-American/Asian/Pacific Islander
Degree and Year: PhD 1957
Major Field: Counseling Psychology
Specialty: Assessment/Diagnosis/Evaluation;School Psychology;School
    Counseling;Special Education

CHANG, Weining C.
National University of Singapore

Department of Psychology
10 Kent Ridge Cresent
Singapore, 119260
SINGAPORE
065-874-6121-**B**, 065-468-4868-**H**, 065-778-1213-**F**
swkweicc@leonis.nus.edu.sg
Ethnicity: Asian-American/Asian/Pacific Islander
Languages: Chinese
Degree and Year: PhD 1973
Major Field: Social Psychology
Specialty: Attribution Theory;Cross Cultural Processes;Cultural &
        Social Processes;Industrial/Organizational
        Psychology;Management & Organization

CHAN, Kenyon S.
Loyola Marymount University
Office of the Dean
College of Liberal Arts
7900 Loyola Boulevard
Los Angeles, CA 90045-8319
(310) 338-2716-**B**, (310) 338-2704-**F**
kchan@lmu.edu
Ethnicity: Asian-American/Asian/Pacific Islander
Degree and Year: PhD 1974
Major Field: Educational Psychology
Specialty: Educational Psychology;Emotional Development;Ethnic
        Minorities

CHAN, Paul K.
1716 Savannah Drive
Rio Ranch, NM 87124-5700
(505) 893-6261-**B**, (505) 867-9051-**H**
Ethnicity: Asian-American/Asian/Pacific Islander
Degree and Year: PhD 1991
Major Field: Industrial/Organizational Psy.
Specialty: Industrial/Organizational Psychology;Work
        Performance;Organizational Development;Survey Theory &
        Methodology;Training & Development

CHAN, Paul K. F.
1716 Savannah Drive
Rio Rancho, NM 87124-5700
(505) 867-9051-**B**, (505) 893-=7741-**H**
Ethnicity: Asian-American/Asian/Pacific Islander
Degree and Year: PhD 1991
Major Field: Industrial/Organizational Psy.
Specialty: Industrial/Organizational Psychology;Survey Theory &
        Methodology;Work Performance;Training &
        Development;Organizational Development

CHAN, Samuel Q.
California School of Professional Psychology
21261 Doble Ave
Torrance, CA 90502-1965
(818) 284-2777-**B**, (213) 328-0396-**H**, (818) 284-0550-**F**
schan@mail.cspp.edu
Ethnicity: Asian-American/Asian/Pacific Islander
Degree and Year: PhD 1979
Major Field: unknown
Specialty: Administration;Ethnic Minorities;Child & Pediatric
        Psychology;Cross Cultural Processes;Leadership;Prevention

CHAO, Christine M.
4770 E Iliff Avenue
Suite #233

Denver, CO 80222
(303) 753-9738-**B**, (303) 399-2567-**H**, (303) 399-8269-**F**
ajones@nova.psy.du.edu
Ethnicity: Asian-American/Asian/Pacific Islander
Degree and Year: PhD 1981
Major Field: Clinical Psychology
Specialty: Cross Cultural Processes;Clinical Psychology;Pastoral
        Psychology;Adult Development;Community Mental Health

CHAO, Georgia T.
Michigan State University
Department of Management
East Lansing, MI 48824-
(517) 353-5418-**B**, (517) 336-1111-**F**
chaog@ pilot.msu.edu
Ethnicity: Asian-American/Asian/Pacific Islander
Languages: Chinese, French
Degree and Year: PhD 1982
Major Field: Industrial/Organizational Psy.
Specialty: Human Resources;Industrial/Organizational Psychology;Job
        Satisfaction;Management & Organization;Training &
        Development

CHAO, Janet
9836 East Evans Drive
Scottsdale, AZ 85260-3850
(608) 493-6354-**B**, (602) 948-9586-**H**
Ethnicity: Asian-American/Asian/Pacific Islander
Degree and Year: EdD 1985
Major Field: School Psychology

CHAPA, Joel R.
13615 W Wesley Avenue
Lakewood, CO 80228-4744
(303) 467-5728-**B**
Ethnicity: Hispanic/Latino
Languages: Spanish
Degree and Year: PsyD 1983
Major Field: Clinical Psychology
Specialty: Cognitive Behavioral Therapy;Ethnic Minorities;Health
        Psychology;Gerontology/Geropsychology;Psychotherapy

CHAPMAN, Nancy G.
Health Promotion and Wellness
CHPPM, U.S. Army
PO Box 164 Gunpowder Drive
Aberdeen, MD 21010
(410) 436-7011-**B**, (410) 297-9769-**H**, (410) 436-7381-**F**
Ethnicity: American Indian/Alaska Native
Degree and Year: PsyD 1994
Major Field: Clinical Psychology
Specialty: Clinical Psychology;Consulting Psychology;Eating
        Disorders;Cognitive Behavioral Therapy;Health
        Psychology;Gender Issues

CHATIGNY, Anita L.
2020 E Acacia Street
Palm Springs, CA 92262
(619) 323-6634-**B**, (619) 322-4478-**H**
Ethnicity: Hispanic/Latino
Languages: Spanish
Degree and Year: PhD 1986
Major Field: Clinical Psychology

Specialty: Rehabilitation;Neuropsychology;Clinical
Neuropsychology;Health Psychology

CHATMAN, Vera A
Meharry Medical College
PO Box 121121
Nashville, TN 37212
615 876-6140-**H**, 615 876-5932-**F**
Ethnicity: African-American/Black
Degree and Year: PhD 1976
Major Field: School Psychology
Specialty: Administration;Curriculum Development/
Evaluation;Management & Organization;Consulting
Psychology;Leadership;Program Evaluation

CHAVES, John F.
46 Carrico Road
Florissant, MO 63034
(618) 474-7203-**B**, (314) 637-2225-**H**, (618) 474-7150-**F**
Ethnicity: Hispanic/Latino
Degree and Year: PhD 1970
Major Field: unknown
Specialty: Hypnosis/Hypnotherapy;Health Psychology;Research
Design & Methodology;Medical Psychology;Rehabilitation

CHAVEZ, Ernest L.
Colorado State University
Department of Psychology
Fort Collins, CO 80523
(970) 491-1354-**B**, (970) 491-0527-**H**, (970) 491-0527-**F**
echavez@lamar.colostate.edu
Ethnicity: Hispanic/Latino
Languages: Spanish
Degree and Year: PhD 1976
Major Field: Clinical Psychology
Specialty: Ethnic Minorities;Administration;Adolescent
Development;Training & Development;Drug
Abuse;Educational Research

CHEN, Eric C
Fordham University
Division of Psychological
& Educational Services
113 West 60th Street
New York, NY 10023-7478
212 636-6474-**B**, 212 283-0204-**H**, 212 636-6416-**F**
echen@mary.fordham.edu
Ethnicity: Asian-American/Asian/Pacific Islander
Languages: Chinese, Taiwanese
Degree and Year: PhD 1995
Major Field: Counseling Psychology
Specialty: Counseling Psychology;Group
Psychotherapy;Psychotherapy;Vocational Psychology

CHENG, W. David
315 Central Park West, 8N
New York, NY 10025
(212) 580-1193-**B**
drdavidnyc@aol.com
Ethnicity: Asian-American/Asian/Pacific Islander
Languages: Chinese, German
Degree and Year: PhD 1976
Major Field: Personality Psychology
Specialty: Clinical Psychology;Counseling Psychology;Industrial/
Organizational Psychology;Psychoanalysis;Psychotherapy

CHEN, Hongjen
425 West Avenue
Wayne, PA 19087
(610) 903-4340-**B**, (610) 971-9563-**H**, (215) 995-4666-**F**
Ethnicity: Asian-American/Asian/Pacific Islander
Languages: Chinese
Degree and Year: PhD 1984
Major Field: Social Psychology
Specialty: Attribution Theory;Clinical Research;Social Behavior;Social
Cognition;Attitudes & Opinions

CHEN, S. Andrew
Slippery Rock University
Department of Counseling and
Educational Psychology
Slippery Rock, PA 16057
(412) 738-2274-**B**, (412) 738-2098-**F**
shiumchen@sru.edu
Ethnicity: Asian-American/Asian/Pacific Islander
Languages: Chinese
Degree and Year: PhD 1970
Major Field: Educational Psychology
Specialty: Research & Training;Educational Research;Ethnic
Minorities;Psycholinguistic;Crime & Criminal Behavior

CHERBOSQUE, Jorge
11911 San Vincente Boulevard
Suite #240
Los Angeles, CA 90049
(310) 207-5100-**B**, (818) 981-2991-**H**
Ethnicity: Hispanic/Latino
Languages: Spanish, Hebrew
Degree and Year: PhD 1984
Major Field: Counseling Psychology
Specialty: Cross Cultural Processes;Drug Abuse;Employee Assistance
Programs;Ethnic Minorities;Stress

CHESNUTT, James H.
875 Wynn Road
Clinton, MD 28328
(910) 533-3517-**H**
Ethnicity: African-American/Black
Degree and Year: PsyD 1980
Major Field: Clinical Psychology
Specialty: Psychotherapy;Religious Psychology;Health
Psychology;Quantitative/Mathematical,
Psychometrics;Personality

CHEW, Marion W.
Center for Multicultural Human Services
701 West Broad Street
Suite 305
Falls Church, VA 22046
(703) 533-3302-**B**, (703) 573-0947-**H**, (703) 237-2083-**F**
cmhs2000@aol.com
Ethnicity: Asian-American/Asian/Pacific Islander
Degree and Year: PhD 1993
Major Field: Clinical Psychology
Specialty: Cross Cultural Processes;Parent-Child Interaction;Child
Development

CHIANG, Grace CT
National Changhua University of
Education

No.1 Gun-Der Road
Changhua, 50058,
TAIWAN
886 4 7211057-**B**, 886 4 7211182-**F**
grace@cc.ncue.edu.tw
Ethnicity: Asian-American/Asian/Pacific Islander
Languages: Chinese
Degree and Year: PhD 1991
Major Field: Cognitive Psychology

CHIA, Rosina
East Carolina University
Department of Psychology
Greenville, NC 27858
(919) 757-6277-**B**, (252) 830-5580-**F**
pschia@ecuum.cis.ecu.edu
Ethnicity: Asian-American/Asian/Pacific Islander
Languages: Chinese
Degree and Year: PhD 1969 BS 1962
Major Field: Social Psychology
Specialty: Cross Cultural Processes;Cultural & Social
Processes;Motivation;Personality;Administration

CHING-YANG HSU, Chris
8025 Falstaff Road
McLean, VA 22102
(202) 692-2331-**B**, (703) 893-3177-**H**
Ethnicity: Asian-American/Asian/Pacific Islander
Languages: Chinese
Degree and Year: PhD 1970
Major Field: Industrial/Organizational Psy.

CHING, June W. J.
Kapiolani Counseling Center
1319 Punahon Street
Suite #648
Honolulu, HI 96826
(808) 983-8368-**B**, (808) 373-9502-**H**, (808) 983-8629-**F**
junec@kapiolani.org
Ethnicity: Asian-American/Asian/Pacific Islander
Languages: Chinese
Degree and Year: PhD 1980
Major Field: Clinical Psychology
Specialty: Child Abuse;Clinical Child Psychology;Clinical
Psychology;Individual Psychotherapy;Psychology of
Women;Learning Disabilities

CHIN, James
92-29 Queens Blvd. #2E
Rego Park, NY 11374
(718) 997-8726-**B**
Ethnicity: Asian-American/Asian/Pacific Islander
Degree and Year: PhD 1981
Major Field: Social Psychology
Specialty: Cognitive Behavioral Therapy;Drug
Abuse;Neuropsychology;Aggression;Alcoholism & Alcohol
Abuse

CHIN, Jean L
CEO Services
614 Dedham Street
Newton, MA 02159
(617) 965-8694-**B**, 617/ 965-0499-**H**, (617) 965-5753-**F**
jlcceoserv@aol.com
Ethnicity: Asian-American/Asian/Pacific Islander

Languages: Chinese, Cantonese, Toisanese
Degree and Year: EdD 1974
Major Field: School Psychology
Specialty: Psychotherapy;Community
Psychology;Administration;Ethnic Minorities

CHIN, Lemin
60 Wes Ridgewood Avenue
Ridgewood, NJ 07450
(201) 689-1899-**B**, (201) 797-3246-**H**
Ethnicity: Asian-American/Asian/Pacific Islander
Languages: Chinese
Degree and Year: PhD 1987
Major Field: Clinical Psychology
Specialty: Health Psychology;Cross Cultural Processes;Clinical
Psychology

CHINN, Roberta N.
113 Farham Drive
Folsom, CA 95630-3505
(916) 322-2703-**B**, (916) 353-1744-**H**, (916) 445-8252-**F**
Ethnicity: Asian-American/Asian/Pacific Islander
Degree and Year: PhD 1984
Major Field: Experimental Psychology
Specialty: Psychometrics;Research Design &
Methodology;Measurement

CHINO, Allan F.
3735 Pacific Street
Las Vegas, NV 89121-4153
(510) 674-2550-**B**, (510) 229-1493-**H**
Ethnicity: Asian-American/Asian/Pacific Islander
Degree and Year: PhD 1984
Major Field: Clinical Psychology
Specialty: Behavior Therapy;Pain & Pain Management;Medical
Psychology;Assessment/Diagnosis/Evaluation;Case
Management

CHIN, Raymond J.
Rural Route 1 Box 22
Lyme, NH 03768
(603) 795-4560-**B**
Ethnicity: Asian-American/Asian/Pacific Islander
Degree and Year: PhD 1986
Major Field: Clinical Psychology

CHIN, Sandra B
Hotel Equatorial
Mid Level Flr, #9
Jalan Sultan Ismail 249
Kuala Lumpur 249,
MALAYSIA
(011) 60 - 261-**B**, (603) 261-9020-**F**
schinby@pc.jaring.my
Ethnicity: Asian-American/Asian/Pacific Islander
Languages: Chinese
Degree and Year: PhD 1987
Major Field: Clinical Psychology
Specialty: Clinical Psychology;Cognitive Behavioral Therapy;Family
Therapy;Eating Disorders;Psychology of Women

CHIRIBOGA, David A.
University of Texas Medical Branch
SAHS, Route, 1028
Galveston, TX 77550
(409) 772-3038-**B**, (409) 740-1648-**H**, (409) 772-3014-**F**

dchiribo@utmb.edu
Ethnicity: Hispanic/Latino
Degree and Year: PhD 1972
Major Field: Developmental Psychology
Specialty: Adult Development;Stress;Health Psychology;Gerontology/
Geropsychology;Ethnic Minorities

CHISUM, Gloria T.
4120 Apalogen Road
Philadelphia, PA 19144-5404
Ethnicity: African-American/Black
Degree and Year: PhD 1960
Major Field: Experimental Psychology
Specialty: Vision;Sensory & Perceptual Processes

CHIU, Lian-Hwam
Indiana University at Kokomo
Kokomo, IN 46902-3500
Ethnicity: Asian-American/Asian/Pacific Islander
Degree and Year: EdD 1968
Major Field: Educational Psychology
Specialty: Cross Cultural Processes

CHIU, Loanne
Medical Towers
1550 W Rosedale (Medical Tower)
Suite #602
Fort Worth, TX 76014-7410
(817) 335-5300-**B**, (817) 731-4790-**H**
Ethnicity: Asian-American/Asian/Pacific Islander
Languages: German, Indoesian, Dutch
Degree and Year: PhD 1971
Major Field: Clinical Psychology
Specialty: Individual Psychotherapy;Assessment/Diagnosis/
Evaluation;Depression;Personality Disorders;Ethnic
Minorities

CHOCA, James
Psychology Service
Roosevelt University
School of Psychology
430 South Michigan Avenue
Chicago, IL 60605
(312) 341-3750-**B**, (773) 472-7791-**H**
Ethnicity: Hispanic/Latino
Languages: Spanish
Degree and Year: PhD 1972
Major Field: Clinical Psychology
Specialty: Personality Measurement;Projective Techniques;Computer
Applications and Programming;Assessment/Diagnosis/
Evaluation;Clinical Neuropsychology

CHOI, George C.
Maui Realty Suites
1885 Main St Ste 104
Wailuku, HI 96793-1827
(808) 243-2218-**B**, (808) 243-9221-**H**
geochoi@gte.net
Ethnicity: Asian-American/Asian/Pacific Islander
Languages: Chinese
Degree and Year: PsyD 1982
Major Field: Clinical Psychology
Specialty: Child Therapy;Individual Psychotherapy;Crisis Intervention
& Therapy;Cross Cultural Processes;Child Abuse

CHONEY, John M.
Oklahoma State University
Department of Psychology
215 North Murray Hall
Stillwater, OK 74078
(405) 744-6027-**B**, (405) 844-3287-**H**, (405) 744-8067-**F**
jachaney@okway.okstate.edu
Ethnicity: American Indian/Alaska Native
Degree and Year: PhD 1991
Major Field: Clinical Psychology
Specialty: Health Psychology;Medical Psychology;Ethnic
Minorities;Rehabilitation

CHOU, Thomas T.
92 Dogwood Road
Williamsville, NY 14221-4628
(716) 634-8015-**B**
Ethnicity: Asian-American/Asian/Pacific Islander
Degree and Year: PhD 1972
Major Field: Social Psychology
Specialty: Mentally Retarded

CHOY, Catherine L.
2652 B No Southport Avenue
Chicago, IL 60614-1262
Ethnicity: Asian-American/Asian/Pacific Islander
Degree and Year: PhD 1974
Major Field: Industrial/Organizational Psy.
Specialty: Management & Organization

CHOY, Stephen S.F.
1314 S King Street
Suite #720
Honolulu, HI 96814-1942
(808) 593-8484-**B**, (808) 947-0017-**H**
Ethnicity: Asian-American/Asian/Pacific Islander
Degree and Year: PhD 1977
Major Field: Clinical Psychology
Specialty: Rational-Emotive Therapy

CHRISS, Gloria M.
El Paso Psychological Center
125 Thunderbird Dr, Ste F
El Paso, TX 79912-4563
(915) 585-7000-**B**, (915) 584-4616-**H**
Ethnicity: Hispanic/Latino
Degree and Year: PhD 1983
Major Field: unknown
Specialty: Family Therapy

CHU, Lily
Route1 Box 377
La Mesa, NM 88044-9768
Ethnicity: Asian-American/Asian/Pacific Islander
Degree and Year: PhD 1973
Major Field: Counseling Psychology
Specialty: Social Behavior;Educational Research

CHUNG, Edith C.
University of Southern California
857 36th Place
YWCA #100
Student Counseling Services
Los Angeles, CA 90089
(213) 740-7711-**B**, (310) 828-0850-**H**, (310) 828-0850-**F**
edithchung@yahoo.com

Ethnicity: Asian-American/Asian/Pacific Islander
Languages: Chinese
Degree and Year: PhD 1994
Major Field: Counseling Psychology
Specialty: Clinical Psychology;Ethnic Minorities;Marriage &
    Family;Counseling Psychology;Group
    Psychotherapy;Personality Disorders

CHUNG, Moon Ja
  Yonsei University
  Department of Child and Family Studies
  #134 Shinchon-dong
  Seoul, 120-749, 218
  SOUTH KOREA
  (011) 8223613-**B**, (011) 82254660-**H**
  mjchung@yansei.ac.kr
Ethnicity: Asian-American/Asian/Pacific Islander
Degree and Year: PhD 1978
Major Field: Developmental Psychology
Specialty: Child Therapy

CHUNG, Rita L.
  The Ohio State University
  College of Education
  283 ARPS Hall, High Street
  Columbus, OH 43210
  (6140) 688-8642-**B**, (6140 292-0102-**F**
  chung.15yc@osu.edu
Ethnicity: Asian-American/Asian/Pacific Islander
Languages: Chinese
Degree and Year: PhD 1989
Major Field: Community Psychology
Specialty: Ethnic Minorities;Gender Issues;Community Mental Health

CHUNG, Y. Barry
  Georgia State University
  CPS Department
  College of Education
  Atlanta, GA 30303
  404/651-3149-**B**, 404/299-1187-**H**, 404/651-1160-**F**
  bchung@gsu.edu
Ethnicity: Asian-American/Asian/Pacific Islander
Languages: Chinese
Degree and Year: PhD 1996
Major Field: Counseling Psychology
Specialty: Vocational Psychology

CHUN, Marvin M.
  Yale University
  PO Box 208205
  New Haven, CT 06520-4629
  (203) 432-4629-**B**, (203) 432-7172-**F**
  marvin.chun@yale.edu
Ethnicity: Asian-American/Asian/Pacific Islander
Languages: Korean
Degree and Year: PhD 1994
Major Field: Cognitive Psychology
Specialty: Cognitive Psychology;Memory;Neurosciences;Experimental
    Psychology;Vision

CHURCH, June S.
  75 Rock Lick Road
  Champanville, WV 25508-9749
  (304) 792-7137-**B**, (304) 752-6808-**H**

Ethnicity: American Indian/Alaska Native
Degree and Year: PhD 1972
Major Field: Clinical Psychology
Specialty: Administration;Clinical Psychology;Cognitive Behavioral
    Therapy;Crisis Intervention & Therapy;Stress

CIMINO, Cynthia R.
  University of South Florida
  Department of Psychology BEH-339
  4202 East Fowler Avenue
  Tampa, FL 33620
  (813) 974-0385-**B**, (813) 974-4617-**F**
  cimino@luna.czs.usf.edu
Ethnicity: Hispanic/Latino
Degree and Year: PhD 1988
Major Field: Clinical Psychology
Specialty: Neuropsychology;Clinical Psychology;Clinical
    Neuropsychology

CIRINO, Gabriel
  University of Puerto Rico
  Suite #1200 Darlington Bldg.
  1007 Munoz Rivera Avenue
  Rio Piedras, PR 00925
Ethnicity: Hispanic/Latino
Degree and Year: PhD 1970
Major Field: Industrial/Organizational Psy.

CLANSY, Pauline A.
  8323 Southwest Freeway
  Suite 105
  Houston, TX 77074
  (713) 777-8633-**B**, (713) 777-9515-**H**, (713) 777-3342-**F**
  linepau@aol.com
Ethnicity: African-American/Black
Degree and Year: EdD 1986
Major Field: Counseling Psychology
Specialty: Counseling Psychology;Crisis Intervention &
    Therapy;Mentally Retarded;School Psychology;Interpersonal
    Processes & Relations;Alcoholism & Alcohol Abuse

CLARK, JR., Eddie M.
  St. Louis University
  Department of Psychology
  221 N Grand Blvd.
  St. Louis, MO 63103
  (314) 977-227-**B**, (314) 977-3677-**F**
Ethnicity: African-American/Black
Degree and Year: PhD 1988 MA 1983
Major Field: Social Psychology
Specialty: Health Psychology;Interpersonal Processes &
    Relations;Attitudes & Opinions

CLARK, Brenda A.
  PO Box 751
  Melville, NY 11704
  (516) 598-6561-**B**, (516) 264-4489-**F**
Ethnicity: African-American/Black
Degree and Year: PhD 1987
Major Field: Clinical Psychology
Specialty: Administration;Adolescent Therapy;Forensic
    Psychology;Psychology of Women;Assessment/Diagnosis/
    Evaluation

CLARKE-PINE, Dora D.
La Sierra University
Eudcational Psychology and
    Counseling Department
4700 Pierce Street
Riverside, CA 92515
(909) 785-2969-**B**, (909) 352-9813-**H**, (909) 785-2205-**F**
dclarke@lasierra.edu
Ethnicity: Asian-American/Asian/Pacific Islander
Degree and Year: PhD 1995
Major Field: Counseling Psychology
Specialty: Assessment/Diagnosis/Evaluation;Crisis Intervention &
    Therapy;Group Psychotherapy;Counseling
    Psychology;Gender Issues;Psychopathology

CLARK, Kenneth B.
17 Pinecrest Drive
Hastings-On-Hudson, NY 10706-3701
Ethnicity: African-American/Black
Degree and Year: PhD 1940
Major Field: Social Psychology
Specialty: Values & Moral Behavior

CLARK, Marie
Behavioral Science Institute, Inc.
111 South Bemiston
Suite G3
Clayton, MO 63105
(314) 725-2667-**B**, (314) 725-2669-**F**
Ethnicity: African-American/Black
Degree and Year: MA 1978
Major Field: Clinical Psychology
Specialty: Sexual Behavior;Aggression;Assessment/Diagnosis/
    Evaluation;Correctional Psychology;Training & Development

CLEVELAND, Adriana F.
62 Sprucewood Blvd.
Central Islip, NY 11722
(516) 544-0939-**B**, (516) 582-1783-**H**
Ethnicity: Hispanic/Latino
Languages: Portuguese, Spanish
Degree and Year: MA 1986
Major Field: Cognitive Psychology
Specialty: Mentally Retarded;Cognitive Behavioral
    Therapy;Stress;Juvenile Delinquency;Eating
    Disorders;Experimental Psychology

COATES, Deborah L.
The Better Babies Project
Institute for Healthier Babies
1275 Mamaroneck Avenue
White Plains, NY 10605-5201
(202) 387-0900-**B**
Ethnicity: African-American/Black
Degree and Year: PhD 1979
Major Field: Developmental Psychology
Specialty: Adolescent Development;Prevention

COATS, Gary L.
2250 South Alibion Street
Denver, CO 80222
(303) 756-5400-**B**, (303) 979-6613-**H**, (303) 753-6498-**F**
Ethnicity: American Indian/Alaska Native
Degree and Year: PhD 1982 AB 1973
Major Field: Clinical Psychology

Specialty: Affective Disorders;Alcoholism & Alcohol Abuse;Family
    Therapy;Adolescent Therapy;Cognitive Psychology;Medical
    Psychology

COELHO, George V.
International Affairs Office
SAMHSA
Parklawn 12C05
5600 Fishers Lane
Rockville, MD 20857
(301) 443-3838-**B**, (301) 443-7590-**H**, (301) 443-7590-**F**
Ethnicity: Asian-American/Asian/Pacific Islander
Languages: French, Italian, Portuguese
Degree and Year: PhD 1956
Major Field: Social Psychology
Specialty: Cross Cultural Processes;Adolescent Development;Ethnic
    Minorities;Health Psychology;Human Relations

COELHO, Richard J.
714 Parkway Drive
Lansing, MI 48910-4629
(517) 887-9059-**B**
Ethnicity: African-American/Black
Degree and Year: PhD 1983
Major Field: Community Psychology
Specialty: Community Psychology;Mentally
    Retarded;Rehabilitation;Mental Health Services;Program
    Evaluation;Research & Training

COES, Maria R.
7509 Calhoun, NE
Albuquerque, NM 87109-6465
(505) 822-7985-**H**
Ethnicity: Hispanic/Latino
Languages: Portuguese
Degree and Year: PhD 1987
Major Field: Educational Psychology
Specialty: Attention Deficit Disorders;Educational
    Psychology;Motivation;Attribution Theory;Gender Issues

COFFEY, Maryann B.
89 Castle Howard Court
Princeton, NJ 08540-0425
(609) 258-1665-**B**, (609) 497-1319-**H**, (609) 258-2502-**F**
Ethnicity: African-American/Black
Languages: German
Degree and Year: PhD 1970
Major Field: Developmental Psychology

COGGINS, Margaret H.
United States Secret Service
950 H Street, NW
Suite 9100
Washington, DC 20223-0001
(202) 436-5470-**B**, (703) 264-0121-**H**
mhcoggins@aol.com
Ethnicity: Asian-American/Asian/Pacific Islander
Degree and Year: PhD 1986
Major Field: Counseling Psychology

COHEN, Isadora
1108 N. LaBrea Avenue
Inglewood, CA 90302
(310) 671-5242-**B**
Ethnicity: African-American/Black
Degree and Year: PhD 1980

Major Field: Clinical Psychology
Specialty: Cognitive Behavioral Therapy;Hypnosis/
Hypnotherapy;Community Mental Health;Crisis Intervention
& Therapy;Depression

COLEBURN, Lila A.
98 Riverside Drive
Suite #14C
New York, NY 10024
(212) 580-2547-**B**, (212) 932-8402-**H**
Ethnicity: African-American/Black
Degree and Year: J.D. 1984
Major Field: Clinical Psychology
Specialty: Psychotherapy;Individual Psychotherapy;Giftedness;Gender
Issues

COLEMAN, Hardin L.
University of Wisconsin, Madison
Department of Counseling Psychology
321 Education Building
1000 Bascom Mall
Madison, WI 53706
(608) 262-2161-**B**, (6080 238-0635-**H**, (608) 265-3347-**F**
hcoleman@facstaff.uisc.edu
Ethnicity: African-American/Black
Degree and Year: PhD 1992
Major Field: Counseling Psychology
Specialty: Adolescent Development;Individual Psychotherapy;Cultural
& Social Processes;Training & Development

COLEMAN, Philip P.
2100 Lakeshore Avenue
Suite B
Oakland, CA 94606
(510) 763-0105-**B**, (510) 933-4962-**F**
Ethnicity: African-American/Black
Degree and Year: PhD 1981
Major Field: Clinical Psychology
Specialty: Individual Psychotherapy;Parent-Child
Interaction;Hypnosis/Hypnotherapy;Family Therapy;Ethnic
Minorities;Stress

COLEMAN, Willie J.
152 Way Road
Salem, CT 06420-3715
(203) 442-3380-**B**, (203) 859-3119-**H**, (203) 437-2153-**F**
Ethnicity: African-American/Black
Degree and Year: PhD 1980
Major Field: Clinical Psychology
Specialty: Alcoholism & Alcohol Abuse;Clinical
Psychology;Community Psychology;Drug Abuse;Adolescent
Therapy

COLLADO, Armando
South Florida Evaluation
and Treatment Center
2200 Northwest Seventh Avenue
Miami, Fl 33128
(305) 637-2547-**B**, (305) 864-3366-**H**, (305) 573-8483-**F**
Ethnicity: Hispanic/Latino
Languages: Spanish
Degree and Year: PhD 1985
Major Field: Clinical Psychology
Specialty: Clinical Psychology;Forensic Psychology

COLLINS, Edsmond J.
390 Doral Drive
Fairfield, CA 94533-7745
(415) 206-8091-**B**
Ethnicity: African-American/Black
Degree and Year: PhD 1992
Major Field: Clinical Psychology
Specialty: Neuropsychology

COLLINS, James F.
Central Washington University
Department of Psychology
Ellensburg, WA 98926-7575
(509) 963-3668-**B**, (509) 962-3757-**H**, (509) 963-2307-**F**
fuji@cwu.edu
Ethnicity: Asian-American/Asian/Pacific Islander
Degree and Year: PhD 1996
Major Field: Clinical Psychology
Specialty: Cross Cultural Processes;Community Mental
Health;Training & Development;Ethnic Minorities;Mental
Health Services;Psychotherapy

COLLINS, William
University of Michigan
1159 Angell Hall
Ann Arbor, MI 48109
(313) 764-9129-**B**, (734) 662-2461-**H**, (734) 763-6359-**F**
wcollins@umich.edu
Ethnicity: African-American/Black
Languages: Spanish
Degree and Year: PhD 1975
Major Field: Personality Psychology
Specialty: Cognitive Psychology;Administration;Death & Dying

COLON, Ana I.
Senorial Mail Station Box #366
Winston Churchill Avenue #138
San Juan, PR 00926-6023
(787) 758-8787-**B**, (787) 731-7909-**H**
Ethnicity: Hispanic/Latino
Languages: Spanish
Degree and Year: PhD 1986
Major Field: Clinical Psychology
Specialty: Forensic Psychology;Program Evaluation;Child Therapy

COLON, Luis H.
352 San Claudio Av-163
San Juan, PR 00926-4107
(809) 758-2420-**H**
Ethnicity: Hispanic/Latino
Degree and Year: EdD 1980
Major Field: Counseling Psychology
Specialty: Clinical Neuropsychology

COLON, R. Phillip
300 Old Country Road
Suite #91
Mineola, NY 11501
(516) 294-8914-**B**, (516) 546-5919-**H**, (516) 294-8532-**F**
Ethnicity: Hispanic/Latino
Degree and Year: PhD 1981
Major Field: Clinical Psychology
Specialty: Clinical Psychology;Marriage & Family;Community Mental
Health;Ethnic Minorities;Chronically Mentally Ill

COLOTLA, Victor A.
Workers Compensation Board
Psychology Department
6951 Westminister Highway
Richmond, BC V7C 1C6
CANADA
(604) 279-7656-**B**, (604) 922-4726-**H**, (604) 279-7405-**F**
Ethnicity: Hispanic/Latino
Languages: Spanish
Degree and Year: PhD 1973
Major Field: Clinical Psychology
Specialty: Clinical Psychology;Experimental Analysis of
    Behavior;Psychopharmacology

COMAS-DIAZ, Lillian
1301 20th Street, NW
Suite #711
Washington, DC 20036
(202) 775-1938-**B**, (202) 223-1146-**F**
Ethnicity: Hispanic/Latino
Languages: Italian, Spanish
Degree and Year: PhD 1979
Major Field: Clinical Psychology
Specialty: Clinical Psychology;Ethnic Minorities;Feminist
    Therapy;Family Therapy;Psychotherapy

CONE-DEKLE, Cynthia A.
600 Marvin Avenue
Statesboro, GA 30458-5451
(912) 681-2401-**B**
Ethnicity: African-American/Black
Degree and Year: PhD 1988
Major Field: Clinical Psychology
Specialty: Community Mental Health

CONGO, Carroll A.
58 Lewis Court
Huntington Station, NY 11746-1143
(516) 421-5664-**B**, (516) 427-0685-**H**
Ethnicity: African-American/Black
Degree and Year: EdD 1980
Major Field: School Psychology
Specialty: School Psychology;Assessment/Diagnosis/
    Evaluation;Community Mental Health;Child
    Therapy;Adolescent Therapy

CONNOR, Michael E.
California State University
Psychology Department
1250 Bellflower Boulevard
Long Beach, CA 90840
(562) 985-5013-**B**, (949) 499-0383-**H**, (562) 985-8004-**F**
mconnor@csulb.edu
Ethnicity: African-American/Black
Degree and Year: PhD 1972
Major Field: Clinical Psychology
Specialty: Cognitive Behavioral Therapy;Clinical Child
    Psychology;Parent-Child Interaction;Parent Education;Ethnic
    Minorities;Sports Psychology

CONSTANTINE, Madonna G.
Teachers College, Columbia University
525 West 120th Street, Box 102
Department of Counseling
    and Clinical Psychology

New York, NY 10027
(212) 678-3398-**B**, (212) 678-3275-**F**
mc816@columbia.edu
Ethnicity: African-American/Black
Languages: French
Degree and Year: PhD 1991
Major Field: Counseling Psychology
Specialty: Cross Cultural Processes;Counseling Psychology;Ethnic
    Minorities

CONSTANZO, Magda S.
One Alhambra Circle
Suite #604
Conal Gables, FL 33134
(305) 461-5185-**B**, (305) 461-5185-**H**, (305) 669-9282-**F**
Ethnicity: Hispanic/Latino
Languages: Spanish
Degree and Year: PhD 1969
Major Field: Clinical Psychology
Specialty: Clinical Psychology;Counseling Psychology;Health
    Psychology;Social Psychology;Gerontology/Geropsychology

CONTRERAS, Raquel J.
Texas Technical University
Counseling Cener
PO Box 45008
Lubbock, TX 79409-5008
(806) 742-3674-**B**, (806) 797-7327-**H**, (806) 742-1735-**F**
Ethnicity: Hispanic/Latino
Languages: Spanish
Degree and Year: PhD 1989
Major Field: Counseling Psychology
Specialty: Cross Cultural Processes;Ethnic Minorities;Research &
    Training;Administration

COOK, Donelda
University of Maryland
Counseling Ctr
Loyola Col/beatty Hall Ste 203
4501 N Charles St
Baltimore, MD 21210-2601
(410) 617-5109-**B**, (301) 604-4722-**H**
Ethnicity: African-American/Black
Degree and Year: PhD 1983
Major Field: Counseling Psychology
Specialty: Counseling Psychology;Ethnic Minorities;Cultural & Social
    Processes;Training & Development;Community Psychology

COOK, Rudolf E.
95 South Market Street
Suite 300
Santa Jose, CA 95113-2391
(408) 994-3215-**B**, (408) 241-5758-**H**, (408) 995-3202-**F**
Ethnicity: African-American/Black
Degree and Year: PhD 1965
Major Field: Counseling Psychology
Specialty: Crisis Intervention & Therapy;Assessment/Diagnosis/
    Evaluation;Counseling Psychology;Cognitive Behavioral
    Therapy;Humanistic Psychology;Psychology & Law

COOPER, Alan
1719 Spring Lake Drive
Arlington, TX 76012
(972) 771-3969-**B**, (817) 265-0644-**H**, (972) 771-8258-**F**
Ethnicity: African-American/Black

Languages: Spanish
Degree and Year: PhD 1987
Major Field: Clinical Psychology
Specialty: Alcoholism & Alcohol Abuse;HIV/AIDS;Sex/Marital
Therapy;Depression;Lesbian & Gay Issuues;Drug Abuse

COOPER, Colin
Bowie State University
5605 Lockwood Road
Cheverly, MD 20785-1126
(301) 322-8936-**H**, (301) 772-5386-**F**
ccooper@bellatlantic.net
Ethnicity: African-American/Black
Degree and Year: PhD 1983
Major Field: Industrial/Organizational Psy.
Specialty: Industrial/Organizational Psychology;Training &
Development;Human Resources;Ethnic
Minorities;Management & Organization;Selection & Placement

COOPER, Donna M.
One Darnall Road
Box 571105
Washington, DC 20057-1105
(202) 687-7060-**B**, (202) 687-7060-**H**
Ethnicity: African-American/Black
Languages: Portuguese, Spanish
Degree and Year: PhD 1983
Major Field: Clinical Psychology
Specialty: Psychotherapy;Psychopathology;Group
Psychotherapy;Clinical Psychology;Family Therapy

COPELAND, JR., E. Thomas
4045 Campbell
Kansas City, MO 64110
(816) 471-3000-**B**, (816) 756-0710-**H**, (816) 234-5915-**F**
Ethnicity: African-American/Black
Degree and Year: PhD 1974
Major Field: Developmental Psychology
Specialty: Alcoholism & Alcohol Abuse;Domestic Violence;Ethnic
Minorities;Family Therapy;Forensic Psychology

COPEMANN, Chester D.
Office of Dr. Chester Copeman
PO Box 1547
Christiansted, VI 00851
340/773-5113-**B**, 340/773-5163-**F**
Ethnicity: African-American/Black
Degree and Year: PhD 1973
Major Field: Clinical Psychology
Specialty: Behavior Therapy;Forensic
Psychology;Rehabilitation;Clinical Psychology

COPHER-HAYNES, Harriett
866 Lenox Avenue
St. Paul, MN 55119-5607
(612) 624-5862-**B**
Ethnicity: African-American/Black
Degree and Year: PhD 1979
Major Field: Counseling Psychology
Specialty: Organizational Development;Consulting Psychology;Clinical
Psychology;Training & Development;Ethnic Minorities

CORDERO, Fernando
PO Box 7742
Santa Maria, CA 93456-7742

(805) 934-6380-**B**, (805) 934-6381-**F**
Ethnicity: Hispanic/Latino
Languages: Spanish
Degree and Year: PhD 1982
Major Field: Clinical Psychology
Specialty: Clinical Psychology;Community Mental Health;Cross
Cultural Processes;Chronically Mentally Ill;Communications/
Journalism;Social Psychology

CORNIDE, Carmen R.
1601 Palm Avenue
Suite 300
Pembrooke Pines, FL 33026
(954) 409-3475-**B**, (954) 436-2864-**H**
Ethnicity: Hispanic/Latino
Languages: Spanish
Degree and Year: PsyD 1995
Major Field: Clinical Psychology
Specialty: Adolescent Therapy;Clinical Psychology;Gerontology/
Geropsychology;Assessment/Diagnosis/Evaluation;Consulting
Psychology;Industrial/Organizational Psychology

CORNWELL, Henry G.
P.O. Box 114
Lincoln, PA 19352
(215) 932-8442-**H**
Ethnicity: African-American/Black
Languages: Portuguese, Spanish
Degree and Year: PhD 1952
Major Field: Experimental Psychology
Specialty: Sensory & Perceptual Processes;Quantitative/Mathematical,
Psychometrics;Personality;Assessment/Diagnosis/Evaluation

CORR, Donald
1806 Merrywood Drive
Edison, NJ 08817-6507
(609) 497-2820-**B**, 908 636-4637-**H**
Ethnicity: African-American/Black
Degree and Year: PsyD 1987
Major Field: School Psychology
Specialty: Cognitive Behavioral Therapy

CORREA, Martha L.
St. Luke's Roosevelt Medical Center
411 West 114 Street
New York, NY 10025
(212) 222-5394-**B**, (212) 222-5719-**H**, (212) 222-5394-**F**
spmc@msn.com
Ethnicity: Hispanic/Latino
Languages: Spanish
Degree and Year: PhD 1993
Major Field: Clinical Psychology

CORTE, Henry E.
Green Valley Development Cener
PO Box 944
Greeneville, TN 37745
(423) 798-6310-**B**, (423) 638-5174-**H**
Ethnicity: Hispanic/Latino
Languages: Spanish
Degree and Year: PhD 1969
Major Field: Clinical Child Psychology
Specialty: Developmental Psychology;Clinical Psychology;Clinical
Child Psychology;Cognitive Behavioral Therapy;Behavior
Therapy

CORTESE, Margaret
250 Citrus Grove
P.O. Box 5184
Suite #210
Oxnard, CA 93031-5184
(805) 485-5445-**B**, (805) 983-6471-**H**, (805) 981-9007-**F**
Ethnicity: Hispanic/Latino
Languages: Spanish
Degree and Year: PhD 1979
Major Field: Clinical Psychology
Specialty: Clinical Psychology;Ethnic Minorities;Psychotherapy

COSTA, Armenio S.
15 Upper College Road
Kingston, RI 02881-1309
401/789-5172-**B**, 401/789-5172-**H**, 401/789-5172-**F**
ascosta@hotmail
Ethnicity: Hispanic/Latino
Languages: Portuguese, Spanish
Degree and Year: PhD 1990 MS 1978
Major Field: Clinical Psychology
Specialty: Clinical Psychology;Schizophrenia;Ethnic
        Minorities;Affective Disorders;Gerontology/
        Geropsychology;Medical Psychology

COTTERELL, Norman
1421 W Fischer Avenue
Philidelphia, PA 19141
(215) 898-4100-**B**, (215) 329-5104-**H**, (215) 898-1865-**F**
Ethnicity: African-American/Black
Degree and Year: PhD 1989
Major Field: Clinical Psychology
Specialty: Cognitive Behavioral Therapy;Drug Abuse;Personality
        Theory;Social Psychology

COTTINGHAM, Alice L.
666 Greenwich Street
New York, NY 10014-6329
Ethnicity: African-American/Black
Languages: Spanish
Degree and Year: PhD 1963
Major Field: Clinical Psychology
Specialty: Psychotherapy;Personality Measurement

CRAIG, U-Shaka
3978 Bent Way
South San Francisco, CA 94080
(650) 878-1976-**H**, (650) 878-1976-**F**
ushaka@juno.com
Ethnicity: African-American/Black
Degree and Year: PhD 1994
Major Field: Clinical Psychology

CRANE, Rosario S.
4144 N Armenia Ave, Ste 301
Tampa, FL 33607-6447
(813) 875-0122-**B**, (813) 839-3071-**H**, (813) 875-0208-**F**
Ethnicity: Hispanic/Latino
Languages: Spanish
Degree and Year: PhD 1981
Major Field: Clinical Psychology
Specialty: Assessment/Diagnosis/Evaluation;Clinical
        Psychology;Depression;Adolescent Development

CRAWFORD, Monica L.
The Barry Robinson Center
443 Kempsville Road
Norfolk, VA 23502
(757)455-6188-**B**, 757/483-5070-**H**, 757/455-6178-**F**
Ethnicity: African-American/Black
Degree and Year: PsyD 1994
Major Field: Clinical Psychology
Specialty: Clinical Psychology;Assessment/Diagnosis/
        Evaluation;Psychotherapy;Clinical Child Psychology;Training
        & Development;Family Therapy

CREDIDIO, Vivian F.
806 Manhattan Beach Blvd.
Suite #209
Manhattan Beach, CA 90266
(310) 376-3388-**B**, (310) 541-9414-**H**, (310) 372-0198-**F**
Ethnicity: Hispanic/Latino
Languages: Spanish
Degree and Year: PhD 1985
Major Field: Clinical Psychology
Specialty: Affective Disorders;Clinical Psychology;Ethnic
        Minorities;Consulting Psychology;Family Therapy

CRESPO, Alfredo E.
12725 Ventura Boulevard
Suite #K
Studio City, CA 91604
(818) 506-1348-**B**, (818) 998-1012-**H**
Ethnicity: Hispanic/Latino
Degree and Year: PhD 1985
Major Field: Clinical Psychology
Specialty: Child Abuse;Child Therapy;Clinical Psychology;Family
        Therapy;Ethnic Minorities

CRESPO, Gloria M.
94 Hemlock Drive
Glen Mills, PA 19342
(302) 428-2110-**B**, (215) 558-3760-**H**
Ethnicity: Hispanic/Latino
Languages: Spanish
Degree and Year: PsyD 1988
Major Field: Clinical Psychology
Specialty: Psychotherapy;Group Psychotherapy;Personality
        Disorders;Training & Development;Affective Disorders

CRITTON, Barbara L.
2839 West 63rd Avenue
Merrillville, IN 46410-2819
(219) 886-4629-**B**, (219) 887-4773-**H**
Ethnicity: African-American/Black
Degree and Year: PhD 1983
Major Field: Clinical Psychology
Specialty: General Psychology;Religious Psychology;Rehabilitation

CROCKETT, Deborah P.
1243 Willis Mill Rd SW
Atlanta, GA 30311-2438
(770) 460-3576-**B**, (404) 758-9887-**H**, (404) 827-8539-**F**
preznasp@aol.com
Ethnicity: African-American/Black
Degree and Year: PhD 1987
Major Field: School Psychology
Specialty: School Psychology;Assessment/Diagnosis/Evaluation;Ethnic
        Minorities;Special Education;Child Development

CROWDER, Virginia B.
4 Washington Square Village
Apartment #17J
New York, NY 10012
(212) 998-5661-**B**, (212) 475-0402-**H**, (212) 995-4193-**F**
virginia.crowder@nyu.edu
Ethnicity: African-American/Black
Languages: French
Degree and Year: PhD 1969
Major Field: Clinical Psychology
Specialty: Mental Health
Services;Administration;Measurement;Counseling
Psychology;Ethnic Minorities

CRUZ-LOPEZ, Miguel
P.O. Box 5575
College Station
Mayaguez, PR 00681
(809) 832-0881-**B**, (809) 834-1592-**H**, (809) 832-6570-**F**
Ethnicity: Hispanic/Latino
Languages: Spanish
Degree and Year: PhD 1979
Major Field: Clinical Psychology
Specialty: Clinical Child Psychology;Health Psychology;Gerontology/
Geropsychology;Child & Pediatric Psychology

CRUZ, Albert R.
4116 Harvard Street
Silver Spring, MD 20906
(301) 942-3859-**H**
Ethnicity: Hispanic/Latino
Languages: Spanish
Degree and Year: MS 1958
Major Field: Clinical Psychology
Specialty: Administration;Consumer Psychology;Psychology & the
Arts;Human Relations;Decision & Choice Behavior;Cultural &
Social Processes

CRUZ, Arnold de la
University of California @ Davis
2 Prestwick Court
Sacramento, CA 95833-1991
(916) 752-0871-**B**
Ethnicity: Hispanic/Latino
Degree and Year: PhD 1986
Major Field: Clinical Psychology

CRUZ, Maria C.
401 Austin Highway #218
San Antonio, TX 78209
(210) 828-8495-**B**, (210) 828-0797-**H**, (210) 828-7534-**F**
Ethnicity: Hispanic/Latino
Languages: Spanish
Degree and Year: PhD 1984
Major Field: Clinical Psychology
Specialty: Learning Disabilities;Attention Deficit
Disorders;Depression;Special Education;Assessment/
Diagnosis/Evaluation;Clinical Psychology

CRUZ, Vivian A.
19741 NW 86th Avenue
Miami, FL 33018
(305) 819-5500-**B**
Ethnicity: Hispanic/Latino
Languages: Spanish

Degree and Year: PsyD 1988
Major Field: School Psychology
Specialty: Child Therapy;Family Therapy;Parent-Child
Interaction;Depression;Psychopathology

CUESTA, George M.
Kingsbrook Jewish Medical Center
David Minkin Rehabilitation Institute
Suite #4321
585 Schenectady Avenue
Brooklyn, NY 11203-1891
(718) 604-5000-**B**, (212) 867-4129-**H**, (718) 604-5272-**F**
Ethnicity: Hispanic/Latino
Languages: Spanish
Degree and Year: Phd 1995
Major Field: Clinical Psychology
Specialty: Assessment/Diagnosis/Evaluation

CUMMINGS, Joseph D.
609 West Mountain Ridge Road
Lake lAlmanor, CA 96137
(530) 251-5100-**B**, (530) 259-3594-**H**
Ethnicity: American Indian/Alaska Native
Languages: Spanish
Degree and Year: PhD 1974
Major Field: Clinical Psychology
Specialty: Clinical Psychology;Drug Abuse;Individual
Psychotherapy;Marriage & Family;Management &
Organization

CUNHA, Maria I.
4817 Sheboygan Avenue #620
Madison, WI 53705
(608) 273-6220-**B**, (608) 288-1818-**H**
Ethnicity: Hispanic/Latino
Languages: French, Portuguese, Spanish
Degree and Year: PhD 1975
Major Field: Clinical Psychology
Specialty: Family Therapy;Clinical Psychology;Consulting
Psychology;Psychotherapy;School Psychology

CUNNINGHAM, Michael
Tulane University
Department of Psychology
2007 Percival Stern Hall
New Orleans, LA 70118
(504)862-3308-**B**, 504/587-7141-**H**, 504/862-8744-**F**
mcunnin1@mailhost.tcs.tulane
Ethnicity: African-American/Black
Degree and Year: PhD 1994
Major Field: Developmental Psychology
Specialty: Developmental Psychology;Human Development & Family
Studies;Prevention

CUNNINGHAM, Wayman B.
9404 Slow Rainway
Columbia, MD 21046-2-01
(202) 832-8936-**B**
Ethnicity: African-American/Black
Degree and Year: MA 1959
Major Field: Clinical Psychology

CURRY, Alpha O.
514 Mockingbird Hill Drive
Boron, CA 93516-2102
Ethnicity: African-American/Black

Degree and Year: PhD 1981
Major Field: Clinical Psychology
Specialty: Humanistic Psychology

CURRY, Bonita Pope
  Michigan State University
  207 Student Services Building
  East Lansing, MI 48824
  (517) 353-4409-**B**
Ethnicity: African-American/Black
Degree and Year: PhD 1978
Major Field: Counseling Psychology
Specialty: Psychotherapy

D'HEURLE, Adma J.
  Mercy College
  Dobbs Ferry, NY 10522
  (914) 693-4500-**B**, (914) 941-2216-**H**, (914) 674-7542-**F**
Ethnicity: Asian-American/Asian/Pacific Islander
Languages: Arabic, French, Swedish
Degree and Year: PhD 1953
Major Field: Developmental Psychology
Specialty: Clinical Child Psychology;Educational Psychology;Systems, Methods & Issues;Social Psychology

DAISY, Fransing
  University of Washington
  Cabrina Medical Tower - HIVNET
  901 Boren Avenye
  Suite 1300
  Seattle, WA 980104
  (206) 521-5817-**B**, (2060 767-3093-**H**, (206) 521-5828-**F**
  fransing@u.washington.com
Ethnicity: American Indian/Alaska Native
Degree and Year: PhD 1989
Major Field: Clinical Psychology
Specialty: Alcoholism & Alcohol Abuse;Cognitive Behavioral Therapy;Health Psychology;Client-Centered Therapy;Ethnic Minorities;HIV/AIDS

DALHOUSE, A. Derick
  Moorhead State University
  Department of Psychology
  Moorhead, MN 56563
  (618) 236-3090-**B**, (618) 233-3970-**H**, (218) 236-2168-**F**
  dalhouse@mhd1.moorehead.msus.e
Ethnicity: African-American/Black
Degree and Year: PhD 1974
Major Field: Physiological Psychology
Specialty: Brain Functions;Central Nervous System;Developmental Psychobiology;Neurosciences;Psychopathology

DALLAS, Mercedes
  4906 Sharon Road
  Temple Hills, MD 20748-2236
Ethnicity: Hispanic/Latino
Degree and Year: PhD 1982
Major Field: Clinical Psychology
Specialty: Psychotherapy

DALY, Frederica Y.
  526 Hermosa NE
  Albuquerque, NM 87108-1030
  (505) 265-2425-**B**
  rica@unm.edu
Ethnicity: African-American/Black

Degree and Year: PhD 1956
Major Field: Counseling Psychology
Specialty: Adolescent Development;Developmental Psychology;Alcoholism & Alcohol Abuse

DARUNA, Jorge H.
  Tulane University @ School of Medicine
  Department of Psychiatry & Neurology
  1430 Tulane Avenue
  New Orleans, LA 70112
  (504) 588-5401-**B**, (504) 738-2095-**H**
Ethnicity: Hispanic/Latino
Languages: Spanish
Degree and Year: PhD 1980
Major Field: Clinical Psychology
Specialty: Alcoholism & Alcohol Abuse;Clinical Child Psychology;Employee Assistance Programs;Psychobiology;Psychoimmunology

DAS, Ajit K.
  University of Minnesota
  Department of Psychology
  Duluth, MN 55812
  (218) 726-8139-**B**
Ethnicity: Asian-American/Asian/Pacific Islander
Degree and Year: PhD 1962
Major Field: Developmental Psychology
Specialty: Personality

DAS, Jagannath P.
  University of Alberta
  Developmental Disabilities Center
  6-123C Ed. North
  Edmonton, Alberta, T6G 2G5
  CANADA
  (403) 492-4505-**B**, (403) 435-6194-**H**, (403) 492-1318-**F**
Ethnicity: Asian-American/Asian/Pacific Islander
Degree and Year: PhD 1957
Major Field: Educational Psychology
Specialty: Child Development;Educational Psychology

DAS, Manju P.
  Seven Trailwood Circle
  Rochester, NY 14618-0527
  (716) 589-5511-**B**, (716) 244-2774-**H**
Ethnicity: Asian-American/Asian/Pacific Islander
Languages: Hindi
Degree and Year: MA 1984
Major Field: Clinical Psychology
Specialty: Clinical Psychology;Personality Psychology

DAVE, Jagdish P.
  Governors State University
  Division of Psychology and Counseling
  University Park, IL 60466-0975
  (708) 534-4903-**B**, (708) 957-4572-**H**, (708) 534-8451-**F**
Ethnicity: Asian-American/Asian/Pacific Islander
Languages: Hindi
Degree and Year: PhD 1964 PsyD 1992
Major Field: Clinical Psychology
Specialty: Client-Centered Therapy;History & Systems of Psychology;Ethnic Minorities;Cross Cultural Processes;Health Psychology;Stress

DAVILA, Joanne
UCLA Department of Psychology
Box 951563
Los Angeles, CA 90095
(310) 825-2880-**B**, (310) 826-7148-**H**, (310) 206-5895-**F**
davila@psych.ucla.edu
Ethnicity: Hispanic/Latino
Degree and Year: PhD 1993
Major Field: Clinical Psychology
Specialty: Adolescent Development;Interpersonal Processes &
        Relations;Personality;Depression;Marriage & Family;Social
        Cognition

DAVIS-RUSSELL, Elizabeth
3127 McKelvy Avenue
Clovis, CA 93611-6029
(209) 456-2777-**B**, (209) 292-5816-**H**, (209) 253-2267-**F**
edavisru@mail.cssp.edu
Ethnicity: African-American/Black
Degree and Year: PhD 1987 EdD 1973
Major Field: Clinical Psychology
Specialty: Assessment/Diagnosis/Evaluation;Cross Cultural
        Processes;Curriculum Development/Evaluation;Ethnic
        Minorities;Individual Psychotherapy

DAVIS, Annette E.
3011 Oregon Knolls Dr Nw
Washington, DC 20015-2211
(202) 806-6701-**B**
Ethnicity: African-American/Black
Degree and Year: PhD 1974
Major Field: Educational Psychology

DAVIS, Bernice M.
North Jersey Developmental Cener
169 Minnisik Road
PO Box 169
Totowa, NJ 07511
(973) 256-1700-**B**, (201) 420-3346-**H**
Ethnicity: African-American/Black
Degree and Year: PsyD 1994
Major Field: Clinical Psychology
Specialty: Mentally Retarded;Community Mental Health;Chronically
        Mentally Ill;Ethnic Minorities;Cognitive Behavioral
        Therapy;Child Abuse

DAVIS, Charles E.
Illinois School of Professional
Psychology - Chicago Campus
Two National Plaza
20 South Clark Street, 3rd Floor
Chicago, IL 60603
(708) 431-2245-**B**, (708) 383-0198-**H**, (312) 201-1907-**F**
Ethnicity: African-American/Black
Degree and Year: PhD 1983
Major Field: Clinical Psychology
Specialty: Adolescent Therapy;Child Therapy;Family
        Therapy;Attention Deficit Disorders;Conduct Disorders;Cross
        Cultural Processes

DAVIS, Cheryl L.
Hathaway Children and Family Services
11500 Eldridge Avenue
Suite 204
Lake View Terrace, CA 91342

(818) 896-2255-**B**, (818) 892-1090-**H**, (818) 892-1090-**F**
Ethnicity: African-American/Black
Degree and Year: PhD 1987 BA 1979
Major Field: Clinical Child Psychology
Specialty: Child Therapy;Adolescent Therapy

DAVIS, Jerry H.
1447 Peachtree Street, NE
Suite #410
Atlanta, GA 30309-3033
(404) 892-0952-**B**
Ethnicity: African-American/Black
Degree and Year: PhD 1974
Major Field: Clinical Psychology
Specialty: Developmental Psychology;Clinical Psychology

DAWIS, Rene V.
229 Bedford Street, SE
Minneapolis, MN 55414
(612) 379-7311-**H**
dawis001@maroon.tc.umn.edu
Ethnicity: Asian-American/Asian/Pacific Islander
Languages: Filipino
Degree and Year: PhD 1956
Major Field: Counseling Psychology
Specialty: Individual Difference;Vocational
        Psychology;Measurement;Counseling Psychology

DAWKINS, Arthur C.
2103 Shiver Drive
Alexandria, VA 22307-1635
(703) 768-4669-**B**
Ethnicity: African-American/Black
Degree and Year: PhD 1973
Major Field: Educational Psychology
Specialty: Educational Research

DAWKINS, Marva P.
807 North Ninth Avenue
Maywood, IL 60153
(312) 236-1498-**B**, (708) 345-1130-**H**
Ethnicity: African-American/Black
Degree and Year: PhD 1975
Major Field: Clinical Psychology
Specialty: Clinical Psychology;Forensic Psychology;Community
        Mental Health;Human Relations;Assessment/Diagnosis/
        Evaluation

DAWSON, Harriett E.
197 Drake Avenue
New Rochelle, NY 10805
(914) 636-3008-**H**
Ethnicity: African-American/Black
Degree and Year: EdD 1974
Major Field: School Psychology
Specialty: Assessment/Diagnosis/Evaluation;Individual
        Psychotherapy;Learning Disabilities;Personality
        Measurement;School Psychology

DE APODACA, Roberto F.
9742 Willo Glenn
Santa Ana, CA 92705
(714) 944-8455-**B**, (714) 858-0360-**H**, (714) 972-9162-**F**
Ethnicity: Hispanic/Latino
Languages: Spanish
Degree and Year: PhD 1979

Major Field: Clinical Psychology
Specialty: Forensic Psychology;Neuropsychology

DE ARMAS, Armando
3605 Long Beach Blvd.
Long Beach, CA 90807-4013
(310) 424-7710-**B**, (310) 494-4916-**H**
Ethnicity: Hispanic/Latino
Degree and Year: PhD 1984
Major Field: Clinical Psychology
Specialty: Psychotherapy

DE FUENTES, Nanette
1809 Verdugo Blvd. #260
Glendale, CA 91298
(818) 790-0628-**B**, (818) 440-9574-**H**
Ethnicity: Hispanic/Latino
Languages: Spanish
Degree and Year: PhD 1986
Major Field: Clinical Psychology
Specialty: Employee Assistance Programs;Death & Dying;Humanistic
Psychology;Hypnosis/Hypnotherapy;Psychotherapy

DE JESUS, Nelson H.
3840 N Via de Cordoba
Tucson, AZ 85749
(602) 885-5116-**B**, (602) 760-0861-**H**, (602) 885-4473-**F**
Ethnicity: Hispanic/Latino
Languages: Spanish
Degree and Year: PhD 1978
Major Field: Educational Psychology
Specialty: Adolescent Therapy;Pain & Pain Management;Hypnosis/
Hypnotherapy;Biofeedback;Family Therapy

DE LA CANCELA, Victor
Salud Management Association
2727 Palisade Avenue
Suite 4H
Riverdale, NY 10463-1020
(718) 796-0971-**B**, (718) 796-2070-**H**, (212) 385-2644-**F**
Ethnicity: Hispanic/Latino
Degree and Year: PhD 1981
Major Field: Clinical Psychology

DE LA PENA, Augustin M.
Sleep Discords Center
San Jose Medical Center
675 E Santa Clara Street
San Jose, CA 95112-1932
(408) 993-7055-**B**, 415 366-6365-**H**, 415 364-1613-**F**
Ethnicity: Hispanic/Latino
Languages: Spanish
Degree and Year: PhD 1971
Major Field: Physiological Psychology
Specialty: Psychophysiology;Health Psychology;Sleep
Disorders;Stress;Cognitive Development

DE LA SERNA, Marcelo
5272 Amhurst Drive
Norcross, GA 30092
(404) 662-5108-**B**
Ethnicity: Hispanic/Latino
Degree and Year: PhD 1977
Major Field: unknown
Specialty: Clinical Neuropsychology;Rational-Emotive Therapy

DE LA SOTA, Elizanda M.
1600 W 38th Street
Suite #428
Austin, TX 78731
(512) 454-3685-**B**, (512) 288-5428-**H**, (512) 454-3689-**F**
Ethnicity: Hispanic/Latino
Languages: Spanish
Degree and Year: PhD 1985
Major Field: Counseling Psychology
Specialty: Marriage & Family;Organizational Development;Hypnosis/
Hypnotherapy;Sexual Dysfunction;Health Psychology

DE LAS FUENTES, Cynthia
Our Lady of the Lake University
411 SW 24th Street
San Antonio, TX 78207
(210)431-3914-**B**, 515/327-2772-**H**, 210/436-0824-**F**
delac@lake.ollusa.edu
Ethnicity: Hispanic/Latino
Languages: American Sign Language, French, Spanish
Degree and Year: PhD 1994 BA 1984
Major Field: Counseling Psychology
Specialty: Counseling Psychology;Gender Issues;Psychotherapy;Ethnic
Minorities;Lesbian & Gay Issuues

DE LEAIRE, Robert
230 East 88th Street
New York, NY 10128
(212) 427-1224-**H**
Ethnicity: African-American/Black
Degree and Year: PhD 1986
Major Field: Counseling Psychology
Specialty: Counseling Psychology;Disadvantaged;Mentally
Retarded;Parent Education;Learning Disabilities

DE LLANO, Carmen
4140 Mt. Alifan Place #E
San Diego, CA 92111-2841
(619) 292-1848-**B**, (619) 292-7914-**H**
Ethnicity: Hispanic/Latino
Languages: Spanish
Degree and Year: PhD 1986
Major Field: Clinical Psychology
Specialty: Alcoholism & Alcohol Abuse;Assessment/Diagnosis/
Evaluation;Ethnic Minorities;Family Therapy;Forensic
Psychology

DE LOUREDES MATTEI, Maria
53 Center Street
Northhampton, MA 01060-3000
(215) 328-3645-**H**
Ethnicity: Hispanic/Latino
Languages: Spanish
Degree and Year: PhD 1983
Major Field: Clinical Psychology
Specialty: Developmental Psychology;Psychoanalysis

DE QUEIROZ, Aidyl M.
Rua Pelagio
Lobo #107
Sao Paulo SP 05 009,
BRAZIL
Ethnicity: Hispanic/Latino
Degree and Year: PhD 1962
Major Field: Clinical Psychology

DE VARONA, M.
414 N Hawthorne Rd
Winston Salem, NC 27104-3223
(910) 725-7777-**B**, (910) 723-7385-**H**
Ethnicity: Hispanic/Latino
Degree and Year: PhD 1980
Major Field: Clinical Psychology
Specialty: Psychotherapy

DEBARDELABEN, Garfield
1803 NE Thompson
Portland, OR 97212-4211
(503) 282-3158-**B**
Ethnicity: African-American/Black
Degree and Year: PhD 1979
Major Field: Clinical Psychology
Specialty: Medical Psychology;Physically Handicapped

DEBLASSIE, III, Paul A.
2201 San Pedro Drive, NE
Building #20
Albuquerque, NM 87110-4155
(505) 884-2292-**B**
Ethnicity: Hispanic/Latino
Degree and Year: PhD 19
Major Field: Clinical Psychology
Specialty: Pastoral Psychology

DEFERREIRE, Mary Elizabeth
Texas Department of
Mental Health Retardation
Austin State Hospital
4110 Guadalupe Street
Austin, TX 78751
512 452-0381-**B**, 512 440-1875-**H**, 512 478-2044-**F**
Ethnicity: Hispanic/Latino
Languages: Spanish
Degree and Year: PhD 1984 MS 1973
Major Field: Clinical Psychology
Specialty: Clinical Psychology;Family Therapy;Behavior
        Therapy;Ethnic Minorities;Feminist Therapy;Individual
        Psychotherapy

DEFOUR, Darlene C.
Hunter College
Department of Psychology
695 Park Avenue
New York, NY 10021
(212) 772-5678-**B**, (212) 926-2150-**H**, (212) 772-5620-**F**
ddefour@shiva.hunter.cuny.edu
Ethnicity: African-American/Black
Degree and Year: PhD 1986
Major Field: Social Psychology
Specialty: Ethnic Minorities;Gender Issues;Community
        Psychology;Cultural & Social Processes;Psychology of Women

DEGRAFF, Christopher D.
343 Fairview Drive
Suite #104
Carson City, NV 89701
(702) 887-1817-**B**
Ethnicity: American Indian/Alaska Native
Degree and Year: PhD 1980

Major Field: Clinical Psychology
Specialty: Medical Psychology;Pain & Pain Management;Sex/Marital
        Therapy

DEHMER-ABALO, Elena M.
LAC/U.S.C. Medical Center
1715 Griffin Avenue
Los Angeles, CA 90033
(2130 226-3237-**B**, (626) 477-4031-**H**
drdehmer@takenote.net
Ethnicity: Hispanic/Latino
Languages: Spanish
Degree and Year: PhD 1991
Major Field: Clinical Psychology
Specialty: Neurological Disorders;Child & Pediatric
        Psychology;Assessment/Diagnosis/Evaluation;Clinical Child
        Neuropsychology

DEL RIO, Augusto B.
15445 Ventura Blvd.
Suite #348
Sherman Oaks, CA 91413
(818) 784-2507-**B**, (818) 990-5143-**F**
Ethnicity: Hispanic/Latino
Languages: Spanish
Degree and Year: PhD 1973
Major Field: Physiological Psychology
Specialty: Clinical Neuropsychology;Clinical Psychology;Assessment/
        Diagnosis/Evaluation;Educational Psychology;Psychometrics

DELEAIRE, Robert N.
230 East 88th Street
New York, NY 10128
(212) 427-1224-**H**
Ethnicity: African-American/Black
Degree and Year: PhD 1986
Major Field: Counseling Psychology
Specialty: Counseling Psychology;Mentally Retarded;Learning
        Disabilities;Disadvantaged;Parent Education

DELGADO-HACHEY, Maria
P.O. Box 940034
Plano, TX 75094-0034
Ethnicity: Hispanic/Latino
Languages: Spanish
Degree and Year: nhD 1984
Major Field: Developmental Psychology
Specialty: Cognitive Development;Child & Pediatric
        Psychology;Infancy;Assessment/Diagnosis/Evaluation

DEMEIS, Debra K.
Hobart & Williams Smith College
Department of Psychology
Geneve, NY 14456
(315) 781-3457-**B**, (315) 789-8741-**H**, (315) 781-3560-**F**
Ethnicity: Asian-American/Asian/Pacific Islander
Degree and Year: PhD 1977
Major Field: Developmental Psychology
Specialty: Infancy;Adult Development;Psychology of
        Women;Preschool & Day Care Issues

DENDALUCE, Inaki
Palacio, 30-3
San Sebastian, 20008 398

SPAIN
(943) 212659-**B**
Ethnicity: Hispanic/Latino
Degree and Year: PhD 1971
Major Field: Experimental Psychology
Specialty: Educational Research

DENNEDY-FRANK, David P.
1025 Camino Redondo
Santa Fe, NM 87505-5219
(719) 589-9233-**B**
Ethnicity: Hispanic/Latino
Degree and Year: PhD 1981
Major Field: Clinical Psychology
Specialty: Community Mental Health

DENNIS, Dothlyn J.G.
340 Claremont Avenue
Mt. Vernon, NY 10552-2351
(914) 664-0982-**B**, (914) 699-3256-**H**, (914) 422-2311-**F**
DD@WPBOL.uhric.org.
Ethnicity: African-American/Black
Degree and Year: PhD 1982
Major Field: School Psychology
Specialty: School Counseling

DENSON, Eric L.
University of Delaware
Counseling Center
261 Perkins Center
Newark, DE 19716
(302) 831-2141-**B**, (302) 831-2148-**F**
Ethnicity: African-American/Black
Degree and Year: PhD 1992
Major Field: Clinical Psychology
Specialty: Sports Psychology;Personality Disorders;Eating
          Disorders;Individual Psychotherapy

DENT, Harold E.
30 Brough Lane
Suite #301
Hampton, VA 23669-3273
(415) 777-9160-**B**, (510) 653-5080-**H**
Ethnicity: African-American/Black, American Indian/Alaska Native
Degree and Year: PhD 1966
Major Field: Community Psychology
Specialty: Community Mental Health

DEROCHER, Terry L.
P O Box 611597
Port Huron, MI 48061-1597
(810) 987-1750-**B**, 810 982-6068-**H**
Ethnicity: American Indian/Alaska Native
Degree and Year: PhD 1987
Major Field: Social Psychology
Specialty: Community Mental Health;Community Psychology;Child
          Abuse;Mental Health Services;Juvenile Delinquency

DERRICK, Sara M.
1323 Johnson Street
Sandusky, OH 44870-4628
Ethnicity: African-American/Black
Degree and Year: PhD 1975
Major Field: Developmental Psychology

DERRICKSON, Kimberly B.
5904 Ayleshire Road
Baltimore, MD 99508-6700
(410) 550- 9808-**H**
Ethnicity: African-American/Black
Languages: Spanish
Degree and Year: PhD 1993
Major Field: Counseling Psychology
Specialty: Family Therapy;Adolescent
          Therapy;Disadvantaged;Administration;Assessment/
          Diagnosis/Evaluation

DESDIN, Roberto
8209 NW 201 Terrace
Hialeah, FL 33015-5934
(305) 458-7329-**B**
Ethnicity: Hispanic/Latino
Degree and Year: PhD 1985
Major Field: Clinical Psychology
Specialty: Clinical Psychology

DESHMUKH, Mukund
5305 Los Estados, #27
Yorba Linda, CA 92687-5104
Ethnicity: Asian-American/Asian/Pacific Islander
Degree and Year: MD 1979
Major Field: unknown
Specialty: Neurosciences

DETRES, Michael P.
Metro New York Developmental
  Disabilities Services Office
416 West 149th Street
New York, NY 10031
(212) 281-8224-**B**, (212) 268-3687-**H**, (212) 268-3687-**F**
71643.2112@compuserve.com
Ethnicity: Hispanic/Latino
Degree and Year: PhD 1994
Major Field: Clinical Psychology
Specialty: Applied Behavior Analysis;Assessment/Diagnosis/
          Evaluation;Instructional Methods;Adult
          Development;Educational Psychology;Learning/Learning
          Theory

DEVEZIN, Armond A.
35324 Camp Salmen Road
Slidell, LA 70460
(504) 523-2018-**B**
Ethnicity: African-American/Black
Degree and Year: PhD 1977
Major Field: Clinical Psychology

DEWINDT-ROBSON, L. Kimberly
4630 Gallant Lane
Winston-Salem, NC 27101-6409
(919) 996-8890-**B**
Ethnicity: African-American/Black
Degree and Year: PhD 1986
Major Field: Clinical Psychology

DHIMITRI, Patricio
295 Campbell Road
North Andover, MA 01845-5700
(508) 794-0276-**B**

Ethnicity: Hispanic/Latino
Degree and Year: D.Mi 1978
Major Field: unknown
Specialty: Psychotherapy

DIAS, Milagres C.
15133 E La Subida Drive
Hacienda Heights, CA 91745
(213) 738-3724-**B**, (562) 945-1393-**H**
Ethnicity: Asian-American/Asian/Pacific Islander
Degree and Year: PhD 1971
Major Field: Counseling Psychology
Specialty: Clinical Psychology

DIAZ-GUERRERO, Rogelio
Apartado Postal 73-B
Morelos
62158
Guernavaca, Morelos,
MEXICO
011 5273131783-**H**
Ethnicity: Hispanic/Latino
Languages: Spanish
Degree and Year: PhD 1947
Major Field: General Psy./Methods & Systems
Specialty: Cross Cultural Processes;Cultural & Social
Processes;Personality Theory;Personality Psychology

DIAZ-MACHADO, Carmen B.
5681 SW Court
Miami, FL 33143-2311
(305) 666-4962-**B**
Ethnicity: Hispanic/Latino
Languages: Spanish
Degree and Year: PhD 1987
Major Field: Neurosciences
Specialty: Alzheimer's Disease;Chronically Mentally Ill;Crisis
Intervention & Therapy;Neuropsychology;Clinical
Neuropsychology

DIAZ, Eduardo I.
Independent Review Panel
140 West Flagler Street
Suite 1101
Miami, FL 33130-1561
(305) 375-4880-**B**, (305) 255-5817-**H**, (305) 375-4880-**F**
irp@co.miami-dade.fl.us
Ethnicity: Hispanic/Latino
Languages: Spanish
Degree and Year: PhD 1979
Major Field: Physiological Psychology
Specialty: Cultural & Social Processes;Policy Analysis;Problem
Solving;Human Relations;Psychology & Law;Prevention

DIAZ, Raul
3900 Woodlake Blvd.
Suite #211
Greenacres, FL 33463-3045
(407) 683-2892-**B**
Ethnicity: Hispanic/Latino
Degree and Year: PhD 1985
Major Field: Clinical Psychology
Specialty: Psychotherapy

DINGUS, C. Mary
VA Health Care System
Seattle Division (111ONE)
1660 South Columbia Way
Seattle, WA 98108
(206) 764-2185-**B**
Ethnicity: African-American/Black
Degree and Year: PhD 1978
Major Field: Clinical Psychology
Specialty: Medical Psychology;Clinical
Psychology;Rehabilitation;Neuropsychology;Health
Psychology

DIXON, Carrie B.
55 Monument Circle
Suite 1334
Indianapolis, IN 46204
Ethnicity: African-American/Black
Degree and Year: PhD 1985
Major Field: Clinical Psychology
Specialty: Clinical Psychology;Individual
Psychotherapy;Stress;Cognitive Behavioral Therapy;Rational-
Emotive Therapy;Motivation

DIXON, J. Faye
Allegheny University of the Health/
Sciences EPPI
3200 Henry Avenue
Philidelphia, PA 19118-3425
(215) 842-4412-**B**, (215) 247-2092-**H**, (215) 843-7384-**F**
dixonj@auhs.edu
Ethnicity: African-American/Black
Degree and Year: PhD 1989
Major Field: Clinical Psychology
Specialty: Clinical Psychology;Depression;Psychopathology;Suicide

DOBBINS, James E.
721 Homewood Avenue
Dayton, OH 45406
(513) 873-3490-**B**, (513) 873-3434-**F**
Ethnicity: African-American/Black
Degree and Year: PhD 1978
Major Field: Clinical Psychology
Specialty: Ethnic Minorities;Individual Psychotherapy;Marriage &
Family;Professional Issues in Psychology

DOCKETT, Kathleen H.
4224 Blagden Avenue, NW
Washington, DC 20011
(202) 282-2152-**B**, (202) 723-0503-**H**, (202) 282-3676-**F**
kdockett@aol.com
Ethnicity: African-American/Black
Degree and Year: EdD 1974
Major Field: Community Psychology
Specialty: Community Psychology;Group Processes;Homelessness &
Homeless Populations;Social Change

DONAHUE, Pamela J.
Slippery Rock University
6558 Turkey Track Road
Conneautville, PA 16406
(814) 587-4187-**H**
Ethnicity: African-American/Black
Degree and Year:
Major Field: unknown

DONATE-BARTFIELD, Evelyn
Marquette University School of Denistry
2117 N 122nd Street
Wauwatosa, WI 53226
(414) 288-7470-**B**, (414) 453-7132-**H**
evilu@aol.com
Ethnicity: Hispanic/Latino
Degree and Year: PhD 1989
Major Field: Clinical Psychology

DONG, Tim T.
Mira Costa College
One Barnard Drive
Oceanside, CA 92056
(706) 795-6610-**B**, (760) 795-6609-**F**
tdong@mee.miracosta.cc.ca.us
Ethnicity: Asian-American/Asian/Pacific Islander
Degree and Year: PhD 1968
Major Field: Cognitive Psychology
Specialty: Ethnic Minorities;Social Cognition

DONNELLA, John
Residence Ferrare Apt. #2082
100 Blvd Massena
Paris, Cedex 13
F-750-12 144,
FRANCE
331 45 83 0657-**B**
Ethnicity: African-American/Black
Degree and Year: PhD 1975
Major Field: Clinical Psychology
Specialty: Psychotherapy

DOOLEY, John A.
Gertrude Levin Pain Center
4727 St. Antoine, Apt # 404
Detroit, MI 48201
(313) 745-7246-**B**, (313) 884-1029-**H**, (313) 993-7197-**F**
jdooley@med.wayne.edu
Ethnicity: Hispanic/Latino
Languages: German
Degree and Year: PhD 1985 MA 1980
Major Field: Clinical Psychology
Specialty: Pain & Pain Management;Health Psychology;Cognitive
        Behavioral Therapy;Stress;Administration

DORIS, Terri M.
Northeastern University Counseling Center
302 Ell Hall
Boston, MA 02115
(6170 373-2142-**B**, (6270 373-4142-**F**
te.davis@nunet.neu.edu
Ethnicity: African-American/Black
Degree and Year: PhD 1995
Major Field: Counseling Psychology
Specialty: Ethnic Minorities;Counseling Psychology;Training &
        Development;Cross Cultural Processes

DONALD, Liz
3001 Lake Brook Blvd.
Knoxville, TN 37909
(615) 588-2933-**B**
Ethnicity: African-American/Black
Degree and Year: PhD 1985
Major Field: Clinical Psychology
Specialty: Affective Disorders;Alcoholism & Alcohol
        Abuse;Personality Disorders;Sex/Marital Therapy;Stress

DORR, Bernadette
Wendy's International, Inc.
PO Box 256
4288 W. Dublin-Granville Road
Dublin, OH 43017
(614) 764-6726-**B**, (614) 766-3919-**F**
Ethnicity: African-American/Black
Degree and Year: PhD 1992
Major Field: Industrial/Organizational Psy.
Specialty: Industrial/Organizational Psychology

DOS SANTOS, John F.
Emeritus Professor of Psychology
University of Notre Dame
Trustee, Retirement Research Foundation
2408 East Merrin Road
Plant City, FL 33567
(813) 759-8303-**H**
Ethnicity: Hispanic/Latino
Languages: Portuguese, Spanish
Degree and Year: PhD 1965
Major Field: Gerontology
Specialty: Suicide;Training & Development;Sensory & Perceptual
        Processes;Gerontology/Geropsychology;Homelessness &
        Homeless Populations

DOSAMANTES-BEAUDRY, Irma
UCLA
Department of World Arts & Cultures
Box 951608
Los Angeles, CA 90095-1608
(310) 825-3951-**B**, (3100 276-0748-**H**, (310) 825-7507-**F**
Ethnicity: Hispanic/Latino
Languages: Spanish
Degree and Year: PhD 1962
Major Field: Clinical Psychology
Specialty: Clinical Psychology;Creativity;Developmental
        Psychology;Psychoanalysis;Cross Cultural
        Processes;Psychotherapy

DOSS, Juanita K.
Burdette & Associates
17352 West Twelve Mile Road
Southfield, MI 48076
(248) 559-0736-**B**, (248) 540-2996-**H**, (248) 569-7626-**F**
Ethnicity: African-American/Black
Degree and Year: PhD 1987 MA 1972
Major Field: Clinical Psychology
Specialty: Marriage & Family;Stress

DOUGLAS, Byron C.
8553 Windsor Court
Ypsilanti, MI 48198-3613

Ethnicity: African-American/Black
Degree and Year: PhD 1985
Major Field: Clinical Psychology

DOZIER, Arthur L.
401 Pennsylvania Avenue
Freeport, NY 11520
(516) 867-5240-**B**, (516) 867-3494-**H**
Ethnicity: African-American/Black
Degree and Year: PhD 1975
Major Field: School Psychology
Specialty: School Psychology;Clinical Psychology;Ethnic
Minorities;Psychotherapy;Assessment/Diagnosis/Evaluation

DRIEBERG, Keith L
12440 Quail Lane
Grand Terrace, CA 92324-5756
(714) 887-2565-**B**
Ethnicity: Asian-American/Asian/Pacific Islander
Degree and Year: PhD 1990
Major Field: Educational Psychology
Specialty: Neuropsychology

DROZ, Elizabeth
University of Pennsylvania
University Counseling Service
133 So. 36th Street, 2nd Floor
Philidelphia, PA 19104
(215 898-7021-**B**, (215) 748-6092-**H**
Ethnicity: Hispanic/Latino
Languages: Spanish
Degree and Year: PhD 1990
Major Field: Counseling Psychology
Specialty: Alcoholism & Alcohol Abuse;Learning Disabilities;Ethnic
Minorities;Vocational Psychology

DUAN, Changming
University of Missouri
215 Education
Kansas City, MO 64110
(816) 235-1481-**B**, (785) 228-1481-**H**, (785) 228-0815-**F**
Ethnicity: Asian-American/Asian/Pacific Islander
Languages: Chinese
Degree and Year: PhD 1992
Major Field: Counseling Psychology
Specialty: Counseling Psychology;Cross Cultural Processes;Cultural &
Social Processes;Consulting Psychology;Social
Psychology;Psychotherapy

DUDLEY-GRANT, G. Rita
Virgin Islands Behavioral Services
P.O. Box 24241
St. Croix, VI 00824-0241
(340) 774-6222-**B**, (342) 773-8384-**H**, (340) 773-7734-**F**
grdg@worldnet.att.net
Ethnicity: African-American/Black
Degree and Year: PhD 1980 MPh 1984
Major Field: Clinical Psychology
Specialty: Drug Abuse;Community Mental Health;Projective
Techniques;Cross Cultural Processes;Disadvantaged;Family
Therapy

DUDLEY, Charma D.
5221 Schenley Avenue
Pittsburgh, PA 15224-1030
Ethnicity: African-American/Black

Degree and Year: PhD 1984
Major Field: Counseling Psychology
Specialty: Child Therapy

DUNBAR, Waldo
83 Spindrift Drive
Portuguese Bend, CA 90274-6049
(213) 377-4771-**B**
Ethnicity: Hispanic/Latino
Degree and Year: PhD 1956
Major Field: Clinical Psychology
Specialty: Psychotherapy

DUNCAN, Bessie A.
498 West End Avenue #1C
New York, NY 10024
(212) 724-0380-**B**, (201) 489-6760-**H**, (212) 724-0380-**F**
Ethnicity: African-American/Black
Degree and Year: PhD 1979
Major Field: Clinical Psychology
Specialty: Clinical Psychology;Cognitive Behavioral
Therapy;Alcoholism & Alcohol Abuse;Adolescent
Therapy;Ethnic Minorities

DUNSTON, Patricia
1366 Tewkesbury Place, NW
Washington, DC 20012-2922
(202) 364-3422-**B**, (202) 829-0605-**H**
dunstonp@receivercmhs.org
Ethnicity: African-American/Black
Degree and Year: PhD 1979
Major Field: Developmental Psychology
Specialty: Values & Moral Behavior

DURAN, Richard P.
University of California
Graduate School of Education
Santa Barbara, CA 93106
(805) 893-3555-**B**, (805) 893-8016-**F**
Ethnicity: Hispanic/Latino
Languages: Spanish
Degree and Year: PhD 1977
Major Field: Educational Psychology
Specialty: Statistics

DURANT, JR., Adrian J.
Consulting Psychologist
1716 Lincoln Road
Champaign, IL 61821-5636
217 359-2283-**B**
Ethnicity: American Indian/Alaska Native
Degree and Year: EdD 1957
Major Field: unknown
Specialty: Consulting Psychology;Clinical Psychology;Assessment/
Diagnosis/Evaluation;School Psychology;Special Education

DYSON, Vida
3319 Maple Lane
Hazel Crest, IL 60429-1566
(312) 413-1231-**B**
Ethnicity: African-American/Black
Degree and Year: PhD 1979
Major Field: Personality Psychology
Specialty: Personality Measurement

EATON, Sheila J.
Wayne State University
Department of Psychiatry & Behavioral
Neuroscience
2880 Ryan Road, Suite 300
Warran, MI 48092
(248) 398-7770-**B**, (313) 259-7052-**H**
Ethnicity: American Indian/Alaska Native
Degree and Year: PhD 1984
Major Field: Clinical Psychology
Specialty: Psychotherapy;Individual Psychotherapy;Clinical
Research;Psychoanalysis;Child Therapy;Aggression

EBERHARDT, Carolyn A.
15200 SW 84th Avenue
Miami, FL 33157-2110
Ethnicity: African-American/Black
Degree and Year: PhD 1980
Major Field: Clinical Psychology
Specialty: Psychotherapy

EBREO, Angela
Department of Behavioral Science
University of Kentucky
College Medicine Office Building
Lexington, KY 40536
(606) 323-5771-**B**, (606) 268-9863-**H**, (606) 323-5350-**F**
aebreo2@pop.uky.edu
Ethnicity: Asian-American/Asian/Pacific Islander
Degree and Year: PhD 1998
Major Field: Social Psychology
Specialty: Ethnic Minorities;Cross Cultural Processes;HIV/AIDS

ECHAVARRIA, David
1490 W 49th Place, South
Suite #265
Hialeah, FL 33012
(305) 826-2754-**B**, (305) 861-4405-**H**, (305) 861-4405-**F**
Ethnicity: Hispanic/Latino
Languages: Spanish
Degree and Year: PhD 1983
Major Field: Clinical Psychology
Specialty: Clinical Child Psychology;School Psychology

ECHEMENDIA, Ruben J.
314 Bruce V Moore Bldg
Penn State Univ
University Park, PA 16802-
(814) 865-2191-**B**, 814353-8340-**H**, (814) 863-7003-**F**
Ethnicity: Hispanic/Latino
Languages: Spanish
Degree and Year: PhD 1984
Major Field: Clinical Psychology
Specialty: Clinical Neuropsychology;Assessment/Diagnosis/
Evaluation;Psychotherapy;Ethnic Minorities

EDELIN, Patricia
9614 Windermere Turn
Ft. Washington, MD 20744-5720
(202) 657-5540-**B**
Ethnicity: African-American/Black
Degree and Year: MA 1959
Major Field: Clinical Psychology

EDWARDS, Henry P.
University of Ottawa
School of Psychology
PO Box 450, Station A
Ottawa
Ontario K1N6N5,
CANADA
(613) 514-2250-**B**, (613) 562-5147-**F**
hedwards@uottawa.ca
Ethnicity: Hispanic/Latino, European/White
Languages: French, Spanish
Degree and Year: PhD 1967
Major Field: Experimental Psychology
Specialty: Curriculum Development/Evaluation;Clinical Research;Labor
& Management Relations

EDWARDS, Karen L.
3806 Williamsburg Road
Cincinnati, OH 45215-5126
(513) 556-0648-**B**, (513) 948-8565-**H**, (513) 948-8565-**F**
Ethnicity: African-American/Black
Degree and Year: PhD 1979
Major Field: Social Psychology
Specialty: Cultural & Social Processes;Humanistic
Psychology;Organizational Development;Psychology of
Women;Psychotherapy

EL-AMIN, Debra El-Amin
University of Toleda
Student Medical Center
2801 West Bancroft
Toledo, OH 43606
(419) 530-3443-**B**, (419) 471-1127-**H**, (419) 530-3499-**F**
Ethnicity: African-American/Black
Degree and Year: PsyD 1995
Major Field: Clinical Psychology
Specialty: Clinical Child Psychology;Child Therapy;Child & Pediatric
Psychology;Cross Cultural Processes

ELDER, Patricia
6800 Stenton Avenue
Philadelphia, PA 19150
Ethnicity: African-American/Black
Degree and Year: PhD 1978
Major Field: Counseling Psychology

ELENA LEE, Karen
3029 North Prospect Road
Peoria, IL 61603
(309) 679-4955-**B**, (309) 682-6278-**H**, (309) 679-0995-**F**
elenalee@sprynet.com
Ethnicity: Hispanic/Latino
Degree and Year: PsyD 1990
Major Field: Clinical Psychology
Specialty: Neuropsychology;Memory;Psychology of Women;Learning
Disabilities;Rehabilitation

ELION, Victor H.
P.O. Box 10897
Alexandria, Va 22310
(703) 691-1326-**B**, (703) 719-6619-**H**
Ethnicity: African-American/Black
Degree and Year: PhD 1978
Major Field: Clinical Psychology

Specialty: Psychotherapy;Forensic Psychology;Child Abuse;Mental
Disorders;Personality Disorders

ELLIGAN, Don G.
Boston University School of Medicine
Dept. of Psychiatry, Center for Multi-
cultural Training in Psych. ,One Boston
Medical Center Place, 7 Dowling North
Boston, MA 02118-2999
(617) 414-4646-**B**, (617)414-4792 -**F**
elligan@bu.edu
Ethnicity: African-American/Black
Degree and Year: PhD 1997
Major Field: Clinical Psychology
Specialty: Clinical Psychology;Social Psychology;Clinical Child
Psychology;Cultural & Social Processes;Cognitive Behavioral
Therapy;Ethnic Minorities

ELLIOTT, Vanessa E.
St. Jude's Children Res. Hospital
Department of Behavioral Medicine
332 North Lauderdale Street
Memphis, TN 38105-2794
(901) 495-3580-**B**
Ethnicity: African-American/Black
Degree and Year: PhD
Major Field: unknown

ELLIS, Edwin E.
1211 Locust Street
Philadelphia, PA 19107
(215) 546-7444-**B**, (609) 435-4546-**H**
Ethnicity: Hispanic/Latino
Languages: French, Spanish
Degree and Year: PhD 1976
Major Field: Clinical Psychology
Specialty: Alcoholism & Alcohol Abuse;Clinical Psychology;HIV/
AIDS;Psychotherapy;Group Psychotherapy

ELLIS, Rosita P.
7416 Alaska Avenue, NW
Washington, DC 20012-1512
(202) 576-6518-**B**
Ethnicity: African-American/Black
Degree and Year: MA 1970
Major Field: unknown
Specialty: Community Mental Health

EMORY, Eugene K.
Emory University
Department of Psychology
Atlanta, GA 30322
(404) 686-7524-**B**, (404) 727-7860-**F**
Ethnicity: African-American/Black
Degree and Year: PhD 1978
Major Field: Clinical Psychology

ENG, Albert M.
164 Marview Way
San Francisco, CA 94131
(415) 668-5955-**B**, (415) 641-9149-**H**
Albert_M_Eng@dph.sf.ca.us
Ethnicity: Asian-American/Asian/Pacific Islander
Languages: Chinese
Degree and Year: PhD 1985
Major Field: Clinical Psychology

Specialty: Psychotherapy;Group Psychotherapy;Organizational
Development

EPPS, Pamela J.
Emory University Counseling Center
Cox Hall, Suite 217
Atlanta, GA 30322
(404) 727-7450-**B**, (404) 296-4041-**H**, (404) 727-2906-**F**
pepps@emory.edu
Ethnicity: African-American/Black
Degree and Year: PhD 1989
Major Field: Clinical Psychology
Specialty: Psychotherapy;Ethnic Minorities;Affective
Disorders;Clinical Psychology;Psychology of Women

ERTZ, Dewey J.
P.O. BOX 5
Dupree, SD 57623-0005
(605) 964-8622-**B**, (605) 365-5396-**H**
Ethnicity: American Indian/Alaska Native
Degree and Year: EdD 1977
Major Field: School Psychology

ERVIN, Betty J.
407 Gonzalez Drive
San Francisco, CA 94132
(510) 637-1221-**B**, (415) 337-9559-**H**
Ethnicity: African-American/Black
Degree and Year: EdS 1981 MA 1978
Major Field: Counseling Psychology
Specialty: Employee Assistance Programs;Rehabilitation;Industrial/
Organizational Psychology;Educational Psychology;Vocational
Psychology;Training & Development

ESCANDELL, Vincent A.
1722 9th Street
Wichita Falls, TX 76301-5003
(817) 322-1075-**B**
Ethnicity: Hispanic/Latino
Degree and Year: PhD 1980
Major Field: unknown
Specialty: Neurological Disorders;Clinical Psychology

ESCOFFERY, Aubrey S.
1236 New Mill Drive
Chesapeake, VA 23320-7047
Ethnicity: African-American/Black
Degree and Year: PhD 1967
Major Field: Clinical Psychology

ESCOVAR, Luis A.
Florida International University
Psychology Department
Miami, FL 33199
(305) 348-2880-**B**
Ethnicity: Hispanic/Latino
Languages: Spanish
Degree and Year: PhD 1975
Major Field: unknown
Specialty: Personality Disorders

ESCUDERO, Micaela
1168 Lake Avenue, Unit #14
Clark, NJ 07066-2746
(908) 527-2170-**B**, (908) 827-0463-**H**
Ethnicity: Hispanic/Latino

Languages: Spanish
Degree and Year: EdD 1986
Major Field: Educational Psychology
Specialty: Developmental Psychology;Cognitive Development;Research Design & Methodology;Special Education;Rehabilitation

ESKANDARI, Esfandiar
California Graduate Institute
  Counseling Center
1100 Glendon Avenue, Suite #1119
Westwood, CA 90024
(310) 208-4240-**B**, (310) 473-2120-**H**, (310) 208-0648-**F**
Ethnicity: Asian-American/Asian/Pacific Islander
Languages: Farsi
Degree and Year: PhD 1997
Major Field: Clinical Psychology
Specialty: Clinical Psychology;Interpersonal Processes & Relations;Group Psychotherapy;Alcoholism & Alcohol Abuse;Affective Disorders

ESPARZA, Ricardo
777 29th Street
Suite 201
Boulder, CO 80303-2316
(303) 447-3122-**B**, (303) 449-5793-**H**, 303 447-0031'-**F**
Ethnicity: Hispanic/Latino
Languages: Spanish
Degree and Year: PhD 1977
Major Field: Clinical Psychology
Specialty: Psychotherapy;Pain & Pain Management;Cross Cultural Processes;Marriage & Family;Rehabilitation

ESPIN, Oliva M.
San Diego State University
Department of Women's Studies
San Diego, CA 92182 -8138
(619) 594-3739-**B**, (619) 594-4998-**F**
Ethnicity: Hispanic/Latino
Languages: French, Spanish
Degree and Year: PhD 1974
Major Field: Counseling Psychology
Specialty: Psychology of Women;Ethnic Minorities;Cultural & Social Processes;Lesbian & Gay Issuues

ESQUIVEL, Giselle B.
106 Dellwood Rd
Edison, NJ 08820-3832
(212) 636-6467-**B**, (732) 549-6525-**H**
Ethnicity: Hispanic/Latino
Languages: Spanish
Degree and Year: PsyD 1981
Major Field: School Psychology
Specialty: Projective Techniques;Creativity;Cross Cultural Processes;Psychotherapy

ESSANDOH, Pius K.
13 Equestrian Drive
Burlington, NJ 08016-3057
(201) 200-2322-**B**, (609) 747-0574-**H**
Ethnicity: African-American/Black
Languages: Fante
Degree and Year: PhD 1992
Major Field: Counseling Psychology
Specialty: Counseling Psychology;Cross Cultural Processes;Ethnic

Minorities;Family Processes;Group Processes

EVANS, Helen L.
1525 E. 53rd Street
Suite #531
Chicago, IL 60615
(312) 752-0531-**B**, (312) 667-8040-**H**
Ethnicity: African-American/Black
Degree and Year: PhD 1981
Major Field: Clinical Psychology
Specialty: Behavior Therapy;Clinical Child Psychology;Cognitive Behavioral Therapy;Health Psychology;Stress

EVERETT, Moses L.
1809 Ferdon Road
Ann Arbor, MI 48104
(313) 429-2531-**B**, (313) 663-3739-**H**
Ethnicity: African-American/Black
Degree and Year: PhD 1982
Major Field: Clinical Psychology
Specialty: Clinical Psychology;Forensic Psychology;Ethnic Minorities

EVERSON, Howard T.
9962 Ft. Hamilton Parkway
Brooklyn, NY 11209-8317
(212) 794-5443-**B**, (212) 745-9219-**H**
Ethnicity: American Indian/Alaska Native
Degree and Year: PhD 1985
Major Field: Educational Psychology
Specialty: Educational Research

EZEILO, Bernice N.
University of Nigeria Nsukka
Department of Psychology
Nsukka 296,
Nigeria
042 771911 x352-**B**, 042 457016-**H**
uninec@aol.com
Ethnicity: African-American/Black
Degree and Year: PhD 1984
Major Field: Clinical Psychology
Specialty: Adolescent Therapy;Behavior Therapy;Clinical Psychology;Clinical Research;Domestic Violence;Stress

FAIN, Thomas C.
The Psychology Group
701 South Acadian Thruway
Baton Rouge, LA 70806-5698
(504) 387-3325-**B**
Ethnicity: American Indian/Alaska Native
Degree and Year: PhD 1978
Major Field: Clinical Psychology
Specialty: Assessment/Diagnosis/Evaluation;Forensic Psychology;Personality Disorders;Pain & Pain Management;Psychopharmacology;Deviant Behavior

FAIRCHILD, Halford H.
2271 West 25th Street
Los Angeles, CA 90018
(323) 734-0809-**B**, (213) 734-0809-**H**, (323) 734-0076-**F**
E2e4mate@aol.com
Ethnicity: African-American/Black
Languages: Spanish
Degree and Year: PhD 1977
Major Field: Social Psychology

Specialty: Ethnic Minorities;Mass Media Communication;Educational Research;Gender Issues

FALICOV, Celia J.
4145 Miller Street
San Diego, CA 92103-1542
(619) 683-7755-**B**, (619) 298-5927-**H**, (619) 296-9407-**F**
celita000@aol.com
Ethnicity: Hispanic/Latino
Languages: Italian, Spanish
Degree and Year: PhD 1971
Major Field: Clinical Psychology
Specialty: Family Therapy;Marriage & Family;Ethnic Minorities;Cross Cultural Processes;Psychotherapy;Parent-Child Interaction

FANIBANDA, Darius K.
P.E.E.R.S. Associates, Inc.
15814 Winchester Boulevard
Suite #102
Los Gatos, CA 95030
(408) 354-5071-**B**, (408) 354-5071-**F**
Ethnicity: Asian-American/Asian/Pacific Islander
Languages: Hindi, Gujarati
Degree and Year: PhD 1976 MS 1972
Major Field: Clinical Psychology
Specialty: Clinical Psychology;Counseling Psychology;Crisis Intervention & Therapy;Cognitive Behavioral Therapy;Family Therapy

FANKHANEL, Edward H.
U.S. Courts/Probabtion Office
134 Zambeze St Rph
San Juan, PR 00926-
(809) 766-5596-**B**, (809) 754-7213-**H**
Ethnicity: Hispanic/Latino
Languages: Spanish
Degree and Year: MA 1985
Major Field: Counseling Psychology
Specialty: Counseling Psychology;Adolescent Therapy;Sexual Behavior;Crime & Criminal Behavior;HIV/AIDS;Juvenile Delinquency

FARACI, Ana M.
1346 South Greenwood
Coral Gables, FL 33134-4767
(305) 820-8505-**B**, (305) 444-7025-**H**, (305) 820-8508-**F**
Ethnicity: Hispanic/Latino
Languages: Spanish
Degree and Year: PhD 1982
Major Field: Clinical Psychology
Specialty: Family Therapy;Child Therapy;Group Psychotherapy;Marriage & Family;Psychotherapy

FARLEY, Florence S.
18 S Little Church Street
Petersburg, VA 23803-4431
Ethnicity: African-American/Black
Degree and Year: PhD 1977
Major Field: Educational Psychology

FAYARD, Carlos
23023 Merle Court
Grand Terrace, CA 92324
(909) 425-7773-**B**, (909) 783-4145-**H**
Ethnicity: Hispanic/Latino

Languages: Spanish
Degree and Year: PhD 1988
Major Field: Clinical Psychology
Specialty: Ethnic Minorities;Attention Deficit Disorders;Chronically Mentally Ill;Clinical Psychology

FAZZANO, Catalina U.
1745 Eagle Trace Blvd., East
Coral Springs, FL 33071-7818
(305) 341-0660-**B**
Ethnicity: Hispanic/Latino
Degree and Year: PhD 1980
Major Field: Clinical Psychology
Specialty: Family Therapy

FELDMAN, Esther
20605 NE 22nd Court
Miami, FL 33180-1346
(305) 547-6862-**B**
Ethnicity: Hispanic/Latino
Degree and Year: PhD 1984
Major Field: Clinical Psychology
Specialty: Clinical Neuropsychology

FERDMAN, Bernardo M.
CA School of Professional Psychology
Organization Psychology Programs
6160 Cornerstone Court
San Diego, CA 92121-3710
(619) 623-2777-**B**, (619) 695-9964-**H**, (619) 552-1974-**F**
bferdman@mail.cspp.edu
Ethnicity: Hispanic/Latino
Languages: Spanish
Degree and Year: PhD 1987
Major Field: Social Psychology
Specialty: Management & Organization;Ethnic Minorities;Cross Cultural Processes;Organizational Development;Industrial/ Organizational Psychology

FERGUS, Esther O.
Michigan State University
Department of Family & Child Ecology
125 West Fee Hall
East Lansing, MI 48824-1315
(517) 355-0166-**B**, (517) 351-3304-**H**
Ethnicity: Asian-American/Asian/Pacific Islander
Languages: Japanese
Degree and Year: PhD 1973
Major Field: Community Psychology
Specialty: Community Mental Health;Community Psychology;Rehabilitation

FERNANDEZ, Ephrem
Southern Methodist University
Psychology Department
Hyer Hall
Dallas, TX 75275-0442
(214) 768-3414-**B**, (2140 696-0699-**H**, (214) 768-3910-**F**
efernandez@mail.smu.edu
Ethnicity: Asian-American/Asian/Pacific Islander, Hispanic/Latino
Degree and Year: PhD 1989
Major Field: Clinical Psychology
Specialty: Cognitive Behavioral Therapy;Emotion;Pain & Pain

Management;Cross Cultural Processes

FERNANDEZ, M. Isabel
NIMH Aids Programs
13835 Dowlais Drive
Rockville, MD 20853-2630
(301) 443-5850-**B**
Ethnicity: Hispanic/Latino
Degree and Year: PhD 1986
Major Field: Community Psychology
Specialty: Prevention

FERNANDEZ, Maria C.
University of Miami
Mailman Center for Child Development
1601 NW 12th Avenue
Miami, FL 33136
(305) 243-6857-**B**, (305) 226-3045-**H**, (305) 243-4512-**F**
Ethnicity: Hispanic/Latino
Languages: Spanish
Degree and Year: PhD 1978
Major Field: Clinical Psychology
Specialty: Autism;Clinical Psychology;Ethnic Minorities;School
Psychology;Assessment/Diagnosis/Evaluation;Clinical Child
Psychology

FERNANDEZ, Peter
1100 N Stanton
Suite #701
El Paso, TX 79902
(915) 541-1100-**B**, (915) 585-3437-**H**, (915) 541-1104-**F**
Ethnicity: Hispanic/Latino
Languages: Spanish
Degree and Year: PhD 1986
Major Field: Clinical Psychology
Specialty: Clinical Psychology;Clinical Neuropsychology;Individual
Psychotherapy;Rehabilitation;Forensic Psychology

FERNANDEZ, Rosemary
Passaic Board of Education
101 Passaic Avenue
Passaic, NJ 07055
(201) 670-6074-**H**
Ethnicity: Hispanic/Latino
Languages: Spanish
Degree and Year: EdD 1988
Major Field: Counseling Psychology
Specialty: School Psychology;Special Education;Intelligence;Cultural &
Social Processes;School Counseling;Counseling Psychology

FERREIRA, Pedro M.
1701 Augustine Cut Off
Suite #26
Wilmington, DE 19803-4495
Ethnicity: Hispanic/Latino
Degree and Year: PhD 1983
Major Field: Clinical Psychology

FICHER, Ilda V.
502 Lombard Street
Philadelphia, PA 19147-1415
(215) 627-3372-**B**
Ethnicity: Hispanic/Latino
Degree and Year: PhD 1977
Major Field: unknown
Specialty: Sex/Marital Therapy;Family Therapy

FIELD, Lucy F.
Private Practice
1145 Indianapolis Road
Greencastle, IN 46135
(765) 653-9698-**B**, (765) 653-8675-**H**
Ethnicity: Asian-American/Asian/Pacific Islander
Degree and Year: PhD 1990 MS 1981
Major Field: Counseling Psychology
Specialty: Counseling Psychology

FIELDS, Amanda H.
Psychology Resources
511 Boulevard Suite 1
Salem, VA 24153
(540) 387-3977-**B**, (540) 951-2938-**H**, (540) 387-3977-**F**
Ethnicity: American Indian/Alaska Native
Languages: Spanish
Degree and Year: PhD 1985
Major Field: Educational Psychology
Specialty: Clinical Child Neuropsychology;Adolescent
Development;Assessment/Diagnosis/Evaluation;Child Therapy

FIELDS, Anika C.
Florida State University
Student Counseling Center, R108-A
Tallahassee, FL 32306-2141
(850) 644-2003-**B**, (850) 562-6810-**H**, (850) 644-3150-**F**
afields@admin.fsu.edu
Ethnicity: African-American/Black
Degree and Year: PhD 1982
Major Field: Clinical Psychology
Specialty: Ethnic Minorities;Pain & Pain Management;Stress;Cognitive
Behavioral Therapy;Religious Psychology

FIELDS, Richard L.
2213 New Castle Road
Greensboro, NC 27406-3232
Ethnicity: African-American/Black
Degree and Year: EdD 1964
Major Field: unknown
Specialty: Mentally Retarded

FIGLER, Clare S.
22 Summit Ave
Winthrop, MA 02152-1036
(617) 846-2169-**B**, (617) 846-3254-**H**
Ethnicity: Hispanic/Latino
Degree and Year: EdD 1980
Major Field: School Psychology
Specialty: School Psychology;Counseling Psychology

FIGUEREDO, Migdalia I.
7241 SW 63rd avenue
Suite 202
South Miami, FL 33143
(305) 666-4853-**B**
Ethnicity: Hispanic/Latino
Languages: Spanish
Degree and Year: PhD 1984
Major Field: Developmental Psychology
Specialty: Psychotherapy;Assessment/Diagnosis/Evaluation;Drug
Abuse;Eating Disorders;Affective Disorders;Parent-Child
Interaction

FIGUEROA, Jorge L.
2001 S Shields
Building K
Ft. Collins, CO 80526-1838
(970) 229-9145-**B**, (970) 568-3110-**H**, (970) 229-9195-**F**
figueroa@healthdistrict.org
Ethnicity: Hispanic/Latino
Degree and Year: PhD 1981   1982
Major Field: Clinical Psychology
Specialty: Medical Psychology;Sexual Dysfunction;Cognitive
        Behavioral Therapy;Pain & Pain Management;Gender
        Issues;Marriage & Family

FIGUEROA, Rolando G.
Athens Behavioral Health
  Consultants, P.C.
1060 Gaines School Road
Suite b-3
Athens, GA 30605-3100
(706) 354-1286-**B**, (706) 354-1258-**F**
athbehcons@prodigy.net
Ethnicity: Hispanic/Latino
Languages: Spanish
Degree and Year: PhD
Major Field: Clinical Psychology
Specialty: Attention Deficit Disorders;Clinical Psychology;Family
        Therapy;Autism;Cognitive Behavioral Therapy;Mentally
        Retarded

FILS, David H.
10650 Holman Avenue
Los Angeles, CA 90024
(213) 114-4700-**B**, (310) 475-3755-**H**
Ethnicity: Hispanic/Latino
Languages: French, Spanish
Degree and Year: PhD 1950
Major Field: Clinical Psychology
Specialty: Brain Damage;Clinical Child Psychology;Individual
        Psychotherapy;Mentally Retarded;Disadvantaged

FINKEL, Eva
63 Redbrook Road
Great Neck, NJ 11024
(718) 628-1083-**B**, (516) 466-6044-**H**
Ethnicity: Hispanic/Latino
Languages: French, Portuguese, Spanish
Degree and Year: PsyD 1985
Major Field: School Psychology
Specialty: Adolescent Development;Aggression;Cross Cultural
        Processes

FINLEY, Laurene Y.
2122 N 18th Street
Philadelphia, PA 19121
(215) 925-4633-**B**, (215) 765-4068-**H**
Ethnicity: African-American/Black
Degree and Year: PhD 1989
Major Field: Counseling Psychology
Specialty: Cognitive Behavioral Therapy;Ethnic Minorities;Mental
        Health Services;Rehabilitation;Depression

FISHER, Patricia A.
3132 W Street, SE

Washington, DC 20020
(202) 5443-0013-**B**, (202) 583-8926-**H**, (202) 584-2699-**F**
Ethnicity: African-American/Black
Degree and Year: PhD 1976
Major Field: Counseling Psychology
Specialty: Psychotherapy;Drug Abuse;Counseling
        Psychology;Managed Care;Employee Assistance Programs

FLACHIER, Roberto
Burgess Medical Center
1521 Gull Road
Kalamazoo, MI 49001
(616) 226-7413-**B**, (616) 323-0180-**H**, (616) 385-0337-**F**
Ethnicity: Hispanic/Latino
Languages: Spanish
Degree and Year: PhD 1982
Major Field: Clinical Psychology
Specialty: Group Psychotherapy;Parent-Child Interaction;Individual
        Psychotherapy;Clinical Child Psychology;Family
        Therapy;Adolescent Therapy

FLAHERTY, Maria Y.
Interaction Psychotherapy and
  Counseling Center
925 West Hedding Street
San Jose, CA 95126
(408) 246-4422-**B**, (408) 395-5752-**H**, (408) 246-5044-**F**
maria_flaherty@hotmail.com
Ethnicity: Hispanic/Latino
Languages: Spanish
Degree and Year: PhD 1989
Major Field: Clinical Psychology
Specialty: Sex/Marital Therapy;Sexual Behavior;Clinical
        Psychology;Sexual Dysfunction;Health
        Psychology;Psychology of Women

FLEISHER, Nancy F.
300 Central Park West
Suite 1K
New York, NY 10024
(212) 875-9595-**B**
Ethnicity: Hispanic/Latino
Languages: Spanish
Degree and Year: PhD 1988
Major Field: Clinical Psychology
Specialty: Child Development;Clinical Child
        Psychology;Infancy;Parent-Child Interaction

FLEMING, Andrea L.
1320 Wynnton Road
Suite D
Columbus, GA 31906
(706) 660-9335-**B**
Ethnicity: African-American/Black
Degree and Year: PhD 1988
Major Field: School Psychology
Specialty: Clinical Child Psychology;Family Therapy;Assessment/
        Diagnosis/Evaluation;Adolescent Therapy

FLEMING, Candace M.
Colorado Health Science Center
4200 E Ninth Avenue
Denver, CO 80220-3706
(303) 270-4600-**B**
Ethnicity: American Indian/Alaska Native

Degree and Year: PhD 1979
Major Field: Clinical Psychology
Specialty: Alcoholism & Alcohol Abuse

FLETCHER, Betty A.
Counseling Center at Towson University
8000 York Road
Towson, MD 21252
(410) 418-8372-**B**, (410) 830-2512-**H**
Ethnicity: African-American/Black
Degree and Year: PhD 1982
Major Field: Clinical Psychology
Specialty: Counseling Psychology;Ethnic Minorities

FLIMAN, Vivian P.
438 Ray Norrish Drive
Cincinnati, OH 45246
(513) 671-7400-**B**, (513) 761-6743-**H**
Ethnicity: Hispanic/Latino
Languages: Spanish, Hebrew
Degree and Year: PhD 1982
Major Field: Clinical Psychology
Specialty: Clinical Psychology;Clinical Child Psychology;Child
Therapy;Assessment/Diagnosis/Evaluation;Stress

FLORES DE APODACA, Roberto
Xerox Centre Building
1851 East First Street
Suite 950
Santa Ana, CA 92705
(714) 972-2939-**B**, (714) 858-0360-**H**, (714) 972-9162-**F**
Ethnicity: Hispanic/Latino
Languages: Spanish
Degree and Year: PhD 1979
Major Field: Clinical Psychology
Specialty: Forensic Psychology;Neuropsychology

FLORES, Elena
University of San Francisco
Counseling Psychology Department
2130 Fulton Street
San Francisco, CA 94117
(415) 422-6901-**B**, (415) 206-1030-**H**, (415) 422-5528-**F**
florese@usfca.edu
Ethnicity: Hispanic/Latino
Languages: Spanish
Degree and Year: PhD 1992 MS 1979
Major Field: Clinical Psychology
Specialty: Family Processes;Parent-Child Interaction;Sexual Behavior

FLORES, Philip J.
4034 Jordan Lake Drive
Marietta, GA 30062-5786
(404) 250-9340-**B**
Ethnicity: Hispanic/Latino
Degree and Year: PhD 1983
Major Field: Clinical Psychology
Specialty: Alcoholism & Alcohol Abuse

FLOWERS, Jana D.
3809 Nash Lane
Plano, TX 75025-2032
(214) 238-6065-**B**, 214 618-0845-**H**
Ethnicity: African-American/Black
Degree and Year: PhD 1980

Major Field: Developmental Psychology

FLOYD, Bridget J.
229 Pebble Brook Dr
Madison, AL 35758-7356
(205) 533-1970-**B**, (205) 837-5039-**H**
Ethnicity: African-American/Black
Languages: Spanish
Degree and Year: PhD 1984
Major Field: Clinical Child Psychology
Specialty: Child & Pediatric Psychology;Child Therapy;Child
Development;Stress;Ethnic Minorities

FLOYD, James A.
23 Quarry Street
Princeton, NJ 08540
jafloyd@hotmail-**B**, (609) 924-6772-**H**
Ethnicity: African-American/Black
Degree and Year: PhD 1976
Major Field: Clinical Psychology
Specialty: Community Psychology;Administration;Institutionalization/
Deinstitutionalization;Clinical Psychology;Individual
Psychotherapy;Mental Health Services

FONG, Donald L.
390 Carmelita Place
Fremont, CA 94539-3605
(510) 438-9891-**H**
Ethnicity: Asian-American/Asian/Pacific Islander
Languages: Chinese
Degree and Year: MA
Major Field: School Psychology
Specialty: Personality Measurement;Learning Disabilities;Consulting
Psychology;Interpersonal Processes & Relations;Research
Design & Methodology

FONG, Geoffrey T.
University of Waterloo
Department of Psychology
Waterloo, Ontario, N2L3G1
CANADA
(519) 888-4567-**B**, (519) 886-4732-**H**, (519) 746-8631-**F**
Ethnicity: Asian-American/Asian/Pacific Islander
Degree and Year: PhD 1984
Major Field: Health Psychology
Specialty: Health Psychology;HIV/AIDS;Decision & Choice
Behavior;Social Cognition

FONG, Jane Y.
2026 Alturas Road
Atascadero, CA 93422-1102
(805)466-2972-**B**, (805) 466-2972-**H**, 805/462-2110-**F**
janefong@msn.com
Ethnicity: Asian-American/Asian/Pacific Islander
Degree and Year: PhD 1973 MA 1968
Major Field: Clinical Psychology
Specialty: Assessment/Diagnosis/Evaluation;Ethnic
Minorities;Cognitive Behavioral Therapy

FONG, Larry
Fong & Associates, Ltd.
Ste #850, 736 6th Ave Sw
Calgary, AB T2P3T-7
CANADA

(403) 233-7533-**B**, (403) 266-4998-**F**
lsfong@urb.net
Ethnicity: Asian-American/Asian/Pacific Islander
Degree and Year: PhD 1987
Major Field: Clinical Psychology
Specialty: Forensic Psychology;Clinical Psychology;Psychology &
    Law;Family Therapy;Industrial/Organizational Psychology

FOO, Koong H.
Nanyan Polytechnic
180 Ang Mo Kio, Avenue 8
Singapre 569830,
SINGAPORE
(650 550-1426-**B**, (650 763-2936-**H**, (65) 459-6811-**F**
foo_kong_hean@nyp.gov.sg
Ethnicity: Asian-American/Asian/Pacific Islander
Languages: Chinese
Degree and Year: MA 1987
Major Field: General Psy./Methods & Systems
Specialty: Child Development;Communication;Health
    Psychology;General Psychology

FOO, Rebecca E.
Switzer Center
1110 Sartori Avenue
Torrance, CA 90501
(310) 328-3611-**B**, (310) 375-3324-**H**, (310) 328-3611-**F**
ref@earthlink.net
Ethnicity: Asian-American/Asian/Pacific Islander
Degree and Year: PhD 1991
Major Field: Clinical Child Psychology
Specialty: Learning Disabilities;Special Education;Adolescent
    Therapy;Assessment/Diagnosis/
    Evaluation;Neuropsychology;Family Therapy

FORD, Deshay D.
Los Angeles County
Children Services
1213 Deodar Avenue
Oxnard, CA 93030
(310) 263-2155-**B**, (805) 487-3033-**H**, (310) 263-7734-**F**
Ethnicity: African-American/Black
Degree and Year: PhD 1998
Major Field: Clinical Psychology
Specialty: Alcoholism & Alcohol Abuse;Counseling
    Psychology;Conditioning, Operant & Classical;Child
    Abuse;Cross Cultural Processes;Behavior Therapy

FORD, Fatima Y
PO Box 11209
Oakland, CA 94611
fyford@aol.com
Ethnicity: African-American/Black
Degree and Year:
Major Field: Clinical Psychology

FORD, Leon I.
5630 Darlington Road
Pittsburgh, PA 15217
(412) 521-7135-**H**
Ethnicity: African-American/Black
Degree and Year: PhD 1956
Major Field: Clinical Psychology
Specialty: Assessment/Diagnosis/Evaluation;Clinical

Psychology;Hypnosis/Hypnotherapy;Individual
    Psychotherapy;Group Psychotherapy

FORRESTER, Bettye J.
1410 Villa Place
Nashville, TN 37212-3023
Ethnicity: African-American/Black
Degree and Year: MA 1961
Major Field: Developmental Psychology
Specialty: Preschool & Day Care Issues

FOSTER, JR., Hilliard G.
P.O. Box 174
West Simsbury, CT 06092-0174
Ethnicity: African-American/Black
Degree and Year: PhD 1978
Major Field: Physiological Psychology
Specialty: Electrophysical Psychology;Forensic Psychology

FOSTER, Daniel V.
P.O. Box 1439
Browning, MT 59417-1439
(406) 338-6146-**B**, (406) 338-7912-**H**
Ethnicity: American Indian/Alaska Native
Degree and Year: PsyD 1980
Major Field: Clinical Psychology
Specialty: Forensic Psychology;Clinical Neuropsychology

FOSTER, Evelyn L.
2465 Swallow Drive
Charleston, SC 29414
(803) 722-7605-**B**, (803) 763-0978-**H**
Ethnicity: African-American/Black
Degree and Year: PhD 1977
Major Field: Clinical Psychology
Specialty: Child Therapy;Adolescent Therapy;Crisis Intervention &
    Therapy;Family Therapy;Psychotherapy

FOSTER, Rachel A.
Central Michigan University
Department of Psychology
Mt. Pleasant, MI 48859
(517) 774-6475-**B**, (517) 773-5070-**H**
3ysrdc5@cmuvm.csv.cmich.edu
Ethnicity: American Indian/Alaska Native
Degree and Year: PhD 1989
Major Field: Social Psychology

FOSTER, Robert
2959 Schoolhouse Circle
Silver Spring, MD 20902-2561
(301) 649-8025-**B**, (301) 933-0008-**H**, (301) 649-8005-**F**
Ethnicity: African-American/Black
Degree and Year: PhD 1992
Major Field: School Psychology
Specialty: Developmental Psychology;Clinical Child
    Psychology;Counseling Psychology

FOSTER, RoseMarie P.
155 East 29th Street
New York, NY 10016
(212) 779-0341-**B**, (914) 241-0660-**H**
Ethnicity: Hispanic/Latino
Languages: Spanish
Degree and Year: PhD 1982
Major Field: Clinical Psychology

Specialty: Psychoanalysis;Individual Psychotherapy;Language
Process;Cross Cultural Processes;Personality Disorders

FOUAD, Nadya A.
University of Wisconsin @ Milwaukee
Department of Educational Psychology
729 Enderis Hall
Po Box 413
Milwaukee, WI 53201-0413
(414) 229-6830-**B**, (414) 332-0419-**H**, (414) 229-4939-**F**
nfouad@soe.uwm.edu
Ethnicity: Hispanic/Latino
Degree and Year: PhD 1984
Major Field: Counseling Psychology
Specialty: Counseling Psychology;Cultural & Social
Processes;Vocational Psychology;Assessment/Diagnosis/
Evaluation

FO, Walter S O
Practitioner
4220 Kahala Avenue
Honolulu, HI 96816-4822
(808) 735-9400-**B**, (808) 735-1316-**H**
Ethnicity: Asian-American/Asian/Pacific Islander
Degree and Year: PhD 1975
Major Field: Clinical Psychology
Specialty: Behavior Therapy;Health Psychology;Professional Issues in
Psychology;Cognitive Behavioral Therapy

FRANCISCO, Richard P.
266-B West Rincon Avenue
Campbell, CA 95008
(408) 924-5910-**B**
Ethnicity: African-American/Black
Languages: Spanish
Degree and Year: PhD 1976
Major Field: Counseling Psychology
Specialty: Assessment/Diagnosis/Evaluation;Counseling
Psychology;Industrial/Organizational Psychology;Cultural &
Social Processes;Forensic Psychology;Consulting Psychology

FRANCOIS, Theodore V.
507 Macon Street
Brooklyn, NY 11233
(718) 245-2580-**B**, (718) 452-0494-**H**
Ethnicity: African-American/Black
Degree and Year: PhD 1977
Major Field: Clinical Psychology
Specialty: Administration;Chronically Mentally Ill;Depression;Ethnic
Minorities;Psychoanalysis

FRASER, Kathryn P.
Halifax Medical Center
Family Practice Residency Program
303 North Clyde Norrise Boulevard
Box 2830
Daytona Beach, FL 32120-2830
(904) 254-4171-**B**, (904) 304-6779-**H**
Ethnicity: African-American/Black
Degree and Year: PhD 94
Major Field: Counseling Psychology
Specialty: Child Therapy

FREEMAN, Charlotte M.
Exchange Club Family Center
2180 Union Avenue

Memphis, TN 38104
(901) 276-2200-**B**, (901) 725-9355-**H**, (901) 276-6828-**F**
cmfreeman@aol.com
Ethnicity: African-American/Black
Degree and Year: PhD 1996
Major Field: Clinical Child Psychology
Specialty: Clinical Child Psychology;Cross Cultural Processes;Religious
Psychology;Behavior Therapy;Domestic Violence;School
Psychology

FREEMAN, James E.
Department of Pschology
University of Virginia
Granville, OH 43023
(614) 587-6673-**B**, (614) 587-2680-**H**
Ethnicity: African-American/Black
Degree and Year: PhD 1976
Major Field: Experimental Psychology
Specialty: Learning/Learning Theory;Conditioning, Operant &
Classical;Ethnic Minorities;Research Design &
Methodology;Statistics

FRESH, Edith M.
Morehouse School of Medicine
Department of Family Medicine
Biopsychosocial Medicine Division
505 Fairburn Road, SW
Atlanta, GA 30331
(404) 756-1246-**B**, (404) 691-5462-**H**, (404) 691-6435-**F**
freshe@msm.edu
Ethnicity: African-American/Black
Degree and Year: PhD 1993
Major Field: Clinical Psychology
Specialty: Cognitive Behavioral Therapy;Clinical Child
Psychology;Psychometrics;Child Therapy;Sex/Marital
Therapy;Family Therapy

FRIDAY, Jennifer C.
Centers for Disease Control
6785 Timbers East Drive
Lithonia, GA 30058
(404) 488-4646-**B**, (404) 482-6781-**H**, (404) 488-4338-**F**
jxf1@cdc.gov
Ethnicity: African-American/Black
Degree and Year: PhD 1983
Major Field: Community Psychology
Specialty: Health Psychology;Sexual Behavior;HIV/AIDS;Homicide

FRIED-CASSORLA, Martha J.
7408 Woodlawn Avenue
Melrose Park, PA 19126
(215) 576-8430-**B**, (215) 635-0461-**F**
Ethnicity: Hispanic/Latino
Languages: French
Degree and Year: PhD 1981
Major Field: Clinical Psychology
Specialty: Clinical Psychology;Death & Dying;Employee Assistance
Programs;Individual Psychotherapy;Marriage & Family

FRISBY, Craig L.
University of Missouri
Department of Educational and
Counseling Psychology
4H Hill Hall
Columbia, MO 65211
(573) 884-2561-**B**, 573/884-5989-**F**

edcoclt@showme.missouri.edu
Ethnicity: African-American/Black
Degree and Year: PhD 1987
Major Field: School Psychology

FRY, Prem S.
University of Victoria
Department of Psychology
Victoria, BC V8N3P-5
CANADA
Ethnicity: Asian-American/Asian/Pacific Islander
Degree and Year: PhD 1963
Major Field: Clinical Psychology

FUENTES, Dainery M.
Asilomar Psychological Services
Suite 450
Coral Gables, FL 33134-5224
(305) 441-2422-**B**, (305) 441-0814-**F**
Ethnicity: Hispanic/Latino
Languages: Spanish
Degree and Year: PhD 1982
Major Field: Clinical Psychology
Specialty: Administration;Chronically Mentally Ill;Forensic
Psychology;Hypnosis/Hypnotherapy

FUGITA, Stephen S.
University of Santa Clara
Department of Psychology
Santa Clara, CA 95053
(408) 554-6880-**B**, (408) 265-5241-**H**, (408) 554-6880-**F**
Ethnicity: Asian-American/Asian/Pacific Islander
Degree and Year: PhD 1969
Major Field: Social Psychology
Specialty: Cross Cultural Processes;Cultural & Social Processes;Ethnic
Minorities;Nonverbal Communication

FUHRMANN, Max E.
3027 E. Hillcrest Drive
Westlake Village, CA 91362
(805) 496-4442-**B**, (805) 373-6822-**F**
Ethnicity: Hispanic/Latino
Degree and Year: PhD 1988
Major Field: Gerontology
Specialty: Gerontology/Geropsychology;Cognitive Behavioral
Therapy;Alzheimer's Disease;Medical Psychology;Memory

FUJII, Daryl E M
Hawaii State Hospital
45-710 Keaahara Road
Kaneohe, HI 96744
(808) 236-8493-**B**, (808) 261-9061-**H**, (808) 247-7335-**F**
Ethnicity: Asian-American/Asian/Pacific Islander
Degree and Year: PhD 1991
Major Field: Clinical Psychology
Specialty: Neuropsychology;Brain Damage;Schizophrenia;Brain
Functions;Clinical Neuropsychology;Alzheimer's Disease

FUJIMURA, Laura E.
2745 Old Oak Lane
Springfield, OH 45503
(513) 225-5847-**B**, (513) 390-9425-**H**
Ethnicity: Asian-American/Asian/Pacific Islander
Degree and Year: PhD 1985

Major Field: Counseling Psychology
Specialty: Assessment/Diagnosis/Evaluation;Forensic Psychology

FUJINAKA, Larry H.
Leeward Community College
96-045 Ala Ike
Pearl City, HI 96782
(808) 455-0374-**B**, (808) 623-9514-**H**, (808) 455-0471-**F**
Ethnicity: Asian-American/Asian/Pacific Islander
Languages: Japanese
Degree and Year: PhD 1971
Major Field: unknown

FUJIOKA, Terry Ann T.
75-5744 Ali Drive
Suite #237
Kaliua-Kona, HI 96740
(808) 329-7050-**B**, (808) 329-1605-**H**
Ethnicity: Asian-American/Asian/Pacific Islander
Degree and Year: PhD 1986
Major Field: Clinical Psychology
Specialty: Adolescent Therapy;Child Therapy;Assessment/Diagnosis/
Evaluation;Psychotherapy;Psychopathology

FUJITA, George T.
2440 Campus Road
Honolulu, HI 96822
(808) 956-7927-**B**, (808) 988-7113-**H**
Ethnicity: Asian-American/Asian/Pacific Islander
Degree and Year: PhD 1961
Major Field: Educational Psychology
Specialty: Psychotherapy;Family Therapy;Family Processes;Marriage
& Family

FUJITSUBO, Lani C.
Southern Oregon University
1250 Siskiyou Building
Ashland, OR 97520
(541) 522-6940-**B**, (541) 552-6988-**F**
fujitsubo@sou.edu
Ethnicity: Asian-American/Asian/Pacific Islander
Degree and Year: PhD 1991
Major Field: Clinical Psychology
Specialty: Cognitive Behavioral Therapy;Individual
Psychotherapy;Psychotherapy;Curriculum Development/
Evaluation;Educational Psychology

FUKUYAMA, Mary A.
University of Florida
Counseling Center
301 Peabody Hall Po Box 114100
University Of Florida
Gainesville, FL 32611-2058
(352) 392-1575-**B**, (352) 371-9136-**H**, (904) 392-8452-**F**
fukuyama@counsel.ufl.edu
Ethnicity: Asian-American/Asian/Pacific Islander
Degree and Year: PhD 1981 MA 1977
Major Field: Counseling Psychology
Specialty: Counseling Psychology;Ethnic Minorities;Training &
Development;Cross Cultural Processes;Religious Psychology

FULLILOVE, Constance
180 N. Michigan
Suite #1130

Chicago, IL 60601
(312) 236-1498-**B**, (312) 288-2070-**H**
Ethnicity: African-American/Black
Degree and Year: PhD 1977
Major Field: Clinical Psychology
Specialty: Clinical Child Psychology;Family Therapy;Adolescent
        Therapy;Ethnic Minorities

FULTON, Aubyn
Pacific Union College
Behavioral Science Department
Angwin, CA 94508
(707) 965-6536-**B**, (707) 965-2991-**H**, (707) 965-6538-**F**
afulton@puc.edu
Ethnicity: African-American/Black
Degree and Year: PhD 1990
Major Field: Clinical Psychology
Specialty: Individual Psychotherapy;Family Therapy;Adolescent
        Development;Forensic Psychology

FULTON, Wayne M.
11516 Badger Colony Court
Wilton, CA 95693-9789
Ethnicity: African-American/Black
Degree and Year: PhD 1980
Major Field: unknown
Specialty: Medical Psychology

FUNABIKI, Dean
P.O. Box 214
Pullman, WA 99163-0214
Ethnicity: Asian-American/Asian/Pacific Islander
Degree and Year: PhD 1977
Major Field: Clinical Psychology

FUNG, Hellen C.
7625 111th Place SE
Renton, WA 90856
(206) 226-8569-**B**, (206) 271-7625-**H**, (206) 226-8569-**F**
Ethnicity: Asian-American/Asian/Pacific Islander
Languages: Chinese
Degree and Year: PhD 1988
Major Field: Clinical Psychology
Specialty: Psychotherapy;Ethnic Minorities;Cross Cultural
        Processes;Interpersonal Processes & Relations;Parent
        Education

FUNG, Samuel
1335 Sun Valley Road
Clarksville, TN 37040
Ethnicity: Asian-American/Asian/Pacific Islander
Degree and Year: PhD 1987
Major Field: Social Psychology

FURUKAWA, James M.
Towson State University
Psychology Department
Towson, MD 21204-7097
(410) 830-3074-**B**, (410) 821-1277-**H**
Ethnicity: Asian-American/Asian/Pacific Islander
Languages: Japanese
Degree and Year: PhD 1969
Major Field: Educational Psychology
Specialty: Special Education;Statistics

FURUNO, Setsu
1460 Kalanikai Place
Honolulu, HI 96821-1202
(808) 373-1424-**B**
Ethnicity: Asian-American/Asian/Pacific Islander
Degree and Year: PhD 1961
Major Field: unknown

GABORIT, Mauricio
Universidad Centroamericana
 Jose Simeon Canas
Apartado Postal (01) 168
San Salvador,
El Salvador
(503) 273-4400-**B**, (503) 2434-6898-**H**, (503) 273-1010-**F**
gaboritm@rdi.uca.edu.sv
Ethnicity: Hispanic/Latino
Languages: French, Italian, Spanish
Degree and Year: PhD 1984
Major Field: Social Psychology
Specialty: Social Cognition;Cross Cultural Processes;Social
        Psychology;Research Design & Methodology

GADSON, Eugene J.
613B Rose Hollow Drive
Yardley, PA 19067-6332
(609) 695-5378-**B**
Ethnicity: African-American/Black
Degree and Year: PsyD 1984
Major Field: School Psychology

GAINES, Stanley O.
Department of Psychology
Pomona College
550 North Harvest Avenue
Claremont, CA 91711
(909) 607-2441-**B**, (909) 624-1284-**H**, (909) 621-8623-**F**
sgaines@pomona.edu
Ethnicity: African-American/Black
Degree and Year: PhD 1991
Major Field: Social Psychology
Specialty: Social Psychology;Cultural & Social Processes;Gender
        Issues;Personality;Ethnic Minorities;Marriage & Family

GALAZ, Alfred
19801 Scenic Loop Road
Helotes, TX 78023-9213
Ethnicity: Hispanic/Latino
Degree and Year: PhD 1972
Major Field: Clinical Psychology
Specialty: Child Therapy

GALLAGHER, Rosina M.
6728 N Francisco
Chicago, IL 60645
(312) 534-8238-**B**, (312) 465-2711-**H**, (312) 534-8205-**F**
Ethnicity: Hispanic/Latino
Languages: French, Italian, Spanish
Degree and Year: PhD 1974
Major Field: Clinical Psychology
Specialty: Assessment/Diagnosis/Evaluation;Counseling
        Psychology;Giftedness;Ethnic Minorities;Parent Education

GALLARDO-COOPER, Maria M.
Circles of Care, Inc.
260 Pompano Drive

Melbourne Beach, FL 32951
(407) 984-5394-**B**, (407) 768-8047-**H**, (407) 676-6680-**F**
cooper@digital.net
Ethnicity: Hispanic/Latino
Languages: Spanish
Degree and Year: MA 1974 PhD 1997
Major Field: School Psychology
Specialty: Mental Health Services;Child Therapy;Assessment/
    Diagnosis/Evaluation;Marriage & Family;Social Skills

GALUE, Alberto I.
A222 Bowser Avenue
Unit A
Dallas, TX 75219-5909
(972) 718-6043-**B**, (214) 521-2441-**H**, (972) 718-4521-**F**
albertogalue@telops.gte.com
Ethnicity: Hispanic/Latino
Languages: French, Spanish
Degree and Year: PhD 1990
Major Field: Industrial/Organizational Psy.
Specialty: Industrial/Organizational Psychology;Management &
    Organization;Leadership

GAMEZ, George L.
Psychological Center for Treatment
    and Evaluation
6360 Wilshire Boulevard
Suite 305
Los Angeles, CA 90048-5601
(213) 655-8777-**B**
Ethnicity: Hispanic/Latino
Languages: Spanish
Degree and Year: PhD 1970
Major Field: Clinical Psychology
Specialty: Creativity;Psychology & the Arts;Cross Cultural
    Processes;Humanistic Psychology

GAM, John
1235 Sanders St
Auburn, AL 36830-2670
(334) 749-3385-**B**, (334) 887-3989-**H**
Ethnicity: Asian-American/Asian/Pacific Islander
Degree and Year: PhD 1980
Major Field: Clinical Psychology

GANT, Bob L.
The Glen Lakes Clinic, Inc.
9400 North Central #1305
Dallas, TX 75231
214/361-6092-**B**, 972/479-9092-**H**, 214/361-5429-**F**
drgrant@aol.com
Ethnicity: American Indian/Alaska Native
Languages: Russian
Degree and Year: PhD 1977
Major Field: Clinical Psychology
Specialty: Neuropsychology;Professional Issues in
    Psychology;Rehabilitation;Medical Psychology;Gerontology/
    Geropsychology;Communications/Journalism

GARCIA-ABID, Calixto
Florida International University
Counseling & Psychology Services Center
University park

Miami, Fl 33199
(305) 919-5808-**B**, (305) 866-9445-**H**, (305) 919-5211-**F**
garcia@fiu.gdu
Ethnicity: Hispanic/Latino
Languages: Spanish
Degree and Year: PhD 1990
Major Field: Clinical Psychology
Specialty: Clinical Psychology;Counseling
    Psychology;Biofeedback;Clinical Neuropsychology;Cultural &
    Social Processes;Cognitive Behavioral Therapy

GARCIA-COLL, Cynthia
Brown University
Department of Education
Box 1938
Providence, RI 02906
(401) 863-3147-**B**, 401 863-1276-**F**
cynthia garcia coll@brown.edu
Ethnicity: Hispanic/Latino
Languages: Spanish
Degree and Year: PhD 1981
Major Field: Developmental Psychology
Specialty: Developmental Psychology

GARCIA-GONZALEZ, Jose A.
Apartado Postal 6056
Caracas,   101-A 455,
Venezula
(212) 989-7513-**B**
Ethnicity: Hispanic/Latino
Degree and Year: PhD 1978
Major Field: Social Psychology

GARCIA-PELTONIEMI, Rosa E.
1730 Dayton Avenue
St. Paul, MN 55104-6108
612626-1400-**B**
Ethnicity: Hispanic/Latino
Degree and Year: PhD 1986
Major Field: Clinical Psychology

GARCIA-SHELTON, Linda M.
1607 Walnut Hts. Drive
East Landsing, MI 48823
(313) 762-8484-**B**, (517) 337-7844-**H**
Ethnicity: Hispanic/Latino
Languages: Spanish
Degree and Year: PhD 1979
Major Field: Counseling Psychology
Specialty: Health Psychology;Family Therapy;Clinical
    Psychology;Management & Organization;Ethnic Minorities

GARCIA, Agustin
IBM Tower
Suite 915
Munoz Rivera Avenue #645
Hato Rey, PR 00918
(809) 756-6230-**B**, (809) 760-8301-**H**
Ethnicity: Hispanic/Latino
Degree and Year: PhD
Major Field: Counseling Psychology

GARCIA, Betty
California State University, Fresno
671 W Ellery Ave
Clovis, CA 93612-5726

(209) 278-2550-**B**, (209) 278-7191-**F**
betty_garcia@csufresno.edu
Ethnicity: Hispanic/Latino
Languages: Spanish
Degree and Year: PhD 1985
Major Field: Social Psychology
Specialty: Child Abuse;Mental Health Services;Cross Cultural
       Processes;Ethnic Minorities;Social Psychology

GARCIA, Hector D.
1020 Alhambra Circle
Coral Gables, FL 33134-3528
(305) 377-7130-**B**, (305) 444-0524-**H**
Ethnicity: Hispanic/Latino
Languages: Spanish
Degree and Year: MS 1979
Major Field: Community Psychology

GARCIA, Jose L.
1091 NW 101st Street
Plantation, FL 33322-6505
(954) 677-6220-**B**, (954) 452-9280-**H**
jlg61!mediaone.net@shlgroup.cm
Ethnicity: Hispanic/Latino
Languages: Spanish
Degree and Year: PhD 1993
Major Field: Industrial/Organizational Psy.
Specialty: Organizational Development;Management &
       Organization;Industrial/Organizational Psychology;Human
       Resources;Training & Development

GARCIA, Lazaro
8720 SW 48th Street
Miami, FL 33165-5907
Ethnicity: Hispanic/Latino
Languages: Spanish
Degree and Year: PhD 1982
Major Field: Cognitive Psychology

GARCIA, Luis T.
Rutgers University
Department of Psychology
Camden, NJ 08102
Ethnicity: Hispanic/Latino
Degree and Year: PhD 1977
Major Field: Social Psychology
Specialty: Sexual Behavior

GARCIA, Margarita
24 Walnut Street
Rutherford, NJ 07070
(973) 655-7395-**B**, (201) 460-1390-**H**, (201) 804-0324-**F**
garciam@saturn.montclair.edu
Ethnicity: Hispanic/Latino
Languages: Spanish
Degree and Year: PhD 1972
Major Field: Experimental Psychology
Specialty: Brain Functions;Cross Cultural Processes;Ethnic Minorities

GARCIA, Melinda A.
2918 Mountain Road, NW
Albuquerque, NM 87104
(505) 247-3303-**B**, 505 764-0403-**H**
Ethnicity: Asian-American/Asian/Pacific Islander, Hispanic/Latino
Languages: Spanish
Degree and Year: PhD 1988 EdM 1908

Major Field: Clinical Psychology
Specialty: Community Mental Health

GARCIA, Michael A.
39 Brittle Lane
Hicksville, NY 11801-6122
(516) 935-6535-**B**
Ethnicity: Hispanic/Latino
Degree and Year: PhD 1979
Major Field: Clinical Psychology

GARCIA, Pedro I.
Centro Psicologico del Atenas
221 Pase Real Montejo
Manati, PR 00674-5710
(809) 884-5591-**B**, (787) 854-3475-**H**, (787) 884-5591-**F**
Ethnicity: Hispanic/Latino
Languages: Spanish
Degree and Year: PhD 1978
Major Field: Clinical Psychology
Specialty: Clinical Psychology;Human Relations;Affective
       Disorders;Ethnic Minorities;Military Psychology;Intelligence

GARCIA, Teresa
University of Texas at Austin
Department of Educational Psychology
SZB 504
Austin, TX 78712
(512) 471-4155-**B**, (512) 331-8962-**H**, (512) 471-1288-**F**
tgarcia@mail.utexas.edu
Ethnicity: Hispanic/Latino
Languages: Spanish
Degree and Year: PhD 1993
Major Field: Educational Psychology
Specialty: Motivation;Quantitative/Mathematical, Psychometrics;Social
       Cognition;Learning/Learning Theory;Survey Theory &
       Methodology;Personality

GARDANO, Anna C.
4450 South Park Avenue
314
Chevy Chase, MD 20815-3633
(301) 986-9489-**H**
Ethnicity: Hispanic/Latino
Languages: French, Spanish
Degree and Year: PhD 1988 MA 1976
Major Field: Clinical Psychology
Specialty: Family Therapy;Adolescent Therapy;Gender Issues;Child
       Therapy;Ethnic Minorities;Training & Development

GARDNER, Lamaurice H.
29845 Rambling Road
Southfield, MI 48076-5729
(313) 489-8860-**B**, (313) 569-3615-**H**
Ethnicity: African-American/Black
Degree and Year: PsyD 1988
Major Field: Clinical Psychology
Specialty: Clinical Neuropsychology;Clinical Psychology;Cognitive
       Behavioral Therapy;Child Therapy

GARG, Mithlesh
Tewksbury Hospital
Hathorne Mental Health Units
365 East Street

Tewsbury, MA 01876
(978) 851-7321-**B**, (617) 489-4281-**H**, (617) 489-3439-**F**
Ethnicity: Asian-American/Asian/Pacific Islander
Languages: Hindi
Degree and Year: PhD 1966
Major Field: Clinical Psychology
Specialty: Chronically Mentally Ill;Clinical Neuropsychology;Clinical Psychology;Assessment/Diagnosis/Evaluation

GARNER, Edward L.
5770 Christopher Street
San Bernardino, CA 92407-2282
(714) 387-7675-**B**
Ethnicity: African-American/Black
Degree and Year: PhD 1980
Major Field: Community Psychology
Specialty: Community Mental Health

GARNES, Delbert F.
Texas Southern University
9314 Riverside Lodge Drive
Houston, TX 77083
(713) 313-7344-**B**, (713) 561-8005-**H**
Ethnicity: African-American/Black
Languages: French
Degree and Year: PhD 1980
Major Field: Clinical Psychology
Specialty: Forensic Psychology;Juvenile Delinquency;Crisis Intervention & Therapy;Values & Moral Behavior;Cross Cultural Processes

GARRETT-AKINSANYA, BraVada
5507 Pipingwood Drive
Houston, TX 77084
(713) 221-8133-**B**, (713) 550-0573-**H**
Ethnicity: African-American/Black
Languages: French, Spanish
Degree and Year: PhD 1990
Major Field: Clinical Psychology
Specialty: Ethnic Minorities;Depression;Assessment/Diagnosis/Evaluation

GARRETT, Aline M.
University of Southwestern Louisiana
Psychology Department
P.O. Box 4-3131
Lafayette, LA 70504-3131
(318) 231-6597-**B**, (318) 856-8419-**H**, (318) 231-6195-**F**
Ethnicity: African-American/Black
Degree and Year: PhD 1971
Major Field: Developmental Psychology
Specialty: Child Development;Cultural & Social Processes;Adult Development;Ethnic Minorities

GARRIDO-CASTILLO, Pedro
19 Grovernor Road #3
Jamaica Plain, MA 02130-1784
(617) 498-1150-**B**, (617) 983-3730-**H**, (617) 421-5876-**F**
garrido@fas.harvard.edu
Ethnicity: Hispanic/Latino
Languages: Spanish
Degree and Year: PhD 1984
Major Field: Counseling Psychology
Specialty: Clinical Neuropsychology;Alcoholism & Alcohol Abuse;Cross Cultural Processes;Ethnic Minorities;Individual Psychotherapy

GARRIDO, Maria C.
Po Box 1576
Christiansted
St. Croix , VI, 00821-1576
(809) 773-7997-**B**, (809) 778-3573-**H**, (809) 773-4640-**F**
Ethnicity: Hispanic/Latino
Languages: Spanish
Degree and Year: MA 1976
Major Field: Clinical Psychology
Specialty: Measurement;Alcoholism & Alcohol Abuse;Psychotherapy;Drug Abuse;School Psychology;Assessment/Diagnosis/Evaluation

GARRIDO, Maria
839 North Main Street
Providence, RI 02904
(401) 272-2288-**B**, (401) 247-2373-**H**, (401) 861-6531-**F**
mgarrido@uriacc.uri.edu
Ethnicity: Hispanic/Latino
Languages: Spanish
Degree and Year: PsyD 1988
Major Field: Clinical Psychology
Specialty: Child Therapy;Cross Cultural Processes;Psychotherapy

GARRIGA-TRILLO, Ana J.
Rosalia De Castro 84, 6
Madrid   398 -,
SPAIN
(011) 34 - 398-**B**, (011) 34 - 373-**H**
Ethnicity: Hispanic/Latino
Degree and Year: PhD 1985
Major Field: unknown

GARY, Juneau M.
Kean University
49 Pine Grove Avenue
Somerset, NJ 08873
(708) 527-2523-**B**, (732) 846-3074-**H**, (732) 846-3074-**F**
juneaux@juno.com
Ethnicity: African-American/Black
Degree and Year: PsyD 1981
Major Field: Clinical Psychology
Specialty: Cross Cultural Processes;Eating Disorders;Ethnic Minorities;Individual Psychotherapy

GARZA, Alicia de la
Col Anahuac San Nicolas
J Manrique #221
Monterrey,
MEXICO
Ethnicity: Hispanic/Latino

Degree and Year: MA 1979
Major Field: unknown
Specialty: Psychometrics;Psychotherapy

GARZA, Joe G.
180 Rudi Lane, West
Golden, CO 80403
(303) 444-8070-**B**, (303) 642-0321-**H**, (303) 449-1883-**F**
Ethnicity: Hispanic/Latino
Languages: Spanish
Degree and Year: PhD 1981
Major Field: Clinical Psychology
Specialty: Child Abuse;Behavior Therapy;Clinical Psychology;Cross Cultural Processes;Cognitive Behavioral Therapy

GASQUOINE, Philip G.
South Texas Neuropsychology
329 Southern Court
Corpus Christi, TX 78404
(512) 854-9596-**B**, (512) 888-7999-**H**, (512) 854-1224-**F**
Ethnicity: Asian-American/Asian/Pacific Islander
Degree and Year: PhD 1983
Major Field: Neurosciences
Specialty: Neuropsychology;Clinical Neuropsychology;Cross Cultural Processes;Rehabilitation;Forensic Psychology;Pain & Pain Management

GAYLE, Michael C.
State University of New York
 at New Paltz
75 South Manheim Boulevard
Department of Psychology
New Paltz, NY 12561
(914) 257-3473-**B**, (914) 257-3474-**H**, (914) 257-3474-**F**
gaylem@npvm.newpaltz.edu
Ethnicity: African-American/Black
Degree and Year: PhD 1992
Major Field: Experimental Psychology
Specialty: Experimental Psychology;Emotion;Cognitive Psychology;Research Design & Methodology

GAYLES, Joyce M.
4331 Wigton
Houston, TX 77096-4428
(713) 667-6047-**B**, (713) 728-1680-**H**, (713) 667-1745-**F**
transworks@aol.com
Ethnicity: African-American/Black
Degree and Year: PhD 1983
Major Field: Clinical Psychology
Specialty: Psychotherapy;Sex/Marital Therapy;Affective Disorders;Lesbian & Gay Issuues;Stress;Job Satisfaction

GAY, Patricia L.
5138 Village Green
Los Angeles, CA 90016-5206
(213) 299-0314-**B**, (213) 294-4047-**H**, (213) 290-0516-**F**
patgay@pacbell.net
Ethnicity: African-American/Black
Degree and Year: PsyD 1994
Major Field: Health Psychology
Specialty: HIV/AIDS;Sexual Behavior;Cognitive Behavioral Therapy;Sex/Marital Therapy;Sexual Dysfunction;Death & Dying

GEE, Carol S.
Psychological & Behavioral Consultation
3799 South Green Road
Beechwood, OH 44122
(216) 831-6611-**B**, (216) 321-5518-**H**, (216) 831-2726-**F**
irsten@apk.net
Ethnicity: Asian-American/Asian/Pacific Islander
Languages: Chinese
Degree and Year: PhD 1987
Major Field: Clinical Psychology
Specialty: Cognitive Behavioral Therapy;Health Psychology;Family Therapy;Adolescent Therapy

GENERO, Nancy P.
Wellesley College
Department of Psychology
Welley, MA 02181
(617) 283-3281-**B**, (617) 283-3646-**F**
Ethnicity: Hispanic/Latino
Languages: Spanish
Degree and Year: PhD 1985
Major Field: Social Psychology
Specialty: Social Development;Social Cognition;Gender Issues;Cultural & Social Processes;Research Design & Methodology

GENHART, Michael J.
555 Pennsylvania Avenue
San Francisco, CA 94107-2913
Ethnicity: Hispanic/Latino
Degree and Year: PhD 1989
Major Field: Clinical Psychology
Specialty: Psychotherapy

GETER-DOUGLAS, Beth
Johns Hopkins University
School of Medicine - BPRU
5510 nathan Shock Drive
Baltimore, MD 20906
(410) 550-3706-**B**, (301) 871-0622-**H**, (410) 550-0030-**F**
bethgd@jhmi.edu
Ethnicity: African-American/Black
Degree and Year: PhD 1993
Major Field: Psychopharmacology
Specialty: Drug Abuse;Clinical Research;Psychopharmacology;Experimental Psychology;Conditioning, Operant & Classical;Neurosciences

GHALIB, Nadeem
House No. N A 213/D 7th Road
Satellite Town
Rawalpindi, 311
Rawalpindi, 311
PAKISTAN
(011) 0512713-**B**, (011) 0514292-**H**
Ethnicity: Asian-American/Asian/Pacific Islander
Languages: Urdu
Degree and Year: PhD 1994
Major Field: Clinical Psychology
Specialty: Clinical Psychology;Psychosomatic Disorders

GHASSEMZADEH, Habib
Roozbeh Hospital
Kargar Avenue
Tehran 13334 185
Tehran, 13334 185

IRAN
Ethnicity: Asian-American/Asian/Pacific Islander
Degree and Year: PhD 1976
Major Field: Developmental Psychology

GIBBONS-CARR, Michele V.
Phoenix Consultants
Four Skyline Drive
Wellesley, MA 02181
phnxmgc@aol.com
Ethnicity: African-American/Black
Degree and Year: PhD 1981
Major Field: Clinical Psychology
Specialty: Consulting Psychology;Industrial/Organizational
Psychology;Training & Development;Human
Relations;Management & Organization

GIBBS, Charles C.
710 NW 199th Avenue
Pembroke Pines, FL 33029-3349
(3050) 362-8326-**B**, (954) 437-2399-**H**
gibbs-i5@unforgettable.com
Ethnicity: African-American/Black
Degree and Year: PhD 1988
Major Field: Clinical Psychology
Specialty: Behavior Therapy;Cognitive Behavioral Therapy;Individual
Psychotherapy;Child Therapy;Stress

GIBBS, Jewelle Taylor
University of California
School of Social Welfare
120 Haviland Hall
Berkeley, CA 94720
(415) 643-6662-**B**
Ethnicity: African-American/Black
Degree and Year: PhD 1980
Major Field: Clinical Psychology
Specialty: Adolescent Therapy

GIBSON, Ralph M.
321 Riverview Drive
Ann Arbor, MI 48104-1847
Ethnicity: African-American/Black
Degree and Year: PhD 1959
Major Field: Clinical Psychology
Specialty: Neurological Disorders

GIBSON, Rose C.
321 Riverview Drive
Ann Arbor, MI 48104-1847
Ethnicity: African-American/Black
Degree and Year: PhD 1977
Major Field: unknown

GILES, Cheryl A.
134 Cliff Avenue
Winthrop, MA 02152-1008
(617) 846-6158-**B**
Ethnicity: African-American/Black
Degree and Year: PsyD 1990
Major Field: Clinical Psychology
Specialty: Child Abuse;Cross Cultural Processes;Child & Pediatric
Psychology;Adolescent Development;Individual
Psychotherapy;Pastoral Psychology

GILLEM, Angela R
Beaver College
450 South Easton Road
Glenside, PA 19038-3215
(215) 572-2184-**B**
Ethnicity: African-American/Black
Degree and Year: PhD 1984
Major Field: Clinical Psychology
Specialty: Ethnic Minorities;Feminist Therapy;Lesbian & Gay
Issuues;Psychology of Women;Individual Psychotherapy

GINORIO, Angela B.
NW Center for Research on Women
University of Washington
NWCROW Box 35-1380
Seattle, WA 98195-1380
(206) 543-9531-**B**, (206) 783-8120-**H**, (206) 685-4490-**F**
ginorio@u.washington.edu
Ethnicity: Hispanic/Latino
Languages: Spanish
Degree and Year: PhD 1979
Major Field: Social Psychology
Specialty: Psychology of Women;Cross Cultural Processes;Cultural &
Social Processes;Ethnic Minorities;Gender Issues;Educational
Research

GIRALDO, Macario
6826 Georgetown Pike
McLean, VA 22101-2147
Ethnicity: Hispanic/Latino
Degree and Year: PhD
Major Field: Clinical Psychology
Specialty: Group Psychotherapy

GIRONELLA, Oliva C.
15103 Rio Terrace Drive
Edmonton, Alberta, T5R5M-6
CANADA
(403) 454-0411-**B**, (403) 487-3419-**H**
Ethnicity: Asian-American/Asian/Pacific Islander
Languages: American Sign Language, Filipino, Spanish
Degree and Year: PhD 1959
Major Field: Counseling Psychology
Specialty: Adolescent Therapy;Alcoholism & Alcohol Abuse;Child
Therapy;Counseling Psychology;Family Therapy

GIST, Marilyn E.
University of Washington
School of Business Administration
Department of Management
and Organization, DJ-10
Seattle, WA 98195
(206) 685-4367-**B**, (206) 685-9392-**F**
Ethnicity: African-American/Black, American Indian/Alaska Native
Degree and Year: PhD 1985
Major Field: unknown
Specialty: Social Cognition;Training & Development;Individual
Difference;Cultural & Social Processes;Research Design &
Methodology

GLADUE, Brian A.
University of Cincinnatti
Institute Health Policy/HSR
ML-0840
Cincinnatti, OH 45267-0001

(513) 558-2753-**B**, (513) 558-2744-**F**
brian.gladue@uc.edu
Ethnicity: American Indian/Alaska Native
Languages: German, Italian, Spanish
Degree and Year: PhD 1979
Major Field: Physiological Psychology
Specialty: Sexual Physiology/Behavior;Aggression;Lesbian & Gay Issuues;Sexual Behavior;Hormones & Behavior;Gender Issues

GLORIA, Alberta M.
University of Wisconsin
Department of Counseling Psychology
321 Education Building
1000 Bascom Mall
Madison, WI 537061398
(608) 262-2669-**B**, (608) 265-3347-**F**
agloria@mail.soemadison.wisc.e
Ethnicity: Hispanic/Latino
Degree and Year: PhD 1993 MA 1989
Major Field: Counseling Psychology
Specialty: Counseling Psychology;Ethnic Minorities

GLOSTER, Janice L.
821 Filly Lane
Temple, TX 76504-4959
(713) 527-1827-**B**
Ethnicity: African-American/Black
Degree and Year: PhD 1980
Major Field: Clinical Psychology
Specialty: Correctional Psychology

GLOVER, O.S.
3150 Hilltop Mall Road
Richmond, CA 94806
(510) 233-8900-**B**, (707) 554-4130-**H**, (707) 554-4308-**F**
Ethnicity: African-American/Black
Degree and Year: PhD 1980
Major Field: Clinical Psychology
Specialty: Social Psychology

GOBURDHUN, Sara S.
1789 Long Lake Shores Drive
Bloomfield Hills, MI 48302-1232
(313) 559-8190-**B**
Ethnicity: Asian-American/Asian/Pacific Islander
Degree and Year: PhD 1987
Major Field: Clinical Psychology

GOCK, Terry S.
Asian Pacific Family Center
Pacific Clinics
9353 East Valley Boulevard
Rosemead, CA 91770-1934
(626) 287-2988-**B**, (323) 221-6411-**H**, (626) 287-1937-**F**
Ethnicity: Asian-American/Asian/Pacific Islander
Languages: Chinese
Degree and Year: PhD 1980 MPA 1990
Major Field: Clinical Psychology
Specialty: Ethnic Minorities;Forensic Psychology;HIV/AIDS;Management & Organization;Psychotherapy;Lesbian & Gay Issuues

GOEBES, Diane D.
6408J Seven Corners Place
Falls Church, VA 22044
(703) 532-6707-**B**, (703) 892-1924-**H**

Ethnicity: Hispanic/Latino
Languages: Spanish
Degree and Year: PhD 1977
Major Field: Clinical Psychology
Specialty: Affective Disorders;Assessment/Diagnosis/Evaluation;Individual Psychotherapy;Psychotherapy;Stress

GOFFIN, Richard D.
Northern Illinois University
Department of Psychology
Dekalb, IL 60115
(519) 679-2111-**B**
Ethnicity: American Indian/Alaska Native
Degree and Year: PhD 1987
Major Field: unknown

GOH, David S.
Queens College of the
City University of New York
Flushing, NY 11367
(718) 997-5230-**H**, (516) 883-4539-**F**
Goh@QCVAXA.EDU.
Ethnicity: Asian-American/Asian/Pacific Islander
Languages: Chinese
Degree and Year: PhD 1973
Major Field: School Psychology
Specialty: Assessment/Diagnosis/Evaluation;Behavior Therapy;Clinical Research;Ethnic Minorities;Psychopathology

GOLTZ, Sonia
University of Notre Dame
Department of Management
Notre Dame, IN 46556
(219) 631-5104-**B**, (219) 233-9378-**H**, (219) 631-5255-**F**
Ethnicity: Hispanic/Latino
Languages: Portuguese
Degree and Year: PhD 1987
Major Field: Industrial/Organizational Psy.
Specialty: Motivation

GOMEZ, JR., Francisco C.
San Diego State University
1120 Fort Stockton Drive
San Diego, CA 92103
1800 800-7759-**B**, (619) 299-3961-**H**, (619) 291-6921-**F**
Ethnicity: Hispanic/Latino
Languages: Spanish
Degree and Year: PhD 1994
Major Field: Clinical Psychology
Specialty: Alcoholism & Alcohol Abuse;Clinical Psychology;Forensic Psychology;Assessment/Diagnosis/Evaluation;Ethnic Minorities

GOMEZ, Ana L
University of Denver
Graduate School of Professional Psych.
2484 South Humboldt Street
Denver, CO 80210
(303) 455-8480-**B**, (303) 755-7950-**H**, (303) 369-5072-**F**
lola70@aol.com
Ethnicity: Hispanic/Latino
Languages: Spanish
Degree and Year: PsyD
Major Field: Clinical Child Psychology

GOMEZ, John P
 Department of Psychology
 411 S.W. 24th Street
 San Antonio TX 78207
 (734) 764-9397-**B**, (734) 677-8886-**H**, (734) 763-0044-**F**
 jgomez@umich.edu
 Ethnicity: Hispanic/Latino
 Degree and Year: PhD 1998 MA 1994
 Major Field: Clinical Psychology
 Specialty: Cultural & Social Processes;Personality Disorders;Ethnic
  Minorities;Measurement

GOMEZ, Madeleine Y.
 1207 Maple Avenue
 Evanston, IL 60202-1216
 (708) 864-4961-**B**
 Ethnicity: Hispanic/Latino
 Degree and Year: PhD 19
 Major Field: Clinical Psychology
 Specialty: Psychotherapy

GONG-GUY, Elizabeth
 1819 Mandeville Canyon Road
 Brentwood, CA 90049-2222
 (213) 476-0397-**B**
 Ethnicity: Asian-American/Asian/Pacific Islander
 Degree and Year: PhD 1985
 Major Field: Clinical Psychology

GONG, Susan M.
 Octagon Psychological Services
 PO box 12889
 Marina del Rey, CA 90295
 (310)823-1324-**B**, 310/823-1324-**F**
 drsgong@aol.com
 Ethnicity: Asian-American/Asian/Pacific Islander
 Degree and Year: PhD 1985
 Major Field: Clinical Psychology
 Specialty: Clinical Psychology;Clinical Child Psychology;Ethnic
  Minorities

GONSALVES, Carlos J.
 1497 Los Rios Drive
 San Jose, CA 95120
 (408) 236-5177-**B**, (408) 268-3432-**H**, (408) 236-5092-**F**
 Ethnicity: Hispanic/Latino
 Languages: Spanish
 Degree and Year: PhD 1979
 Major Field: Clinical Psychology
 Specialty: Cross Cultural Processes;Ethnic Minorities

GONZALES, Linda R.
 Portland VA Medical Center
 13133 Brookside Drive, NE
 Aurora, OR 97002
 (503) 220-8262-**B**
 Ethnicity: Hispanic/Latino
 Languages: Spanish
 Degree and Year: PhD 1984
 Major Field: Gerontology
 Specialty: Training & Development;Cognitive Behavioral
  Therapy;Consulting Psychology

GONZALES, Michael
 4010 Barranca Parkway
 Suite #252
 Irvine, CA 92714
 (714) 259-7160-**B**, (714) 733-1438-**F**
 Ethnicity: Hispanic/Latino
 Degree and Year: PhD 1981
 Major Field: Clinical Psychology
 Specialty: Sex/Marital Therapy;Alcoholism & Alcohol Abuse;Gender
  Issues;Cross Cultural Processes;Sexual Dysfunction

GONZALES, Ricardo R.
 3364 La Ave De San Marcos
 Santa Fe, NM 87505-9209
 (505)-988-9821-**B**, (505) 473-9885-**H**
 Ethnicity: Hispanic/Latino
 Languages: Spanish
 Degree and Year: PhD 1982
 Major Field: Clinical Psychology
 Specialty: Clinical Psychology;Ethnic Minorities;Medical
  Psychology;Drug Abuse;Alcoholism & Alcohol Abuse

GONZALEZ-FORESTIER, Tomas
 906 W Jefferson
 Knoxville, IA 50138-3015
 (515) 828-7092-**B**
 Ethnicity: Hispanic/Latino
 Degree and Year: PhD 1983
 Major Field: Clinical Psychology

GONZALEZ-HUSS, Mary
 8 Florence Pl
 Salinas, CA 93905-3318
 (408) 751-3459-**B**, (408) 422-9987-**H**
 Ethnicity: Hispanic/Latino
 Languages: Spanish
 Degree and Year: PhD 1984
 Major Field: Clinical Psychology
 Specialty: Adolescent Therapy;Child Therapy;Family
  Therapy;Assessment/Diagnosis/Evaluation;Training &
  Development

GONZALEZ-PABON, Jose F.
 University of Puerto Rico
 Department of Social Science
 Mayaguez Campus
 Mayaguez, PR 00681
 (809) 265-1209-**B**, (809) 254-2674-**H**
 Ethnicity: Hispanic/Latino
 Languages: Spanish
 Degree and Year: PhD 1971
 Major Field: Clinical Psychology
 Specialty: Psychotherapy;Individual
  Psychotherapy;Neuroses;Personality Disorders

GONZALEZ-SORENSEN, Anna G.
 4131 Spicewood Springs Road
 Suite #E-3
 Austin, TX 78759
 (512) 345-8195-**B**, (512) 452-6157-**H**, (512) 345-2102-**F**
 Ethnicity: Hispanic/Latino
 Languages: Spanish
 Degree and Year: PhD 1978

Major Field: Counseling Psychology
Specialty: Group Psychotherapy;Psychotherapy;Marriage & Family;Hypnosis/Hypnotherapy;Crisis Intervention & Therapy

GONZALEZ, Alexander
California State University
@ Fresno
5241 North Maple
Fresno, CA 93740-0054
(209) 278-2636-**B**, (209) 434-8042-**H**, (209) 278-7987-**F**
Ethnicity: Hispanic/Latino
Languages: Spanish
Degree and Year: PhD 1979
Major Field: Social Psychology

GONZALEZ, Fernando
Center of Excellence for
Research on Training
Morris Brown College
643 ML King Jr., Drive
Atlanta, GA 30314
(404) 220-0350-**B**, (404) 220-0339-**F**
Ethnicity: Hispanic/Latino
Languages: Spanish
Degree and Year: PhD 1973
Major Field: Cognitive Psychology
Specialty: Cognitive Psychology;Experimental Psychology

GONZALEZ, Gerardo M
California State University
Department of Psychology
San Marcos, CA 92069
(760) 750-4094-**B**, (760) 750-4030-**F**
ggonz@mailhost1.csusm.edu
Ethnicity: Hispanic/Latino
Languages: Spanish
Degree and Year: PhD 1989
Major Field: Clinical Psychology

GONZALEZ, Haydee M.
85 Columbia Terrace
Weehawken, NJ 07087
(427) 9003x3641-**B**, (201) 866-8848-**H**, (212) 427-7349-**F**
Ethnicity: Hispanic/Latino
Languages: French, Portuguese, Spanish
Degree and Year: PsyD 1986
Major Field: Clinical Psychology
Specialty: Forensic Psychology;Cultural & Social Processes;Mental Health Services;Labor & Management Relations;Homelessness & Homeless Populations

GONZALEZ, Hector P.
8600 SW 92nd Street
Suite #106
Miami, FL 33156-7377
(305) 274-7053-**B**
Ethnicity: Hispanic/Latino
Degree and Year: PhD 1978
Major Field: Clinical Psychology
Specialty: Psychotherapy

GONZALEZ, John
Lubbock I.S.D.
1628 19th Street
Lubbock, TX 79401
(806) 766-1761-**B**, (806) 745-0589-**H**
Ethnicity: Hispanic/Latino
Languages: Spanish
Degree and Year: EdD 1994
Major Field: Educational Psychology
Specialty: Counseling Psychology;Educational Psychology;General Psychology

GONZALEZ, Laura A.
Edif Bogoricin
1606 Ave Ponce De Leon
Ste 700
San Jaun, PR 00909-1827
(787) 721-6850-**B**, (787) 726-8819-**H**
Ethnicity: Hispanic/Latino
Degree and Year: MA 1981
Major Field: Clinical Psychology
Specialty: Psychotherapy

GONZALEZ, Maria L.
One Marineview Plaza
Hoboken, NJ 07030
(201) 420-6770-**B**
Ethnicity: Hispanic/Latino
Languages: Spanish
Degree and Year: PhD 1986
Major Field: Clinical Psychology
Specialty: Assessment/Diagnosis/Evaluation;Clinical Psychology;Cross Cultural Processes;Psychotherapy;Research & Training

GONZALEZ, Matthew B.
148 Fort Dearborn Street
Dearborn, MI 48124-1031
(313) 565-2660-**B**, 313 561-4852-**H**
Ethnicity: Hispanic/Latino
Languages: Spanish
Degree and Year: PsyD 1989
Major Field: Clinical Psychology
Specialty: Clinical Neuropsychology;Attention Deficit Disorders;Pain & Pain Management;Adolescent Therapy;Child Therapy

GONZALEZ, Max A.
Nogal Aven IL-32
Royal Palm
Bayamon, PR 00956
(809) 786-1313-**B**, (809) 780-5446-**H**
Ethnicity: Hispanic/Latino
Languages: Spanish
Degree and Year: PhD 1976
Major Field: Clinical Child Psychology
Specialty: Clinical Child Psychology;Mental Health Services;Child & Pediatric Psychology

GONZALEZ, Rocio R
Edelman Westside Mental Health Center
PO Box 65615
Los Angeles, CA 90065-0615
(323) 255-3494-**B**, (3230 255-3494-**H**
arevelta@juno.com
Ethnicity: Hispanic/Latino

Languages: Spanish
Degree and Year: PhD 1988
Major Field: Clinical Psychology

GORDON, Kimberly A.
805 Emerald Lane
Apartment D2
Carbondale, IL 62901-2429
(618) 536-2441-**B**, 618 457-1635-**H**, 618 453-4244-**F**
KAGORDON@SIU.EDU
Ethnicity: African-American/Black
Languages: French
Degree and Year: PhD 1993 ED.S 1990
Major Field: Developmental Psychology
Specialty: Adolescent Development;Cognitive Development;Ethnic
Minorities;Human Development & Family Studies;Preschool
& Day Care Issues

GORDON, LaFaune Y.
1525 Aviation Boulevard #389
Redondo Beach, CA 90278
(310) 281-7359-**B**, (310) 379-5610-**F**
lygflash@aol.com
Ethnicity: African-American/Black
Degree and Year: PhD 1993
Major Field: Clinical Child Psychology
Specialty: Assessment/Diagnosis/Evaluation;Child & Pediatric
Psychology;Ethnic Minorities;Child Development;Child
Therapy;Clinical Child Psychology

GORDON, Rhea J.
1130 Banbury Cross
Avondale Estates, GA 30002-1507
(404) 378-9444-**B**, (404) 299-7686-**H**, (404) 378-9499-**F**
Ethnicity: African-American/Black
Degree and Year: PhD 1989
Major Field: Clinical Psychology
Specialty: Child Abuse;Psychology of Women;Feminist
Therapy;Individual Psychotherapy;Gender Issues;Cross
Cultural Processes

GORDON, Ruth H.
301 East Riding Road
Montogmery, AL 36116-3741
(919) 334-7750-**B**, (919) 292-0912-**H**
Ethnicity: African-American/Black
Degree and Year: PhD 1974
Major Field: Counseling Psychology
Specialty: Community Mental Health;Curriculum Development/
Evaluation

GRABAU, David
10916 Gillette Avenue
Temple Terrace, FL 33627-3115
(813) 974-9319-**B**, (813) 985-3356-**H**
Ethnicity: Hispanic/Latino
Languages: Spanish
Degree and Year: PsyD 1985
Major Field: Clinical Psychology
Specialty: Depression;Individual Psychotherapy;Psychoanalysis

GRADDICK, Miriam M.
AT&T
233 Mount Airy Road

Room #1A07
Basking Ridge, NJ 07920
(908) 204-4242-**B**, (201) 292-2336-**H**, (908) 204-4115-**F**
Ethnicity: African-American/Black
Degree and Year: PhD 1981
Major Field: Industrial/Organizational Psy.
Specialty: Social Psychology

GRAHAM, Quentin
6929 Georgia Avenue, NW
Washington, DC 20012
(202) 726-6062-**B**, (202) 726-0032-**F**
Ethnicity: African-American/Black
Degree and Year: PhD 1984
Major Field: Clinical Psychology
Specialty: Individual Psychotherapy;School Psychology;Learning
Disabilities;Assessment/Diagnosis/Evaluation;Group Processes

GRAHAM, Sandra
University of California, Los Angeles
Department of Education
Los Angeles, CA 90095-1521
(310) 206-12-**B**, (213) 318-5234-**H**, (310) 206-6293-**F**
Ethnicity: African-American/Black
Degree and Year: PhD 1982
Major Field: Developmental Psychology
Specialty: Educational Psychology;Social Psychology;Social
Cognition;Aggression

GRAJALES, Elisa M.
The University of Iowa
University Counseling Service
330 Westlawn South
Iowa City, IA 52242-1100
(319) 335-7294-**B**, (319) 358-7754-**H**, (319) 335-7298-**F**
elisa-grajales@uiowa.edu
Ethnicity: Hispanic/Latino
Languages: Spanish
Degree and Year: PhD 1987
Major Field: Counseling Psychology
Specialty: Cognitive Behavioral Therapy;Individual
Psychotherapy;Cross Cultural Processes;Ethnic
Minorities;Feminist Therapy

GRANBERRY, Dorothy
1705 Beechwood Avenue
Nashville, TN 37212
(615) 963-5149-**B**, (615) 297-4836-**H**, (615) 963-5140-**F**
granberry@harpo.tnstate.edu
Ethnicity: African-American/Black
Degree and Year: PhD 1972
Major Field: Social Psychology
Specialty: Cultural & Social Processes;Ethnic
Minorities;Aggression;Performance Evaluation;Human
Resources

GRANT, Kim D.
530 Slane Trace
Roswell, GA 30076-4455
(303) 399-8020-**B**
Ethnicity: African-American/Black
Degree and Year: PhD 1983
Major Field: Clinical Psychology
Specialty: Chronically Mentally Ill;Clinical Psychology;Feminist
Therapy;Psychotherapy

GRANT, Swadesh S.
South Beach Psychiatric Center
120 Stuyvesant Place
Staten Island, NY 10301
(718) 727-6500-**B**, (212) 316-4262-**H**, (718) 720-2444-**F**
Ethnicity: Asian-American/Asian/Pacific Islander
Languages: Hindi
Degree and Year: PhD 1971
Major Field: Social Psychology
Specialty: Individual Psychotherapy;Forensic Psychology;Personality Disorders;Affective Disorders;Drug Abuse;Cultural & Social Processes

GRANT, Wanda F.
Institute for the Study of Child Development
Robert Wood Johnson Medical School
97 Paterson Street
New Brunswick, NJ 08903
(732) 235-7903-**B**, (782) 235-6189-**F**
grantwf@umdnj.edu
Ethnicity: African-American/Black
Languages: French
Degree and Year: PhD 1993
Major Field: Clinical Child Psychology
Specialty: Developmental Psychology;Neuropsychology

GRAVES-COOPER, Phyllis J.
Board of Education
New York City
516 West 181 Street
New York, NY 10033
(914) 278-9070-**H**
Ethnicity: African-American/Black
Languages: Spanish
Degree and Year: PhD 1991
Major Field: Clinical Psychology
Specialty: Adolescent Development;Assessment/Diagnosis/ Evaluation;Learning Disabilities;Clinical Child Psychology;School Psychology;Aggression

GRAVES, Kenneth J.
Huntsville Madison County MHC
660 Gallatin Street
Huntsville, AL 35801
(205) 533-1970-**B**
Ethnicity: African-American/Black
Degree and Year: PhD 1982
Major Field: Clinical Psychology

GRAVES, Sherryl B.
Hunter College
695 Park Avenue
New York, NY 10021-5024
(212) 772-4710-**B**, (203) 625-0948-**H**, (212) 650-3959-**F**
Ethnicity: African-American/Black
Languages: Spanish
Degree and Year: PhD 1975
Major Field: Clinical Psychology
Specialty: Mass Media Communication;Child Development;Ethnic Minorities;Educational Technology;Gender Issues

GRAY-LITTLE, Bernadette
Department of Psychology-258 Davie Hall
University of North Carolina
Chapel Hill, NC 27599-3270

(919) 962-3088-**B**, (919) 962-2537-**F**
bernadet@email.unc.edu
Ethnicity: African-American/Black
Degree and Year: PhD 1970
Major Field: Clinical Psychology
Specialty: Psychopathology;Ethnic Minorities;Psychotherapy;Persoanality & Experimental Psychopathology

GRAY, Arthur A.
8 Gramercy Park, South
Suite #2J
New York, NY 10003-1764
(212) 228-8434-**B**
Ethnicity: African-American/Black
Degree and Year: PhD 1979
Major Field: Clinical Psychology

GREEN, Charles A.
Detroit Board of Education
5035 Woodward
Detroit, MI 48202
(313) 494-2022-**B**, (313) 821-1311-**H**
Ethnicity: African-American/Black
Degree and Year: PhD 1974
Major Field: Clinical Psychology
Specialty: Clinical Psychology;Program Evaluation;Educational Research;Individual Psychotherapy

GREENE, Anthony F.
University of Florida
Box J-165 Health Sciences
Gainesville, FL 32602
Ethnicity: African-American/Black
Degree and Year: PhD 1988
Major Field: Health Psychology
Specialty: Psychosomatic Disorders

GREENE, Beverly
St. Johns University
Department of Psychology
26 St. Johns Place
Brooklyn, NY 11217
(718) 990-1538-**B**, (718) 638-6451-**H**, (718) 638-6451-**F**
bgreene203@aol.com
Ethnicity: African-American/Black
Degree and Year: PhD 1983
Major Field: Clinical Psychology
Specialty: Ethnic Minorities;Lesbian & Gay Issuues;Psychology of Women;Feminist Therapy;Individual Psychotherapy

GREENE, Clifford
329 Murray Ave
Englewood, NJ 07631-1418
(201) 648-5806-**B**, (201) 569-2332-**H**
Ethnicity: African-American/Black
Degree and Year: PhD 1984
Major Field: Clinical Psychology
Specialty: Cognitive Behavioral Therapy;Depression;Individual Psychotherapy;Psychotherapy;Ethnic Minorities

GREENE, Karen J.
215 West 88th Street
Suite 1B
New York, NY 10024

(212) 781-3967-**B**, (212) 781-9427-**F**
kjgreene@erols.com
Ethnicity: African-American/Black, European/White
Degree and Year: PhD 1988
Major Field: Clinical Psychology
Specialty: Clinical Psychology;Feminist Therapy;Psychology of
Women

GREENE, Lorraine
1900 Church Street
Suite 500
Nashville, TN 37203
(615) 862-7887-**B**, (615) 327-0329-**H**
lgreene@nashville.org
Ethnicity: African-American/Black
Degree and Year: PhD
Major Field: Clinical Psychology

GREEN, Theophilus E.
Psychological Solutions, P.C.
225 West Washington
Suite 2200
Chicago, IL 60606
(773) 262-3680-**B**, (773) 262-3601-**H**
73363.1577@compuserve.com
Ethnicity: African-American/Black
Languages: Portuguese, Spanish
Degree and Year: PsyD 1982
Major Field: Clinical Psychology
Specialty: Psychotherapy

GREGORY, Robert A.
1324 Santa Fe Drive
Encinitas, CA 92024-4009
(619) 453-4774-**B**
Ethnicity: American Indian/Alaska Native
Degree and Year: EdD 1974
Major Field: Industrial/Organizational Psy.

GRIER, Priscilla E.
Behavior Science Institute, Inc.
225 Meramex Avenue
411
St. Louis, MO 63105-3511
(314) 725-2667-**B**, (314) 725-2669-**F**
Ethnicity: African-American/Black
Degree and Year: PhD 1986
Major Field: Clinical Psychology
Specialty: Clinical Psychology;Deviant Behavior;Child Abuse;Cognitive
Behavioral Therapy;Ethnic Minorities

GRIFFIN, Patricia L.
18 Corporate Hill
Suite 205
Little Rock, AR 72205
(501) 223-8883-**B**, (501) 224-7832-**H**, (501) 227-6095-**F**
Ethnicity: African-American/Black
Degree and Year: PhD 1978
Major Field: Clinical Psychology
Specialty: Assessment/Diagnosis/Evaluation;Cognitive Behavioral
Therapy;Eating Disorders;Hospital Care;Marriage & Family

GRIFFITH, Albert R.
270 Everett Place
Englewood, NJ 07631
(973) 624-4315-**B**, (201) 568-7789-**H**, (973) 624-4315-**F**

arg.edd@worldnet.net
Ethnicity: African-American/Black
Degree and Year: EdD 1975
Major Field: Counseling Psychology
Specialty: Alcoholism & Alcohol Abuse;Cognitive Behavioral
Therapy;Assessment/Diagnosis/Evaluation;Employee
Assistance Programs;Drug Abuse

GRIFFITH, Marlin S.
6453 Westover Drive
Oakland, CA 94611-1605
(510) 287-5324-**B**, (510) 770-4452-**F**
Ethnicity: African-American/Black
Degree and Year: PhD 1975
Major Field: Clinical Psychology
Specialty: Clinical Psychology;Forensic Psychology;Employee
Assistance Programs;Individual Psychotherapy

GRIFFITH, Stanford
166-05 Highland Avenue, L1
Jamaica, NY 11432
(718) 297-2672-**B**, (718) 526-2521-**H**
Ethnicity: African-American/Black
Degree and Year: PhD 1983
Major Field: Clinical Psychology
Specialty: Family Therapy;Clinical Psychology;Case
Management;Ethnic Minorities;Individual Psychotherapy

GRIMES, Tresmaine R
South Carolina State University
300 College Street, NE
PO Box 7003
Orangeburg, SC 29117
(803) 536-8169-**B**, 803 534-9926-**H**, (803) 533-3714-**F**
tgrimes@scsu.scsu.edu
Ethnicity: African-American/Black
Degree and Year: PhD 1990
Major Field: Developmental Psychology
Specialty: Adolescent Development

GRINSTEAD, Olga A.
UCSF Center for AIDS Prevention Studies
Center for AIDS Prevention Study
74 New Montgomery Street #600
San Francisco, CA 94105
(415) 597-9168-**B**, (415) 597-9213-**F**
ogrinstead@psg.ucsf.edu
Ethnicity: African-American/Black
Degree and Year: PhD 1981
Major Field: Clinical Psychology
Specialty: HIV/AIDS;Research Design &
Methodology;Prevention;Program Evaluation

GROSSO, Federico C.
2020 Alameda Padre Serra #227
Santa Barbara, CA 93103-1756
(805) 962-3628-**B**
fcgt@concentric.net
Ethnicity: Hispanic/Latino
Languages: Portuguese, Spanish
Degree and Year: PhD 1992
Major Field: Clinical Psychology

GRUBB, Henry J.
Behavioral Consultants
103 Wilson Avenue

Johnson City, TN 37604
(423) 928-6500-**B**, (423) 928-3737-**H**, (423) 928-5659-**F**
rocdeisel@aol.com
Ethnicity: African-American/Black, American Indian/Alaska Native
Degree and Year: PhD 1986
Major Field: Clinical Psychology
Specialty: Child Abuse;Child & Pediatric Psychology;Clinical Child
    Psychology;Cognitive Behavioral Therapy;Cultural & Social
    Processes

GRUNHAUS-BELZER, Rosa
    3251 Third Ave
    San Diego, CA 92103-5615
    (619) 297-4355-**B**, (619) 481-6027-**H**, (619) 297-1422-**F**
Ethnicity: Hispanic/Latino
Languages: Spanish, Hebrew
Degree and Year: PhD 1984
Major Field: Clinical Psychology
Specialty: Assessment/Diagnosis/
    Evaluation;Psychotherapy;Depression;Training &
    Development;Ethnic Minorities

GRYCH, Diane S.
    208 North 2nd Street
    Princeton, WV 24740-3356
    (304) 384-6077-**B**, (304) 425-3444-**H**
Ethnicity: African-American/Black
Degree and Year: EdS 1979
Major Field: Developmental Psychology
Specialty: Infancy;Parent Education;Special Education;Mentally
    Retarded;Child Development

GUANIPA, Carmen L.
    San Diego State University
    College of Education
    5500 Campanile Drive
    San Diego, CA 92182
    (619) 594-7727-**B**, (619) 673-0809-**H**, (619) 594-7025-**F**
    guanipa@mail.sdsu.edu
Ethnicity: Hispanic/Latino
Languages: Spanish
Degree and Year: PhD 1992
Major Field: Clinical Psychology

GUBLER, Lyle W.
    232 Jackson Avenue
    Syosset, NY 11791-4208
Ethnicity: Hispanic/Latino
Degree and Year: PhD 1978
Major Field: School Psychology
Specialty: Counseling Psychology

GUERRA, Anna Maria
    Child Guidance Centers, Inc.
    2050 Youth Way
    Fullerton, CA 92635
    (7140) 871-9264-**B**, (6260 791-7572-**H**
Ethnicity: Hispanic/Latino
Languages: Spanish
Degree and Year: PhD 1992
Major Field: Clinical Psychology
Specialty: Clinical Child Psychology;Adolescent Therapy;Child Abuse

GUERRA, Julio J.
    4825 East First Street
    Long Beach, CA 90803

(714) 891-7301-**B**, (310) 439-3684-**H**, (310) 439-1514-**F**
Ethnicity: Hispanic/Latino
Languages: Spanish
Degree and Year: PhD 1970
Major Field: Clinical Psychology
Specialty: Adolescent Therapy;Behavior Therapy;Child
    Therapy;Clinical Psychology;Family Therapy

GUEVARRA, Josephine S.
    406 Bergen Street
    Brooklyn, NY 11217-2010
Ethnicity: African-American/Black
Degree and Year: PhD 1991
Major Field: Social Psychology
Specialty: Health Psychology;Personality Psychology;Social
    Psychology

GUI, Chui-Liu Serena
    Florida Hospital Family Practice
      Residency Program
    2501 North Orange Avenue
    Suite 235
    Orland, FL 32804
    (407) 897-1514-**B**, (407) 304-5665-**H**, (407) 897-1885-**F**
Ethnicity: Asian-American/Asian/Pacific Islander
Languages: Chinese
Degree and Year: PhD 1984
Major Field: Counseling Psychology
Specialty: Eating Disorders;Group Psychotherapy;Psychology of
    Women;Psychotherapy;Health Psychology;Domestic Violence

GUILLORY, Paul T.
    4315 Piedmont Avenue
    Oakland, CA 94611-4715
Ethnicity: African-American/Black
Degree and Year: PhD 1985
Major Field: Clinical Psychology
Specialty: Family Therapy;Psychotherapy

GULAR, Enrique
    State University of New York
    Health Science Center, Brooklyn
    450 Clarkson Avenue
    Box 1241
    Brooklyn, NY 11203-2098
    (212) 741-2522-**B**, (212) 741-2522-**H**
    egular@mindspring.com
Ethnicity: Hispanic/Latino
Languages: French, Spanish
Degree and Year: PhD 1995
Major Field: Clinical Psychology
Specialty: Clinical Psychology;HIV/AIDS;Parent-Child
    Interaction;Health Psychology;Mental Health
    Services;Preschool & Day Care Issues

GULLEY, Silas
    8005 Marsannay Way
    Sacramento, CA 95829
    (916) 732-9600-**B**
Ethnicity: African-American/Black
Degree and Year: PhD 1980
Major Field: Clinical Psychology
Specialty: Assessment/Diagnosis/Evaluation;Child Therapy;Crisis
    Intervention & Therapy;Forensic Psychology;Mental Health
    Services

GUMP, Janice P.
4545 42nd Street
Suite #304
Washington, DC 20016
(202) 966-2321-**B**, (301) 299-7564-**H**, (202) 363-1434-**F**
Ethnicity: African-American/Black
Degree and Year: PhD 1967
Major Field: Clinical Psychology
Specialty: Psychoanalysis;Individual Psychotherapy;Child
    Abuse;Cultural & Social Processes;Ethnic
    Minorities;Hypnosis/Hypnotherapy

GUNN, Robert L.
17252 Van Gogh
Granada Hills, CA 91344-1220
(818) 360-6725-**B**
Ethnicity: African-American/Black
Degree and Year: PhD 1956
Major Field: Industrial/Organizational Psy.

GUO, Trudy Narikiyo
Kapiolani Counseling Center
1319 Punahou Street
Honolulu, HI 96826
(808) 983-8368-**B**
trudyg@kapiolani.org
Ethnicity: Asian-American/Asian/Pacific Islander
Degree and Year: PhD 1991
Major Field: Clinical Psychology
Specialty: Ethnic Minorities;Cognitive Behavioral Therapy;Affective
    Disorders;Domestic Violence;Sex/Marital Therapy;Eating
    Disorders

GURRI GLASS, Margarita E.
8415 Bellona Lane
Suite #214
Towson, MD 21204
(410) 337-0193-**B**, (410) 337-0290-**F**
Ethnicity: Hispanic/Latino
Languages: American Sign Language, Spanish
Degree and Year: PhD 1983
Major Field: Clinical Psychology
Specialty: Psychotherapy;Child Abuse;Sex/Marital Therapy;Sleep
    Disorders;Hypnosis/Hypnotherapy

GUTIERREZ, Manuel J.
OMG Center for Collaborative Learning
1528 Walnut Street
Suite 805
Philadelphia, PA 19102
(215) 732-2200-**B**, (215) 732-8132-**F**
omgmanual@aol.com
Ethnicity: Hispanic/Latino
Languages: Spanish
Degree and Year: PhD 1975
Major Field: Clinical Psychology
Specialty: Program Evaluation;Community Psychology;Ethnic
    Minorities;Family Therapy;Cross Cultural Processes

GUTTERMAN, Carmen Y.
6209 St Johns Ave
Edina, MN 55424-1855
(612) 832-2509-**B**, (612) 560-6994-**H**
Ethnicity: Asian-American/Asian/Pacific Islander
Languages: Spanish

Degree and Year: PhD 19
Major Field: Clinical Child Psychology
Specialty: Clinical Child Psychology;Clinical Child
    Neuropsychology;Psychopathology;Family Therapy;Behavior
    Therapy

GUZMAN, L. Philip
Child Counseling Center
Of Greater Bridgeport
1081 Iranistan Avenue
Bridgeport, CT 06604
(203) 367-5361-**B**, 203 795-6221-**H**, 203 339-452-**F**
Ethnicity: Hispanic/Latino
Languages: Spanish
Degree and Year: PhD 1976
Major Field: Clinical Psychology
Specialty: Clinical Child Psychology;Cross Cultural Processes;Mental
    Health Services;Community Mental Health;Ethnic Minorities

GUZMAN, Milagros
304-B Domenech Avenue
Hato Rey, PR 00918
(809) 764-5145-**B**, (809) 720-4966-**H**, (809) 763-8754-**F**
Ethnicity: Hispanic/Latino
Languages: Spanish
Degree and Year: MA 1963
Major Field: Industrial/Organizational Psy.
Specialty: Industrial/Organizational Psychology;Research &
    Training;Cross Cultural Processes;Interpersonal Processes &
    Relations;Organizational Development

HADDOCK, Dean M.
Community Counseling and
  Psychological Services
4800 Easton Drive
Suite #109
Bakersfield, CA 93309
(805) 326-8167-**B**, (805) 326-8221-**F**
dhaddock@netxn.com
Ethnicity: American Indian/Alaska Native
Degree and Year: PsyD 1982
Major Field: Clinical Psychology
Specialty: Administration;Neuropsychology;Marriage & Family;Child
    Abuse;Attention Deficit Disorders

HAGGINS, Kristee L.
UC Davis Counseling Center
219 North Hill
One Shields Avenue
Davis, CA 95616
(530) 752-0871-**B**, (916) 689-0889-**H**, (530) 752-9923-**F**
klhaggins@uscadavis.edu
Ethnicity: African-American/Black
Degree and Year: PhD 1994
Major Field: Counseling Psychology
Specialty: Counseling Psychology;Ethnic Minorities;Vocational
    Psychology;Cross Cultural Processes;Training & Development

HALEY, Adriana R.
Five Wakeman Road
South Salem, NY 10598
(914) 533-5198-**B**, (914) 533-5049-**H**, (914) 533-5538-**F**
ahaley@bestweb.net

Ethnicity: Hispanic/Latino
Languages: Italian, Spanish
Degree and Year: PhD 1993
Major Field: Counseling Psychology
Specialty: Assessment/Diagnosis/Evaluation;Stress;Mentally Retarded;Industrial/Organizational Psychology;Parent-Child Interaction

HALL, Christine I.
Glendale Community College
Senior Associate Dean of Instruction
6000 West Olive Avenue
Glendale, AZ 85302
(602) 435-3877-**B**
hall@gc.maricopa.edu
Ethnicity: Asian-American/Asian/Pacific Islander
Degree and Year: PhD 1980 MA 1975
Major Field: Social Psychology
Specialty: Ethnic Minorities;Gender Issues;Social Psychology;Psychotherapy;Training & Development

HALL, Howard
Rainbow Babies and Children's Hospital
Division of Behavioral Pediatrics
11100 Euclid Avenue
Cleveland, OH 44106-6038
(216) 844-3230-**B**, (216) 991-6737-**H**, (216) 844-7601-**F**
hrh@po.curu.edu
Ethnicity: African-American/Black
Degree and Year: PsyD 1982 PhD 1978
Major Field: Clinical Psychology
Specialty: Health Psychology;Pain & Pain Management;Hypnosis/ Hypnotherapy

HALL, Juanita L.
1640 E. 50th Street
Suite #7B
Chicago, IL 60615
(312) 535-0807-**B**, (312) 324-2286-**H**
Ethnicity: African-American/Black
Degree and Year: PhD 1974
Major Field: General Psy./Methods & Systems
Specialty: Clinical Psychology;Family Therapy;Individual Psychotherapy;Marriage & Family;Physically Handicapped

HALL, M. Elizabeth L.
A Child's Point of View
3186 Old Tunnel Road
Lafayette, CA 94549
(925) 988-9456-**B**, (510) 988-9456-**H**, (925) 847-5537-**F**
beth@ninestones.com
Ethnicity: Hispanic/Latino
Languages: Spanish
Degree and Year: EdD
Major Field: Clinical Psychology

HALL, Ruth L.
The College of New Jersey
Department of Psychology
PO Box 7718
Ewing, NJ 08628-0718
(609) 771-2643-**B**, (215) 925-4794-**H**, (609) 637-5178-**F**
ruthhall@voicenet.com
Ethnicity: African-American/Black

Degree and Year: M.Ed 1996 PhD 1979
Major Field: Clinical Psychology
Specialty: Ethnic Minorities;Gender Issues;Cultural & Social Processes;Affective Disorders

HALL, William A.
1008 W Nolcrest
Silver Springs, MD 20903
(301) 681-8219-**H**
Ethnicity: African-American/Black
Degree and Year: EdD 1981
Major Field: unknown
Specialty: Psychotherapy

HAMADA, Roger S.
Kapi'olani Medical Specialists
1319 Punahou Street, 6th Floor
Honolulu, HI 96826
(808) 983-8368-**B**, (808) 672-4865-**H**, (808) 983-8629-**F**
rogerh@kapiolani.org
Ethnicity: Asian-American/Asian/Pacific Islander
Degree and Year: PhD 1987
Major Field: Clinical Child Psychology
Specialty: Child & Pediatric Psychology;Behavior Therapy;Crisis Intervention & Therapy;Death & Dying

HAMBRICK-DIXON, Priscilla J.
1002 King Street
Chappaqua, NY 10514-3906
(212) 960-8204-**B**
Ethnicity: African-American/Black
Degree and Year: PhD 1976
Major Field: Developmental Psychology

HAMBRIGHT, Jerold E.
Lakeside Village, Unit #21
RFD 2 Box 7290
Winthrop, ME 04364
(207) 621-2625-**B**, (207) 395-4754-**H**
Ethnicity: African-American/Black
Degree and Year: PhD 1988
Major Field: Counseling Psychology
Specialty: Counseling Psychology

HAMDANI-RAAB, Asma J.
20778 Silverthistle Court
Ashburn, VA 22011-4426
(212) 420-1981-**B**
ajhamdani@aol.com
Ethnicity: Asian-American/Asian/Pacific Islander
Languages: Urdu
Degree and Year: PhD 1974
Major Field: Counseling Psychology
Specialty: Religious Psychology;Personality Disorders;Rational-Emotive Therapy;Marriage & Family

HAMER, Forrest M.
5305 College Ave
Oakland, CA 94618-1416
(510) 652-2150-**B**, (510) 601-6334-**H**
Ethnicity: African-American/Black
Degree and Year: PhD 1987
Major Field: Clinical Psychology
Specialty: Assessment/Diagnosis/ Evaluation;Psychoanalysis;Psychotherapy

HAMID, Mohammad
Elgin Mental Health Center
750 S State Street
Elgin, IL 60123-7612
(708) 742-1040-**B**, (708) 742-7124-**H**, (708) 742-7726-**F**
Ethnicity: Asian-American/Asian/Pacific Islander
Languages: Hindi, Urdu
Degree and Year: PhD 1973
Major Field: Clinical Psychology
Specialty: Behavior Therapy;Biofeedback;Cross Cultural
    Processes;Hypnosis/Hypnotherapy;Mental Health Services

HAM, MaryAnna D.
University of Massachusetts at Boston
54 Bridge Street
Lexington, MA 02421
(617) 287-7617-**B**, (781) 861-9803-**H**, (617) 287-7664-**F**
ham@umbsky.cc.umb.edu
Ethnicity: Asian-American/Asian/Pacific Islander
Degree and Year: PhD 1980
Major Field: Counseling Psychology
Specialty: Counseling Psychology;Cross Cultural Processes;Family
    Processes;Cross Cultural Processes;Family Therapy;Marriage
    & Family

HAMMOND, Evelyn S.
7320 Mopac
Suite #402
Austin, TX 78731
(512) 346-5251-**B**, (512) 454-6420-**H**
Ethnicity: Hispanic/Latino
Languages: Spanish
Degree and Year: PhD 1976
Major Field: Educational Psychology
Specialty: Psychotherapy;Clinical Psychology;Individual
    Psychotherapy

HAMMOND, Gladys
6192 Oxon Hill Road
Suite 506
Fort Washington, MD 20744-5403
(301) 292-0550-**B**, (301) 292-2868-**H**
Ethnicity: African-American/Black
Degree and Year: EdD
Major Field: Counseling Psychology
Specialty: Adolescent Therapy;Child Therapy;Hypnosis/
    Hypnotherapy;Assessment/Diagnosis/Evaluation;Ethnic
    Minorities

HAMMOND, W. Rodney
Center for Disease Control
Division of Violence Prevention
Mail Stop K-60
1600 Clifton Road NE
Atlanta, GA 30333
(770) 488-4362-**B**, (770) 248-9820-**H**, 770 488-4349-**F**
rih2@cdc.gov
Ethnicity: African-American/Black
Degree and Year: PhD 1974
Major Field: School Psychology
Specialty: Applied Behavior Analysis;Health Psychology;Mentally
    Retarded;Professional Issues in Psychology;Social Skills

HAMPTON, Juanita R.
8948 S Oglesby Ave
Chicago, IL 60617-3047
(312) 535-3800-**B**, (312) 221-3421-**H**
Ethnicity: African-American/Black
Degree and Year: MA 1969
Major Field: School Psychology
Specialty: School Psychology;Educational Psychology

HANLEY, Jerome H.
13 Fairleaf Court
Columbia, SC 29212
(803) 734-7859-**B**, (803) 781-9025-**H**, (803) 734-7848-**F**
Ethnicity: African-American/Black
Degree and Year: PhD 1977 MSR 1975
Major Field: Clinical Child Psychology
Specialty: Clinical Child Psychology;Community Mental Health;Ethnic
    Minorities;Mental Health Services

HAN, Yu Ling
University of Maryland @ Baltimore
Department of Psychiatry
645 West Redwood Street
Baltimore, MD 21201-1549
(401) 396-0032-**B**, 301 495-2646-**H**, 410 328-1749-**F**
yham@umpsy.ab.umd.edu
Ethnicity: Asian-American/Asian/Pacific Islander
Languages: French, Dutch, Indonesian
Degree and Year: PhD 1995 MA 1990
Major Field: Clinical Psychology
Specialty: Adolescent Therapy;Death & Dying;Ethnic Minorities;Cross
    Cultural Processes;Interpersonal Processes & Relations

HAO, Judy Y.
13950 Milton Avenue #303
Westminster, CA 92683
(714) 906-1969-**B**, (213) 724-5484-**H**, (213) 724-5484-**F**
jyhao@aol.com
Ethnicity: Asian-American/Asian/Pacific Islander
Degree and Year: PhD 1994
Major Field: Clinical Psychology
Specialty: Chronically Mentally Ill;Community Mental
    Health;Schizophrenia;Gerontology/
    Geropsychology;Depression;Psychotherapy

HARDIN, JR., Oscar A.
8647 South Forest Drive
Tempe, AZ 85284-2379
(602) 435-3733-**B**, (602) 831-5992-**H**
docoz@starlink.com
Ethnicity: African-American/Black
Degree and Year: PhD 1977
Major Field: Counseling Psychology
Specialty: Juvenile Delinquency

HARE, Nathan
503 Plaza Drive
Vestal, NY 13850-3670
(607) 797-1652-**B**, (607) 754-4670-**H**
Ethnicity: African-American/Black
Degree and Year: PhD 1975
Major Field: Clinical Psychology

HARGROVE, JR., Jerry E.
206 New York Ave., NW
Washington, DC 20001-1232

(202) 806-7908-**B**, (202) 638-3214-**H**, (202) 638-3213-**F**
hunemancr@aol.com
Ethnicity: African-American/Black, American Indian/Alaska Native
Languages: American Sign Language
Degree and Year: PhD 1997
Major Field: Counseling Psychology
Specialty: Pastoral Psychology;Cross Cultural Processes;Individual
 Psychotherapy;Counseling Psychology;Ethnic Minorities;Sex/
 Marital Therapy

HARGROW, Mary E.
 1016 S Keniston Avenue
 Los Angeles, CA 90019-1707
 (323) 857-0691-**B**, (323) 857-0691-**F**
Ethnicity: African-American/Black, Asian-American/Asian/Pacific
Islander
Degree and Year: PhD 1985
Major Field: Counseling Psychology
Specialty: Clinical Psychology;Psychotherapy;Child Abuse;Adolescent
 Therapy;Affective Disorders;Ethnic Minorities

HARLESTON, Bernard W.
 University of Massachusetts
 @ Boston
 Graduate College of Education
 Boston, MA 02125
 (617) 287-7601-**B**, (617) 287-7664-**F**
Ethnicity: African-American/Black
Languages: French
Degree and Year: PhD 1955
Major Field: Experimental Psychology
Specialty: Creativity;Motivation;Problem Solving;Disadvantaged

HARPER, Frederick
 3564 S George Mason Drive
 Alexandria, VA 22302-1034
 (703) 998-6948-**B**
Ethnicity: African-American/Black
Degree and Year: PhD 19
Major Field: Counseling Psychology

HARPER, Mary S.
 1362 Greysstone Drive
 Tuscaloosa, AL 35406-3222
 (205) 758-1561-**B**, (205) 758-1561-**H**
Ethnicity: African-American/Black
Languages: French
Degree and Year: PhD 1963
Major Field: Clinical Psychology
Specialty: Clinical Psychology;Gerontology/Geropsychology

HARPER, Renuka R.
 Little and Harper
 18 Lavinia Avenue
 Greenville, SC 29601
 (864) 233-3277-**B**, 9864) 244-2006-**H**, (864) 233-3706-**F**
 Rrharper@aol.com
Ethnicity: Asian-American/Asian/Pacific Islander
Degree and Year: PhD 1992
Major Field: Clinical Psychology
Specialty: Clinical Psychology;Eating Disorders;Assessment/Diagnosis/
 Evaluation;Health Psychology;Affective Disorders

HARRELL, Shelly P.
 Graduate School of Education
  and Psychology

Pepperdine University Plaza
400 Corporate Pointe
Culver City, CA 90230
(310) 568-5755-**B**, (310) 568-5600-**H**, (626) 284-0550-**F**
sharrell@pepperdine.edu
Ethnicity: African-American/Black
Degree and Year: PhD 1988 BA 1982
Major Field: Clinical Psychology
Specialty: Community Psychology;Health Psychology;Stress;Program
 Evaluation;Cultural & Social Processes;Psychotherapy

HARRIS, Jasper W.
 11945 Pennsylvania Avenue
 Kansas City, MO 64145
 (816) 224-1300-**B**, (816) 942-4825-**H**, (816) 224-1310-**F**
Ethnicity: African-American/Black
Degree and Year: PhD/ 1981
Major Field: Developmental Psychology
Specialty: Special Education

HARRIS, Josette G.
 University of Colorado
 School of Medicine
 Dept. of Psychiatry -Box C268-71
 4200 East Ninth Avenue
 Denver, CO 80262
 303 315-4610-**B**, 303 315-5347-**F**
 josette.harris@uchsc.edu
Ethnicity: Hispanic/Latino
Degree and Year: PhD 1992
Major Field: Neurosciences
Specialty: Neuropsychology;Schizophrenia;Clinical Neuropsychology

HARRIS, Michelle F.
 2460 Fairmount Blvd, Ste 207
 Cleveland Hgts, OH 44106-3125
 (216) 229-1333-**B**
Ethnicity: African-American/Black
Degree and Year: PhD 1986
Major Field: Clinical Psychology
Specialty: Psychotherapy

HARRIS, Shanette M.
 University of Rhode Island
 19 Indian Trail
 Wakefield, RI 02879
 (401)874-4591-**B**, 401/789-7200-**H**, (401) 874-2157-**F**
 sharris@arc.uri.edu
Ethnicity: African-American/Black
Degree and Year: PhD 1989
Major Field: Clinical Psychology
Specialty: Ethnic Minorities;Health Psychology;Behavior
 Therapy;Gender Issues;Cross Cultural Processes;Clinical
 Psychology

HARRIS, William W.
 20 Yaun Avenue
 Liberty, NY 12754
 (914)292-1235-**B**, (914) 292-8839-**H**, (914) 292-8839-**F**
Ethnicity: Asian-American/Asian/Pacific Islander
Degree and Year: MA 1947
Major Field: Clinical Psychology
Specialty: Clinical Psychology; Counseling Psychology

HARRIS, William G.
9701 Ridgemore Drive
Charlotte, NC 28277-2310
Ethnicity: African-American/Black
Degree and Year: PhD 1980
Major Field: Clinical Psychology
Specialty: Computer Applications and Programming;Psychometrics

HART, Allen J.
Department of Psychology
329 Merrill Science Center
Amherst, MA 01002
(413) 542-2791-**B**, (410) 542-2145-**F**
ajhart@amherst.edu
Ethnicity: African-American/Black
Degree and Year: PhD 1991
Major Field: Social Psychology
Specialty: Interpersonal Processes & Relations;Social
Behavior;Psychology & Law;Nonverbal Communication

HARTANTO, Frans
Jalan Bosscha 29
Bandung, 184
INDONESIA
(011) 62227083-**B**, (011) 6222349-**H**
fhar@ibm.net
Ethnicity: Asian-American/Asian/Pacific Islander
Degree and Year: PhD 1986
Major Field: Industrial/Organizational Psy.

HART, Anton H.
235 West End Avenue
Apartment #2E
New York, NY 10023
(212) 595-3704-**B**
Ethnicity: African-American/Black, American Indian/Alaska Native
Degree and Year: PhD 1989
Major Field: Clinical Psychology
Specialty: Psychoanalysis;Individual Psychotherapy;Family
Therapy;Child Therapy;Adolescent Therapy

HARTE, Lisa M.
Yonkers Public School
Five Tudor City Place
#1411
New York, NY 10017-6872
(212) 856-9585-**H**, (212) 856-9885-**F**
Ethnicity: African-American/Black
Degree and Year: PhD 1996
Major Field: School Psychology
Specialty: Aggression;Emotion;Crisis Intervention & Therapy;Cognitive
Development;Ethnic Minorities;Special Education

HARTKA, Elizabeth
American Institutes for Research
P.O. Box 1113
Palo Alto, CA 94302
(415) 493-3550-**B**, (415) 359-5776-**H**, (415) 858-0958-**F**
Ethnicity: Asian-American/Asian/Pacific Islander
Degree and Year: PhD 1989
Major Field: Quan/Math & Psychometrics/Stat
Specialty: Alcoholism & Alcohol Abuse;Educational
Research;Measurement;Psychometrics;Research Design &
Methodology

HARTZELL, Richard E.
1608 Earlham Avenue
Crofton, MD 21114
(410) 721-7625-**B**, (410) 721-5206-**H**
Ethnicity: American Indian/Alaska Native
Degree and Year: EdD 1970
Major Field: Counseling Psychology
Specialty: Cognitive Behavioral Therapy;Stress;Depression;Health
Psychology;Human Relations

HASHIMOTO, Jerry S.
Cherry Creek School District
Smoky Hill High School
16100 East Smoky Hill Road
Aurora, CO 80015
(303) 693-1700-**B**
Ethnicity: Asian-American/Asian/Pacific Islander
Degree and Year: PsyD 1986
Major Field: Clinical Child Psychology
Specialty: Clinical Child Psychology;Child Development;Adolescent
Therapy;Cultural & Social Processes;Child Therapy;Special
Education

HASS, Giselle A
American School of
Professional Psychology
1400 Wilson Boulevard
Suite 110
Arlington, VA 22209
(703) 243-5300-**B**, 703 691-8973-**H**, 703 243-8973-**F**
Ethnicity: Hispanic/Latino
Languages: Spanish
Degree and Year: Psy 1992
Major Field: Clinical Psychology

HASS, Giselle A.
American School of Professional
Psychology
1400 Wilson Boulevard
Suite 110
Arlington, VA 22209
703/243-5300-**B**, 703/444-5808-**H**, 703/243-8973-**F**
ghass@erols. com
Ethnicity: Asian-American/Asian/Pacific Islander
Languages: Spanish
Degree and Year: PsyD 1992
Major Field: Clinical Psychology
Specialty: Domestic Violence;Policy Analysis

HATSUKAMI, Dorothy K.
2250 Lee Avenue North
Golden Valley, MN 55422-3637
Ethnicity: Asian-American/Asian/Pacific Islander
Degree and Year: PhD 1980
Major Field: Clinical Psychology
Specialty: Psychopharmacology

HAWKINS, Ioma L.
25550 Hawthorne Blvd.
Suite #212
Torrance, CA 90505
(310) 903-6000-**B**, (213) 321-6290-**H**
Ethnicity: African-American/Black
Degree and Year: PhD 1979

Major Field: Clinical Psychology
Specialty: Attribution Theory;Cognitive Behavioral Therapy;Crisis
    Intervention & Therapy;Ethnic Minorities;Marriage & Family

HAWKINS, James Leon
    Bank of America
    333 S Beaudry Avenue
    #Box-6
    Los Angeles, CA 90017-1466
Ethnicity: African-American/Black
Degree and Year: MA 1931
Major Field: Counseling Psychology

HAYES, Forrest L.
    13761 Arne Erickson Circle
    Anchorage, AK 99515-3953
Ethnicity: American Indian/Alaska Native
Degree and Year: PhD 1979
Major Field: Counseling Psychology
Specialty: School Counseling

HAYLES, V. Robert
    1449 Colleen Avenue
    Arden Hills, MN 55112
    (651) 628-9332-**B**, (651) 633-5578-**H**, (651) 628-9067-**F**
Ethnicity: African-American/Black
Degree and Year: PhD 1974
Major Field: Social Psychology
Specialty: Training & Development;Organizational
    Development;Industrial/Organizational Psychology

HEALY, James M.
    P.O. Box 1816
    Tallahassee, FL 32302-1816
Ethnicity: Hispanic/Latino
Degree and Year: PhD 1979
Major Field: Counseling Psychology
Specialty: Psychotherapy

HEARN, Kathleen E.
    7624 S Painter
    Suite #C
    Whittier, CA 90602
    (310) 636-7993-**B**, (310) 694-3598-**H**
Ethnicity: Hispanic/Latino
Languages: Spanish
Degree and Year: PhD 1985
Major Field: Clinical Psychology
Specialty: Clinical Psychology;Chronically Mentally Ill;Ethnic
    Minorities;Individual Psychotherapy

HELLER, Beatriz
    3636 Fourth Avenue
    Suite #304
    San Diego, CA 92103
    (619) 294-4200-**B**, (619) 692-1968-**H**, (619) 294-6606-**F**
Ethnicity: Hispanic/Latino
Languages: Spanish
Degree and Year: PhD 1979
Major Field: Clinical Psychology
Specialty: Forensic Psychology;Cognitive Behavioral
    Therapy;Domestic Violence;Family Therapy;Pain & Pain
    Management

HENDERSON DANIEL, Jessica
    Judge Baker Children's Center/
    Children's Hospital
    Three Blackfan Circle
    Boston, MA 02115
    (617) 232-8390-**B**, (617) 738-5420-**H**, (617) 232-8399-**F**
    DANIEL_J@A1.TCH.HARVARD.EDU
Ethnicity: African-American/Black
Degree and Year: PhD 1969
Major Field: Educational Psychology
Specialty: Adult Development;Prevention;Parent-Child
    Interaction;Religious Psychology;Ethnic
    Minorities;Psychology of Women

HENDERSON, Brenda A.
    7958 South Michigan Avenue
    Chicago, IL 60619-3509
    (312) 791-4443-**B**
Ethnicity: African-American/Black
Degree and Year: PhD 1992
Major Field: Clinical Child Psychology
Specialty: Child Abuse;Child & Pediatric Psychology;Parent-Child
    Interaction;Child Development;Infancy;Clinical Child
    Neuropsychology

HENRY, Rolando R.
    Vanderbilt University
    Department of Psychology
    324 Wilson Hall
    Nashville, TN 37240
    (615) 322-0054-**B**, (615) 343-8449-**H**, (615) 343-8449-**F**
Ethnicity: African-American/Black
Degree and Year: PhD 1977
Major Field: Physiological Psychology
Specialty: Clinical Neuropsychology;Neuropsychology;HIV/AIDS

HENRY, Vincent dePaul
    Vincent dePaul Henry, PsyD
    901 Old Matlton Pike W.
    Marlton, NJ 08053
    (609) 983-3891-**B**
Ethnicity: African-American/Black
Languages: Latin
Degree and Year: PsyD 1981
Major Field: Clinical Psychology
Specialty: Clinical Psychology;Hypnosis/Hypnotherapy;Projective
    Techniques;Pastoral Psychology

HENSON, Ramon M.
    Merck and Company, Inc.
    One Whitehouse Drive
    Whitehouse Station, NJ 08502
    (908) 904-1561-**B**, (908) 423-4704-**H**, (908) 423-1516-**F**
    ramon_henson@merck.com
Ethnicity: Asian-American/Asian/Pacific Islander
Languages: Filipino, Spanish
Degree and Year: PhD 1973
Major Field: Industrial/Organizational Psy.
Specialty: Industrial/Organizational Psychology;Job
    Satisfaction;Management & Organization;Organizational
    Development

HERAS, Patricia
    637 Third Avenue #F
    Chula Vista, CA 91910

(619) 425-9312-**B**
pheras@aol.com
Ethnicity: Asian-American/Asian/Pacific Islander
Languages: Filipino, Spanish, Tagalog
Degree and Year: PhD 1985
Major Field: Clinical Psychology
Specialty: Cross Cultural Processes;Depression;Child Abuse;Ethnic
Minorities

HERMENET, Argelia B.
37 Westernview Street
Springfield, MA 01108-1615
(413) 737-7013-**B**
Ethnicity: Hispanic/Latino
Degree and Year: EdD 1970
Major Field: unknown

HERNANDEZ, Cibeles
Western Miami Psychological Services
8370 W Flagler Street
Suite #234
Miami, FL 33144
(305) 553-2723-**B**, (305) 867-1810-**H**, (305) 553-0010-**F**
Ethnicity: Hispanic/Latino
Languages: Spanish
Degree and Year: PhD 1982
Major Field: Clinical Psychology
Specialty: Affective Disorders;Death & Dying;Feminist
Therapy;Clinical Psychology;Depression;Individual
Psychotherapy

HERNANDEZ, Maria G.
2454 Cameron Drive
Union City, CA 94587
(510) 487-2776-**B**, (510) 487-4172-**F**
mariah1052@aol.com
Ethnicity: Hispanic/Latino
Languages: Spanish
Degree and Year: PhD 1985
Major Field: Community Psychology
Specialty: Community Mental Health;Cross Cultural Processes;Policy
Analysis;Human Resources;Consulting Psychology

HERNANDEZ, Michael
7100 N. High St.
Suite 201
Worthington, OH 43085
(614) 888-4752-**B**, (614) 888-1014-**F**
Ethnicity: African-American/Black
Degree and Year: PhD 1984
Major Field: Clinical Psychology

HERNANDEZ, Vivian O.
2115 North Anthony Boulevard
Fort Wayne, IN 46805-4539
(219) 481-2888-**B**, (219) 483-0606-**H**
Ethnicity: Hispanic/Latino
Languages: Spanish
Degree and Year: PhD 1981
Major Field: Counseling Psychology
Specialty: Counseling Psychology;Depression;Feminist Therapy;Ethnic
Minorities;Managed Care

HERRANS, Laura L.
ICPE de P.R., Inc.
Urb. HNAS. Davila, CalleK - #97

Bayaman, PR 00959
(809) 785-2455-**B**, (809) 785-2455-**F**
Ethnicity: Hispanic/Latino
Languages: Spanish
Degree and Year: PhD 1969
Major Field: Educational Psychology
Specialty: Assessment/Diagnosis/Evaluation;Intelligence;Projective
Techniques;Measurement;Quantitative/Mathematical,
Psychometrics

HERRERA-PINO, Jorge A.
Neurobehavioral Institute of Miami
238 Palermo Ave
Coral Gables, FL 33134-6606
(305) 445-3222-**B**, (305) 856-8233-**H**, (3050 448-7539-**F**
nim@icanect.net
Ethnicity: Hispanic/Latino
Languages: French, Spanish
Degree and Year: PhD 1979 MD 1997
Major Field: Clinical Psychology
Specialty: Learning Disabilities;Neurological
Disorders;Neuropsychology

HESTICK, Henrietta
Morgan State University
1700 East Cold Spring Lane
Baltimore, MD 21239
(410) 319-3061-**B**, (410) 655-3068-**H**, (410) 319-3914-**F**
hhestick@moac.morgan.edu
Ethnicity: African-American/Black
Degree and Year: PhD 1992
Major Field: Developmental Psychology
Specialty: Clinical Research;Ethnic Minorities;Attention Deficit
Disorders;Developmental Psychology;Measurement;Parent
Education

HEVIA, Modesto J.
Florida Hospital
Center for Behavioral Health
400 Celebration Place A250
Celebration, FL 34747
(407) 303-4040-**B**, (407) 259-9710-**H**
modesto_hevia_@flmis.nct
Ethnicity: Hispanic/Latino
Degree and Year: PsyD 1988
Major Field: Clinical Psychology
Specialty: Psychotherapy

HICKS, Laurabeth
13611 Ector Drive
Baker, LA 70714-4659
Ethnicity: African-American/Black
Degree and Year: PhD 1968
Major Field: Counseling Psychology

HICKS, Leslie H.
Howard University
Psychology Department
Washington, DC 20059
(202) 806-6805-**B**, (202) 806-4873-**F**
Ethnicity: African-American/Black
Degree and Year: PhD 1954
Major Field: Physiological Psychology
Specialty: Brain Functions;Brain
Damage;Memory;Neuropsychology;General Psychology

HIGASHI, Wilfred H.
4527 S 2300, East
Suite #104
Salt Lake City, UT 84117
(801) 277-8025-**B**, (801) 278-0644-**H**
Ethnicity: Asian-American/Asian/Pacific Islander
Languages: Japanese, Spanish
Degree and Year: PhD 1958
Major Field: Clinical Psychology
Specialty: Clinical Child Psychology;Alcoholism & Alcohol
Abuse;Health Psychology;Mental Health Services;Pain & Pain
Management

HIGA, William R.
415 Huali Place
Hilo, HI 96720
(808) 961-3318-**B**, (808) 969-7951-**H**
Ethnicity: Asian-American/Asian/Pacific Islander
Degree and Year: PhD 1973
Major Field: Clinical Psychology
Specialty: Behavior Therapy;Cognitive Behavioral Therapy;Individual
Psychotherapy

HIGHTOWER, Eugene
4167 24th St, #1
San Francisco, CA 94114-3645
(510) 881-3484-**B**, (415) 282-4176-**H**, (510) 727-2035-**F**
Ethnicity: African-American/Black, American Indian/Alaska Native
Degree and Year: PhD 1981
Major Field: Clinical Psychology
Specialty: Research & Training;Adult Development;Clinical
Psychology;Developmental Psychology

HILL, JR., Sam S.
Texas A&M Univerity, Corpus Christi
6300 Ocean Drive
Corpus Christi, TX 78412
(512) 985-6670-**B**, (512) 814-8617-**H**, (512) 994-6098-**F**
shill@ciris.net
Ethnicity: Hispanic/Latino
Languages: Spanish
Degree and Year: PsyD 1992
Major Field: Clinical Child Psychology
Specialty: Child & Pediatric Psychology;Ethnic Minorities;Medical
Psychology;Clinical Child Psychology;Health
Psychology;Psychotherapy

HILLABRANT, Walter J.
1927 38th Street, NW
Washington, DC 20007
(301) 587-9006-**B**, (202) 338-6519-**H**, (301) 587-9007-**F**
Ethnicity: American Indian/Alaska Native
Languages: Spanish
Degree and Year: PhD 1972
Major Field: Social Psychology
Specialty: Attitudes & Opinions;Cross Cultural Processes;Group
Processes;Nonverbal Communication;Research Design &
Methodology

HILL, Anthony L
US General Accounting Office
Federal Management Issues
441 G Street, NW

Washington, DC 20548
(202) 512-9604-**B**, 301 963-4152-**H**
Ethnicity: African-American/Black
Degree and Year: PhD 1977
Major Field: Educational Psychology
Specialty: Counseling Psychology

HILTON, William F.
NYC Board of Education - D.A.A.
21 Saint James Pl, #9-k
Brooklyn, NY 11205-5024
(718) 935-5609-**B**, (718) 857-7597-**H**, (718) 935-5490-**F**
Ethnicity: African-American/Black
Degree and Year: PhD 1988
Major Field: Environmental Psychology
Specialty: Program Evaluation;Educational Research;Health
Psychology;Environmental Psychology;Statistics;Stress

HINES, Laura M.
156-20 Riverside Drive, West
Apartment #13A
New York, NY 10032
(718) 430-3850-**B**, (212) 928-2317-**H**
Ethnicity: African-American/Black
Degree and Year: PhD 1978
Major Field: School Psychology
Specialty: Assessment/Diagnosis/Evaluation;Child Therapy;Ethnic
Minorities;Giftedness;Disadvantaged

HINES, Paulette M.
2 Woodgate Drive
Monmouth Jct., NJ 08852
(908) 463-4136-**B**, (908) 297-5493-**H**, (908) 463-5134-**F**
Ethnicity: African-American/Black
Degree and Year: PhD 1978
Major Field: Clinical Psychology
Specialty: Prevention;Family Therapy;Cross Cultural
Processes;Community Mental Health;Parent Education

HIROTO, Donald S.
11980 San Vicente Blvd.
Suite #707
Los Angeles, CA 90049-6605
(213) 820-5120-**B**
Ethnicity: Asian-American/Asian/Pacific Islander
Degree and Year: PhD 1972
Major Field: Clinical Psychology

HO, Chin-Chin
1820 St. Charles Avenue
Suite #211
New Orleans, LA 70130-5248
(504) 525-5070-**B**, (504) 866-0239-**H**, (504) 525-5070-**F**
Ethnicity: Asian-American/Asian/Pacific Islander
Degree and Year: PhD 1976
Major Field: Clinical Psychology
Specialty: Psychotherapy

HO, Christine K.
2910 E Madison St.
Suite #304
Seattle, WA 98112-4214
(206) 329-6414-**B**, (206) 524-7273-**H**, (206) 860-2411-**F**
ckho@uwashington.edu
Ethnicity: Asian-American/Asian/Pacific Islander

Languages: Chinese
Degree and Year: PhD 1985
Major Field: Clinical Psychology
Specialty: Domestic Violence;Death & Dying

HOFER, Ricardo
1070 Via Alta
Lafayette, CA 94549-2916
(510) 283-3949-**B**, (510) 283-3226-**H**, (510) 283-8132-**F**
Ethnicity: Hispanic/Latino
Languages: Italian, Portuguese, Spanish
Degree and Year: PhD 1968
Major Field: Clinical Psychology
Specialty: Assessment/Diagnosis/Evaluation;Clinical
 Psychology;Forensic Psychology;Projective
 Techniques;Psychotherapy

HOJAT, Mohammadr
Jefferson Medical College
Residency in Medical Education and
 Health Care
1025 Walnut Street
Philadelphia, PA 19107-5001
(215) 955-8907-**B**, (215) 677-7634-**H**
hojatm@jeflin.tju.edu
Ethnicity: Asian-American/Asian/Pacific Islander
Degree and Year: PhD 1981
Major Field: unknown
Specialty: Personality Measurement

HO, John E.
525 Washington Street
Westfield, NJ 07090
(908) 232-8860-**B**
Ethnicity: Asian-American/Asian/Pacific Islander
Languages: Chinese
Degree and Year: PhD 1972
Major Field: Clinical Psychology
Specialty: Clinical Psychology;Clinical Child Psychology;Child
 Abuse;Ethnic Minorities;Cross Cultural Processes

HO, Kay
Coastal A/P Mental Health Services
14112 South Kinsley Drive
Gardena, LA 90249
(310) 217-7312-**B**, (310) 377-3097-**H**, (310) 377-3097-**F**
ckkho@aolcom
Ethnicity: Asian-American/Asian/Pacific Islander
Languages: Chinese
Degree and Year: PhD 1983
Major Field: Cognitive Psychology
Specialty: Clinical Psychology;Cognitive Behavioral Therapy;Affective
 Disorders;Child Therapy;Alzheimer's Disease;Religious
 Psychology

HOLLIDAY, Bertha G.
1719 First St., NW
Washington, DC 20001
(202) 336-6029-**B**, (202) 265-8308-**H**, (202) 336-6040-**F**
bholliday@apa.org
Ethnicity: African-American/Black
Degree and Year: PhD 1978
Major Field: Community Psychology

Specialty: Policy Analysis;Ethnic Minorities;Program
 Evaluation;Mental Health Services;Human Development &
 Family Studies

HOLMES, Dorothy E.
4601 Connectivut Avenue, NW
Suite #20
Washington, DC 20008-5700
(202) 966-7437-**B**, (202) 966-7437-**H**, (202) 966-7437-**F**
holmesdo@erols.com
Ethnicity: African-American/Black
Degree and Year: PhD 1968
Major Field: Clinical Psychology
Specialty: Psychotherapy

HOLSEY, Chandra V.
8348 Traford Lane
Suite #201
Springfield, VA 22152
(703) 912-7421-**B**
Ethnicity: African-American/Black
Degree and Year: PhD 1979
Major Field: Clinical Psychology
Specialty: Child Abuse;Attention Deficit Disorders;Individual
 Psychotherapy;Parent-Child Interaction

HOM, Harry L.
SW Missouri State University
Department of Psychology
Springfield, MO 65804
(417) 836-4790-**B**, (417) 864-5364-**H**, (417) 836-4884-**F**
HarryHom@mail.smsu.edu
Ethnicity: Asian-American/Asian/Pacific Islander
Degree and Year: PhD 1972
Major Field: Experimental Psychology
Specialty: Motivation;Developmental Psychology;Sports Psychology

HOM, Jim
6347 Danbury Lane
Dallas, TX 75214
(214) 688-3353-**B**, (214) 696-1931-**H**, (214) 688-2450-**F**
jhom@neuropsych.com
Ethnicity: Asian-American/Asian/Pacific Islander
Languages: Chinese
Degree and Year: PhD 1981
Major Field: Physiological Psychology
Specialty: Alzheimer's Disease;Brain
 Damage;Neuropsychology;Neurological Disorders

HONG, Barry A.
Washington University
School of Medicine
4940 Childrens Place
St. Louis, MO 63110
(314) 256-8796-**B**, (314) 362-4270-**H**
Ethnicity: Asian-American/Asian/Pacific Islander
Degree and Year: PhD 1978
Major Field: Health Psychology
Specialty: Medical Psychology;HIV/AIDS

HONG, Eunsook
University of Nevada
@ Las Vegas
Counseling & Educational Psych.
PO Box 453003

Las Vegas, NV 89154-3003
(702) 895-3246-**B**, (702) 897-2851-**H**
Ethnicity: Asian-American/Asian/Pacific Islander
Languages: Korean
Degree and Year: PhD 1990
Major Field: Educational Psychology
Specialty: Cognitive Psychology;Educational
Psychology;Creativity;Giftedness;Educational Research

HONG, George K.
California State University @ Los Angeles
Division of Administration & Counseling
5151 State University Drive
Los Angeles, CA 90032
(323) 343-4378-**B**, (323) 343-4253-**F**
ghong@calstatela.edu
Ethnicity: Asian-American/Asian/Pacific Islander
Languages: Chinese, Cantonese
Degree and Year: PhD 1982
Major Field: Clinical Psychology
Specialty: Clinical Psychology;Ethnic Minorities;School
Psychology;Child Therapy;Family Therapy;Research &
Training

HOOKER, Olivia J.
Fred S. Keller School of Behavior Analysis
42 Juniper Hill
White Plains, NY 10607-2104
(718) 817-3797-**B**, (914) 949-2981-**H**, (718) 817-3785-**F**
Ethnicity: African-American/Black
Languages: Spanish
Degree and Year: PhD 1962
Major Field: Clinical Psychology
Specialty: Clinical Psychology;Parent-Child Interaction;Clinical Child
Psychology;Preschool & Day Care Issues;Forensic
Psychology

HOPKINS, Kenneth
NIA Psychological Association,Inc.
Nia Psychol Assoc Inc
245 W Chelten Ave
Philadelphia, PA 19144-3802
(215) 843-5559-**B**
Ethnicity: African-American/Black
Degree and Year: EdM 1976
Major Field: School Psychology

HOPSON, Ronald E.
7737 Queensbury Drive
Knoxville, TN 37919-8053
(615) 974-3423-**B**, (615) 525-1825-**H**
Ethnicity: African-American/Black
Degree and Year: PhD 1988
Major Field: Clinical Psychology
Specialty: Drug Abuse

HORSFORD, Bernard I.
Sankofa Exchange, Limited
Africa House
21 Shornell Road
Bakersfield
Nottingham,
UNITED KINGDOM
0115 9110111-**B**, 0 115 9110033-**H**

sanleota@innotts.co.uk
Ethnicity: African-American/Black
Degree and Year: MSc 1996 MBA 1994
Major Field: Industrial/Organizational Psy.
Specialty: Vocational Psychology;Training & Development;Industrial/
Organizational Psychology;Human Resources

HORTON, Carrell
2410 Buchanan Street
Nashville, TN 37208-1937
(615) 329-8681-**B**, (615) 244-6310-**H**, (615) 329-8802-**F**
chorton@dubois.fisk.edu
Ethnicity: African-American/Black
Degree and Year: PhD 1972
Major Field: Developmental Psychology
Specialty: Child Development;Developmental Psychobiology;Statistics

HORVAT, JR., Joseph J.
Weber State University
Department of Psychology
1202 University Center
Ogden, UT 84408-1202
(801) 626-6248-**B**, (801) 626-7130-**F**
jhorvat@weber.edu
Ethnicity: American Indian/Alaska Native
Degree and Year: PhD 1979
Major Field: unknown

HOSHIKO, Michael
707 O James Street
Carbondale, IL 62901
(618)-453-4301-**B**, (618) 549-5129-**H**, 618-453-7714-**F**
Ethnicity: Asian-American/Asian/Pacific Islander
Languages: Japanese
Degree and Year: PhD 1957
Major Field: Physiological Psychology
Specialty: Audition;Biofeedback;Speech Disorders;Ethnic
Minorities;Nonverbal Communication

HOSHINO, Frank
Pob 1840
Atascadero, CA 93423-1840
(805) 461-2000-**B**
Ethnicity: Asian-American/Asian/Pacific Islander
Degree and Year: PhD 1985
Major Field: unknown
Specialty: Humanistic Psychology

HOSHMAND, Lisa T.
Lesley College
Division of Counseling & Psychology
29 Everett Street
Cambridge, MA 02138
(617) 349-8157-**B**, (781) 721-7429-**H**, (671) 349-3333-**F**
lhoshman@mail.lesley.edu
Ethnicity: Asian-American/Asian/Pacific Islander
Languages: Chinese
Degree and Year: PhD 1974
Major Field: Clinical Psychology
Specialty: Philosophy of Science;Counseling Psychology;Clinical
Research;Cultural & Social Processes

HOSSAIN, Ziarat
Fort Lewis College
100 Rim Drive
Department of Psychology

Durangio, CO 81301
(970) 247-7515-**B**, (970) 385-5866-**H**, (970) 247-7623-**F**
hossain-z@fortlewis.edu
Ethnicity: Asian-American/Asian/Pacific Islander
Degree and Year: PhD 1992
Major Field: Developmental Psychology
Specialty: Child Development;Parent-Child Interaction;Cross Cultural
Processes;Infancy;Human Development & Family
Studies;Gender Issues

HOUGH, Sigmund
100 Vantage Terr, #402
Swampscott, MA 01907-1264
(781) 581-8030-**B**
Ethnicity: American Indian/Alaska Native, European/White
Degree and Year: PhD 1987
Major Field: Clinical Psychology
Specialty: Psychotherapy;Clinical
Neuropsychology;Rehabilitation;Assessment/Diagnosis/
Evaluation;Administration

HOUSTON, Holly O.
8951 W 151st Street
Orland Park, IL 60462
(708) 349-5434-**B**, (708) 957-7718-**H**, (708) 747-7681-**F**
Ethnicity: African-American/Black
Degree and Year: PhD 1988
Major Field: Clinical Psychology
Specialty: Cognitive Behavioral Therapy;Depression;Stress;Psychology
of Women;Psychotherapy

HOUSTON, Lawrence N.
379 Tall Meadow Lane
Yardley, PA 19067
(609) 392-5611-**B**, (609) 391-2472-**H**
Ethnicity: African-American/Black
Degree and Year: EdD 1963
Major Field: Counseling Psychology
Specialty: Assessment/Diagnosis/Evaluation;Clinical
Psychology;Behavior Therapy;Cognitive Behavioral Therapy

HOWARD, Mary T.
Veterans Affairs Medical Center
110 N 32 Avenue
St. Cloud, MN 56303
(320) 252-1670-**B**, (320) 252-8627-**H**, (320) 255-6494-**F**
Ethnicity: African-American/Black
Degree and Year: PhD 1967
Major Field: Counseling Psychology
Specialty: Alcoholism & Alcohol Abuse;Domestic Violence;Ethnic
Minorities;Psychology of Women;Vocational Psychology

HSER, Yih-Ing
2012 Greenfield Avenue
Los Angeles, CA 90025
(310) 825-9057-**B**, (310) 478-3324-**H**
Ethnicity: Asian-American/Asian/Pacific Islander
Degree and Year: PhD 1986
Major Field: Social Psychology

HSIA, Heidi
11137 Broad Green Drive
Potomac, MD 20854
(301) 217-1335-**B**, (301) 983-8643-**H**, (301) 217-1494-**F**
Ethnicity: Asian-American/Asian/Pacific Islander
Languages: Chinese

Degree and Year: PhD 1970
Major Field: Clinical Psychology
Specialty: Administration;Clinical Child Psychology;Family
Therapy;Ethnic Minorities;Psychotherapy

HSU, Louis M.
Fairleigh Dickinson University
205 Lakeview Avenue
Teaneck, NJ 07666
(201) 692-2309-**B**, (973) 962-0756-**H**, (201) 692-2304-**F**
Ethnicity: Asian-American/Asian/Pacific Islander
Languages: French
Degree and Year: PhD 1971
Major Field: Quan/Math & Psychometrics/Stat
Specialty: Statistics;Clinical Research;Quantitative/Mathematical,
Psychometrics;Research Design &
Methodology;Psychometrics

HSU, Shang H.
National Chiao-Tung University
Department of Industrial Engineering
1001 Ta Hsueh Road
Hsinchu, 300
TAIWAN
(011) 886-3 57-**B**, (011) 886-2 70-**H**
shhsu@cc.nctu.edu.tw
Ethnicity: Asian-American/Asian/Pacific Islander
Degree and Year: PhD 1980
Major Field: unknown

HUANG, Karen H C
4075 Kozy Korner Lane
Center Valley, PA 18034
(610) 965-5894-**H**
phc2@lehigh.edu
Ethnicity: Asian-American/Asian/Pacific Islander
Degree and Year: PhD 1986
Major Field: Clinical Psychology
Specialty: Eating Disorders;Cultural & Social Processes;Management &
Organization;Individual Psychotherapy

HUANG, Larke N.
Georgetown University
National T.A. Center for Children's
Mental Health
3307 M Street
Washington, DC 20007
(202) 687-5000-**B**, (301) 340-2278-**H**, (202) 687-1954-**F**
huangl@gunet.georgetown
Ethnicity: Asian-American/Asian/Pacific Islander
Degree and Year: PhD 1980
Major Field: Clinical Psychology
Specialty: Child Development;Cross Cultural Processes;Ethnic
Minorities;Psychotherapy;Community Psychology

HUANG, Wei-Jen William
2350 Riverwoods Road
Riverwoods, IL 60015-1967
(312) 996-3490-**B**, (312) 996-7645-**F**
Ethnicity: Asian-American/Asian/Pacific Islander
Languages: Chinese
Degree and Year: PhD 1989
Major Field: Clinical Psychology
Specialty: Clinical Psychology;Ethnic Minorities;Marriage &
Family;Group Psychotherapy;Cross Cultural Processes

HUDLEY, Cynthia
University of California
@ Santa Barbara
Graduate School of Education
Santa Barbara, CA 93106-9490
(805) 893-8324-**B**, 805 648-1086-**H**, 805 893-7264-**F**
hudley@education.ucsb.edu
Ethnicity: African-American/Black
Degree and Year: PhD 1991
Major Field: Educational Psychology
Specialty: Developmental Psychology;Aggression;Social
    Development;Motivation;Attribution Theory;Child Therapy

HUERGO, Mayra
Jardines Metropolitanos
Calle Volta #975
Rio Piedras, PR 00927
(809) 725-1135-**B**
Ethnicity: Hispanic/Latino
Degree and Year: PsyD 1984
Major Field: Clinical Psychology

HUFANO, Linda D.
Diamond Head Child & Adolescent
 Mental Health Center
3627 Kilauea Avenue
Honolulu, HI 96816
Ethnicity: Asian-American/Asian/Pacific Islander
Degree and Year: PhD 1982
Major Field: School Psychology

HUGHES-WHEATLAND, Roxanne
Kennedy Krieger Institute
Department of Neuropsychology
707 North Broadway
Baltimore, MD 21205
(410) 502-9556-**B**, (410) 992-7872-**H**, (410) 502-8196-**F**
wheatland@kennedy.krieger.org
Ethnicity: African-American/Black
Degree and Year: PhD 1989
Major Field: Neurosciences
Specialty: Assessment/Diagnosis/Evaluation;Brain Functions;Cognitive
    Behavioral Therapy;Brain Damage;Clinical
    Neuropsychology;Cross Cultural Processes

HUGHES, Anita L.
1250 4th Street, S.W., W106
Washington, DC 20024
(202) 673-7140-**B**, (202) 479-4073-**H**
Ethnicity: African-American/Black
Degree and Year: EdD 1967
Major Field: unknown
Specialty: Cross Cultural Processes;Psychology & Law;School
    Counseling

HUI, Len Dang
Miami Dade Community College
11380 NW 27th Avenue
Room 8324
Miami, FL 33167-3495
(305) 237-8012-**B**, (954) 430-1941-**H**, (954) 430-1941-**F**
Ethnicity: American Indian/Alaska Native
Languages: Spanish

Degree and Year: PhD 1994
Major Field: Industrial/Organizational Psy.
Specialty: Industrial/Organizational Psychology

HU, Li-Tze
University of California
@ Santa Cruz
Department of Psychology
Clark Kerr Hall
Santa Cruz, CA 95064
(408) 459-3819-**B**, (408) 457-0465-**H**
Ethnicity: Asian-American/Asian/Pacific Islander
Degree and Year: PhD 1988
Major Field: Social Psychology
Specialty: Social Psychology;Social Cognition;Health
    Psychology;Quantitative/Mathematical,
    Psychometrics;Measurement

HUNTER, Knoxice C
United Behavioral Systems of GA
3390 Peachtree Road
Suite 700
Atlanta, GA 30326
(404) 364-8900-**B**, 404 987-2449-**H**, 404 364-8942-**F**
Ethnicity: African-American/Black
Degree and Year: PhD 1984
Major Field: Clinical Psychology
Specialty: Managed Care;Clinical Psychology;Ethnic Minorities;Case
    Management

HUNT, Portia
607 E Sedgwick Street
Philadelphia, PA 19119
(215) 204-1586-**B**, (215) 248-2917-**H**
Ethnicity: African-American/Black
Degree and Year: PhD 1975
Major Field: Counseling Psychology
Specialty: Counseling Psychology;Cultural & Social Processes;Ethnic
    Minorities;Gender Issues

HUNT, William K.
Claremont McKenna College
1340 N Hills Dr
Upland, CA 91784-1762
(714) 621-8000-**B**, (714) 920-3056-**H**
Ethnicity: African-American/Black
Degree and Year: PhD 1989
Major Field: Clinical Psychology
Specialty: Health Psychology;Rehabilitation

HUNT, Wilson L.
Clinical Psychologist
9 Kent Square
Brookline, MA 02146
(617) 277-1825-**B**, (617) 232-9753-**H**
Ethnicity: African-American/Black
Degree and Year: PhD 1955
Major Field: Clinical Psychology
Specialty: Assessment/Diagnosis/Evaluation;Clinical Child
    Psychology;Consulting Psychology;Gerontology/
    Geropsychology;Group Psychotherapy

HURST, Jurlene
18508 Roselawn
Detroit, MI 48221
(313) 270-0340-**B**, (313) 863-4946-**H**, (313) 342-1469-**F**

Ethnicity: African-American/Black
Degree and Year: EdD 1974
Major Field: School Psychology

HUSET, Martha K.
1231 13th Avenue West
Williston, ND 58801-3811
Ethnicity: Asian-American/Asian/Pacific Islander
Degree and Year: MA 1961
Major Field: School Psychology

HUTCHINSON, Kim M.
3771 Barnwell Drive
Winston-Salem, NC 27105
(336) 750-2299-**B**, (336) 748-8666-**H**, (336) 750-2599-**F**
khutch1@ibm.net
Ethnicity: African-American/Black
Degree and Year: EdD 1996
Major Field: Educational Psychology
Specialty: Educational Psychology;Health Psychology;Drug
Abuse;Alcoholism & Alcohol Abuse;Sexual Behavior

HU, Trudy HC
University of Texas @ Austin
1221 Felsmere Drive
Pflugerville, TX 78660
(512) 471-3515-**B**, 512 990-0891-**H**, 512 471-8875-**F**
Ethnicity: Asian-American/Asian/Pacific Islander
Languages: Chinese, Mandarin, Taiwanese
Degree and Year: PhD 1993
Major Field: Counseling Psychology
Specialty: Cognitive Psychology;Depression;Ethnic Minorities;Cross
Cultural Processes;Emotion;Marriage & Family

HWEE, Elsa
2744 NE 140th Street
Seattle, WA 98125-8208
206 546-7215-**B**, 206 935-5603-**H**
Ethnicity: Asian-American/Asian/Pacific Islander
Degree and Year: PsyD 1989
Major Field: Clinical Psychology
Specialty: Attention Deficit Disorders;Child Abuse;Child
Therapy;Individual Psychotherapy;Parent Education

HYDE, Elsie HA
825 12th Avenue
Honolulu, HI 96816
(808) 455-0361-**B**, (808) 735-3630-**H**
hyde2hawaii.edu
Ethnicity: Asian-American/Asian/Pacific Islander
Degree and Year: PhD 1992
Major Field: Personality Psychology
Specialty: Developmental Psychology;Statistics;Quantitative/
Mathematical, Psychometrics;Personality Measurement

HYMAN, Edward J.
Center for Social Research, Berkeley
1315 Star Route
Sausalito, CA 94965
(510) 841-6566-**B**, (415) 388-4479-**H**
debed@ix.netcome.com
Ethnicity: Hispanic/Latino
Languages: Spanish, Hebrew
Degree and Year: PhD 1975

Major Field: Clinical Psychology
Specialty: Clinical Psychology;Child Abuse;Depression;Family
Therapy;Stress;Forensic Psychology

IBRAHIM, Farah A.
University of Connecticut
School of Education
PO Box U-64
249 Glenbrook Road
Storrs, CT 06268
(860) 486-0199-**B**, (860) 487-7540-**H**, (860) 486-0180-**F**
Fibrahim@uconnum.uconn.edu
Ethnicity: Asian-American/Asian/Pacific Islander
Degree and Year: PhD 1979
Major Field: Counseling Psychology
Specialty: Cross Cultural Processes;Psychology of Women;Values &
Moral Behavior;Cultural & Social Processes;Stress

ICHIYAMA, Michael A.
University of San Diego
Department of Psychology
5998 Alcala Park
San Diego, CA 92110-2429
(619) 260-4164-**B**, (619) 637-9057-**H**, (619) 260-4619-**F**
ichiyama@eudoramail.com
Ethnicity: Asian-American/Asian/Pacific Islander
Degree and Year: PhD 1989
Major Field: Clinical Psychology
Specialty: Clinical Research;Interpersonal Processes &
Relations;Alcoholism & Alcohol Abuse;Group
Processes;Ethnic Minorities;Social Behavior

IGUCHI, Martin Y.
Rand
1700 Main Street
PO Box 2138
Santa Monica, CA 90407-2138
(310) 393-0411-**B**, ((310) 391-2234-**H**, (310) 451-70040-**F**
iguchi@rand.org
Ethnicity: Asian-American/Asian/Pacific Islander
Degree and Year: PhD 1986
Major Field: unknown
Specialty: Drug Abuse;Psychopharmacology;Ethnic Minorities;Applied
Behavior Analysis;Behavior Therapy

IKE, Chris A.
PO Box 36279
Fayetteville, NC 28303-1279
(910) 486-1576-**B**
ike@chi1.unsfsu..edu
Ethnicity: African-American/Black
Languages: Ibo, Hausa, Yoruba
Degree and Year: PhD 1979
Major Field: Clinical Psychology
Specialty: Assessment/Diagnosis/Evaluation;Community Mental
Health;Cultural & Social Processes;Homelessness & Homeless
Populations;Psychopathology;Stress

INCERA, Armando
7600 Red Road
P.W. Suite 300
South Miami, FL 33143
(305) 668-6018-**B**, (305) 444-7227-**H**, (3050 668-6016-**F**
Ethnicity: Hispanic/Latino
Languages: Spanish

Degree and Year: PhD 1983
Major Field: Clinical Psychology
Specialty: Cognitive Behavioral Therapy;Hospital Care;Medical Psychology;Health Psychology;Managed Care;Rehabilitation

INCLAN, Jaime
85 Fifth Avenue
Suite #901
New York, NY 10003
(212) 741-3448-**B**, (212) 924-7621-**H**, (212) 727-3714-**F**
Ethnicity: Hispanic/Latino
Languages: Spanish
Degree and Year: PhD 1979
Major Field: Clinical Psychology
Specialty: Family Therapy;Adolescent Therapy;Ethnic Minorities;Community Mental Health

INGRAM, Jesse C.
Behavioral Medical Clinic
Po Box 8300354
Dallas, TX 75205-
(214) 943-8454-**B**, (214) 230-4573-**H**
Ethnicity: African-American/Black
Degree and Year: PhD 1981
Major Field: Counseling Psychology
Specialty: Community Mental Health

INGRAM, Winifred
2106 Beverly Beach Drive, NW
Olympia, WA 98502-3430
(206) 866-6000-**B**, (206) 866-4991-**H**
Ethnicity: African-American/Black
Degree and Year: PhD 1951
Major Field: Clinical Psychology
Specialty: Assessment/Diagnosis/Evaluation;Child & Pediatric Psychology;Clinical Child Psychology;Cross Cultural Processes;Cultural & Social Processes

INOUE, Sachi
10950 International Boulevard
#214
Oakland, CA 94603
(510) 814-8583-**B**, (510) 562-4454-**H**
welltop@pacbell.net
Ethnicity: Asian-American/Asian/Pacific Islander
Languages: Japanese
Degree and Year: PhD 1998
Major Field: Clinical Psychology
Specialty: Ethnic Minorities;Psychology of Women;Feminist Therapy

INSUA, Ana Maria
Lafinur 3165
1425 033 -,
Argentina
54-1-802-9825-**H**, 54-1-803-4637-**F**
Ethnicity: Hispanic/Latino
Languages: Spanish
Degree and Year: PhD 1970
Major Field: Quan/Math & Psychometrics/Stat
Specialty: Clinical Research;Measurement;Memory;Projective Techniques

IP, Sau Mei V.
Saskatchewan Hospital
1916B Foley Drive
N. Battleford, SK S9A 3G9

Canada
(306) 446-6879-**B**, (306) 445-9244-**H**
Ethnicity: Asian-American/Asian/Pacific Islander
Languages: Chinese
Degree and Year: PhD 1991
Major Field: Clinical Psychology
Specialty: Chronically Mentally Ill;Mentally Retarded;Behavior Therapy;Cognitive Behavioral Therapy;Schizophrenia

IQBAL, S. Mohammed
109 Dutton Drive
New Castle, DE 19720
(302) 322-2689-**B**, (302) 322-2689-**H**, (302) 322-2689-**F**
Ethnicity: Asian-American/Asian/Pacific Islander
Languages: Hindi, Urdu
Degree and Year: PhD 1975
Major Field: Clinical Psychology
Specialty: Forensic Psychology;Mental Health Services;Mental Disorders;Personality Measurement;Consulting Psychology

IRELAND HURD, Evelyn C.
1305 Fourth Street, SW
Washington, DC 20024-2201
Ethnicity: African-American/Black
Degree and Year: PhD 1969
Major Field: Clinical Psychology
Specialty: Group Psychotherapy;Health Psychology;Mental Health Services;Family Therapy;Individual Psychotherapy;School Psychology

IRUESTE-MONTES, Ana M.
1 Normandy Circle #1
Colorado Springs, CO 80906-3033
(719) 473-7444-**B**, (719) 578-0069-**H**
Ethnicity: Hispanic/Latino
Languages: Spanish
Degree and Year: PhD 1974
Major Field: Clinical Psychology
Specialty: Child Abuse

ISAACS, Owen K.
P.O. Box 113
Edison, NJ 08818-0113
(201) 247-2468-**B**
Ethnicity: African-American/Black
Degree and Year: EdD 1979
Major Field: Counseling Psychology
Specialty: Psychotherapy

ISHIDA, Taeko H.
1205 Waterview Dr
Mill Valley, CA 94941-3412
(415) 454-1460-**B**, (415) 383-7520-**H**
Ethnicity: Asian-American/Asian/Pacific Islander
Languages: Japanese
Degree and Year: PhD 1978
Major Field: Clinical Psychology
Specialty: Assessment/Diagnosis/Evaluation;Individual Psychotherapy;Group Psychotherapy;Deviant Behavior;Correctional Psychology

ISHIKAWA-FULLMER, Janet
1750 Kalalaua Avenue
Suite #809
Honolulu, HI 96826
(808) 845-9158-**B**, (808) 373-9580-**H**

Ethnicity: Asian-American/Asian/Pacific Islander
Languages: Japanese
Degree and Year: PhD 1976
Major Field: Clinical Psychology
Specialty: Family Therapy;Depression;Individual
    Psychotherapy;Personality Disorders;Neuroses

ISHIYAMA, Toaru
    7703 Howard Street
    Parma, OH 44134
    (216) 842-2068-**H**
Ethnicity: Asian-American/Asian/Pacific Islander
Languages: Japanese
Degree and Year: PhD 1958
Major Field: Clinical Psychology
Specialty: Community Psychology;Social Psychology

ITATANI, Robert M.
    Rio Hondo College
    Psychological Services
    3600 Workman Mill Road
    Whittier, CA 90608
    (562) 692-0921-**B**, (562) 943-2902-**H**
Ethnicity: Asian-American/Asian/Pacific Islander
Degree and Year: PhD 1974
Major Field: Clinical Psychology
Specialty: Individual Psychotherapy;Forensic
    Psychology;Biofeedback;Stress

ITO, Elaine S.
    Baystate Medical Center
    3300 Main Street
    Fourth Floor , Suites A & B
    Springfield, MA 01199
    (413)794-7380-**B**, 413/534-1823-**H**
    elaineito@bbs.org
Ethnicity: Asian-American/Asian/Pacific Islander
Degree and Year: PhD 1996
Major Field: Clinical Child Psychology
Specialty: Health Psychology;Child & Pediatric Psychology;Affective
    Disorders;Behavior Therapy;Endocrine Systems

IWAI, Charles T.
    4487 Smith Hill Road
    Golden, CO 80403-8871
Ethnicity: Asian-American/Asian/Pacific Islander
Degree and Year: PhD 1972
Major Field: School Psychology
Specialty: School Counseling

IWAMASA, Gayle Y.
    University of Indianapolis
    Graduate Psychology Department
    1400 East Hanna Avenue
    Indianapolis, IN 46227
    (317) 788-3353-**B**
Ethnicity: Asian-American/Asian/Pacific Islander
Degree and Year: PhD 1992
Major Field: Clinical Psychology
Specialty: Ethnic
    Minorities;Psychopathology;Psychotherapy;Community
    Mental Health;Gerontology/Geropsychology;Psychology of
    Women

IYENGAR, Shanto
    University of California
    @ Los Angeles
    4289 Bunche Hall
    Los Angeles, CA 90024-1301
Ethnicity: Asian-American/Asian/Pacific Islander
Degree and Year: PhD 1972
Major Field: Social Psychology
Specialty: Mass Media Communication

IZAWA, Chizuko
    Tulane University
    Department of Psychology
    New Orleans, LA 70118
    (504) 862-3329-**B**, (504) 865-1467-**H**, (504) 862-8744-**F**
    izawa@mailhost.tcs.tulane.edu
Ethnicity: Asian-American/Asian/Pacific Islander
Languages: Japanese
Degree and Year: PhD 1965
Major Field: Experimental Psychology
Specialty: Verbal Learning;Memory;Learning/Learning Theory;Cognitive
    Psychology;Cross Cultural Processes;Experimental
    Psychology

IZUTSU, Satoru
    1350 Ala Moana Boulevard
    Suite #611
    Honolulu, HI 96814-4208
    (808) 956-5505-**B**
Ethnicity: Asian-American/Asian/Pacific Islander
Degree and Year: PhD 1963
Major Field: Educational Psychology

JACKSON-DAVIS, Brandi
    3403 74th St
    Lubbock, TX 79423-1105
    (806) 797-7272-**B**, (806) 797-7797-**H**
Ethnicity: African-American/Black
Degree and Year: PhD 1988
Major Field: Clinical Psychology
Specialty: Clinical Psychology

JACKSON, Anna M.
    Meharry Medical College
    1005 D.B. Todd Building
    Box A2
    Nashville, TN 37208
    (615) 327-6182-**B**, (615) 646-6192-**H**, (615) 327-6213-**F**
    jackson82@ccvax.mmc.edu
Ethnicity: African-American/Black
Degree and Year: PhD 1967
Major Field: Clinical Psychology

JACKSON, Helen L.
    6000 Summer, NE
    Albuquerque, NM 87110
    (505) 266-4226-**B**, (505) 899-8938-**H**
Ethnicity: African-American/Black
Degree and Year: PhD 1980
Major Field: Clinical Psychology
Specialty: Adolescent Therapy;Child Therapy;Clinical
    Psychology;Ethnic Minorities;Family Therapy

JACKSON, Jacquelyne F.
    Institute of Human Development
    UC Berkeley

1203 Tolman Hall
Berkeley, CA 94702
(510) 642-3447-**B**, (510) 841-2671-**H**, (510) 642-7969-**F**
Ethnicity: African-American/Black
Degree and Year: PhD 1983
Major Field: Developmental Psychology
Specialty: Adolescent Development;Cultural & Social Processes;Human
Development & Family Studies;Infancy;Interpersonal
Processes & Relations

JACKSON, James S.
University of Michigan
Institute for Social Research
5006
PO Box 1248
Ann Arbor, MI 48109-1248
(734) 763-2491-**B**, (734) 434-5434-**H**, (743) 763-0044-**F**
Ethnicity: African-American/Black
Degree and Year: PhD 1972
Major Field: Social Psychology
Specialty: Family Processes;Human Development & Family
Studies;Mental Health Services;Gerontology/
Geropsychology;Political Psychology

JACKSON, John H.
Wisconsin School of Professional Psycholgy
9120 West Hampton Avenue
Suite 212
Wauwatosa, WI 53222-2205
(414) 464-6924-**B**, (414) 464-6924-**H**
Ethnicity: African-American/Black
Degree and Year: PhD 1957
Major Field: School Psychology
Specialty: Administration;Child Therapy;School Psychology

JACKSON, Joyce Taborn
J Taborn Associates
1219 Marquette Avenue South
Suite 80
Minneapolis, MN 55403-2488
(612) 338-9012-**B**, (612) 545-3287-**H**, (612) 338-9020-**F**
Ethnicity: African-American/Black
Degree and Year: PhD 1969
Major Field: Counseling Psychology
Specialty: Educational Psychology;Ethnic Minorities;Individual
Psychotherapy;Mental Health Services;Adolescent Therapy

JACKSON, Leslie C.
CSPP
1000 S. Fremont Avenue
Los Angeles, CA 91803-1360
(818) 284-2777-**B**, (213) 294-5379-**H**, (818) 284-0550-**F**
Ethnicity: African-American/Black
Degree and Year: PhD 1981
Major Field: Clinical Psychology
Specialty: Psychotherapy;Affective Disorders;Ethnic
Minorities;Cultural & Social Processes;Personality Disorders

JACKSON, Ronald A.
Iowa State University
Student Services Bldg.
Third Floor
Ames, IA 50011

(515) 294-5056-**B**
Ethnicity: African-American/Black
Degree and Year: PhD 1982
Major Field: Counseling Psychology

JACOBS-JR., Walter R.
The College Board
2970 Clairmont Road
Suite #250
Atlanta, GA 30329
Ethnicity: African-American/Black
Degree and Year: MA 1965
Major Field: Educational Psychology

JA, Davis Y.
362 Victoria Street
San Francisco, CA 94132
(510) 523-2300-**B**, (415) 585-2773-**H**, (415) 239-4511-**F**
Ethnicity: Asian-American/Asian/Pacific Islander
Languages: Chinese
Degree and Year: PhD 1981
Major Field: Clinical Psychology
Specialty: Drug Abuse;Community Psychology;Ethnic
Minorities;Consulting Psychology;Family Therapy

JAIMEZ, T. Lanac
191 Clearview Drive
Vallejo, CA 94591
(707) 643-5011-**B**, (707) 643-4355-**H**
tljaimez@i_cafe.net
Ethnicity: Hispanic/Latino
Degree and Year: PhD 1995
Major Field: Clinical Psychology
Specialty: Clinical Psychology;Cognitive Behavioral Therapy

JAIN, Sharat K.
3109 West 199th Street
Leawood, KS 66211-3059
(913) 469-0675-**H**, (913) 469-**F**
Ethnicity: Asian-American/Asian/Pacific Islander
Languages: Hindi
Degree and Year: PhD 1967
Major Field: Clinical Psychology
Specialty: Cognitive Behavioral Therapy;Family Therapy;Health
Psychology;Hypnosis/Hypnotherapy;Sexual Dysfunction

JAITLY, Kailash N.
3003 E Springlake Cir
Colorado Spgs, CO 80906-3729
(719) 520-1711-**B**, (719) 576-1003-**H**
Ethnicity: Asian-American/Asian/Pacific Islander
Degree and Year: PsyD 1978
Major Field: Clinical Psychology
Specialty: Adolescent Therapy;Rational-Emotive Therapy

JAMES, JR., Earnest
5586 Suncrest Court
Parma, OH 44134-2042
(216) 443-4215-**B**, (216) 741-4982-**H**, (216) 443-4878-**F**
Ethnicity: African-American/Black
Degree and Year: PhD 1981
Major Field: Industrial/Organizational Psy.
Specialty: Industrial/Organizational Psychology;Organizational
Development;Management & Organization;Job
Satisfaction;Training & Development;Selection & Placement

JAMES-PARKER, Magna M.
Medlin Treatment Center
175 Corporate Center Drive
Suite D
Stockbridge, GA 30281
(770) 507-6044-**B**, (770) 968-1307-**H**, (770) 507-5284-**F**
Ethnicity: African-American/Black
Degree and Year: PhD 1988
Major Field: Counseling Psychology
Specialty: Adolescent Development;Depression;Religious
Psychology;Cognitive Behavioral Therapy;Ethnic Minorities

JAMES, Lainee M.
5275 Lee Highway
Suite #104
Arlington, VA 22207-1619
(703) 533-1038-**B**
Ethnicity: African-American/Black
Degree and Year: PhD 1982
Major Field: Counseling Psychology

JAMES, Larry C.
Tripler Army Medical Center
Tripler AMC, HI 96859
(808) 433-6060-**B**, (808) 624-2964-**H**, (808) 433-1801-**F**
ljames@hawaii.edu
Ethnicity: African-American/Black
Degree and Year: PhD 1987
Major Field: Counseling Psychology
Specialty: Health Psychology;Pain & Pain Management;Cross Cultural
Processes;Assessment/Diagnosis/Evaluation;Forensic
Psychology

JAMES, Michelle D.
Illinois School of Professional Psychology
20 South Clark Street
3rd Floor
Chicago, IL 60603
(312) 201-0200-**B**, (773) 561-8207-**H**
mjames@uic.edu
Ethnicity: African-American/Black
Degree and Year: PhD 1995
Major Field: Clinical Psychology
Specialty: Group Psychotherapy;Ethnic Minorities;Community Mental
Health;Psychotherapy;Chronically Mentally Ill;Clinical
Psychology

JAMES, Norman L.
University of St. Thomas
1000 LaSalle Street
Minneapolis, MN 55403
(612) 962-4653-**B**, (612) 420-9705-**H**
Ethnicity: African-American/Black
Degree and Year: PhD 1982
Major Field: Educational Psychology
Specialty: Counseling Psychology;Personality;Social
Psychology;Statistics;Group Processes

JAMES, Steven E
Goddard College
11 River Street
Byfield, MA 01922
(508) 463-9022-**H**, 508 463-3644-**F**

steve813@delphi.com
Ethnicity: American Indian/Alaska Native
Languages: French
Degree and Year: PhD 1990
Major Field: Clinical Psychology
Specialty: Family Therapy;Ethnic Minorities;Gender Issues;Death &
Dying;HIV/AIDS;Developmental Psychology

JANI, Aurobindo J.
709 Gateway Lane
Tampa, FL 33613
(813) 962-7993-**B**
Ethnicity: Asian-American/Asian/Pacific Islander
Degree and Year: MA 1964
Major Field: Personality Psychology
Specialty: Personality Theory;History & Systems of Psychology

JAPZON GILLUM, Debra
HHC Seventh CSG Unit 27503
Box 34116
APO, AE 09139-7503
(949) 9522-70661-**H**
dgillum@ba.blitz.net
Ethnicity: Asian-American/Asian/Pacific Islander
Degree and Year: PhD 1989
Major Field: Clinical Child Psychology
Specialty: Clinical Child Psychology;Family Therapy;Cognitive
Behavioral Therapy;Ethnic Minorities;Client-Centered
Therapy

JARAMA, S. Lisbeth
Virginia Commonwealth University
Center for Public Policy
Survey & Evaluation Research Laboratory
921 West Franklin Street
Richmond, VA 232804-3016
(804) 828-1839-**B**, (804) 254-7649-**H**
sljarama@saturn.vcu.edu
Ethnicity: Hispanic/Latino
Languages: Spanish
Degree and Year: PhD 1996 BA 1989
Major Field: Social Psychology
Specialty: Health Psychology

JAVIER, Rafael A.
St. Johns University
Center for Psychological Services
 and Clinical Studies
8000 Utopia Parkway
Jamaica, NY 11439
(718) 990-6331-**B**, (212) 254-0230-**H**, (718) 990-1586-**F**
Ethnicity: Hispanic/Latino
Languages: Spanish
Degree and Year: PhD 1982
Major Field: Clinical Psychology
Specialty: Clinical
Psychology;Psychoanalysis;Psycholinguistic;Psychopathology;Ethnic
Minorities

JAY, Milton T.
211 Bellevue Street
Newton, MA 02458
(617) 928-3446-**B**, (617) 964-4091-**H**, (617) 928-3446-**F**
miltonjay@aol.com

Ethnicity: Asian-American/Asian/Pacific Islander
Degree and Year: EdD 1980
Major Field: Neurosciences
Specialty: Alcoholism & Alcohol Abuse;Drug Abuse;Gerontology/
Geropsychology;Neuropsychology;Brain Damage

JEMAIL, Jay A.
8 Southview Path
Chadds Ford, PA 19317-9180
Ethnicity: Hispanic/Latino
Degree and Year: PhD 1975
Major Field: Clinical Psychology
Specialty: Family Therapy;Sexual Behavior

JEMMOTT, III, John B.
Princeton University
Department of Psychology
Green Hall
Princeton, NJ 08544-1010
(609) 258-4448-**B**, (609) 924-4262-**H**, (609) 258-1275-**F**
jemmott@princeton.edu
Ethnicity: African-American/Black
Degree and Year: PhD 1982
Major Field: Social Psychology
Specialty: HIV/AIDS;Health Psychology;Prevention;Sexual Behavior

JENKINS-MONROE, Valata
5534 Golden Gate Avenue
Oakland, CA 94618-2111
(510) 547-7756-**B**, (510) 652-9516-**H**, (510) 652-7756-**F**
vmonroe@mail.cspp.edu
Ethnicity: African-American/Black
Degree and Year: PhD 1978
Major Field: Clinical Psychology

JENKINS, Adelbert H
New York University
715 Broadway
Room 203
New York, NY 10003
(212) 998-7937-**B**, (212) 690-7473-**H**, 212 995-4687-**F**
jenkins@psych.nyu.edu
Ethnicity: African-American/Black
Degree and Year: PhD 1963 BA 1957
Major Field: Clinical Psychology
Specialty: Clinical Psychology;Ethnic Minorities;Individual
Psychotherapy;Psychotherapy;Humanistic
Psychology;Projective Techniques

JENKINS, Sheila A.
Sheila A. Jenkins, PhD & Associates
2630 Fountainview
Suite 350
Houston, TX 77057
(713) 266-9837-**B**, (281) 403-6056-**H**, (713) 266-9838-**F**
Ethnicity: African-American/Black
Degree and Year: PhD 1992
Major Field: Counseling Psychology
Specialty: Counseling Psychology;Juvenile Delinquency;Group
Processes;Adolescent Development;Ethnic Minorities

JENKINS, Susan M.
Caliber Associates
10530 Rosehaven Street
Fairfax, VA 22030
(703) 385-3200-**B**, (301) 336-5577-**H**, (703) 385-3206-**F**

jenkins@calib.com
Ethnicity: African-American/Black
Degree and Year: PhD 1993
Major Field: Social Psychology
Specialty: Computer Applications and Programming;Drug Abuse;Policy
Analysis;Curriculum Development/Evaluation;Research &
Training

JENKINS, Yvonne M
Boston College
University Counseling Service
Fulton Hall
Room 254
Chestnut Hill, MA 02467
(617) 552-3927-**B**, (617) 254-6861-**H**
jenkinsy@bc.edu
Ethnicity: African-American/Black
Degree and Year: PhD 1981 MEd 1973
Major Field: Counseling Psychology
Specialty: Counseling Psychology;Ethnic
Minorities;Psychopathology;Clinical Psychology;Feminist
Therapy;Cross Cultural Processes

JENNINGS, JR., Wilmar A.
1201 Hollywood Drive
Building #26
Apartment #567
Anchorage, AK 99501-1312
(907) 753-5588-**B**, (907) 278-1410-**H**
Ethnicity: African-American/Black
Degree and Year: PhD 1968
Major Field: Environmental Psychology
Specialty: Psychology & the Arts;Environmental Psychology

JENNINGS, Lesajean M.
The Great Southwest Building
1314 Texas Avenue
Suite 1600
Houston, TX 77002
(713) 225-2280-**B**, (713) 747-8136-**H**, (713) 225-5787-**F**
LjJENNINGS@aol.com
Ethnicity: African-American/Black
Degree and Year: PsyD 1995
Major Field: Clinical Psychology
Specialty: Adolescent Therapy;Ethnic Minorities;Juvenile
Delinquency;Cultural & Social Processes;Forensic
Psychology;Psychotherapy

JENNINGS, Valdea D.
333 W Mt. Airy Avenue
Philadelphia, PA 19119-2941
(215) 248-5228-**B**
Ethnicity: African-American/Black
Degree and Year: EdD 1973
Major Field: Educational Psychology

JETTE, Carmen CB
590 Lowell Street
Lexington, MA 02420-1939
(978) 250-6259-**B**, (781) 861-2978-**H**, (7781) 676-7942-**F**
Ethnicity: Hispanic/Latino
Languages: Spanish
Degree and Year: PhD 1987

Major Field: Clinical Psychology
Specialty: Clinical Psychology;Depression;Cross Cultural
　　　　Processes;Cognitive Behavioral Therapy;Ethnic
　　　　Minorities;Child & Pediatric Psychology

JEW, Cynthia L.
　University of Redlands
　1200 East Colton Avenue
　Redland, CA 92373
　(909) 793-2121-**B**, (909) 430-6231-**H**, (909) 335-5204-**F**
　jew@uor.edu
Ethnicity: Asian-American/Asian/Pacific Islander, Hispanic/Latino
Degree and Year: PhD 1991
Major Field: School Psychology
Specialty: Neuropsychology;Information Processing;Family
　　　　Therapy;Learning Disabilities;Lesbian & Gay
　　　　Issuues;Adolescent Development

JEW, Wing
　3612 Harpers Ferry Drive
　Stockton, CA 95219-3657
　(209) 951-7511-**B**
Ethnicity: Asian-American/Asian/Pacific Islander
Degree and Year: EdD 1970
Major Field: Counseling Psychology

JIMENEZ-SAFIR, Paula B.
　7710 Balboa Avenue
　#2270
　San Diego, CA 92111-2253
　(619) 279-4079-**B**
Ethnicity: Hispanic/Latino
Languages: Spanish
Degree and Year: PhD 1989
Major Field: Clinical Psychology
Specialty: Affective Disorders;Child Therapy;Crisis Intervention &
　　　　Therapy;Family Therapy;Ethnic Minorities

JIN, Young-Sun
　Department of Psychology
　Kyungpook National University
　Taegu,
　KOREA
　053-950-5249-**B**, 053-950-5206-**F**
Ethnicity: Asian-American/Asian/Pacific Islander
Languages: Japanese, Korean
Degree and Year: PhD 1988
Major Field: Cognitive Psychology
Specialty: Brain Functions;Cognitive Psychology;Experimental
　　　　Psychology;Information Processing;Neuropsychology

JOESTING-GOODWOMAN, Joan A.
　415 Rutgers Avenue
　Melbourne, FL 32901-7738
　(813) 977-9396-**B**
Ethnicity: American Indian/Alaska Native
Degree and Year: EdD 1970
Major Field: Educational Psychology
Specialty: Alcoholism & Alcohol Abuse;Drug Abuse

JOFFE, Vera
　Vera Joffe, PhD, P.A.
　9441 West Sample Road
　Suite 210
　Coral Springs, FL 33068
　(54) 341-4441-**B**, (954) 341-4440-**F**

　pitinin@aol.com
Ethnicity: Hispanic/Latino
Languages: Portuguese
Degree and Year: PhD
Major Field: Clinical Psychology
Specialty: Attention Deficit Disorders;Child Therapy;Adolescent
　　　　Therapy

JOHNSON, David L.
　10999 Reed Hartman Hwy Ste 127
　Cincinnati, OH 45242-8302
　(513) 745-5658-**B**, (513) 984-2858-**H**
Ethnicity: African-American/Black
Degree and Year: EdD 1984
Major Field: Educational Psychology
Specialty: School Psychology;Psychoanalysis

JOHNSON, Denise MW
　185 Central Avenue
　Suite 615
　East Orange, NJ 07018
　(973) 675-9200-**B**, (973) 678-8432-**F**
Ethnicity: African-American/Black
Degree and Year: PhD 1989
Major Field: Clinical Psychology
Specialty: Assessment/Diagnosis/Evaluation;Cross Cultural
　　　　Processes;Forensic Psychology;Clinical Psychology;Ethnic
　　　　Minorities;Religious Psychology

JOHNSON, Edward E.
　PO Box 597
　East Brunswick, NJ 08816-0597
　(753) 235-4600-**B**, (732) 257-4885-**H**
Ethnicity: African-American/Black
Degree and Year: PhD 1952
Major Field: Experimental Psychology
Specialty: Persoanality & Experimental Psychopathology;Assessment/
　　　　Diagnosis/Evaluation;Cross Cultural Processes;Alcoholism &
　　　　Alcohol Abuse;Community Psychology;Forensic Psychology

JOHNSON, Eugene H.
　12269 Carroll Mill Road
　Ellicott City, MD 21042
　(202) 673-7021-**B**, (301) 596-9114-**H**, (202) 673-2141-**F**
Ethnicity: African-American/Black
Degree and Year: PhD 1971
Major Field: Educational Psychology
Specialty: Administration;Educational Psychology;Family
　　　　Therapy;Mental Health Services;Psychotherapy

JOHNSON, Fern M.
　21516 Sutcliff Terrace
　Brookeville, MD 20833
　(202) 645-5947-**B**, (301) 260-0649-**H**, (202) 645-0531-**F**
　FernJohnsno@yahoo.com
Ethnicity: African-American/Black
Degree and Year: PhD 1990
Major Field: Neurosciences
Specialty: Statistics;Epidemiology & Biometry;Brain
　　　　Functions;Neuropsychology;Research Design & Methodology

JOHNSON, Fred A.
　5505 Seminary Road
　Falls Church, VA 22041-3532
　(202) 282-2152-**B**, (703) 845-8891-**H**, (202) 282-3676-**F**
Ethnicity: African-American/Black

Degree and Year: PhD 1977
Major Field: Clinical Psychology
Specialty: Assessment/Diagnosis/Evaluation;Child Abuse;Adolescent Therapy;Cognitive Behavioral Therapy

JOHNSON, Joan J.
East Lansing Center for the Family
425 West Grand River
East Lansing, MI
(517) 332-8900-**B**, (517) 371-5385-**H**, (517) 332-8149-**F**
Ethnicity: African-American/Black
Degree and Year: PhD 1975 MA 1971
Major Field: Clinical Psychology

JOHNSON, Johnny
773 Margie Dr
Memphis, TN 38127-2727
(901) 357-5613-**B**, (901) 357-5613-**H**
Ethnicity: African-American/Black
Languages: French, Spanish
Degree and Year: MS 1974
Major Field: Counseling Psychology
Specialty: Social Psychology;Training & Development;Lesbian & Gay Issuues;Attitudes & Opinions;Human Resources

JOHNSON, Lawrence B.
531 Randolph Road
Apartment 341A
Silver Spring, MD 20904
(301) 625-9006-**H**, (301) 625-9011-**F**
Ethnicity: African-American/Black
Degree and Year: PhD 1964
Major Field: Experimental Psychology
Specialty: Human Factors;Engineering Psychology;Performance Evaluation;Management & Organization;Military Psychology

JOHNSON, Marjorie
1795 Coventry Road
Decatur, GA 30030-1011
(404) 508-8889-**B**
Ethnicity: African-American/Black
Degree and Year: PhD 1989
Major Field: Clinical Psychology
Specialty: Psychotherapy

JOHNSON, Matthew B.
99 Northfield Avenue
West Orange, NJ 07052
(201) 731-2334-**B**, (201) 763-0363-**H**, (201) 982-6594-**F**
Ethnicity: African-American/Black
Degree and Year: PhD 1984
Major Field: Clinical Psychology
Specialty: Forensic Psychology;Personality Disorders;Psychology & Law

JOHNSON, Melissa R.
236 Beachers Brook Lane
Cary, NC 27511-5598
(919) 755-8527-**B**
Ethnicity: Hispanic/Latino
Degree and Year: PhD 1980
Major Field: Clinical Psychology

JOHNSON, Paul W.
150 Nickerson #301
Seattle, WA 90109

(206) 281-7381-**B**, (206) 284-5267-**H**, (206) 286-1025-**F**
Ethnicity: Hispanic/Latino
Degree and Year: PhD 1981
Major Field: Gerontology
Specialty: Gerontology/Geropsychology;Alzheimer's Disease;Counseling Psychology;Crime & Criminal Behavior

JOHNSON, Sylvia T
Journal of Negro Education
Howard University
2900 Van Ness Street, NW
Washington, DC 20008
(202) 806-8120-**B**, (301) 593-2495-**H**, (202) 806-8434-**F**
sjohnson@fac.howard.edu
Ethnicity: African-American/Black
Degree and Year: PhD 1974
Major Field: Quan/Math & Psychometrics/Stat

JOHNSON, W. Roy
Iowa State University
College of Business
Department of Management
343 Carver Hall
Ames, IA 50011-2063
(515) 294-8267-**B**, (515) 292-3291-**H**, (515) 294-6060-**F**
wrjohn@iastate.edu
Ethnicity: African-American/Black
Degree and Year: PhD 1986
Major Field: Industrial/Organizational Psy.
Specialty: Selection & Placement;Management & Organization;Organizational Development;Employee Assistance Programs;Labor & Management Relations

JOHNSON, William L.
300 Mercer Street
Suite #3K
New York, NY 10003-6732
(212) 982-4094-**B**
Ethnicity: African-American/Black
Degree and Year: PhD 1964
Major Field: unknown
Specialty: Psychotherapy

JOHNSON, Zonya
Saybrook Research Institute
and Graduate School
450 Pacific, Third Floor
San Francisco, CA 94133
(925) 254-2027-**B**, (925) 254-2027-**H**
Ethnicity: African-American/Black
Degree and Year: PhD 1974
Major Field: Clinical Psychology
Specialty: Cross Cultural Processes;Feminist Therapy;Individual Psychotherapy;Psychoanalysis;Psychopathology

JONES-SAUMTY, Deborah J.
American Indian Associates
302 Fourth Street
Route 1, Box 9261
Talihina, OK 74571
(918) 567-3087-**B**, (918) 567-3575-**H**, (918) 567-3087-**F**
sndjs@aol.com
Ethnicity: American Indian/Alaska Native
Degree and Year: PhD 1994
Major Field: Counseling Psychology

Specialty: Alcoholism & Alcohol Abuse;Clinical
    Neuropsychology;Community Psychology;Drug
    Abuse;Cultural & Social Processes;Management &
    Organization

JONES, Annie Lee
    Clinical Psychologist
    86-75 Midland Parkway #5J
    Jamaica Estates, NY 11432
    (718) 297-4883-**B**, (718) 658-4648-**H**
    annielee.jones@med.gov
Ethnicity: African-American/Black
Degree and Year: PhD 1976
Major Field: Clinical Psychology
Specialty: Child Abuse;Decision & Choice
    Behavior;Psychoanalysis;Psychology of
    Women;Depression;Values & Moral Behavior

JONES, Arthur C.
    University of Denver
    Department of Psychology
    2155 Race Street
    Denver, CO 80208
    (303) 871-3795-**B**, (303) 399-2567-**H**, (303) 399-8269-**F**
    ajones@nova.psy.du.edu
Ethnicity: African-American/Black
Degree and Year: PhD 1974
Major Field: Clinical Psychology
Specialty: Psychology & the Arts;Consulting Psychology;Cultural &
    Social Processes;Cross Cultural Processes;Ethnic Minorities

JONES, Cynthia A.
    The Loudon Counseling Center
    224 Cornwall Street, NW
    Leesburg, VA 20176-2701
Ethnicity: African-American/Black
Degree and Year: PhD 1987
Major Field: Clinical Psychology
Specialty: Family Therapy

JONES, Elaine F.
    Saint Louis University
    Psychology Department
    Shannon Hall
    221 North Grand Boulevard
    St. Louis, MO 63103
    (314)977-2287-**B**, 314/361-1565-**H**, 314/977-3679-**F**
    jonesef@slu.edu
Ethnicity: African-American/Black
Degree and Year: PhD 1991
Major Field: Developmental Psychology
Specialty: Child Development;Ethnic Minorities;Social
    Cognition;Developmental Psychology;Moral
    Development;Social Development

JONES, Ferdinand
    30 Langham Road
    Providence, RI 02906
    (401) 863-7586-**B**, (401) 331-1039-**H**, (401) 863-1300-**F**
    fjones@brownvm.brown.edu
Ethnicity: African-American/Black
Degree and Year: PhD 1959
Major Field: General Psy./Methods & Systems
Specialty: Clinical Psychology;Psychotherapy;Mental Health
    Services;Cultural & Social Processes;Consulting Psychology

JONES, George L.
    150 Howell Circle
    Suite #411
    Greenville, SC 29615
    (803) 656-2239-**B**, (803) 292-9164-**H**, (803) 656-0760-**F**
Ethnicity: African-American/Black
Degree and Year: PhD 1986
Major Field: Clinical Psychology
Specialty: Clinical Child Psychology;Cognitive Behavioral
    Therapy;Cross Cultural Processes;Family Therapy;Ethnic
    Minorities

JONES, Hugh E.
    7130 Medallion Drive
    East Lansing, MI 48917-8530
    (616) 247-3212-**B**
Ethnicity: African-American/Black
Degree and Year: PhD 1975
Major Field: Clinical Psychology
Specialty: Employee Assistance Programs

JONES, James M.
    705 Quaint Acres Drive
    Silver Spring, MD 20904
    (301) 831-2271-**B**, (301) 680-0532-**H**
    jjones@apa.org
Ethnicity: African-American/Black
Degree and Year: PhD 1970
Major Field: Social Psychology
Specialty: Ethnic Minorities;Cultural & Social Processes;Personality
    Measurement;Training & Development;Giftedness

JONES, Paulette
    New York City Board of Education
    36 Court Street
    Brooklyn, NY 11201
    (212) 297-0210-**H**
Ethnicity: African-American/Black
Degree and Year: EdM 1992
Major Field: Cognitive Psychology

JONES, Reginald
    1217 Salem Avenue
    Suite #8
    Dayton, OH 45406
    (513) 277-8961-**B**, (513) 278-0026-**H**
Ethnicity: African-American/Black
Degree and Year: PhD 1990
Major Field: Clinical Psychology

JONES, Reginald L.
    Hampton University
    Department of Psychology
    Hampton, VA 23668
    (757) 727-5104-**B**, (804) 838-1980-**H**, (757) 827-1060-**F**
Ethnicity: African-American/Black
Degree and Year: PhD 1959
Major Field: Educational Psychology

JONES, Ruby M.
    Comprehensive Outpatient
      Psychological Expertise (C.O.P.E.)
    337 Brightseat Raod, Suite 101
    Landover, MD 20785
    (301) 925-4855-**B**, (301) 773-8219-**H**, (301) 423-6206-**F**

copez@pop.erols.com
Ethnicity: African-American/Black
Degree and Year: PhD 1986
Major Field: Clinical Psychology
Specialty: Depression;Alcoholism & Alcohol Abuse;Drug Abuse;Cross Cultural Processes;Family Processes

JONES, Russell T.
Virginia Tech. University
Dept. of Psychology
7092 B. Depring Hall
Blacksburg, VA 24060
(703) 231-5934-**B**, (703) 552-3926-**H**, (703) 231-3652-**F**
Ethnicity: African-American/Black
Degree and Year: PhD 1976
Major Field: Clinical Child Psychology
Specialty: Accident Prevention/Safety;Behavior Therapy;Child & Pediatric Psychology;Ethnic Minorities;Stress

JORDAN, Albert K.
Oaklawn Hospital
330 Lakeview Drive
PO Box 809
Goshen, IN 46527
(219) 533-1234-**B**, (219) 537-2673-**F**
Ethnicity: African-American/Black
Degree and Year: PsyD 1987
Major Field: unknown
Specialty: Assessment/Diagnosis/Evaluation;Community Mental Health;Group Psychotherapy;Clinical Psychology;Family Therapy;Individual Psychotherapy

JOSEPH, JR., Herbert M.
9505 Nightson Lane
Columbia, MD 21046
(617) 414-4646-**B**, (301) 362-5993-**H**, (617) 44-4792-**F**
herbjoseph@aol.com
Ethnicity: African-American/Black
Degree and Year: PhD 1982 MPH 1996
Major Field: Clinical Psychology
Specialty: Clinical Psychology;Ethnic Minorities;Smoking;Community Psychology;Community Mental Health;Training & Development

JOSHI, Sheila
1947 Divisadero Street
Suite 1
San Francisco, CA 94115
(510) 869-5021-**B**, (510) 658-2142-**H**, (510) 658-2142-**F**
drsjoshi@ccnet.com
Ethnicity: Asian-American/Asian/Pacific Islander
Languages: Spanish
Degree and Year: PhD 1992
Major Field: Clinical Psychology
Specialty: Consulting Psychology

JOURE, Sylvia A.
4646 Popluar Circle
Suite 335
Memphis, TN 38115-4433
(901) 683-7792-**B**, (901) 360-8229-**F**
Ethnicity: American Indian/Alaska Native
Degree and Year: PhD 1970
Major Field: Industrial/Organizational Psy.

Specialty: Industrial/Organizational Psychology;Selection & Placement;Training & Development;Survey Theory & Methodology;Systems, Methods & Issues

JOVE-ALTMAN, Jacqueline
20 Stuyvesant oval #12H
New York, NY 10009
212/253-8496-**B**, 212/995-0914-**H**
bja52994@aol.com
Ethnicity: Hispanic/Latino
Languages: Spanish
Degree and Year: PhD 1995
Major Field: School Psychology
Specialty: Child Development

JUAREZ, Reina M.
P.O. Box 12771
La Jolla, CA 92039-2771
(619) 452-7136-**B**
Ethnicity: Hispanic/Latino
Degree and Year: PhD 1982
Major Field: Clinical Psychology
Specialty: Psychotherapy

JUE, Ronald W.
PO Box 5805
Fullerton, CA 92635
(714) 738-8889-**B**, (714) 526-0417-**H**, (714) 447-4701-**F**
Ethnicity: Asian-American/Asian/Pacific Islander
Degree and Year: PhD 1976
Major Field: Clinical Psychology
Specialty: Hypnosis/Hypnotherapy;Adult Development;Clinical Psychology;Psychosomatic Disorders;Religious Psychology

JUNE, Lee N.
Michigan State University
Office of Provost
153 Student Services Building
East Lansing, MI 48824
(517) 355-2264-**B**, (517) 372-2821-**H**, (517) 432-2855-**F**
leejune@pilot.msu.edu
Ethnicity: African-American/Black
Degree and Year: PhD 1974
Major Field: Clinical Psychology
Specialty: Administration;Ethnic Minorities;Vocational Psychology;Clinical Psychology;Marriage & Family

JUN, Heesoon
Evergreen State College
Olympia, WA 98505
(360) 866-6000-**B**
junh@elwha.evergreen.edu
Ethnicity: American Indian/Alaska Native
Languages: Korean
Degree and Year: PhD 1982
Major Field: Counseling Psychology
Specialty: Clinical Psychology;Cross Cultural Processes;Ethnic Minorities;Counseling Psychology;Developmental Psychology;Individual Psychotherapy

JUNN, Ellen
California State University
Child & Adolescence Studies
California State University @ Fullerton

PO Box 6868
Fullerton, CA 92634-6868
(714) 773-4285-**B**, (714) 998-3708-**H**, (714) 773-3314-**F**
Ethnicity: Asian-American/Asian/Pacific Islander
Degree and Year: PhD 1984
Major Field: Developmental Psychology
Specialty: Cognitive Psychology;Child Development;Social
    Cognition;Preschool & Day Care Issues

JURILLA-PASTRANA, Lina L.
Department of Youth Authority
13200 South Bloomfield
Norwalk, CA 90650
(562) 868-9979-**B**, (714) 994-4101-**F**
Ethnicity: Asian-American/Asian/Pacific Islander
Languages: Filipino
Degree and Year: PhD 1985
Major Field: Clinical Psychology
Specialty: Adolescent Therapy;Cognitive Behavioral Therapy;Forensic
    Psychology;Affective Disorders;Correctional
    Psychology;Group Psychotherapy

KAGEHIRO, Dorthy K.
3304 Jefferson Court
Alpharetta, GA 30005-3833
(215) 787-1643-**B**
Ethnicity: Asian-American/Asian/Pacific Islander
Degree and Year: PhD 1981
Major Field: Social Psychology
Specialty: Social Psychology

KAHAN, Harry
98 Liberty Avenue
Rockville Centre, NY 11570
(516) 764-7820-**B**, (516) 764-2387-**H**
Ethnicity: Hispanic/Latino
Languages: Spanish
Degree and Year: PhD 1991
Major Field: Clinical Psychology
Specialty: Psychoanalysis;Educational Psychology;Crisis Intervention
    & Therapy;School Psychology;Psychotherapy;Cross Cultural
    Processes

KAKAIYA, Divya
11739 Thomas Hayes Lane
San Diego, CA 92126-1144
(619) 622-0221-**B**, (619) 578-8975-**H**, (619) 622-0201-**F**
divya@flash.net
Ethnicity: Asian-American/Asian/Pacific Islander
Languages: Hindi, Urdu, Gurajati, Punjabi
Degree and Year: PhD 1991
Major Field: Clinical Psychology
Specialty: Eating Disorders;Family Therapy;Alcoholism & Alcohol
    Abuse;Depression;Ethnic Minorities;Cross Cultural Processes

KAMANO, Dennis K.
731 N Academy Street
Galesburg, IL 61401-2638
(309) 343-4564-**B**
Ethnicity: Asian-American/Asian/Pacific Islander
Degree and Year: PhD 1957
Major Field: Clinical Psychology
Specialty: Psychotherapy

KAME'ENUI, Edward J.
University of Oregon
IDEA
170 College of Education
Eugene, OR 97403-1211
(541) 346-1644-**B**, (541) 344-9506-**H**, (541) 346-3581-**F**
Ethnicity: Asian-American/Asian/Pacific Islander
Degree and Year: PhD
Major Field: Educational Psychology
Specialty: Educational Research;Learning Disabilities;Research &
    Training;Instructional Methods

KAMESHIMA, Shinya
Kansai University of Welfare Science
Department of Social Work
3-11-1 Asahigaoka
Kashiwara City
Oska, 582-0026
JAPAN
011 81729780088-**B**, 011 81729702151-**H**, 011 81729780377-**F**
la,esjo,a@filso-kagk-u.ac.jp
Ethnicity: Asian-American/Asian/Pacific Islander
Languages: Japanese
Degree and Year: PhD 1989
Major Field: Developmental Psychology
Specialty: Child Development;Computer Applications and
    Programming;Human Development & Family Studies;Parent-
    Child Interaction;Research Design & Methodology

KAMII, Constance
University of Alabama
@ Birmingham
University Station
Birmingham, AL 35205-3617
Ethnicity: Asian-American/Asian/Pacific Islander
Degree and Year: PhD 1965
Major Field: unknown
Specialty: Curriculum Development/Evaluation

KAM, Sherilyn M.
The Permanente Medical Group
1800 Harrison Street
7th Floor
Oakland, CA 94612
(510) 267-4230-**B**
sherilyn.m.kam@ncal.kaiperm.or
Ethnicity: Asian-American/Asian/Pacific Islander
Degree and Year: PhD 1995
Major Field: Industrial/Organizational Psy.
Specialty: Industrial/Organizational Psychology

KANESHIGE, Edward
University of Hawaii
Counseling & Student Development Center
240 Campus Road
Honolulu, HI 96822
(808) 956-7927-**B**, (808) 732-6292-**H**, (808) 956-5076-**F**
Ethnicity: Asian-American/Asian/Pacific Islander
Degree and Year: EdD 1959
Major Field: unknown
Specialty: Counseling Psychology;Psychotherapy;Vocational
    Psychology;Administration

KANG, Tai Lydia
3354 Cardoza Avenue
Marina, CA 93933-2132
(309) 827-6026-**B**
Ethnicity: Asian-American/Asian/Pacific Islander
Degree and Year: MA 1982
Major Field: Clinical Psychology
Specialty: Psychotherapy

KANNARKAT, Joy P.
Norfolk State University
Department of Psychology
2401 Corprew Avenue
Norfolk, VA 23504
(804) 486-4061-**B**, (804) 683-8573-**H**
Ethnicity: Asian-American/Asian/Pacific Islander
Languages: Malayalam
Degree and Year: PhD 1975
Major Field: Personality Psychology
Specialty: Adolescent Therapy;Attention Deficit Disorders;Child Therapy;Clinical Psychology;Family Therapy

KANUNGO, Rabindra
McGill University
Faculty of Management
1001 Sherbrooke Street, West
Montreal
Quebec H3A 1G5,
CANADA
(514) 398-4040-**B**, (514) 745-0666-**H**, (514) 398-3876-**F**
Ethnicity: Asian-American/Asian/Pacific Islander
Languages: Hindi, Oriya
Degree and Year: PhD 1962
Major Field: Industrial/Organizational Psy.
Specialty: Attitudes & Opinions;Cross Cultural Processes;Leadership;Motivation;Social Psychology

KAO, Barbara T.
Rhode Island Hospital
593 Eddy Street
Providence, RI 02903
(401) 444-5609-**B**, (401) 351-2922-**H**, (401) 444-6115-**F**
bkao@webtv.net
Ethnicity: Asian-American/Asian/Pacific Islander
Degree and Year: PhD 1991
Major Field: Clinical Psychology
Specialty: Child & Pediatric Psychology;School Psychology;Clinical Child Psychology

KARSON, Samuel
6737 Fairfax Road
Chevy Chase, MD 20815-6518
(301) 656-3960-**B**, (301) 652-3960-**H**
Ethnicity: American Indian/Alaska Native
Degree and Year: PhD 1952
Major Field: Clinical Psychology
Specialty: Personality Measurement

KASHIKAR-ZUCK, Susmita M.
University of Florida
Department of Clinical & Health Psych.
1600 SW Archer Road
Room DG-91
Gainesville, FL 32610
(352) 395-0680-**B**, (352) 379-5896-**H**, (352) 395-0468-**F**

szuck@hp.ufl.edu
Ethnicity: Asian-American/Asian/Pacific Islander
Languages: Hindi
Degree and Year: PhD 1995
Major Field: Clinical Psychology
Specialty: Medical Psychology;Pain & Pain Management

KATO, Takashi
Faculty of Informatics
Kansai University
Takatsuki-Shi
Osaka,   179,
JAPAN
Ethnicity: Asian-American/Asian/Pacific Islander
Degree and Year: PhD 1983
Major Field: Cognitive Psychology
Specialty: Memory

KAU, Alice S. M.
Kennedy Krieger Institute
Johns Hopkins Hospital
10405 Blue Arrow Road
Columbia, MD 21044
(410) 502-8103-**B**, (410) 964-0530-**H**, (410) 509-9383-**F**
hagaman@kennedykrieger.org
Ethnicity: Asian-American/Asian/Pacific Islander
Languages: Chinese
Degree and Year: PhD 1985
Major Field: Developmental Psychology
Specialty: Child Development;Child & Pediatric Psychology;Chronically Mentally Ill;Mentally Retarded;Mental Disorders

KAWAHARA, Yoshito
6128 Tamilynn Street
San Diego, CA 92122
(619) 627-2954-**B**, (619) 458-1710-**H**
Ethnicity: Asian-American/Asian/Pacific Islander
Degree and Year: PhD 1978
Major Field: Physiological Psychology
Specialty: Biofeedback;Stress;Learning/Learning Theory;Cross Cultural Processes;Health Psychology

KEE, Daniel W.
California State University
Department of Psychology
Fullerton, CA 92634
Ethnicity: Asian-American/Asian/Pacific Islander
Degree and Year: PhD 1974
Major Field: Developmental Psychology
Specialty: Neuropsychology

KEEFE, Keunho
734 East Chapman Avenue
Orange, CA 92866
(714) 324-4215-**B**, (714) 992-0688-**F**
Ethnicity: Asian-American/Asian/Pacific Islander
Languages: Korean
Degree and Year: PhD 1989
Major Field: Developmental Psychology
Specialty: Adolescent Development;Developmental Psychology;Forensic Psychology;Ethnic Minorities;Clinical Child Psychology

KEE, PooKong
Bureau of Immigration Research

22 Wimba Avenue
Kew,
AUSTRALIA
(03)3 42-1103-**B**
Ethnicity: Asian-American/Asian/Pacific Islander
Degree and Year: PhD 1980
Major Field: unknown
Specialty: Cross Cultural Processes

KEGLAR, Shelvy H.
3676 N Washington Boulevard
Indianapolis, IN 46205-3560
(317) 923-3930-**B**, (317) 872-9727-**H**, (317) 923-2441-**F**
Ethnicity: African-American/Black
Degree and Year: PhD 1979
Major Field: Clinical Psychology
Specialty: Alcoholism & Alcohol Abuse;Group Psychotherapy;Clinical
    Psychology;Neuropsychology;Group Psychotherapy

KEITA, Gwendolyn P.
American Psychological Association
750 First Street, NE
Washington, DC 20002-4242
(202) 336-6044-**B**, (202) 726-7290-**H**, (202) 336-6117-**F**
gkeita@apa.org
Ethnicity: African-American/Black
Degree and Year: PhD 1977
Major Field: Personality Psychology
Specialty: Gender Issues;Stress;Cross Cultural Processes;Social
    Psychology;Ethnic Minorities

KELLY-RADFORD, Lily M.
8 Gwyn Ln
Greensboro, NC 27403-1088
(919) 288-7210-**B**, (919) 299-6203-**H**
Ethnicity: African-American/Black
Degree and Year: PhD 1982
Major Field: Clinical Psychology

KELLY, Jennifer F.
Atlanta Center for Behavioral Medicine
3280 Howell Mill Road Suite 100
Atlanta, GA 30327
404 351-6789-**B**, 404 319-0541-**H**, 404 351-2932-**F**
jfkphd@aol.com
Ethnicity: African-American/Black
Degree and Year: PhD 1987
Major Field: Clinical Psychology
Specialty: Medical Psychology;Pain & Pain
    Management;Stress;Psychosomatic Disorders

KELLY, Tara L.
12304 Santa Monica, Blvd.
Suite #106
Los Angeles, CA 90025
(310) 559-3620-**B**, (310) 204-1793-**H**
Ethnicity: Hispanic/Latino
Degree and Year: PhD 1988
Major Field: Clinical Psychology
Specialty: Adolescent Therapy;Crisis Intervention & Therapy;Eating
    Disorders;Parent-Child Interaction;Marriage & Family

KELTON-BRAND, Ana
9641 NW 49th Place
Coral Springs, FL 33076-2452

(407) 498-3133-**B**
Ethnicity: Hispanic/Latino
Degree and Year: PhD 1985
Major Field: Clinical Psychology
Specialty: Psychotherapy

KEMP, Arthur D.
910 Conventry Ct
Warrensburg, MO 64093-
(660) 543-8166-**B**, (660) 429-5237-**H**
Ethnicity: African-American/Black
Degree and Year: PhD 1989
Major Field: Counseling Psychology
Specialty: Clinical Neuropsychology;Ethnic
    Minorities;Administration;Medical Psychology;Pain & Pain
    Management

KENNEDY, Clive D.
6090 South Sepulveda Boulevard
Suite #330
Culver City, CA 90230
(310) 216-0329-**B**, (213) 299-5540-**H**, (805) 943-3871-**F**
clivekennedy@msn.com
Ethnicity: African-American/Black
Degree and Year: PhD 1981
Major Field: Clinical Psychology
Specialty: Assessment/Diagnosis/Evaluation;HIV/AIDS;Alcoholism &
    Alcohol Abuse;Drug Abuse;Family Therapy;Forensic
    Psychology

KHALILI, Hassan
Waterford Hospital
Waterford Bridge Road
St. John's, NF A1E 4J8
CANADA
(709) 738-5665-**B**, (709) 745-8405-**H**, (709) 738-5667-**F**
hkhalili@morgan.ucs.mun.ca
Ethnicity: Asian-American/Asian/Pacific Islander
Languages: Farsi
Degree and Year: PhD 1982
Major Field: Clinical Psychology
Specialty: Clinical Psychology;Health Psychology;Developmental
    Psychology

KHAN, Badrul A.
Huronia Regional Center
P.O. Box 1000
Orillia, Ontario, L3V 6L2
CANADA
(705) 326-7361-**B**, (705) 721-5049-**H**, (705) 721-1797-**F**
akhan@barint.on.ea
Ethnicity: Asian-American/Asian/Pacific Islander
Languages: Bengali
Degree and Year: PhD 1971
Major Field: Clinical Psychology
Specialty: Assessment/Diagnosis/Evaluation;Psychotherapy;Employee
    Assistance Programs;Clinical Psychology;Hypnosis/
    Hypnotherapy;Cognitive Behavioral Therapy

KHAN, Kanwar H.
C/O Papago Agency
Department of Interior
Indian Education Programs

PO Box 38
Sells, AZ 95634
011 23321228440-**B**, 011 23321776953-**H**
Ethnicity: Asian-American/Asian/Pacific Islander
Degree and Year: PhD 1976
Major Field: Educational Psychology

KHANNA, Jaswant L.
474 McElroy Road
Memphis, TN 38120-1513
(901) 528-6628-**B**, (901) 767-8114-**H**
Ethnicity: Asian-American/Asian/Pacific Islander
Languages: Hindi, Urdu, Punjabi
Degree and Year: PhD 1956
Major Field: Clinical Psychology
Specialty: Psychotherapy;Group Psychotherapy;Ethnic
    Minorities;Hypnosis/Hypnotherapy;Humanistic Psychology

KHANNA, Mukti
474 McElroy Road
Memphis, TN 38120
(970) 247-7637-**B**, (901) 767-8114-**H**, (970) 247-7623-**F**
khannam@fortlewis.edu
Ethnicity: Asian-American/Asian/Pacific Islander
Degree and Year: PhD 1989
Major Field: Clinical Psychology
Specialty: Hypnosis/Hypnotherapy;Nonverbal
    Communication;Psychology & the Arts;Clinical
    Psychology;Social Psychology;Ethnic Minorities

KHORAKIWALA, Durriyah
Horizons Family Counseling
1112 South Livermore Avenue
Livermore, CA 914550
(9250) 485-1252-**B**, (925) 426-7472-**H**, (925) 485-1252-**F**
durriyah@msn.com
Ethnicity: Asian-American/Asian/Pacific Islander
Languages: Hindi, Urdu, Gujerah
Degree and Year: PhD 1991
Major Field: Clinical Psychology
Specialty: Psychotherapy;Behavior Therapy;Family Therapy;Forensic
    Psychology

KICH, George K.
1678 Shattuck Avenue
Berkeley, CA 94709
(510) 528-7732-**B**
Ethnicity: Asian-American/Asian/Pacific Islander
Degree and Year: PhD 1982
Major Field: Clinical Psychology
Specialty: Ethnic Minorities;Marriage & Family;Gender
    Issues;Research & Training;Individual Psychotherapy

KICH, George Kitahara
National Jury Project/West
One Kaiser Plaze, Suite 1410
Oakland, CA 94612-3604
(510) 832-2583-**B**, (510) 528-7732-**H**, (510) 839-8642-**F**
georgekk@dnai.com
Ethnicity: Asian-American/Asian/Pacific Islander
Degree and Year: PhD 1982
Major Field: Clinical Psychology
Specialty: Ethnic Minorities;Gender Issues;Crime & Criminal
    Behavior;Psychology & Law;Crime & Criminal
    Behavior;Cultural & Social Processes

KIMBAUER, Elli M.
St. Timothy Lutheran Church
52 Soledad Drive
Monterey, CA 93940
(408) 375-2042-**B**, (408) 375-7636-**H**, (408) 375-2036-**F**
StTimLuth@aol.com
Ethnicity: Asian-American/Asian/Pacific Islander
Degree and Year: PsyD 1993
Major Field: Clinical Psychology
Specialty: Pastoral Psychology

KIM, Chang-Dai
Keimyung University
Department of Education
School of Education
100 Shin Dang-Dong Dahlseo-Gu
Daegu, 218
South Korea
011820535805593-**B**, 011820535868542-**H**, 01182535868542-**F**
edkim@kmucc.keimyung.qc.kr
Ethnicity: Asian-American/Asian/Pacific Islander
Languages: Korean
Degree and Year: EdD 1994
Major Field: unknown
Specialty: Adolescent Therapy;Counseling Psychology;Cross Cultural
    Processes;Psychotherapy;Creativity

KIM, Elizabeth J.
16211 East Promontory Place
La Mirada, CA 90638
(714) 761-0203-**B**, (310) 761-5156-**H**, (714) 761-0283-**F**
Ethnicity: Asian-American/Asian/Pacific Islander
Languages: Korean
Degree and Year: PhD 1990
Major Field: Counseling Psychology
Specialty: Child Abuse;Ethnic Minorities;Gender Issues;Managed
    Care;Marriage & Family

KIM, Mary Ann Y.
2443 Fillmore, #138
San Francisco, CA 94115
(415) 905-9680-**B**, (415) 905-9680-**H**, (415) 383-3929-**F**
Ethnicity: Asian-American/Asian/Pacific Islander
Degree and Year: PhD 1984
Major Field: Clinical Psychology
Specialty: Neuropsychology;Forensic Psychology;Assessment/
    Diagnosis/Evaluation;Pain & Pain Management

KIM, Randi I.
Humboldt State University
Department of Psychology
1 Harps Street
Arcata, CA 95521
(707) 826-3270-**B**, (707) 825-7851-**H**, (707) 826-4993-**F**
rlk1@axe.humboldt.edu
Ethnicity: Asian-American/Asian/Pacific Islander
Languages: Korean
Degree and Year: PhD 1992
Major Field: Counseling Psychology
Specialty: Counseling Psychology;Ethnic Minorities;Client-Centered
    Therapy;Cultural & Social Processes;Vocational
    Psychology;Interpersonal Processes & Relations

KIM, Seock-Ho
  The University of Georgia
  325 Aderhold Hall
  Athens, GA 30602
  (706) 542-4224-**B**, (7060 354-0431-**H**, (706) 542-4240-**F**
  skim@coe.uga.edu
Ethnicity: Asian-American/Asian/Pacific Islander
Languages: Korean
Degree and Year: PhD 1991
Major Field: Quan/Math & Psychometrics/Stat
Specialty: Educational
      Psychology;Measurement;Psychometrics;Quantitative/
      Mathematical, Psychometrics;Research Design &
      Methodology;Statistics

KIM, Sook K.
  The University of Texas at Dallas
  PO Box 830688
  EC 3.4
  Richardson, TX 75083-0688
  (972) 883-2993-**B**
Ethnicity: Asian-American/Asian/Pacific Islander
Degree and Year: PhD 1998
Major Field: Developmental Psychology
Specialty: Ethnic Minorities;Social Cognition;Program Evaluation;Cross
      Cultural Processes;Measurement;Statistics

KIM, Sung C.
  2477 Washington Street
  San Francisco, CA 94115
  (415) 441-1233-**B**
Ethnicity: Asian-American/Asian/Pacific Islander
Languages: Korean
Degree and Year: PhD 1980
Major Field: Clinical Psychology
Specialty: Cognitive Behavioral Therapy;Ethnic Minorities;Psychology
      & Law;Sex/Marital Therapy

KIM, Yang Ja
  108 Pershing Road
  Englewood Cliffs, NJ 07632
  (212) 865-2002-**B**, (201) 894-1675-**H**, (201) 541-1267-**F**
Ethnicity: Asian-American/Asian/Pacific Islander
Languages: Korean
Degree and Year: PhD 1980
Major Field: Educational Psychology
Specialty: Assessment/Diagnosis/Evaluation;Clinical
      Psychology;General Psychology;Personality Theory

KIM, Yung Che
  MIRINEI Apt., #5-307
  Bong-Duck-Dong San 89-3
  SOUTH KOREA
  (53) 580-5429-**B**, (53) 471-5989-**H**, 82-53-580-5313-**F**
  kimyung@kmcc.keimyung.ac.kr
Ethnicity: Asian-American/Asian/Pacific Islander
Languages: Korean
Degree and Year: PhD 1971
Major Field: Cognitive Psychology
Specialty: Cognitive Psychology;Educational Psychology;Information
      Processing;Problem Solving;Memory

KING, Valerie
  297 Prospect Place
  Brooklyn, NY 11238-3902
  (718) 857-5838-**B**, (718) 638-5826-**F**
  valerieking@compuserve.com
Ethnicity: African-American/Black
Degree and Year: PhD 1983
Major Field: Clinical Psychology
Specialty: Child Development;Family Therapy;Parent-Child
      Interaction;Cross Cultural Processes;Mental Health
      Services;Community Mental Health

KIRKLEN, Leonard E.
  5125 Sterling Mnaor Drive
  Tampa, FL 33647-2010
  (813) 974-2831-**B**
Ethnicity: African-American/Black
Degree and Year: PhD 1982
Major Field: Clinical Psychology
Specialty: Psychotherapy

KIRST, Stephen P.
  941 Westwood Boulevard
  Suite #215
  Westwood Village, CA 90024
  (310) 208-6244-**H**, (310) 998-9141-**F**
Ethnicity: Hispanic/Latino
Degree and Year: PhD 1975
Major Field: Clinical Psychology
Specialty: Clinical Psychology;Eating Disorders;Individual
      Psychotherapy;Social Change

KITANO, Margie K.
  San Diego State University
  Department of Special Education
  San Diego, CA 92182-0001
  (619) 594-0731-**B**, (619) 229-0523-**H**, (619) 594-6628-**F**
  kitano@mail.sdsu.edu
Ethnicity: Asian-American/Asian/Pacific Islander
Degree and Year: PhD 1976
Major Field: Educational Psychology

KITAYAMA, Shinobu
  University of Kyoto
  Department of Psychology
  Faculty of Integrated Human Service
  Kyoto,
  JAPAN
  81-782-753-6557-**B**
Ethnicity: Asian-American/Asian/Pacific Islander
Degree and Year: PhD 1987
Major Field: Social Psychology
Specialty: Cultural & Social Processes

KLOPNER, Michele C.
  PO 6245
  Laredo, TX 78042
  (210) 723-2256-**H**
Ethnicity: African-American/Black
Languages: French, Haitian,Creole
Degree and Year: PhD 1985
Major Field: Clinical Psychology
Specialty: Assessment/Diagnosis/Evaluation;Community Mental
      Health;Cross Cultural Processes;HIV/AIDS;Forensic
      Psychology

KNAPP, W. Mace
Nevada State Prison
PO Box 6
Silver City, NV 89428
(702) 887-3406-**B**, (702) 847-0368-**H**
Ethnicity: American Indian/Alaska Native
Languages: French, Spanish
Degree and Year: PhD 1970
Major Field: Social Psychology
Specialty: Correctional Psychology;Drug Abuse;Alcoholism & Alcohol
    Abuse;HIV/AIDS;Sexual Dysfunction

KOBAYASHI, Steve K.
23505 Crenshaw Bl. #220
Torrance, CA 90505
(310) 257-9486-**B**, (310) 832-7008-**H**, (310) 832-6885-**F**
Ethnicity: Asian-American/Asian/Pacific Islander
Languages: Japanese
Degree and Year: PhD 1982
Major Field: Clinical Psychology
Specialty: Psychotherapy;Clinical Neuropsychology;Cross Cultural
    Processes;Neuropsychology;Forensic Psychology;Personality
    Disorders

KOCHEVAR-SUKKARIE, Renee J.
Harvard School of Public Health
Department of Health and Social Behavior
1637 Tremont Street
Boston, MA 02128
(617) 432-3231-**B**, (617) 738-7771-**H**, (617) 432-2061-**F**
Ethnicity: Hispanic/Latino
Degree and Year: PhD 1990
Major Field: Clinical Psychology
Specialty: Cognitive Behavioral Therapy;Clinical
    Research;Epidemiology & Biometry;Cardiovascular Processes

KOH, Tong-He
Independent Practice
6007 N Sheridan Road
Apartment 10-B
Chicago, IL 60660
(773) 907-9344-**B**, (773) 878-4109-**H**, (773) 907-9568-**F**
tonghekoh@aol.com
Ethnicity: Asian-American/Asian/Pacific Islander
Languages: Japanese, Korean
Degree and Year: PhD 1960
Major Field: Clinical Psychology
Specialty: Clinical Psychology;Clinical Child Psychology;Cognitive
    Behavioral Therapy;Assessment/Diagnosis/Evaluation;Cross
    Cultural Processes;Ethnic Minorities

KO, Hwawei
National Chung Cheng University
Department of Psychology
Ming-Shiung
Chia-Yi,
TAIWAN
05-272-0411-**B**, 05-272-0837-**F**
psyhwk@ccunix.ccu.edu.tw
Ethnicity: Asian-American/Asian/Pacific Islander
Languages: Chinese
Degree and Year: PhD 1982
Major Field: Developmental Psychology
Specialty: Learning/Learning Theory;Child Development

KOLT, Laurie
1030 Pearl Street
Suite 3
La Jolla, CA 92037-1704
(619) 456-2005-**B**, (619) 592-9121-**H**
ljkolt@aol.com
Ethnicity: Hispanic/Latino
Degree and Year: PhD 1982
Major Field: Clinical Psychology
Specialty: Industrial/Organizational Psychology;Psychology of
    Women;Stress;Market Analysis;Psychotherapy;Professional
    Issues in Psychology

KONDO, Charles Y.
907 S. Fariview Avenue
Salt Lake City, UT 84105-1703
(801) 350-4981-**B**, (801) 582-5588-**H**
Ethnicity: Asian-American/Asian/Pacific Islander
Degree and Year: PhD 1979
Major Field: Clinical Psychology

KOP, Tim M.
Century Center
1750 Kalakaua Avenue
Suite #3-520
Honolulu, HI 96826-3766
(808) 942-3786-**B**
Ethnicity: Asian-American/Asian/Pacific Islander
Languages: Japanese, Korean, Hawaiin
Degree and Year: PhD 1991
Major Field: Industrial/Organizational Psy.
Specialty: Cross Cultural Processes;Human
    Factors;Neurosciences;Artificial Intelligence;Information
    Processing

KOSHINO, Hideya
California State University, San Bernardino
5500 University Parkway
San Barnardino, CA 92407
(909) 880-5435-**B**, (909) 784-5446-**H**, (909) 880-7003-**F**
hkoshino@wiley.csusb.edu
Ethnicity: Asian-American/Asian/Pacific Islander
Degree and Year: PhD 1994
Major Field: Cognitive Psychology
Specialty: Cognitive Psychology;Experimental Psychology;Sensory &
    Perceptual Processes;Vision

KOTHANDAPANI, Virupaksha
5757 Chester Court
Mobile, AL 36609
(205) 666-7765-**B**, (205) 344-1902-**H**
Ethnicity: Asian-American/Asian/Pacific Islander
Languages: Hindi, Urdu, Telugu, Tamil
Degree and Year: PhD 1970
Major Field: Social Psychology
Specialty: Assessment/Diagnosis/Evaluation;Cognitive Behavioral
    Therapy;Hypnosis/Hypnotherapy;Clinical
    Neuropsychology;Rational-Emotive Therapy

KRAMER, Diana R.
One Colonial Way
Chatham, NJ 07928
(201) 635-6867-**B**, (201) 635-6867-**H**
Ethnicity: Hispanic/Latino
Degree and Year: PhD 1976

Major Field: Industrial/Organizational Psy.
Specialty: Human Resources;Organizational Development;Management
& Organization;Leadership;Cultural & Social Processes

KRAMER, Harry M. O.
121 Frost Mountain Drive
Ellensbury, WA 98926
(509) 925-9861-**B**, (509) 962-2112-**H**
Ethnicity: Hispanic/Latino
Degree and Year: PhD 1983
Major Field: Counseling Psychology
Specialty: Forensic Psychology;Alcoholism & Alcohol
Abuse;Assessment/Diagnosis/Evaluation;Correctional
Psychology;Psychotherapy

KRANAU, Edgar J.
2021 South Lewis Avenue
Suite 725
Tulsa, OK 74104
(918) 712-9020-**B**, (918) 747-7643-**H**
Ethnicity: Hispanic/Latino
Degree and Year: PhD 1983
Major Field: Clinical Psychology
Specialty: Psychotherapy;Adolescent Therapy

KUAN, Yie-Wen Y.
3025 NE 194th Street
Seattle, WA 98155
(206) 543-1240-**B**
Ethnicity: Asian-American/Asian/Pacific Islander
Languages: Chinese
Degree and Year: PhD 1990
Major Field: Clinical Psychology
Specialty: Clinical
Psychology;Psychotherapy;Psychopathology;Mental Health
Services

KUMAR, Santosh
Rancho Los Amigos Medical Center
7601 E Imperial Highway
Downey, CA 90242-3456
Ethnicity: Asian-American/Asian/Pacific Islander
Degree and Year: PhD 1970
Major Field: unknown
Specialty: Clinical Psychology;Rehabilitation

KUMAR, V. K.
602 W Nields Street
West Chester, PA 19382
Ethnicity: Asian-American/Asian/Pacific Islander
Degree and Year: PhD 1972
Major Field: Educational Psychology

KUNITAKE, Yutaka
13286 Glencliff Way
San Diego, CA 92130-1309
Ethnicity: Asian-American/Asian/Pacific Islander
Degree and Year: PhD 1965
Major Field: Educational Psychology
Specialty: Statistics

KUPUR, Veena
4615 Morgan Drive
Chevy Chase, MD 20815
(301) 951-9612-**B**, (301) 986-0214-**H**
Ethnicity: Asian-American/Asian/Pacific Islander

Languages: Hindi, Urdu, Punjabi
Degree and Year: PhD 1973
Major Field: Clinical Psychology
Specialty: Psychotherapy;Assessment/Diagnosis/Evaluation;Marriage
& Family;Adolescent Therapy;Child Therapy

KURATO, Yoshiya
Osaka City University
3-138 Sugimoto 3-Chome
Sumiyoshi-Ku
Osaka,
JAPAN
(0886)87-1311-**B**, (078) 842-2898-**H**
Ethnicity: Asian-American/Asian/Pacific Islander
Degree and Year: EdD 1975
Major Field: unknown

KUROSAWA, Kaoru
Chiba University
Faculty of Letters
1-33 Yayoi-Cho, Inage-Ku
Chiba City, JAPAN
043-251-1111-**B**, 043-462-4273-**H**, 043-290-2285-**F**
kurosawa@bun.l.chiba.u.ac.jp
Ethnicity: Asian-American/Asian/Pacific Islander
Languages: Japanese
Degree and Year: PhD 1986
Major Field: Social Psychology
Specialty: Communication;Cultural & Social
Processes;Emotion;Personality Psychology

KWEI-LEVY, Carol
638 Newton-Yardley Road
Suite #1G
Newtown, PA 18940-1738
(215) 860-0938-**B**, (215) 860-9758-**H**
clevy@viocenet.com
Ethnicity: Asian-American/Asian/Pacific Islander
Degree and Year: PhD 1986
Major Field: Clinical Psychology
Specialty: Neurosciences;Psychotherapy;Neuropsychology;Parent-
Child Interaction;Learning Disabilities;Stress

KWON, Paul H.
Washington State University
PO Box 644820
Pullman, WA 99164-4820
(509) 335-4633-**B**, (509) 332-2810-**H**, (509) 335-5043-**F**
kwonp@wsu.edu
Ethnicity: Asian-American/Asian/Pacific Islander
Degree and Year: PhD 1996
Major Field: Clinical Psychology
Specialty: Assessment/Diagnosis/Evaluation;Depression;Projective
Techniques;Cultural & Social Processes;Learning
Disabilities;Psychotherapy

LABARTA, Margarita M.
P.O. Box 141072
Gainesville, FL 32614-1072
(904) 374-5640-**B**
Ethnicity: Hispanic/Latino
Languages: Spanish

Degree and Year: PhD 1982
Major Field: Clinical Psychology
Specialty: Clinical Psychology;Clinical Child Psychology;Assessment/
Diagnosis/Evaluation;Individual Psychotherapy

LABBE, Elise E.
University of South Alabama
Department of Psychology
Mobile, AL 36688
(205) 460-7149-**B**, (205) 844-6849-**H**
elabbe@jaguar1.usouthal.edu
Ethnicity: Hispanic/Latino
Languages: Spanish
Degree and Year: PhD 1983
Major Field: Clinical Psychology
Specialty: Health Psychology;Clinical Child Psychology;Cognitive
Behavioral Therapy;Psychobiology;Child & Pediatric
Psychology

LADUE, Robin A.
1500 Benson Road, South
Suite #201
Renton, WA 98055
(425) 277-5616-**B**, (206) 782-8312-**F**
71524.2541@compuserve.com
Ethnicity: American Indian/Alaska Native
Degree and Year: PhD 1982
Major Field: Clinical Psychology
Specialty: Child Abuse;Cross Cultural Processes;Eating
Disorders;Clinical Psychology;Alcoholism & Alcohol Abuse

LAFARGA-CORONA, Juan B.
U Iberoamericana
Depto Psciologia
P Paseo de la Reforma 880
Lomas de Santa Fe
Mexico City, DF01210
MEXICO
011 525273-3667-**B**, 011 525812-3523-**H**, 011 525273-3667-**F**
Ethnicity: Hispanic/Latino
Degree and Year: PhD 1967
Major Field: Clinical Psychology
Specialty: Client-Centered Therapy;Group Psychotherapy

LAFROMBOISE, Teresa
Stanford University
School of Education
485 Lasuen Mall
Stanford, CA 94305-3009
(650) 723-1202-**B**, (650) 366-6756-**H**, (608)262-9074-**F**
lafromboise@leland.stanford.ed
Ethnicity: American Indian/Alaska Native
Degree and Year: PhD 1980
Major Field: Counseling Psychology
Specialty: Cross Cultural Processes;Community Mental
Health;Cognitive Behavioral Therapy;Suicide

LAGOMASINO, Andrew J.
48 Marion Street
Somerville, MA 02143
(617) 498-1150-**B**, (617) 625-3759-**H**
Ethnicity: Hispanic/Latino
Languages: Spanish
Degree and Year: PsyD 1993

Major Field: Clinical Psychology
Specialty: Clinical Psychology;Cross Cultural Processes;Individual
Psychotherapy

LAGUNA, John N.
Life Span Psychological Services
2819-0 Willow Street Pike
Willow Street, PA 17584
(717) 464-1464-**B**, (717) 464-0877-**H**, (717) 464-4348-**F**
doclags@aol.com
Ethnicity: Hispanic/Latino
Languages: Spanish
Degree and Year: PhD 1983
Major Field: Clinical Psychology
Specialty: Drug Abuse;HIV/AIDS;Gerontology/
Geropsychology;Psychotherapy;Ethnic Minorities

LAMBERT, Michael C.
Michigan State University
Department of Psychology
East Lansing, MI 48824-1117
(517) 432-1625-**B**, (517) 699-1695-**H**
Ethnicity: African-American/Black
Degree and Year: PhD 1988
Major Field: Clinical Psychology
Specialty: Child & Pediatric
Psychology;Disadvantaged;Measurement;Cross Cultural
Processes

LAM, Chow S.
Illinois Institute of Technology
Institute of Psychology
Chicago, IL 60616
(312) 567-3514-**B**, (708) 362-0735-**H**, 312-567-3493-**F**
lam@charlie.cns.iit.edu
Ethnicity: Asian-American/Asian/Pacific Islander
Languages: Chinese
Degree and Year: PhD 1985
Major Field: Counseling Psychology
Specialty: Counseling Psychology;Rehabilitation;Special
Education;Vocational Psychology

LAMPKIN, Emmett C.
1731 Quincent St
Iowa City, IA 52245-5711
(319) 338-0229-**B**, (319) 337-9976-**H**
Ethnicity: African-American/Black
Degree and Year: PhD 1976 MA 1969
Major Field: Social Psychology
Specialty: Mass Media Communication;Developmental Psychology

LANCASTER, JoAnn
St. James Condominiums
3704 N Charles Street
Suite #105
Baltimore, MD 21218
(410) 235-4145-**B**, (410) 235-4146-**H**
Ethnicity: Hispanic/Latino
Degree and Year: PhD 1982
Major Field: Clinical Psychology
Specialty: Clinical Psychology;Biofeedback;Cognitive
Psychology;Personality Psychology;Pain & Pain Management

LANGLEY, Merlin R
Lesley College Graduate School
7 Mellen Street

Cambridge, MA 02138
(617) 349-8336-**B**, 617 860-9132-**H**
Ethnicity: African-American/Black
Degree and Year: PhD 1992
Major Field: Clinical Psychology
Specialty: Adult Development;Assessment/Diagnosis/
Evaluation;Clinical Psychology;Cross Cultural
Processes;Ethnic Minorities;Gender Issues

LANGROD, John
2109 Broadway
Suite #506
New York, NY 10023-2130
(718) 409-9450-**B**, (212) 877-0662-**H**, (718) 931-1432-**F**
Ethnicity: Hispanic/Latino
Languages: French, Portuguese, Spanish, Polish
Degree and Year: PhD 1978
Major Field: Psychopharmacology
Specialty: Drug Abuse;HIV/AIDS;Ethnic Minorities;Mental
Disorders;Psychopharmacology;Religious Psychology

LAOSA, Luis M.
Educational Testing Service
Research Building 8-R
Rosedale Road
Princeton, NJ 08541
(609) 734-5524-**B**, (609) 734-1090-**F**
Ethnicity: Hispanic/Latino
Languages: French, Portuguese, Spanish
Degree and Year: PhD 1971
Major Field: General Psy./Methods & Systems
Specialty: Child Development;Measurement;Educational
Psychology;Program Evaluation;Research Design &
Methodology

LASAGA, Agueda M.
10300 Coral Way
Suite #E-33
Miami, FL 33165-7966
(305) 221-6905-**B**
Ethnicity: Hispanic/Latino
Degree and Year: PhD 1959
Major Field: Clinical Psychology
Specialty: Psychotherapy;Group Psychotherapy

LASAGA, Jose I.
10300 Coral Way
Suite #E 33
Miami, FL 33165-7966
(305) 221-6905-**B**
Ethnicity: Hispanic/Latino
Degree and Year: PhD 1940
Major Field: Clinical Psychology
Specialty: Psychotherapy;Projective Techniques

LASHLEY, Karen H.
PO Box 574
Bethany, OK 73008-0574
(405) 495-6340-**B**, (405) 348-1118-**H**
Ethnicity: American Indian/Alaska Native
Degree and Year: PhD 1989
Major Field: Counseling Psychology
Specialty: Clinical Child Psychology;Child Therapy;Counseling
Psychology;Depression;Family Therapy

LATORRE, Miriam D.
178 W. 9th Street
Bayonne, NJ 07002
(201) 676-1000-**B**, (201) 823-9648-**H**
Ethnicity: Hispanic/Latino
Languages: Spanish
Degree and Year: PsyD 1981
Major Field: Clinical Psychology
Specialty: Individual Psychotherapy;Pain & Pain Management;Cross
Cultural Processes;Death & Dying;Psychoanalysis

LAU, Godwin
88 Charnwood Pl
Thornhill, ON L3T5H-3
CANADA
(416) 495-2582-**B**, (905) 881-8017-**H**, (416) 495-2582-**F**
Ethnicity: Asian-American/Asian/Pacific Islander
Languages: Chinese
Degree and Year: PhD 1985
Major Field: Clinical Psychology
Specialty: Psychotherapy;Pain & Pain Management;Marriage &
Family;Program Evaluation;Religious Psychology

LAU, Lavay
1600 Kapiolani Boulevard
Suite 620
Honolulu, HI 96814-3802
(808) 942-5778-**B**, (808) 373-2424-**H**, (808) 942-5232-**F**
Ethnicity: Asian-American/Asian/Pacific Islander
Languages: Chinese
Degree and Year: PsyD 1979
Major Field: Clinical Psychology
Specialty: Child Therapy;Clinical Psychology;Cross Cultural
Processes;Family Therapy;Marriage & Family

LAVIENA, Luis
201 east 28th Street, 4K
New York, NY 10016
(212) 260-7679-**B**, (212) 252-0396-**H**
laviena@mail.ldt.net
Ethnicity: Asian-American/Asian/Pacific Islander
Languages: Filipino, German, Hindi, Portuguese
Degree and Year: PhD 1991
Major Field: Cognitive Psychology
Specialty: Individual Psychotherapy;Cognitive Psychology;Ethnic
Minorities;Health Psychology

LAWRENCE, Stephen N.
4811 Stonebrick Drive
Lawrence, KS 66047-3341
(212) 878-7766-**B**, (201) 525-1715-**H**
Ethnicity: African-American/Black
Degree and Year: PhD 1982
Major Field: unknown

LAWRENCE, Valerie W.
Kenneaw State University
Department of Psychology (PO Box 444)
Marietta, GA 30061
(404) 423-6603-**B**, (404) 333-9743-**H**, (404) 423-6432-**F**
Ethnicity: African-American/Black
Degree and Year: PhD 1985
Major Field: Developmental Psychology
Specialty: Social Development;Parent-Child Interaction;Cognitive
Development;Language Development

LAWSON, Gary W.
254 Carmelita Drive
Moutain View, CA 94040
(408) 253-8600-**B**, (415) 965-2758-**H**, (408) 253-6909-**F**
Ethnicity: Hispanic/Latino
Degree and Year: PsyD 1982
Major Field: Clinical Psychology
Specialty: Clinical Psychology;Managed Care;Management &
Organization

LAWSON, Jasper J.
28 Thorndike Street
Somerville, MA 02144
(508) 256-2250-**B**, (617) 776-7129-**H**, (617) 776-7129-**F**
jasper j. lawson,phd@aol.com
Ethnicity: African-American/Black
Languages: Spanish
Degree and Year: PhD 1980
Major Field: Clinical Psychology
Specialty: Mental Health Services;HIV/
AIDS;Psychometrics;Psychotherapy;School Psychology

LE-XUAN-HY, G. M.
37000 Highland Place
Fairfax, VA 22033
(202) 512-6167-**B**, (703) 385-8860-**H**, (202) 512-0622-**F**
Ethnicity: Asian-American/Asian/Pacific Islander
Languages: Vietnamese
Degree and Year: PhD 1986
Major Field: Social Psychology
Specialty: Personality;Cross Cultural Processes;Statistics;Social
Development;Developmental Psychology

LEARY, Kimberlyn
527 East Liberty Street
Suite 209D
Ann Arbor, MI 48104
(313) 665-4827-**B**, (313) 761-7606-**H**
Ethnicity: African-American/Black
Degree and Year: PhD 1988
Major Field: Clinical Psychology
Specialty: Psychotherapy;Psychoanalysis;HIV/
AIDS;Psychopathology;Child Abuse

LEDESMA, Lourdes K.
Legaspi Village, Makati
117 Gamboa Street - Suite 806
Manila,
PHILIPPINES
(632) 85-72-05-**B**, (632) 818-5097-**F**
Ethnicity: Asian-American/Asian/Pacific Islander
Languages: Filipino
Degree and Year: PhD 1979
Major Field: Counseling Psychology
Specialty: Neuropsychology;Assessment/Diagnosis/Evaluation;Learning
Disabilities;Mentally Retarded;Autism

LEE-RICHTER, Julie
8414 S. Painted Sky
Highlands Ranch, CO 80126
(303) 470-7708-**B**, (303) 791-2148-**H**
Ethnicity: Asian-American/Asian/Pacific Islander

Languages: Chinese
Degree and Year: PhD 1984
Major Field: Clinical Child Psychology
Specialty: Child Therapy;Marriage & Family;Adolescent
Therapy;Parent-Child Interaction;Professional Issues in
Psychology

LEE, Anna C.
Costa do Guia, Lote 21-4B
Cascaus 2750, 332
PORTUGAL
351-1-483-5910-**B**, 351-1-483-5902-**F**
aclee@mail.telepac.pt
Ethnicity: Asian-American/Asian/Pacific Islander
Languages: Chinese, Portuguese
Degree and Year: PhD 1980
Major Field: Clinical Psychology
Specialty: Physically Handicapped

LEE, C. Jarnie W J
101 Aupuni Street - Suite 119
Hilo, HI 96720
(808) 961-3616-**B**, (808) 961-3616-**F**
Ethnicity: Asian-American/Asian/Pacific Islander
Degree and Year: EdD 1975
Major Field: Counseling Psychology
Specialty: Counseling Psychology;Stress;Psychotherapy;Child
Therapy;Adolescent Therapy;Prevention

LEE, D. John
D.J. Lee & Associates
58 Lincoln Lake, SE
Lowell, MI 49331
(616) 752-8019-**H**
leedj@iserv.net
Ethnicity: Asian-American/Asian/Pacific Islander
Degree and Year: PhD 1987
Major Field: Counseling Psychology
Specialty: Counseling Psychology;Cognitive Psychology;Consulting
Psychology;Cross Cultural
Processes;Psychodrama;Organizational Development

LEE, Daniel D.
2021 E. Fourth Street - Suite 102
Santa Ana, CA 92705
(714) 834-1074-**B**, (714) 495-3267-**H**
Ethnicity: Asian-American/Asian/Pacific Islander
Languages: Vietnamese
Degree and Year: PhD 1979
Major Field: Clinical Psychology
Specialty: Clinical Neuropsychology;Clinical Psychology;Death &
Dying;Ethnic Minorities;Forensic Psychology

LEE, David Y. K.
33 Abbott Road
Bradford, PA 16701-1056
(814) 368-6076-**B**, (814) 368-5958-**H**, (814) 362-2552-**F**
dal5+@pitt.edu
Ethnicity: Asian-American/Asian/Pacific Islander
Languages: Chinese
Degree and Year: MA 1970
Major Field: School Psychology

LEE, Hing-Chu B.
Flat A, 17/F
No. 53 Broadway

Mei Fo Sun Chuen
Kowloon, 177,
HONG KONG
(011) 852-859-**B**
Ethnicity: Asian-American/Asian/Pacific Islander
Languages: Chinese
Degree and Year: PhD 1983
Major Field: Clinical Psychology
Specialty: Clinical Neuropsychology;Clinical
 Psychology;Depression;Gerontology/Geropsychology;Health
 Psychology

LEE, Howard B.
 Department of Psychology-CSUN
 18111 Nordhoff Street
 Northridge, CA 91330
 (818) 885-2827-**B**, (818) 704-5316-**H**, (818) 885-2829-**F**
Ethnicity: Asian-American/Asian/Pacific Islander
Degree and Year: PhD 1979
Major Field: Quan/Math & Psychometrics/Stat
Specialty: Computer Applications and
 Programming;Psychometrics;Measurement;Statistics;Operations
 Research

LEE, Jerome
 Albright College
 Department of Psychology
 Reading, PA 19612
 (215) 921-7586-**B**, (215) 796-1933-**H**
Ethnicity: Asian-American/Asian/Pacific Islander
Degree and Year: PhD 1980
Major Field: Physiological Psychology
Specialty: Physiological Psychology;Experimental
 Psychology;Psychobiology;Learning/Learning
 Theory;Comparative Psychology

LEE, Jo Ann
 Deparment of Psychology
 University of N.C.-Charlotte
 Charlotte, NC 28223
 (704) 547-4753-**B**, (704) 563-2713-**H**, (704) 547-3096-**F**
 jolee@email.uncc.edu
Ethnicity: Asian-American/Asian/Pacific Islander
Degree and Year: PhD 1980 MS 1977
Major Field: Industrial/Organizational Psy.
Specialty: Industrial/Organizational Psychology;Individual
 Difference;Human Resources;Measurement;Performance
 Evaluation

LEE, Julie C.
 Children's Health Council
 700 Sand Hill Road
 Palo Alto, CA 94304
Ethnicity: Asian-American/Asian/Pacific Islander
Languages: Korean
Degree and Year: PhD 1996
Major Field: Clinical Psychology
Specialty: Clinical Child Psychology;Autism;Child
 Development;Parent-Child Interaction

LEE, Jung K.
 27745 Royal Forest Drive
 Westlake, OH 44145
 (216) 941-8800-**B**, (216) 871-0581-**H**

Ethnicity: Asian-American/Asian/Pacific Islander
Degree and Year: PhD 1985
Major Field: Clinical Psychology
Specialty: Mental Health Services;Mentally Retarded;Forensic
 Psychology;Assessment/Diagnosis/Evaluation;Clinical
 Psychology

LEE, Margaret
 12257 County Road #9 NE
 Spicer, MN 56288
 (320) 235-4613-**B**, (320) 796-6821-**H**
Ethnicity: Asian-American/Asian/Pacific Islander
Languages: Chinese
Degree and Year: PhD 1969
Major Field: Counseling Psychology
Specialty: Individual Psychotherapy;Group Psychotherapy;Crisis
 Intervention & Therapy

LEE, Ronald W.
 Cherry Creek School District
 Smoky Hill Road
 16100 East Smoky Hill Road
 Aurora, CO 80015
 (303) 693-1700-**B**, (303) 698-3840-**H**, (303) 693-1700-**F**
Ethnicity: Asian-American/Asian/Pacific Islander
Degree and Year: PsyD 1987
Major Field: Clinical Psychology
Specialty: Educational Psychology;Emotional Development;Ethnic
 Minorities

LEE, See-Woo S.
 Children and Youth Services
 Orange County Health Care Agency
 1200 North Main Street
 Suite 500
 Santa Ana, CA 92701
 (714) 568-4378-**B**
 seewoo@hotmail.com
Ethnicity: Asian-American/Asian/Pacific Islander
Languages: Korean
Degree and Year: PhD 1974
Major Field: Developmental Psychology
Specialty: Clinical Child Psychology;Clinical Psychology;Cognitive
 Behavioral Therapy;Child Therapy

LEE, Seong S.
 University of the British of Columbia
 Department of Educational Psychology
 and Special Education
 Vancouver, BC V6T1Z4
 CANADA
Ethnicity: Asian-American/Asian/Pacific Islander
Degree and Year: PhD 1967
Major Field: Educational Psychology
Specialty: Thought Processes

LEE, Thomas W.
 University of Washington
 School of Business, Room DJ-10
 Box 353200
 Seattle, WA 98195-3200
 (206) 543-4389-**B**, (206) 685-9392-**F**
Ethnicity: Asian-American/Asian/Pacific Islander

Languages: Chinese, Norwegian
Degree and Year: PhD 1984
Major Field: Industrial/Organizational Psy.
Specialty: Industrial/Organizational Psychology;Management &
　　Organization;Selection & Placement;Vocational
　　Psychology;Statistics

LEE, Wanda M. L.
　San Francisco State University
　Department of Psychology, BH524
　1600 Holloway Avenue
　San Francisco, CA 94132
　(415) 338-1707-**B**, (415) 338-0594-**F**
　walee@sfsu.edu
Ethnicity: Asian-American/Asian/Pacific Islander
Degree and Year: PhD 1979
Major Field: Clinical Psychology
Specialty: Counseling Psychology;Ethnic Minorities;Organizational
　　Development;Depression;Gender Issues

LEE, William W.
　2645 Washington Street
　Suite 445
　Wankegan, IL 60085
Ethnicity: Asian-American/Asian/Pacific Islander
Degree and Year: EdD 1977
Major Field: Social Psychology
Specialty: Clinical Psychology;Health
　　Psychology;Rehabilitation;Medical Psychology;Affective
　　Disorders

LEE, Yolanda W.
　14600 Onaway Road
　Shaker Heights, OH 44120-2845
　(216) 561-7760-**B**
Ethnicity: African-American/Black
Degree and Year: MA 1946
Major Field: Clinical Psychology

LEE, Yueh-Ting
　Westfield State College
　Department of Psychology
　Westfield, MA 01086
　(413) 572-5748-**B**, (413) 668-6610-**H**, (413) 562-3613-**F**
Ethnicity: Asian-American/Asian/Pacific Islander
Languages: Chinese
Degree and Year: PhD 1991
Major Field: Social Psychology
Specialty: Cross Cultural Processes;Social
　　Psychology;Personality;Industrial/Organizational
　　Psychology;Health Psychology

LEIN, H. Beatriz
　3407 W. Sixth Street
　Suite 800
　Los Angeles, CA 90020
　(213) 382-1664-**B**, (310) 652-9750-**H**, (310) 652-9750-**F**
Ethnicity: Hispanic/Latino
Languages: Spanish
Degree and Year: PhD 1983
Major Field: Clinical Child Psychology
Specialty: Child Abuse;Clinical Child Psychology;Adolescent Therapy

LEMOS-METTEL, Thereza P. De
　University of Brasilia
　SQN 115, Bloco G
　Apartment #610
　Brasila,　70772,
　BRAZIL
　0672724576-**B**
Ethnicity: Hispanic/Latino
Degree and Year: PhD 1963
Major Field: Developmental Psychology

LEONG, Che K.
　University of Saskatchewan
　College of Education
　Dept. of Education for Except. Children
　Saskatoon, SK S7N0W-0
　CANADA
　(306) 966-5257-**B**, (306) 934-4732-**H**
Ethnicity: Asian-American/Asian/Pacific Islander
Degree and Year: PhD 1974
Major Field: Educational Psychology

LEONG, Deborah J.
　Metropolitan State College
　5288 Crawford Gulch
　Golden, CO 80403-8112
　(303) 556-3028-**B**
Ethnicity: Asian-American/Asian/Pacific Islander
Degree and Year: PhD 1977
Major Field: Educational Psychology
Specialty: Preschool & Day Care Issues;Developmental Psychology

LEONG, Frederick T. T.
　Ohio State University
　Department of Psychology
　1885 Neil Avenue
　Columbus, OH 43210
　(614) 292-8219-**B**, (614) 847-4257-**H**, (614) 292-4537-**F**
　leong.10@osu.edu
Ethnicity: Asian-American/Asian/Pacific Islander
Languages: Chinese
Degree and Year: PhD 1988
Major Field: Counseling Psychology
Specialty: Counseling Psychology;Vocational Psychology;Ethnic
　　Minorities;Cross Cultural Processes;Industrial/Organizational
　　Psychology

LEON, Ruben
　2079 Barnett Road
　Los Angeles, CA 90032-4131
　(213) 383-1300-**B**
Ethnicity: Hispanic/Latino
Degree and Year: PhD 1973
Major Field: Clinical Psychology
Specialty: Psychotherapy;Psychotherapy

LEON, Yolanda C.
　1509 West Swann Avenue #255
　Tampa, FL 33606
　(813) 251-8856-**B**, (813) 872-4895-**H**
Ethnicity: Hispanic/Latino
Languages: Spanish
Degree and Year: PhD 1993 EdS 1989
Major Field: Clinical Child Psychology

Specialty: Clinical Psychology;Child & Pediatric Psychology;Clinical
Neuropsychology;Assessment/Diagnosis/Evaluation;Learning
Disabilities;Clinical Child Neuropsychology

LEQUERICA, Martha
1199 Egret Circle South
Jupiter, FL 33458
(561) 744-2637-**B**, (561) 744-2637-**H**
Ethnicity: Hispanic/Latino
Languages: Spanish
Degree and Year: PhD 1982
Major Field: Educational Psychology
Specialty: Child & Pediatric Psychology;Child Therapy;Parent
Education;School Psychology;Preschool & Day Care
Issues;Training & Development

LERMA, Joe L.
P.O. Box 270082
Corpus Christi, TX 78427
(512) 993-0346-**B**, (512) 993-9408-**F**
Ethnicity: Hispanic/Latino
Languages: French, Italian, Spanish
Degree and Year: PhD 1983
Major Field: Counseling Psychology
Specialty: Counseling Psychology;Depression;Marriage &
Family;Psychotherapy;Medical Psychology

LESSING, Elise E.
1103 S Lyman Avenue
Oak Park, IL 60304
(312) 794-3992-**B**, (708) 848-4643-**H**, (708) 848-4643-**F**
Ethnicity: African-American/Black
Degree and Year: PhD 1955
Major Field: Clinical Child Psychology
Specialty: Administration;Clinical Child Psychology;Clinical
Research;Mental Health Services;Psychopathology

LESURE-LESTER, G. Evelyn
Chapman
Department of Psychology
333 North Glasswell
Orange, CA 92866
(818) 512-6322-**B**, (626) 852-0392-**H**, (626) 852-0393-**F**
gell@webtv.net
Ethnicity: African-American/Black
Degree and Year: PhD 1975
Major Field: Clinical Psychology
Specialty: Clinical Psychology;Ethnic Minorities

LE, Trinh To
17819 Mossy Ridge Ln
Houston, TX 77095-4422
(281) 985-7109-**B**, (281) 463-2566-**H**
Ethnicity: Asian-American/Asian/Pacific Islander
Degree and Year: MA 1989
Major Field: Clinical Psychology
Specialty: Cognitive Behavioral Therapy;Child Development;Family
Therapy;Individual Psychotherapy;Projective Techniques

LEUNG, Alex C. N.
Mills Estate Office Building
1838 El Camino Real
Suite #105
Burlingame, CA 94010
(415) 692-6648-**B**, (415) 286-9608-**F**
Ethnicity: Asian-American/Asian/Pacific Islander

Languages: Chinese
Degree and Year: PhD 1984
Major Field: Clinical Psychology
Specialty: Assessment/Diagnosis/Evaluation;Cultural & Social
Processes;Ethnic Minorities;Forensic Psychology;Hospital
Care

LEUNG, Paul
Deakin University
22 Burwood Highway
Australia
+61 3 9244 6480-**B**, +61 3 9244 6671-**F**
pleung@deakin.edu.au
Ethnicity: Asian-American/Asian/Pacific Islander
Degree and Year: PhD 1970
Major Field: Counseling Psychology
Specialty: Physically Handicapped

LEUNG, S. Alvin
University of Houston
491 Farish Hall
Houston, TX 77204
(402) 472-6948-**B**
Ethnicity: Asian-American/Asian/Pacific Islander
Degree and Year: PhD 1988
Major Field: Counseling Psychology

LEVERMORE, Monique A.
Florida Institute of Technology
School of Psychology
150 West University Boulevard
Melbourne, FL 32901-6975
(407) 674-8104-**B**, (407) 647-7105-**F**
levermo@fit.edu
Ethnicity: African-American/Black
Languages: Spanish
Degree and Year: PhD 1995 MsEd 1990
Major Field: Clinical Psychology
Specialty: Ethnic Minorities;Psychotherapy;Forensic
Psychology;Clinical Psychology;Consulting
Psychology;Group Processes

LEWIS, Brenda J.
28935 San Carlos
Southfield, MI 48076
(313) 875-4434-**B**, (313) 352-2969-**H**, (313) 875-4435-**F**
Ethnicity: African-American/Black
Degree and Year: PhD 1976
Major Field: Educational Psychology
Specialty: School Psychology;Group Psychotherapy;Individual
Psychotherapy;Consulting Psychology;Clinical Child
Psychology;Child Abuse

LEWIS, Carmelita M.
Hunter Medical Center
Hunter Behavioral Health
2100 Wescott Drive
Flemington, NJ 08822
(908) 788-6401-**B**, (215) 860-8792-**H**
Ethnicity: Hispanic/Latino
Degree and Year: PhD 1985
Major Field: Clinical Psychology
Specialty: Hypnosis/Hypnotherapy;Affective
Disorders;Depression;Pain & Pain Management;Cognitive
Behavioral Therapy;Marriage & Family

LEWIS, George R.
Oakbrook Professional Building
120 Center Mall
Suite #624
Oak Brook, IL 60521
(708) 574-0480-**B**
Ethnicity: African-American/Black
Degree and Year: PhD 1959
Major Field: Clinical Psychology
Specialty: Forensic Psychology

LEWIS, Marva L
Louisiana State University Medical Center
Department of Psychiatry
1542 Tulane Avenue
New Orleans, LA 70126
504 568-4451-**B**, 504 241-4722-**H**, 504 568-6842-**F**
qdops2@uno.edu
Ethnicity: African-American/Black
Degree and Year: PhD 1993 MA 1993
Major Field: Developmental Psychology
Specialty: Parent-Child Interaction;Cultural & Social Processes;Cross
   Cultural Processes;Developmental Psychology

LEWIS, Page
7150 Gila Court
Palmeda, CA 93551-4701
(661) 726-9924-**B**
Ethnicity: African-American/Black, Asian-American/Asian/Pacific
Islander
Degree and Year: PhD 1988
Major Field: Clinical Psychology
Specialty: Eating Disorders;Cognitive Behavioral Therapy;Affective
   Disorders;Clinical Psychology;Managed Care

LEW, Wei M.
Chinatown Child Development Center
San Francisco Community Health Services
615 Grant Avenue
Fifth Floor
San Francisco, CA 94108
(415) 393-4453-**B**
Ethnicity: Asian-American/Asian/Pacific Islander
Languages: Chinese
Degree and Year: PhD 1970
Major Field: Clinical Psychology
Specialty: Clinical Child Psychology;Quantitative/Mathematical,
   Psychometrics

LICUANAN, Patricia
Miriam College
Office of the President
UP PO Box 110
1104 Dilimau
Quelon City,
PHILIPPINES
011 632924-6769-**B**, 011 632921-3367-**H**, 011 632426-0169-**F**
licuanan@mc.edu.ph
Ethnicity: Asian-American/Asian/Pacific Islander
Degree and Year: PhD 1970
Major Field: Social Psychology
Specialty: Cultural & Social Processes

LIEM, Ramsay
81 Greenough Street
Brookline, MA 02146

(617) 552-4108-**B**, (617) 277-3378-**H**, (617) 552-3199-**F**
Ethnicity: Asian-American/Asian/Pacific Islander
Degree and Year: PhD 1970
Major Field: Clinical Psychology
Specialty: Community Psychology;Cross Cultural Processes;Cultural &
   Social Processes;Ethnic Minorities;Social Problems

LIE, Rudolph T.B
205 Portchester Road
Holland, MT 49424
(616) 393-5600-**B**, (616)7 86-2499-**H**
Ethnicity: Asian-American/Asian/Pacific Islander
Languages: Japanese, Indonesian, Dutch
Degree and Year: PhD 1973
Major Field: Clinical Psychology
Specialty: Community Mental Health;Administration;Managed
   Care;Psychopathology;Clinical Psychology

LIFUR-BENNETT, Linda
Town & Country Office Park
956 Town & Country Road
Orange, CA 92668-4601
(714) 680-8388-**B**
Ethnicity: Hispanic/Latino
Degree and Year: PhD 1982
Major Field: Clinical Psychology
Specialty: Family Therapy

LIJTMAER, Ruth M
88 W Ridgewood Avenue
Ridgewood, NJ 07450-3141
(201) 445-5522-**B**, (210) 444-9174-**H**, (201) 444-2598-**F**
hlijtmaer@pol.net
Ethnicity: Hispanic/Latino
Languages: Italian, Spanish
Degree and Year: PhD 1978
Major Field: Clinical Psychology
Specialty: Psychoanalysis;Cross Cultural Processes;Continuing
   Education;Individual Psychotherapy;Psychology of Women

LIM, Hoili C.
4132-4 Keanu Street
Honolulu, HI 96816
(808) 621-9122-**B**
Ethnicity: Asian-American/Asian/Pacific Islander
Degree and Year: PhD 1984
Major Field: Clinical Psychology
Specialty: Mentally Retarded

LIM, Patricia J.
Rehabilitation Associates of the Midwest, SC
909 East Palatine Road
Suite A
Palatine, IL 60067
(847) 776-1400-**B**, (847) 776-1864-**F**
patilim@chicagonet.net
Ethnicity: Asian-American/Asian/Pacific Islander
Degree and Year: PsyD 1996
Major Field: Health Psychology
Specialty: Rehabilitation;Clinical Psychology;Brain Damage;Clinical
   Neuropsychology;Health Psychology;Cardiovascular
   Processes

LINARES, Lourdes O.
67 Dana St Apt 3
Cambridge, MA 02138-4323

(617) 534-3694-**B**, (617) 868-4525-**H**, (617) 534-3690-**F**
oriana.linares@bu.org
Ethnicity: Hispanic/Latino
Languages: Spanish
Degree and Year: PhD 1986
Major Field: Developmental Psychology
Specialty: Child Abuse;Drug Abuse;Parent-Child Interaction

LINEBERGER, Marilyn H.
Kensington Office Park
4151 Memorial Drive
Suitte #208-E
Decatur, GA 30032-1515
(404) 508-8889-**B**
Ethnicity: African-American/Black
Degree and Year: PhD 1979
Major Field: Clinical Psychology
Specialty: Cultural & Social Processes

LIN, Hsin-Tai
F10, #8 Alley 1 Lane 16
20 Chang Road, Hsintien
Taipei, 419 23123
TAIWAN
(011) n88622356-**B**
t14001@cc.ntnu.edu.tw
Ethnicity: Asian-American/Asian/Pacific Islander
Languages: Chinese
Degree and Year: EdD 1981
Major Field: Educational Psychology
Specialty: Creativity;Giftedness;School Counseling;Quantitative/
    Mathematical, Psychometrics;Counseling Psychology

LIN, J.C. Gisela G.
Student Counseling Service
Texas A&M University
College Station, TX 77843-1263
(409) 845-4427-**B**, (409) 862-4383-**F**
gisela@scs.tamu.edu
Ethnicity: Asian-American/Asian/Pacific Islander
Languages: Chinese
Degree and Year: PhD 1993
Major Field: Counseling Psychology
Specialty: Counseling Psychology;Cognitive Behavioral Therapy;Crisis
    Intervention & Therapy;Cross Cultural Processes;Problem
    Solving;Prevention

LIN, Jeanne L.
University of San Francisco
Counseling Center
2130 Fulton Street
San Francisco, CA 94705
(415) 422-6452-**B**, (415) 440-1694-**H**, (415) 922-8038-**F**
linj@usfca.edu
Ethnicity: Asian-American/Asian/Pacific Islander
Degree and Year: PhD 1990
Major Field: Clinical Psychology
Specialty: Ethnic Minorities;Adult Development;Depression;Cultural &
    Social Processes

LIN, Marie K.
1317 Chesterton Way
Walnut Creek, CA 94596-6463

(510) 688-8310-**B**
Ethnicity: Asian-American/Asian/Pacific Islander
Degree and Year: PhD 1978
Major Field: Clinical Psychology

LINN, Nancy SC
18 Echo H1
Moraga, CA 94556-1317
Ethnicity: Asian-American/Asian/Pacific Islander
Degree and Year:
Major Field: Quan/Math & Psychometrics/Stat

LIN, Thung-Rung
Personnel Selection & Training Branch
315 East 21st Street
Los Angeles, CA 90011-1005
(213) 743-3608-**B**, (213) 748-3608-**F**
trl@aol.com
Ethnicity: Asian-American/Asian/Pacific Islander
Languages: Chinese
Degree and Year: PhD 1983
Major Field: Industrial/Organizational Psy.

LIPSON, Diane R.
4419 Van Nuys Blvd Ste 404
Sherman Oaks, CA 91403
(818) 990-1190-**B**
Ethnicity: African-American/Black
Degree and Year: PhD 1984
Major Field: Counseling Psychology
Specialty: Psychotherapy;Medical Psychology

LISTON, Hattye H.
1213 Eastside Drive
Greensboro, NC 27406
(919) 334-7970-**B**, (919) 274-4064-**H**
Ethnicity: African-American/Black
Degree and Year: PhD 1973
Major Field: Clinical Psychology
Specialty: Clinical Psychology;Biofeedback;Alcoholism & Alcohol
    Abuse;Community Mental Health;Health Psychology

LIU, An-Yen
Jackson State University
Department of Psychology
113 Pebble Brook Drive
Clinton, MS 39056
(601) 968-2371-**B**, (601) 924-0613-**H**
Ethnicity: Asian-American/Asian/Pacific Islander
Languages: Chinese
Degree and Year: PhD 1971
Major Field: Quan/Math & Psychometrics/Stat
Specialty: Adolescent Development;Educational Research;Social
    Psychology

LIU, Joseph C.
11406 Avenida Del Gato
San Diego, CA 92126-1204
(619) 586-7364-**H**
Ethnicity: Asian-American/Asian/Pacific Islander
Languages: Chinese
Degree and Year: PhD 1977
Major Field: Clinical Psychology
Specialty: Adolescent Development;Affective Disorders;Assessment/
    Diagnosis/Evaluation;Behavior Therapy;Cognitive Behavioral
    Therapy

LI, Xiaoming
University of Maryland School of Medicine
700 West Lombard Street
Second Floor
Baltimore, MD 21201-1069
(410) 706-1783-**B**, (410) 750-3382-**H**, (410) 706-0653-**F**
kiliAumaryland.edu
Ethnicity: Asian-American/Asian/Pacific Islander
Languages: Chinese
Degree and Year: PhD 1992
Major Field: Quan/Math & Psychometrics/Stat
Specialty: Statistics;Quantitative/Mathematical,
   Psychometrics;Research Design & Methodology;Adolescent
   Development

LLADO, Sarah L.
Turabo I-4
Las Haciendas
Caguas, PR 00725
(809) 724-0303-**B**, (809) 258-4298-**H**
Ethnicity: Hispanic/Latino
Languages: Spanish
Degree and Year: PsyD 1988
Major Field: Clinical Psychology
Specialty: Child Abuse;Clinical Psychology;Community Mental
   Health;Crisis Intervention & Therapy;Family Therapy

LLANOS, Aracely B.
First Federal Building
1519 Ponce de Leon Avenue
Suite #607-609
Santurce, PR 00909
(809) 723-5825-**B**, (809) 727-7163-**H**, (809) 723-5825-**F**
Ethnicity: Hispanic/Latino
Languages: Spanish
Degree and Year: PhD 1982
Major Field: Clinical Psychology
Specialty: Clinical Psychology

LLORCA, Arthur L.
Psychological Services
Box 1074
Wrightsville Beach, NC 28480
(919) 799-6470-**B**, (919) 799-3491-**H**, (910) 313-0479-**F**
Ethnicity: Hispanic/Latino, European/White
Languages: French, Spanish
Degree and Year: MTID 1975 MA 1980
Major Field: Clinical Psychology
Specialty: Assessment/Diagnosis/Evaluation;Clinical
   Neuropsychology;Clinical Psychology;Mental
   Disorders;Psychology & Law

LLORENTE, Antolin M.
Baylor College of Medicine, Texas
Children's Hospital
6621 Fanning Street
Suite 530
Houston, TX 77030
(713) 770-3400-**B**, (713) 668-0494-**H**, (713) 770-3399-**F**
llorente@bcm.tmc.edu
Ethnicity: Hispanic/Latino
Languages: Spanish
Degree and Year: PhD 1993

Major Field: Clinical Psychology
Specialty: Clinical Neuropsychology;Neuropsychology;Affective
   Disorders;Child & Pediatric Psychology;Clinical Child
   Neuropsychology;Cross Cultural Processes

LONDON, Dyanne P.
80 Howard Street
Cambridge, MA 02139
(617) 547-2399-**H**
dianne-england@usu.net
Ethnicity: African-American/Black
Degree and Year: PhD 1990
Major Field: Clinical Psychology
Specialty: Alcoholism & Alcohol Abuse;Child & Pediatric
   Psychology;HIV/AIDS;Training & Development;Assessment/
   Diagnosis/Evaluation

LONDON, Lorna H.
Loyola University, Chicago
Department of Counseling Psychology
1041 Ridge Road
Wilmette, IL 60091
(847) 853-3347-**B**, (847) 733-8334-**H**, (847) 853-3375-**F**
llondon@luc.edu
Ethnicity: African-American/Black
Degree and Year: PhD 1995
Major Field: Clinical Psychology
Specialty: Family Therapy;Community Psychology;Ethnic
   Minorities;Child Therapy;Marriage & Family;Health
   Psychology

LOO, Chalsa M.
Pacific Center for PTSD
1132 Bishop Street
Suite #307
Honolulu, HI 96813
(808) 956-7557-**B**, (808) 396-0565-**H**, (808) 956-4700-**F**
Ethnicity: Asian-American/Asian/Pacific Islander
Degree and Year: PhD 1971
Major Field: Clinical Psychology
Specialty: Ethnic Minorities;Psychotherapy;Clinical Psychology;Stress

LOONG, James
4571 W 10520 N
Highland, UT 84003
(805) 541-4920-**B**
Ethnicity: Asian-American/Asian/Pacific Islander
Languages: Chinese
Degree and Year: PhD 1984
Major Field: Clinical Psychology
Specialty: Neuropsychology;Brain Damage;Brain Functions;Clinical
   Neuropsychology;Neurosciences

LOO, Russell
98-644 Puailima Street
Aiea, HI 96701-2231
(808) 486-6060-**B**, (808) 487-1135-**H**
Ethnicity: Asian-American/Asian/Pacific Islander
Degree and Year: PhD 1971
Major Field: Clinical Psychology
Specialty: Child Therapy;Adolescent Therapy;Cognitive Behavioral
   Therapy;Personality Measurement

LOPEZ-BAEZ, Sandra I.
Walsh University
Graduate Program

2020 Easton Street, NW
North Canton, OH 44720
(330) 490-7231-**B**, (330) 490-7165-**F**
lopezbaez@alex.walsh.edu
Ethnicity: Hispanic/Latino
Languages: Spanish
Degree and Year: PhD 1980
Major Field: Counseling Psychology
Specialty: Counseling Psychology;Cross Cultural
    Processes;Biofeedback;Hypnosis/Hypnotherapy;Lesbian &
    Gay Issuues;HIV/AIDS

LOPEZ-REYES, Ramon
139 Kuulei Road
Kailua, HI 96734-2719
(808) 263-4015-**H**
Ethnicity: Hispanic/Latino
Degree and Year: PhD 1961
Major Field: Clinical Psychology

LOPEZ, Anthony A.
Neighborhood Center
9255 Pioneer Blvd.
Santa Fe Spring, CA 90670-2380
(213) 692-0261-**B**
Ethnicity: Hispanic/Latino
Degree and Year: PhD 1979
Major Field: Clinical Psychology
Specialty: Community Mental Health;Prevention

LOPEZ, Emilia
Queens College @ CUNY
Education & Community Programs
165-30 Kissena Boulevard
Flushing, NY 11367
(718) 997-5234-**B**
lopez@qcvaxa.qc.edu
Ethnicity: Hispanic/Latino
Languages: Spanish
Degree and Year: PhD 1989
Major Field: School Psychology
Specialty: School Psychology;Assessment/Diagnosis/Evaluation;Ethnic
    Minorities

LOPEZ, Martita A.
Rush-Presbyterian
@ St. Luke's Medical Center
Department of Psychology
1653 West Congress Parkway
Chicago, IL 60612
(312) 942-2003-**B**, (708) 251-4829-**H**, (312) 942-2387-**F**
Ethnicity: Hispanic/Latino
Degree and Year: PhD 1977
Major Field: Clinical Psychology
Specialty: Gerontology/Geropsychology;Health Psychology;Medical
    Psychology;Rehabilitation

LOPEZ, Sarah C.
1 Corporate Square
Suite #220
Atlanta, GA 30329
(404) 321-2990-**B**, (404) 876-2216-**H**, (404) 325-2897-**F**
Ethnicity: Hispanic/Latino
Languages: Spanish

Degree and Year: PhD 1982
Major Field: Clinical Psychology
Specialty: Ethnic Minorities;Group Psychotherapy;HIV/
    AIDS;Interpersonal Processes & Relations;Marriage & Family

LOPEZ, Steven R.
University of California
Department of Psychology
Los Angeles, CA 90095-1563
(310) 206-8752-**B**, (818) 831-9899-**H**, (310) 206-5895-**F**
lopez@psych.ucla.edu
Ethnicity: Hispanic/Latino
Languages: Spanish
Degree and Year: PhD 1983
Major Field: Clinical Psychology
Specialty: Assessment/Diagnosis/Evaluation;Cross Cultural
    Processes;Ethnic Minorities;Psychopathology;Psychotherapy

LOPEZ, Thomas W.
27 Baylor Circle
White Plains, NY 10605-3005
(914) 949-9639-**B**
Ethnicity: Hispanic/Latino
Degree and Year: PhD 1970
Major Field: unknown

LOREDO, Carlos M.
Carlos M. Loredo, PhD, P.C.
2111 Montclaire Street
Austin, TX 78704
(512) 443-0190-**B**, (512) 440-8417-**H**, (512) 326-4818-**F**
Ethnicity: Hispanic/Latino
Languages: Spanish
Degree and Year: PhD 1977
Major Field: Clinical Psychology
Specialty: Sexual Behavior;Child & Pediatric Psychology;Adolescent
    Therapy;Child Abuse;Forensic Psychology;Family Therapy

LORENZO, Gladys
14410 Sabal Drive
Miami Lake, FL 33014-2543
(305) 820-8505-**B**
Ethnicity: Hispanic/Latino
Degree and Year: PhD 1973
Major Field: Clinical Psychology
Specialty: Clinical Neuropsychology

LOSADA-PAISEY, Gloria
81 Wopowog Road
East Hampton, CT 06424
(806) 262-6225-**B**, (203) 267-8101-**H**
Ethnicity: Hispanic/Latino
Languages: Spanish
Degree and Year: PhD 1984
Major Field: Clinical Psychology

LOUDEN, Delroy M.
159-34 Riverside Drive West #4E
New York, NY 10032
1 800 669-9656-**B**, (212) 795-9723-**H**, (212) 795-6513-**F**
Tennarch@aol.com
Ethnicity: African-American/Black
Degree and Year: PhD 1977
Major Field: Health Psychology
Specialty: Health Psychology;Clinical Child
    Psychology;Statistics;Research Design & Methodology

LOUREDES MATTEI, Maria De
325 Dartmouth Avenue
Apartment I-6
Swarthmore, PA 19081
(215) 328-3645-**B**, (215) 328-3645-**H**
Ethnicity: Hispanic/Latino
Languages: Spanish
Degree and Year: PhD 1983
Major Field: Clinical Psychology
Specialty: Developmental Psychology;Psychoanalysis

LOVE, Craig T.
Center for Alcohol & Addiction Studies
Box G-BH, Brown University
Providence, RI 02912
(401) 444-1829-**B**, (203) 657-4274-**H**, (401) 444-1850-**F**
Ethnicity: American Indian/Alaska Native
Degree and Year: PhD 1978
Major Field: Educational Psychology
Specialty: Correctional Psychology

LOVELACE, Valeria O.
Children's Television Workshop
1 Lincoln Plaza
New York, NY 10023
(212) 595-3456-**B**
Ethnicity: African-American/Black
Degree and Year: PhD 1980
Major Field: Social Psychology
Specialty: Mass Media Communication;Social Behavior

LOW, Benson P.
2107 Elliott Avenue
Suite #206
Seattle, WA 98121-2139
(206) 448-0561-**B**, (206) 441-4536-**F**
Ethnicity: Asian-American/Asian/Pacific Islander
Degree and Year: PhD 1979
Major Field: Clinical Child Psychology
Specialty: Adolescent Development;Adolescent Therapy;Ethnic
    Minorities;Family Therapy

LOWE, Susana M.
Boston College
Campion 209
Chestnut Hill, MA 02167
(617) 552-4079-**B**, (617) 482-0473-**H**, (617) 552-1981-**F**
lowesa@bc.edu
Ethnicity: Asian-American/Asian/Pacific Islander
Languages: Chinese
Degree and Year: PhD 1998
Major Field: Counseling Psychology
Specialty: Cross Cultural Processes;Ethnic Minorities;Social
    Change;Cultural & Social Processes;Interpersonal Processes &
    Relations

LOWMAN, Rodney
Cspp-san Diego
6160 Corner Stone Ct E
San Diego, CA 92121-
(619) 623-2777-**B**, (713) 527-8130-**F**
Ethnicity: Hispanic/Latino
Languages: Spanish

Degree and Year: PhD 1979
Major Field: Industrial/Organizational Psy.
Specialty: Vocational Psychology;Consulting Psychology;Clinical
    Psychology;Work Performance

LOYOLA, Jaime L.
Philadelphia Board of Education
12 Parkview Road
Cheltenham, PA 19012
(215) 291-5680-**B**, (215) 635-2237-**H**, (215) 635-5377-**F**
Ethnicity: Hispanic/Latino
Languages: Spanish
Degree and Year: PhD 1985
Major Field: School Psychology
Specialty: Assessment/Diagnosis/Evaluation;School Psychology;Ethnic
    Minorities;Special Education;Drug Abuse;Child Abuse

LOZANO, Irma
1913 E. 17th Street, #202
Santa Ana, CA 92701
(714) 569-0067-**B**, (714) 638-4345-**H**
Ethnicity: Hispanic/Latino
Languages: Spanish
Degree and Year: PhD 1987
Major Field: Clinical Psychology
Specialty: Adolescent Therapy;Affective Disorders;Child
    Therapy;Clinical Psychology;Sex/Marital Therapy

LUCAS, Jay H.
5025 W. Frontage Road
Highway 52 North
Rochester, MN 55901
(507) 285-0401-**B**, (507) 282-6595-**H**, (507) 285-0083-**F**
Ethnicity: American Indian/Alaska Native
Degree and Year: PhD 1971
Major Field: Clinical Psychology
Specialty: Psychotherapy;Forensic Psychology;Sex/Marital
    Therapy;Hypnosis/Hypnotherapy;Stress

LUDMER, Alba
88 West Ridgewood Avenue
Ridgewood, NJ 07450
(201) 670-1870-**B**, (201) 652-5491-**H**
ludalb@aol.com
Ethnicity: Hispanic/Latino
Languages: Spanish
Degree and Year: PhD 1988
Major Field: Counseling Psychology
Specialty: Adolescent Therapy;Child Therapy;Individual
    Psychotherapy;Counseling Psychology;Adult
    Development;Family Therapy

LU, Elsie G.
IDEA, Inc.
1300-Pioneer Street
Brea, CA 92821
(562) 697-4332-**B**, (562) 697-3382-**H**, (310) 690-1352-**F**
Ethnicity: Asian-American/Asian/Pacific Islander
Languages: Chinese
Degree and Year: PhD 1966
Major Field: Clinical Psychology
Specialty: Administration;Chronically Mentally Ill;Community Mental
    Health;Mental Health Economics and
    Financing;Institutionalization/Deinstitutionalization

LUGO, Daisy R.
3601 Consohocken Avenue
Philadelphia, PA 19131-5353
(215) 568-0860-**B**, (215) 424-3240-**H**
Ethnicity: Hispanic/Latino
Languages: Spanish
Degree and Year: MS
Major Field: Clinical Psychology

LUI, Barbara J.
2910 East Madison
SAE 305
Seattle, WA 98112
(206) 860-2446-**B**, (206) 725-1115-**F**
bjlui@aol.com
Ethnicity: Asian-American/Asian/Pacific Islander
Degree and Year: PhD 1990
Major Field: Clinical Child Psychology
Specialty: Clinical Child Psychology

LUJAN, Cleo C.
7500 West Mississippi
E-124
Lakewood, CO 80226
(303) 922-2079-**B**, (303) 984-2836-**H**
Ethnicity: Hispanic/Latino
Degree and Year: PsyD 1980
Major Field: Clinical Psychology
Specialty: Individual Psychotherapy;Affective Disorders;Family
    Therapy;Ethnic Minorities;Adolescent
    Development;Counseling Psychology

LUKE, Equilla
University of California
@ San Diego
Psychological & Counseling Svc.
Room #MUIR-0106
La Jolla, CA 92093
(619) 534-3585-**B**, (619) 552-9245-**H**
Ethnicity: African-American/Black
Degree and Year: PhD 1986
Major Field: Counseling Psychology
Specialty: Psychotherapy;Counseling Psychology;Cross Cultural
    Processes;Eating Disorders

LUKMAN, Roy L.
Florida Hospital Medical Education
2501 N Orange
Suite #235
Orlando, FL 32804-4641
(407) 897-1514-**B**
Ethnicity: Asian-American/Asian/Pacific Islander
Degree and Year: PhD 1983
Major Field: unknown
Specialty: Human Development & Family Studies

LUM, Rodger G.
22 Woodford Drive
Moraga, CA 94556
(510) 268-2100-**B**, (510) 376-4889-**H**
rlum@ssa.mail.co.alemeda.ca.us
Ethnicity: Asian-American/Asian/Pacific Islander
Languages: Chinese

Degree and Year: PhD 1979
Major Field: Clinical Psychology
Specialty: Community Mental Health;Cultural & Social
    Processes;Disadvantaged;HIV/AIDS;Mental Health Services

LUNA, Donna J.
Sonoma State University
1079 Santa Barbara Dr
Santa Rosa, CA 95404-6148
(707) 664-2677-**B**, (707) 523-0242-**H**
Ethnicity: Hispanic/Latino
Degree and Year: MA 1983
Major Field: General Psy./Methods & Systems
Specialty: Social Psychology;Counseling Psychology;Developmental
    Psychobiology

LUTHAR, Suniya S.
Teachers College
Columbia University, Box 133
525 West 120th Street
New York, NY 10027-6696
(212) 678-3798-**B**, (914) 381-4579-**H**, (212) 678-3483-**F**
suniya.luthar@columbia.edu
Ethnicity: Asian-American/Asian/Pacific Islander
Languages: Hindi, Punjai
Degree and Year: PhD 1990
Major Field: Clinical Child Psychology
Specialty: Adolescent Development;Drug Abuse;Child
    Development;Psychopathology;Stress

LYLES, William B.
285 E. Los Flores Avenue
Altadena, CA 91001
(213) 268-1861-**B**, (818) 398-1650-**H**, (213) 269-2541-**F**
Ethnicity: African-American/Black
Degree and Year: PhD 1987
Major Field: General Psy./Methods & Systems
Specialty: Administration;Adolescent Therapy;General
    Psychology;Social Psychology;Group Psychotherapy

MACARANAS, Eduarda A.
407 Church Street, NE
Suite One
Vienna, VA 22180-4737
(703) 356-1330-**B**, (703) 323-0448-**H**, (703) 356-34855-**F**
Ethnicity: Asian-American/Asian/Pacific Islander
Languages: Filipino, Tagalog
Degree and Year: PhD 1971
Major Field: Clinical Psychology
Specialty: Affective Disorders;Individual Psychotherapy;Mental
    Disorders;Personality Disorders;Crisis Intervention &
    Therapy

MACHABANSKI, Hector
43 E Ohio
Suite #615
Chicago, IL 60611
(312) 222-1830-**B**, (708) 673-4826-**H**
Ethnicity: Hispanic/Latino
Languages: Spanish
Degree and Year: PhD 1985
Major Field: Clinical Psychology
Specialty: Ethnic Minorities;Cross Cultural Processes;Assessment/
    Diagnosis/Evaluation;Clinical Psychology;School Psychology

MACHIDA, Sandra K.
California State University at Chico
Psychology Department
Chico, CA 95929
(916) 895-6253-**B**
Ethnicity: Asian-American/Asian/Pacific Islander
Degree and Year: PhD 1983
Major Field: Developmental Psychology

MACK, Delores E.
Monsour Counseling Center
Claremont University Center
735 North Dartmouth
Claremont, CA 91711
(909) 621-8202-**B**, (909) 621-8482-**F**
deloresm@cuc.claremont.edu
Ethnicity: African-American/Black
Degree and Year: PhD 1970
Major Field: Clinical Psychology
Specialty: Cross Cultural Processes;Ethnic Minorities;Family
Therapy;Psychotherapy

MACK, Faite R. P.
Grand Valley State University
301 W. Fulton Street
Grand Rapids, MI 49504
(616) 771-6650-**B**, 616) 458-0800-**H**, (616) 771-6515-**F**
Ethnicity: African-American/Black
Degree and Year: PhD 1972
Major Field: School Psychology
Specialty: Assessment/Diagnosis/Evaluation;Special
Education;Psychometrics;Ethnic Minorities;School
Psychology

MADISON, James K.
5306 Izard Street
Omaha, NE 68132-2143
(402) 559-5524-**B**
Ethnicity: Hispanic/Latino
Degree and Year: PhD 1983
Major Field: Clinical Psychology
Specialty: Eating Disorders

MADRAZO-PETERSON, Rita
Executive Park N
Albany, NY 12203-3746
(518) 458-2070-**B**
Ethnicity: Hispanic/Latino
Degree and Year: PhD 1977
Major Field: Counseling Psychology

MADRID, Raul P.
1417 Manorwood Drive, SE
Kentwood, MI 49508
(616) 247-3212-**B**, (616) 281-9702-**H**, (616) 247-3113-**F**
Ethnicity: Hispanic/Latino
Languages: Spanish
Degree and Year: PsyD 1988
Major Field: Clinical Psychology
Specialty: Ethnic Minorities;Cross Cultural Processes;Alcoholism &
Alcohol Abuse;Clinical Psychology;Crisis Intervention &
Therapy

MAGRAN, Betty A.
1001 Valley Road
Melrose Park, PA 19126

(215) 635-0371-**B**, (215) 635-0371-**H**
Ethnicity: Hispanic/Latino
Languages: Portuguese, Spanish
Degree and Year: MA 1963
Major Field: Clinical Psychology
Specialty: Child Therapy;Ethnic Minorities;Family Therapy;Marriage
& Family;Psychotherapy

MAHABEE-HARRIS, Marilyn M.
Rockdale Center
977A Taylor Street
Conyers, GA 30012
(770) 918-6677-**B**, (404) 299-6812-**H**, (770) 918-6686-**F**
Ethnicity: African-American/Black, Hispanic/Latino
Languages: Spanish
Degree and Year: PhD 1986
Major Field: Clinical Child Psychology
Specialty: Clinical Child Psychology;Family Therapy;Juvenile
Delinquency;Adolescent Therapy;Assessment/Diagnosis/
Evaluation;Parent-Child Interaction

MAHY, Yvonne C.
Bethune-Cookman College
640 Dr. Mary McLeod-Bethune Boulevard
Daytona Beach, FL 32117
(904) 255-1401-**B**, (904) 673-1258-**H**
mahyy@cookman.edu
Ethnicity: African-American/Black
Languages: French, Spanish
Degree and Year: PhD 1980
Major Field: Educational Psychology
Specialty: Psychology of Women;School Counseling;Social
Psychology;Child Development;Adolescent
Development;Environmental Psychology

MAJESTY, Melvin S.
216 Gifford Way
Sacramento, CA 95864
Ethnicity: Hispanic/Latino
Degree and Year: PhD 1967
Major Field: Industrial/Organizational Psy.
Specialty: Industrial/Organizational Psychology;Selection &
Placement;Research Design & Methodology;Human
Resources;Ethnic Minorities

MAJUMDER, Ranjit K.
West Virginia University
P.O. Box 6122
Morgantown, WV 26506-6122
Ethnicity: Asian-American/Asian/Pacific Islander
Degree and Year: PhD 1966
Major Field: unknown
Specialty: Clinical Neuropsychology;Sensory & Perceptual Processes

MALANCHARUVIL, Joseph M.
3137 Valencia
San Bernadino, CA 92404
(909) 381-1041-**B**
Ethnicity: Asian-American/Asian/Pacific Islander
Languages: Malayalam
Degree and Year: PhD 1982
Major Field: Clinical Psychology
Specialty: Schizophrenia;Psychopathology;Psychotherapy

MALDONADO, Loretto
  2727 North Ocean Boulevard #203A
  Boca Raton, FL 33431-7172
  (561) 367-9997-**B**, (561) 391-8935-**H**, (561) 391-3574-**F**
Ethnicity: Hispanic/Latino
Languages: French, Spanish
Degree and Year: PhD 1985
Major Field: Clinical Psychology
Specialty: Clinical Psychology;Rehabilitation;Health Psychology;Eating
    Disorders;Psychoimmunology

MALLISHAM, Ivy J.
  Direct Counseling Center
  Columbus State University
  4225 University Avenue
  Columbus, GA 31907-5645
  (706) 568-2233-**B**
  mallisham_ivy@colstate.edu
Ethnicity: African-American/Black
Degree and Year: PsyD 1983
Major Field: Clinical Psychology
Specialty: Clinical Psychology;Psychotherapy

MANCILLAS, Paul
  5005 Burnaby Drive
  Covina, CA 91724
  (818) 331-0990-**B**, (818) 964-2367-**H**
Ethnicity: Hispanic/Latino
Languages: Spanish
Degree and Year: PhD 1986
Major Field: Clinical Psychology
Specialty: Drug Abuse;Measurement;Mentally Retarded;Personality
    Measurement;Stress

MANE, Kamille L.
  5032 Laurel Park Drive
  Camarillo, CA 93012-5305
  (805) 484-3661-**B**
Ethnicity: Asian-American/Asian/Pacific Islander
Degree and Year: PhD 1972
Major Field: Clinical Psychology

MANESE, Jeanne E.
  University of California @ San Diego
  Psychological & Counseling Services
  Room #0509
  La Jolla, CA 92093-0509
  (619) 534-3035-**B**, (619) 458-0822-**H**, (619) 534-8931-**F**
Ethnicity: Asian-American/Asian/Pacific Islander
Degree and Year: PhD 1987
Major Field: Counseling Psychology
Specialty: Individual Psychotherapy;Cross Cultural Processes;Health
    Psychology;Stress;Training & Development;Counseling
    Psychology

MANESE, Wilfredo R.
  US West, Inc.
  188 Iverness Drive, West
  Suite #800
  Englewood, CO 80112-5207
  (303) 741-8536-**B**
Ethnicity: Asian-American/Asian/Pacific Islander
Degree and Year: PhD 1971

Major Field: Industrial/Organizational Psy.
Specialty: Labor & Management Relations

MANGHI, Elina R.
  The Family Institute
  47 S 6th Avenue, South
  Suite #132
  La Grange, IL 60525
  (708) 482-8812-**B**, (708) 383-7458-**H**
Ethnicity: Hispanic/Latino
Languages: Spanish
Degree and Year: PsyD 1988
Major Field: Clinical Psychology
Specialty: Assessment/Diagnosis/Evaluation;Child Therapy;Cross
    Cultural Processes;Depression;Family Therapy

MANN, Coramae R.
  Indiana University
  324 Sycamore
  Bloomington, IN 47401
Ethnicity: African-American/Black
Degree and Year: PhD 1976
Major Field: unknown

MANRUQUE-REICHARD, Marta E.
  University of Miami,
  Behavioral Medicine
  1450 NW 10th Avenue (M870)
  Cardiac Rehabilitation
  Miami, FL 33136
  (305) 243-2046-**B**, (305) 597-4331-**H**, (305) 243-2055-**F**
  mreichar@mednet.med.miami.edu
Ethnicity: Hispanic/Latino
Languages: Spanish
Degree and Year: PhD 1996
Major Field: Clinical Psychology
Specialty: Cardiovascular Processes;Cross Cultural Processes;Health
    Psychology;Clinical Psychology;Depression

MANUEL, Gerdenio M.
  Jesuit Comun, Santa Clara Univ
  500 El Camino Real
  Santa Clara, CA 95050-4345
  (408) 554-6896-**B**, (408) 554-4124-**H**, (408) 354-6465-**F**
Ethnicity: Asian-American/Asian/Pacific Islander
Degree and Year: PhD 1985
Major Field: Clinical Psychology
Specialty: Clinical Psychology;Psychotherapy;Religious Psychology

MANZANARES, Dan L.
  4770 E Iliff Avenue
  Suite #115
  Denver, CO 80222
  (303) 397-0545-**B**, (303) 393-6128-**H**, (303) 757-7994-**F**
Ethnicity: Hispanic/Latino
Degree and Year: PsyD 1983
Major Field: Clinical Psychology
Specialty: Alcoholism & Alcohol Abuse;Cognitive Psychology;Drug
    Abuse;Ethnic Minorities;Gender Issues

MARGARIDA, Maria T.
  Geranio 40
  San Juan, PR 00927
  (787) 754-3193-**B**, (809) 766-4750-**H**, (787) 754-4148-**F**

Ethnicity: Hispanic/Latino
Languages: Spanish
Degree and Year: PsyD 1987
Major Field: Clinical Psychology
Specialty: Child Abuse;Neuropsychology;Forensic Psychology

MAR, Harvey H.
St. Luke's
Roosevelt Hospital Center
428 W 59th Street
New York, NY 10019
(212) 523-6230-**B**, (212) 523-6241-**F**
Ethnicity: Asian-American/Asian/Pacific Islander
Degree and Year: PhD 1977
Major Field: Clinical Child Psychology
Specialty: Child Development;Mentally Retarded;Child & Pediatric Psychology;Special Education;Communication

MARIANO, Tomas V.
5406 N Lake Drive
Roanoke, VA 24019-2628
(703) 772-2866-**B**
Ethnicity: Asian-American/Asian/Pacific Islander
Degree and Year: PhD 1973
Major Field: Clinical Psychology
Specialty: Stress;Biofeedback

MARINA, Dorita
Miami Psychological Services
8500 West Flagler Street
Suite #B-206
Miami, FL 33144
(305) 551-3995-**B**, (305) 553-0403-**H**, (305) 551-3913-**F**
Ethnicity: Hispanic/Latino
Languages: Spanish
Degree and Year: PhD 1975
Major Field: Clinical Psychology
Specialty: Psychoanalysis;Projective Techniques;Forensic Psychology;Clinical Child Psychology;Neuropsychology;Mental Disorders

MARIN, Gerardo
University of Psychology
Department of Psychology
2130 Fulton Street
San Francisco, CA 94117-1080
(416) 422-2199-**B**, (415) 479-2621-**H**, (415) 422-5700-**F**
marin@usfca.edu
Ethnicity: Hispanic/Latino
Languages: Spanish
Degree and Year: PhD 1979
Major Field: Social Psychology
Specialty: Cross Cultural Processes;Attitudes & Opinions;Survey Theory & Methodology;Smoking;Health Psychology

MA, Rita J.
Metropolitan State Hospital
11400 Norwalk Boulevard
Program IV, Unite 401
Norwalk, CA 90650
(562) 651-3217-**B**, (626) 355-5232-**H**
Ethnicity: Asian-American/Asian/Pacific Islander
Degree and Year: PhD 1983
Major Field: Clinical Psychology

Specialty: Chronically Mentally Ill;Clinical Psychology;Psychopathology

MARMOL, Leonardo M.
George Fox University
Grad School of Clinical Psychology
414 N. Meridian Street
Newberg, OR 97132-2697
(503) 554-2762-**B**, (503) 537-3834-**F**
lmarmol@georgefox.edu
Ethnicity: Hispanic/Latino
Languages: Spanish
Degree and Year: PhD 1973
Major Field: Clinical Psychology
Specialty: Forensic Psychology;Neuropsychology;Clinical Psychology;Assessment/Diagnosis/Evaluation;Psychology & Law

MAR, Norman J.
8141 6th Avenue, SW
Seattle, WA 98106
(206) 684-8775-**B**
Ethnicity: Asian-American/Asian/Pacific Islander
Degree and Year: PhD 1979
Major Field: Clinical Psychology
Specialty: Community Psychology;Crisis Intervention & Therapy;Clinical Psychology;Stress

MAROTTA, Sylvia A.
George Washington University
2134 G Street, NW
#323
Washington, DC 20052
(202) 994-6642-**B**, (703) 548-6241-**H**, (202) 994-3436-**F**
syl@gwu.edu
Ethnicity: Hispanic/Latino
Languages: Spanish
Degree and Year: PhD 1992
Major Field: Counseling Psychology
Specialty: Clinical Research;Psychotherapy;Ethnic Minorities;Counseling Psychology;Group Psychotherapy;Family Therapy

MARQUEZ, E. Mario
9316 Freedom Way, NE
Alberquerque, NM 87109
(505) 864-2173-**B**, (505) 821-4998-**H**
Ethnicity: Hispanic/Latino
Languages: Spanish
Degree and Year: PhD 1990
Major Field: Counseling Psychology
Specialty: Counseling Psychology;School Psychology;Special Education;Child Therapy;Adolescent Therapy

MARQUEZ, Steven
Western State Hospital
2928 Lybarger Street, SE
Olympia, WA 98501-3649
(253) 756-2890-**B**, (360) 534-0318-**H**, (253) 756-2681-**F**
Ethnicity: Hispanic/Latino
Degree and Year: PhD 1983
Major Field: Clinical Child Psychology
Specialty: Forensic Psychology

MARRACH, Alexa
Federal Correctional Institute Seagoville
Seagoville, TX 75159
(972) 287-2911-**B**, (214) 827-6805-**H**
Ethnicity: Hispanic/Latino
Degree and Year: PhD 1994
Major Field: Clinical Psychology
Specialty: Correctional Psychology;Personality Disorders;Individual
    Psychotherapy;Crisis Intervention & Therapy

MARRERO, Bernie
Shands Rehabilitation Hospital
8900 NW 39th Avenue
Gainesville, FL 32606
(352) 338-0091-**B**, (352) 331-6965-**H**, (352) 376-4743-**F**
marreb.vpreach@shands.ufl.edu
Ethnicity: Hispanic/Latino
Languages: Spanish
Degree and Year: PhD 1986
Major Field: Educational Psychology
Specialty: Rehabilitation;Neuropsychology;Psychotherapy

MARROQUIN, Arthur R.
PO Box 2060
Ann Arbor, MI 48106
(734) 429-0862-**B**, (734) 971-1085-**H**, (734) 429-1817-**F**
marroquina@state.mi.us
Ethnicity: Hispanic/Latino
Languages: Spanish
Degree and Year: PhD 1983
Major Field: Clinical Psychology
Specialty: Psychotherapy;Assessment/Diagnosis/Evaluation;Forensic
    Psychology;Psychoses;Consulting Psychology

MARS, Raymond G.
Memphis Police Department
4371 OK Robertson Road
Memphis, TN 38127
(901) 354-1704-**B**, (901) 756-6966-**H**, (901) 354-1735-**F**
Ethnicity: African-American/Black
Degree and Year: PhD 1995
Major Field: Counseling Psychology
Specialty: Stress;Marriage & Family;Mental Disorders

MARTINEZ, JR., Joe L.
University of Texas
San Antonio
Division of Life Sciences
6900 North Loop 1604W
San Antonio, TX 78249-1130
210 458-4457-**B**, 210 458-5658-**F**
jmartinez@utsa.edu
Ethnicity: Hispanic/Latino
Degree and Year: PhD 1971
Major Field: Neurosciences
Specialty: Psychopharmacology;Psychobiology;Memory;Cross
    Cultural Processes;Drug Abuse

MARTINEZ-LUGO, Miguel E.
San Jorge 277
Apartment #303
Santurce, PR 00912
(809) 725-6500-**B**
Ethnicity: Hispanic/Latino

Languages: Spanish
Degree and Year: PhD 1983
Major Field: Industrial/Organizational Psy.
Specialty: Job Satisfaction;Measurement;Motivation;Stress

MARTINEZ-URRUTIA, Angel C.
61 West 62nd Street
Suite #4-H
New York, NY 10023
(212) 246-0088-**B**, (212) 246-0088-**H**, (212) 246-0088-**F**
Ethnicity: Hispanic/Latino
Languages: Spanish
Degree and Year: PhD 1972
Major Field: Clinical Psychology
Specialty: Psychoanalysis;Consulting Psychology;Cultural & Social
    Processes;Psychometrics

MARTINEZ, Alejandro M.
Stanford University
Cowell Student Health Service
670 Campus Drive
Stanford, CA 94305-8580
(650) 725-4120-**B**, (650) 494-6969-**H**, (651) 725-2887-**F**
amartinez@stanford.edu
Ethnicity: Hispanic/Latino
Languages: Spanish
Degree and Year: PhD 1980
Major Field: Clinical Psychology
Specialty: Administration;Crisis Intervention & Therapy;Cultural &
    Social Processes;Ethnic Minorities;Research & Training

MARTINEZ, Cynthia
California State University, Northridge
18111 Nordhoff Street
Northridge, CA 91330-8217
(818) 677-2366-**B**, (626) 331-6015-**H**, (818) 677-2371-**F**
cynthia.martinez@csun.edu
Ethnicity: Hispanic/Latino
Degree and Year: PhD 1994 MS 1987
Major Field: Counseling Psychology
Specialty: Drug Abuse;Counseling Psychology

MARTINEZ, Eduardo M.
23 SO St Las Lomas #772
Rio Piedras, PR 00921
809 721-3220-**B**, 809 727-162469-**H**
Ethnicity: Hispanic/Latino
Languages: Spanish
Degree and Year: PhD 1986
Major Field: Clinical Psychology
Specialty: Alcoholism & Alcohol Abuse;Rehabilitation;Community
    Psychology;Ethnic Minorities;Gerontology/Geropsychology

MARTINEZ, Floyd H.
1933 E Elm Street
Tucson, AZ 85719
(602) 884-9920-**B**, (602) 881-2906-**H**, (602) 792-0654-**F**
Ethnicity: Hispanic/Latino
Languages: Spanish
Degree and Year: PhD 1969
Major Field: Counseling Psychology
Specialty: Administration;Managed Care;Mental Health
    Services;Operations Research;Cross Cultural Processes

MARTINEZ, Gabriel P.
2615 Montebello
Waterford, MI 48329
(313) 858-0089-**B**, (313) 673-1619-**H**
Ethnicity: Hispanic/Latino
Degree and Year: MA 1970
Major Field: Clinical Psychology
Specialty: Forensic Psychology;Juvenile
　　Delinquency;Psychometrics;Psychotherapy;Drug Abuse

MARTINEZ, Maria J.
New York City Board of Education
600 East 6th Street
PS-64 Robert Simon School
Manhattan, NY 11373
(212) 505-6923-**B**, (718) 699-3076-**H**
Ethnicity: Hispanic/Latino
Languages: Spanish
Degree and Year: M
Major Field: School Psychology
Specialty: School Counseling;Assessment/Diagnosis/
　　Evaluation;Projective Techniques;School Psychology;Special
　　Education;Cross Cultural Processes

MARTINEZ, Raul
944 Ruiz Street
San Antonio, TX 78207
(210) 532-8811-**B**, (210) 222-0827-**H**
Ethnicity: Hispanic/Latino
Languages: Spanish
Degree and Year: PhD 1982
Major Field: Clinical Psychology
Specialty: Affective Disorders;Chronically Mentally Ill;Clinical Child
　　Psychology;Clinical Psychology;Death & Dying

MARTINEZ, Sergio I.
4650 North Cerritos Drive
Tucson, AZ 85745-9558
(602) 740-6201-**B**, (602) 743-3331-**H**
Ethnicity: Hispanic/Latino
Degree and Year: PhD 1981
Major Field: unknown

MARTIN, Laura P.
4172 Forest Hill Drive
La Canada, CA 91011
(818) 339-5545-**B**, (818) 790-4699-**H**, (619) 456-2144-**F**
Ethnicity: Hispanic/Latino
Languages: Spanish
Degree and Year: PhD 1974
Major Field: Clinical Psychology
Specialty: Adolescent Therapy;Feminist Therapy;Clinical
　　Psychology;Family Therapy;Gerontology/Geropsychology

MARTIN, William F.
4604 Brightwater Court #1
Owings Mills, MD 21117-4982
(504) 483-7315-**B**, (504) 895-3530-**H**
Ethnicity: African-American/Black, Hispanic/Latino
Degree and Year: PsyD 1989
Major Field: Clinical Psychology
Specialty: Health Psychology;Employee Assistance Programs;Training
　　& Development;Cognitive Behavioral Therapy;Administration

MARTORELL, Mario F.
20 49th Street
Weehawkea, NJ 07087
(212) 927-1916-**B**, (201) 348-4156-**H**
Ethnicity: Hispanic/Latino
Languages: Spanish
Degree and Year: PhD 1991
Major Field: School Psychology
Specialty: Assessment/Diagnosis/Evaluation;School
　　Psychology;Educational Research;Creativity;Learning
　　Disabilities

MARUYAMA, Geoffrey
University of Minnesota
Department of Educational Psychology
210 Burton
178 Pillsbury Drive, SE
Minneapolis, MN 55455
(612) 624-5861-**B**, (612) 699-6782-**H**, (612) 624-8241-**F**
geofmar@tc.umn.edu
Ethnicity: Asian-American/Asian/Pacific Islander
Degree and Year: PhD 1977
Major Field: Social Psychology
Specialty: Social Psychology;Educational Psychology;Cultural & Social
　　Processes;Social Change;Research Design & Methodology

MARUYAMA, Magoroh
Kokusai Seiji Keizai Department
Shibuya 4-4-25
Shibuya-Ku,
JAPAN
Ethnicity: Asian-American/Asian/Pacific Islander
Degree and Year: PhD 1959
Major Field: unknown
Specialty: Management & Organization

MASINI, Angela
4877 Chambliss Avenue
Knoxville, TN 37919
(615) 588-1923-**B**
Ethnicity: Hispanic/Latino
Languages: Spanish
Degree and Year: PhD 1973
Major Field: Clinical Psychology
Specialty: Psychotherapy;Alcoholism & Alcohol Abuse;Hypnosis/
　　Hypnotherapy;Family Therapy

MASTRAPA, Selma A.
Takoma Academy
8120 Carroll Avenue
Takoma Park, MD 20912
(301) 434-4700-**B**, (301) 434-4814-**F**
Ethnicity: Hispanic/Latino
Languages: Spanish
Degree and Year: PhD 1982
Major Field: Counseling Psychology
Specialty: School Counseling;Religious Psychology;Ingestive Behavior
　　& Nutrition;Counseling Psychology;Adult Development

MATE-KOLE, C. Charles
Central Connecticut State University
1615 Stanley Street
New Britain, CT 06050
(860) 832-3105-**B**, (860) 826-1929-**H**, (860) 832-3123-**F**

matekolec@ccsu.edu
Ethnicity: African-American/Black
Degree and Year: PhD 1986
Major Field: Clinical Psychology
Specialty: Cross Cultural Processes;Clinical Research;Gerontology/
Geropsychology;Clinical Neuropsychology;Alzheimer's
Disease;Psychopathology

MATHESON, Charlene
2412 N. 30th, Suite 102
Tacoma, WA 98407
(206) 756-8119-**B**
Ethnicity: American Indian/Alaska Native
Degree and Year: PhD 1981
Major Field: Clinical Psychology
Specialty: Adult Development;Individual Psychotherapy;Adolescent
Therapy;Affective Disorders;Cognitive Behavioral Therapy

MATSUI, Wesley T.
135 Columbia Turnpike
Suite #303
Florham Park, NJ 07932
(201) 377-3116-**B**, (201) 836-2108-**H**
Ethnicity: Asian-American/Asian/Pacific Islander
Degree and Year: PhD 1986
Major Field: Clinical Psychology
Specialty: Family Therapy;Marriage & Family;Training &
Development;Gender Issues;Alcoholism & Alcohol Abuse

MATSUMIYA, Yoichi
Brown University
Box 1853
Providence, RI 02912
(401) 863-2041-**B**, (617) 444-7344-**H**, (401) 863-1300-**F**
Ethnicity: Asian-American/Asian/Pacific Islander
Languages: Japanese
Degree and Year: PhD 1963
Major Field: Physiological Psychology
Specialty: Neurophysiology;Neurological Disorders;Sensory Motor
Processes;Neurosciences;Conditioning, Operant & Classical

MATSUMOTO, David
San Francisco State University
Psychology Department
1600 Holloway Avenue
San Francisco, CA 94132-1722
(415) 338-1114-**B**, (510) 236-9171-**H**, (415) 338-2584-**F**
dm@sfsu.edu
Ethnicity: Asian-American/Asian/Pacific Islander
Languages: Japanese
Degree and Year: PhD 1986
Major Field: Social Psychology
Specialty: Emotion;Cross Cultural Processes;Cultural & Social
Processes;Nonverbal Communication

MATSUMOTO, Gregory Y.
2180 Jefferson Street
Suite #209
Napa, CA 94559
(707) 252-7811-**B**, (707) 226-2147-**H**, (707) 224-8631-**F**
Ethnicity: Asian-American/Asian/Pacific Islander
Degree and Year: PhD 1986
Major Field: Clinical Psychology
Specialty: Psychotherapy;Assessment/Diagnosis/Evaluation;Child
Abuse;Cross Cultural Processes;Marriage & Family

MATSUMOTO, Roy T.
California State @ Hayward
Hayward, CA 94542
(510) 881-3485-**B**, (510) 236-9173-**H**
Ethnicity: Asian-American/Asian/Pacific Islander
Degree and Year: PhD 1965
Major Field: Experimental Psychology
Specialty: Classical Conditioning;Experimental
Psychology;Conditioning, Operant & Classical;Learning/
Learning Theory

MATSUURA, Larry N.
Alamoana Counseling Service
1441 Kapiolani Blvd.
Suite #905
Honolulu, HI 96814-4402
(808) 949-5055-**B**
Ethnicity: Asian-American/Asian/Pacific Islander
Degree and Year: EdD 19
Major Field: Counseling Psychology

MATTHEWS, Belvia W.
115 Fairington Road
Huntsville, AL 35806
(205) 726-7047-**B**, (205) 830-4099-**H**, (205) 726-7409-**F**
Ethnicity: African-American/Black
Degree and Year: PhD 1977
Major Field: Clinical Psychology
Specialty: Psychotherapy;Personality Measurement;Clinical
Psychology;Marriage & Family;Industrial/Organizational
Psychology

MAUNG, Iqbal T.
4055 Coolidge Avenue
Los Angeles, CA 90066-5411
(909) 860-2166-**B**, (310) 539-3086-**H**
Ethnicity: Asian-American/Asian/Pacific Islander
Degree and Year: MA 1986
Major Field: Clinical Psychology
Specialty: Family Therapy;Biofeedback

MA, Yat-Ming C.
The Family Institute
of Northwestern University
618 Library Place
Evanston, IL 60201-2908
(8470) 733-9301-**B**, (847) 732-0390-**F**
yma@nwu.edu
Ethnicity: Asian-American/Asian/Pacific Islander
Degree and Year: PsyD
Major Field: unknown

MAYNARD, Edward S.
RD 7, Box 370
Monroe, NY 10950
(212) 749-6691-**B**, (914) 783-1552-**H**, (212) 749-6691-**F**
Ethnicity: African-American/Black
Languages: Spanish
Degree and Year: PhD 1984
Major Field: Clinical Psychology
Specialty: Clinical Psychology;Counseling Psychology;Cross Cultural
Processes;Pastoral Psychology

MAYO, Benjamin F.
Bear Institute
3450 West 43rd Street #101

Los Angeles, CA 90008
(213) 294-9101-**B**, (213) 292-9810-**H**, (213) 294-5254-**F**
bmayo11397@aol.com
Ethnicity: African-American/Black
Degree and Year:
Major Field: Personality Psychology

MAYS, Vickie M.
University of California @ LA
Department of Psychology
285 Franz Hall
Hilgard Avenue
Los Angeles, CA 90095-1563
(310) 206-5159-**B**
mays@ucla.edu
Ethnicity: African-American/Black
Degree and Year: PhD 1979
Major Field: Clinical Psychology
Specialty: Ethnic Minorities;HIV/AIDS;Policy Analysis;Sexual
         Behavior;Research Design & Methodology

MCCAIN, Lillie W.
11377 Grand Oak
Grand Blanc, MI 48439-2204
(313) 732-2003-**B**
Ethnicity: African-American/Black
Degree and Year: PhD 1975
Major Field: Community Psychology
Specialty: Community Psychology

MCCANDIES, Terry T
Duke University Medical Center
PO Box 2917
Durham, NC 27710
(919) 684-8723-**B**, 919 286-0330-**H**
Ethnicity: African-American/Black
Degree and Year:
Major Field: unknown

MCCANN, Robin S.
CMHIP-IFP
1600 W 24th Street
Pueblo, CO 81003
(719) 546-4965-**B**
Ethnicity: Asian-American/Asian/Pacific Islander
Degree and Year: PhD 1989
Major Field: Clinical Psychology
Specialty: Cognitive Behavioral Therapy;Domestic Violence;Forensic
         Psychology;Clinical Psychology;Psychology of Women

MCCARLEY, Victor J.
McCarley & Associates, Inc.
PO Box 252
Dayton, OH 45406
(513) 461-0386-**B**
Ethnicity: African-American/Black
Degree and Year: PhD 1981
Major Field: Clinical Psychology
Specialty: Assessment/Diagnosis/Evaluation;Drug Abuse;Cognitive
         Behavioral Therapy;Marriage & Family;Adolescent Therapy

MCCLURE, Faith H.
CCU San Bernardino
Psychology Department
5500 University Parkway
San Bernardino, CA 92407

(909) 880-5598-**B**, (909) 799-9572-**H**
Ethnicity: African-American/Black
Degree and Year: PhD 1989
Major Field: Clinical Psychology
Specialty: Clinical Psychology;Community Mental Health;Stress;Child
         Abuse;Psychotherapy

MCCOMBS, Daniel
30 Elmwood Drive
North Kingstown, RI 02852-1722
(401) 874-2288-**B**, (401) 874-5010-**F**
Ethnicity: African-American/Black, American Indian/Alaska Native
Degree and Year: PhD 1981
Major Field: Clinical Psychology
Specialty: Clinical Psychology;Psychotherapy;Community Mental
         Health;Forensic Psychology;Ethnic Minorities

MCCOMBS, Harriet G.
Bureau of Primary Health Care
Health Resources and Services Administration (HRSA)
4350 East West Highway, 11th Floor
Bethesda, MD 20814
(301) 594-4457-**B**, (301) 594-4989 -**F**
Hmccombs@hrsa.gov.
Ethnicity: African-American/Black
Degree and Year: PhD 1978
Major Field: Social Psychology
Specialty: Program Evaluation;Mental Health Services;Ethnic
         Minorities;Homelessness & Homeless Populations;Policy
         Analysis

MCCOY, George F.
Parklawn Building
5600 Fishers Lane, Room 6A-38
Rockville, MD 20857
(301) 443-2334-**B**, (301) 990-6520-**H**, (301) 227-6213-**F**
Ethnicity: American Indian/Alaska Native
Degree and Year: PhD 1960
Major Field: School Psychology

MCDONALD, II, Ozzie H.
2650 Burnet Avenue
Cincinnati, OH 45219-2550
(513) 281-6663-**B**
Ethnicity: African-American/Black
Degree and Year: PhD 1982
Major Field: Clinical Psychology
Specialty: Psychotherapy

MCDONALD, Arthur L.
Box 326
Lame Deer, MT 59043
(406) 748-3634-**B**, (406) 477-6441-**H**, (406) 477-8157-**F**
amcdonald@mci.net
Ethnicity: American Indian/Alaska Native
Degree and Year: PhD 1966
Major Field: Experimental Psychology
Specialty: Human Factors;Alcoholism & Alcohol Abuse;Cross Cultural
         Processes

MCGOWAN, Eugene
1630 Wilmington Road
New Castle, DE 19720-3673
Ethnicity: African-American/Black
Degree and Year: PhD 1960
Major Field: School Psychology

Specialty: School Counseling

MCINTYRE, Lorna A.
899 Orlando Avenue
West Hempstead, NY 11552-3940
(718) 217-5398-**B**
Ethnicity: African-American/Black
Degree and Year: PhD 1985
Major Field: Clinical Psychology

MCKENZIE, JR., Loratuis L.
4316 Sturtevant
Detroit, MI 48204
(313) 349-1800-**B**, (313) 933-0476-**H**
Ethnicity: African-American/Black
Degree and Year: PhD
Major Field: Clinical Psychology
Specialty: Psychoses;Projective Techniques;Neuroses;Mental Health
Services;Affective Disorders

MCLEAN, JR, Alvin
Paradigm Health Corporation
1001 Galaxy Way
Suite 300
Concord, CA 94520
Ethnicity: African-American/Black
Degree and Year: PhD 1981
Major Field: unknown
Specialty: Clinical Neuropsychology;Rehabilitation

MCLOYD, Vonnie C.
University of Michigan
Center for Human Growth & Development
300 North Ingalls
Tenth Floor
Ann Arbor, MI 48109
(734) 764-2443-**B**, (734) 669-9202-**H**, (734) 936-9288-**F**
vcmcloyd@umich.edu
Ethnicity: African-American/Black
Degree and Year: PhD 1975
Major Field: Developmental Psychology
Specialty: Child Development;Ethnic Minorities;Social
Behavior;Disadvantaged;Family Processes;Stress

MCMILLAN, Robert
30 Shanley Avenue
Newark, NJ 07108
(201) 546-0990-**B**, (201) 744-3843-**H**
Ethnicity: African-American/Black
Degree and Year: EdD 1978
Major Field: Counseling Psychology
Specialty: Assessment/Diagnosis/Evaluation;Psychotherapy;Clinical
Neuropsychology;Child Abuse;Educational Psychology

MCNEAL, Meryl
Morehouse School of Medicine
720 Westview Drive
Atlanta, GA 30310
(404) 752-1638-**B**
Ethnicity: African-American/Black
Degree and Year: PhD 1991
Major Field: Community Psychology

MCNEILL, Brian

Washington State University
Department of Education
Leadership and Counseling Psychology
Pullman, WA 99164-2136
(509) 335-6477-**B**, (208) 883-8483-**H**, (509) 335-7977-**F**
mcniell@mail.wsu.edu
Ethnicity: Hispanic/Latino, European/White
Degree and Year: PhD 1984
Major Field: Counseling Psychology
Specialty: Thought Processes;Professional Issues in Psychology;Ethnic
Minorities;Cultural & Social Processes

MCNEILL, Earle
4000 Gypsy Lane, Unit #235
Philadelphia, PA 19144
(215) 732-9573-**B**, (215) 849-3312-**H**, (215) 732-8005-**F**
exm23@mail.voicenet.com
Ethnicity: African-American/Black
Degree and Year: EdD 1973
Major Field: Counseling Psychology
Specialty: Ethnic Minorities;Alcoholism & Alcohol Abuse;Counseling
Psychology;Group Psychotherapy;Human Relations

MCNEILL, Elizabeth M.
2600 Denali Street
Suite #701
Anchorage, AK 99503
(907) 278-6732-**B**, (907) 248-2350-**H**, (907) 278-9909-**F**
Ethnicity: Hispanic/Latino
Languages: Spanish
Degree and Year: PhD 1993
Major Field: Clinical Psychology
Specialty: Marriage & Family;Depression;Eating Disorders;Group
Psychotherapy;Lesbian & Gay Issuues

MCRAE, Mary B.
351 W. 114th Street
New York, NY 10026
(212) 998-5552-**B**
Ethnicity: African-American/Black
Degree and Year: PhD 1987
Major Field: Counseling Psychology
Specialty: Counseling Psychology;Cross Cultural Processes;Cultural &
Social Processes;Human Relations;Group Processes

MCWILLIAMS, Junko O.
5734 Mineral Hill Road
Sykesvelle, MD 21784
(301) 233-1400-**B**, (410) 795-8455-**H**
Ethnicity: Asian-American/Asian/Pacific Islander
Languages: Japanese
Degree and Year: PhD 1978
Major Field: Clinical Psychology
Specialty: Adolescent Therapy;Behavior Therapy;Clinical Child
Psychology;Cognitive Behavioral Therapy;Family Therapy

MEADOWS-YANCEY, Dorothy
3338 Greenland Avenue, NW
Roanoke, VA 24012
(540) 563-1511-**B**, (508) 756-8822-**H**
Ethnicity: African-American/Black
Languages: German
Degree and Year: C.A. 1979
Major Field: Educational Psychology

Specialty: School Psychology;School Counseling;Counseling Psychology;Consulting Psychology;Child Therapy

MEHROTRA, Chandra M.N.
The College of Scholastica
Duluth, MN 55811
(218) 723-6161-**B**, (218) 728-4882-**H**, (218) 723-6796-**F**
cmehrotr@css.edu
Ethnicity: Asian-American/Asian/Pacific Islander
Languages: Hindi
Degree and Year: PhD 1968
Major Field: Gerontology
Specialty: Gerontology/Geropsychology;Program Evaluation;Performance Evaluation;Selection & Placement;Ethnic Minorities

MEHTA, Kripal K.
26 Lancashire Way
Pittsford, NY 14534
(716) 473-3230-**B**, (716) 383-8015-**H**, (716) 586-4916-**F**
Ethnicity: Asian-American/Asian/Pacific Islander
Languages: Hindi, Punjabi
Degree and Year: PhD 1973
Major Field: Clinical Psychology
Specialty: Adolescent Therapy;Assessment/Diagnosis/Evaluation;Child Therapy;Family Therapy;Group Psychotherapy

MEHTA, Sheila
Auburn University @ Montgomery
Department of Psychology
7300 University Drive
Montgomery, AL 36117-3596
(334) 244-3312-**B**, 334 887-5490-**H**, 334 244-3762-**F**
mehta@sciences.aum.edu
Ethnicity: Asian-American/Asian/Pacific Islander, European/White
Degree and Year: PhD 1993
Major Field: Clinical Psychology
Specialty: Clinical Psychology;Ethnic Minorities;Mental Disorders;Cultural & Social Processes;Gender Issues

MEJIA, Juan A.
136 East South Temple
Suite #2200
Salt Lake City, UT 84111
(801) 328-4500-**B**
Ethnicity: Hispanic/Latino
Languages: Spanish
Degree and Year: PhD 1981
Major Field: Clinical Psychology
Specialty: Clinical Psychology;Assessment/Diagnosis/Evaluation;Clinical Neuropsychology;Forensic Psychology;Juvenile Delinquency

MELGOZA, Bertha
8515 Cliffridge Avenue
La Jolla, CA 92037
(619) 457-1264-**B**, (619) 450-1296-**H**, (619) 546-9884-**F**
grantbaker@aol.com
Ethnicity: Hispanic/Latino
Languages: Spanish
Degree and Year: PhD 1980
Major Field: Clinical Psychology
Specialty: Psychotherapy;Family Therapy;Ethnic Minorities;Marriage & Family;Physically Handicapped

MELLOR-CRUMMEY, Cynthia A.
101 Southwestern Boulevard
Suite
Sugarland, TX 77478
(713) 813-6740-**B**, (713) 721-7174-**F**
Ethnicity: Hispanic/Latino
Languages: Spanish
Degree and Year: PhD 1990
Major Field: Clinical Psychology
Specialty: Clinical Child Psychology;Family Therapy;Drug Abuse;Mental Health Services;Parent-Child Interaction

MELLOR, Catherine A.
6821 Baile Road
Las Vegas, NV 89146-6550
(702) 799-1591-**B**, (702) 873-6725-**H**
Ethnicity: American Indian/Alaska Native
Degree and Year: MS 1975
Major Field: Educational Psychology
Specialty: Administration;Special Education;Counseling Psychology;Assessment/Diagnosis/Evaluation;Physically Handicapped

MELLOT, Ramona N.
Northern Arizona University
CEE Box 5774
Flagstaff, AZ 86002
(520) 523-6534-**B**, 520 774-4658-**H**, 520 523-1929-**F**
ramona.mellot@nau.edu
Ethnicity: Asian-American/Asian/Pacific Islander
Languages: Hindi
Degree and Year: PhD 1991
Major Field: Counseling Psychology
Specialty: Assessment/Diagnosis/Evaluation;Alcoholism & Alcohol Abuse;Child Abuse;Counseling Psychology;Cognitive Behavioral Therapy;Mental Disorders

MENCHACA, Victoria A.
11845 W Olympic Blvd.
Suite 1155
Los Angeles, CA 90064-5025
(310) 575-3505-**B**, (310) 575-4007-**H**
vmenchaca@worldnet.att.net
Ethnicity: Hispanic/Latino
Degree and Year: PhD 1986
Major Field: Clinical Psychology
Specialty: Child Therapy;Marriage & Family;Parent-Child Interaction;Individual Psychotherapy;Adolescent Therapy

MENDELBERG, Hava E.
2577 N Downer Avenue
Suite #215
Milwaukee, WI 53211
(414) 964-9200-**B**, (414) 332-3432-**H**
Urimendelber@aol.com
Ethnicity: Hispanic/Latino
Languages: Spanish, Hebrew
Degree and Year: PhD 1981
Major Field: Clinical Psychology
Specialty: Affective Disorders;Clinical Psychology;Depression;Group Psychotherapy;Psychotherapy

MENDEZ-CALDERON, Luis M.
University of the Sacred Heart
Street A

Villa Caparra Tower
Guayana, PR 00966
(809) 728-1515-**B**, (809) 782-6944-**H**, (809) 728-1515-**F**
Ethnicity: Hispanic/Latino, European/White
Languages: Spanish
Degree and Year: PhD 1979
Major Field: Educational Psychology
Specialty: Educational Psychology

MENDEZ, Gloria I.
Christiansted
P.O. Box 1416
St. Croix, VI 00821
(809) 773-3322-**B**, (809) 773-3577-**H**, (809) 773-2566-**F**
Ethnicity: Hispanic/Latino
Languages: Spanish
Degree and Year: PhD 1979
Major Field: Educational Psychology
Specialty: Assessment/Diagnosis/Evaluation;Intelligence;Vocational
    Psychology;Personality Measurement;School Psychology

MENDOZA, Jorge L.
University of Oaklahoma
Psychology Department
Dale Hall
Norman, OK 73019
(405) 325-4511-**B**, (405) 321-4676-**H**, (405) 325-4737-**F**
jmendoza@ou.edu
Ethnicity: Hispanic/Latino
Languages: Spanish
Degree and Year: PhD 1974
Major Field: Quan/Math & Psychometrics/Stat
Specialty: Industrial/Organizational
    Psychology;Psychometrics;Statistics

MERRITT, Marcellus M.
Duke University Medical Cener
Department of Psychiatry
2212-F Elder Street, Building F
Durham, NC 27705
(919) 684-2792-**B**, (919) 477-1588-**H**, (919) 681-8960-**F**
mmerritt@duke.edu
Ethnicity: African-American/Black
Degree and Year: PhD 1997 MS 1994
Major Field: Personality Psychology
Specialty: Cardiovascular Processes;Psychophysiology;Personality
    Psychology;Health Psychology;Quantitative/Mathematical,
    Psychometrics;Stress

MICCIO-FONSECA, L. C.
591 Camino De La Reina
Suite 533
San Diego, CA 92108-3107
(619) 293-3330-**B**, (619) 294-3322-**F**
lcmf@ix.netcom.com
Ethnicity: Hispanic/Latino
Languages: Spanish
Degree and Year: PhD 1982
Major Field: Clinical Psychology
Specialty: Forensic Psychology;Adolescent Therapy;Child
    Therapy;Sexual Dysfunction

MIKAMO, Akiko
U.S. Japan Psychological Services
3750 Convoy Street #318

San Diego, CA 92111
(619) 505-0085-**B**, (619) 505-0095-**F**
usjpnpsych@aol.com
Ethnicity: Asian-American/Asian/Pacific Islander
Languages: Japanese
Degree and Year: PsyD 1995
Major Field: Clinical Psychology
Specialty: Assessment/Diagnosis/Evaluation;Child Therapy;Cognitive
    Behavioral Therapy;Consulting Psychology;Family
    Therapy;Individual Psychotherapy

MILBURN, Norweeta G.
3680 Shadow Grove Road
Pasadena, CA 91107-2112
(516) 463-5295-**B**
Ethnicity: African-American/Black
Degree and Year: PhD 1982
Major Field: Community Psychology
Specialty: Community Psychology;Homelessness & Homeless
    Populations;Drug Abuse

MILES, Gary T.
Po Box 52053
Palo Alto, CA 94303-0748
(408) 275-7600-**B**, (415) 967-3510-**H**, (408) 275-7606-**F**
Ethnicity: African-American/Black
Degree and Year: PhD 1988
Major Field: Clinical Psychology
Specialty: Neuropsychology;HIV/AIDS;Cognitive Behavioral
    Therapy;Ethnic Minorities;Lesbian & Gay Issuues

MILLAN, Fred
State University of New York
Psychol Dept, Suny Col
Po Box 210
Old Westbury, NY 11568-0210
(516) 876-3198-**B**, (718) 224-9786-**H**
Ethnicity: Hispanic/Latino
Languages: Spanish
Degree and Year: PhD 1990
Major Field: Counseling Psychology
Specialty: HIV/AIDS;Counseling Psychology;Psychotherapy;Ethnic
    Minorities;Group Psychotherapy;Cultural & Social Processes

MILLARD, Wilbur A.
3228 13th Street, N.W.
Washington, DC 20010
(202) 332-0336-**B**
Ethnicity: African-American/Black
Degree and Year: EdD 1968
Major Field: School Psychology
Specialty: Mental Health Services;Clinical Psychology;Educational
    Psychology;Developmental Psychology;Special Education

MILLER, Fayneese
Brown University
Department of Education
Providence, RI 02912
Ethnicity: African-American/Black
Degree and Year: PhD 1981
Major Field: Social Psychology
Specialty: Attitudes & Opinions;Cultural & Social Processes

MILLER, Robin L.
University of Illinois at Chicago
Department of Psychology (M/C 285)

1007 West Harrison Street
Chicago, IL 60607-7137
(312) 413-2638-**B**, (312) 413-4122-**F**
rlmiller@uic.edu
Ethnicity: African-American/Black
Degree and Year: PhD 1994
Major Field: Community Psychology
Specialty: HIV/AIDS;Lesbian & Gay Issuues;Community
Psychology;Program Evaluation;Prevention

MILLER, S. Walden
University of California, San Diego
2760 5th Avenue Suite 100
San Diego, CA 92103
(619) 543-4742-**B**, (760) 739-8429-**H**, (619) 543-1235-**F**
Ethnicity: African-American/Black
Degree and Year: PhD 1974
Major Field: Neurosciences
Specialty: Assessment/Diagnosis/Evaluation;Neuropsychology;HIV/
AIDS;Brain Functions;Physiological Psychology;Ethnic
Minorities

MILLER, Sarah S.
1447 4th Street Suite A
Napa, CA 94559
(707) 258-8500-**B**, (707) 258-8500-**F**
sarahbe@ibm.net
Ethnicity: American Indian/Alaska Native
Degree and Year: PhD 1978
Major Field: Health Psychology
Specialty: Medical Psychology;Emotional Development;Clinical
Neuropsychology;Research & Training

MILLS, Marcia C.
1808 Via Estudillo
Palos Verdes Ests., CA 90274
(310) 378-6082-**B**, (310) 373-7852-**H**, (310) 378-6082-**F**
Ethnicity: African-American/Black
Degree and Year: PhD 1980
Major Field: Clinical Psychology
Specialty: Forensic Psychology;Administration;Assessment/Diagnosis/
Evaluation;Ethnic Minorities;Endocrine Systems

MILNER, Joel S.
Northern Illinois University
Department of Psychology
De Kalb, IL 60115
(815) 753-0739-**B**, (815) 753-8088-**F**
jmilner@niu.edu
Ethnicity: American Indian/Alaska Native
Degree and Year: PhD 1970
Major Field: Clinical Psychology
Specialty: Psychotherapy;Personality Measurement

MINAGAWA, Rahn Y.
827 Leppert Street
San Diego, CA 92114-3039
Ethnicity: Asian-American/Asian/Pacific Islander
Degree and Year: PhD 1983
Major Field: Clinical Psychology
Specialty: Psychotherapy

MINDINGALL, Marilyn P.
Mercer University
1400 Coleman Avenue
Macon, GA 31207-0001

(912) 752-4151-**B**, (912) 750-8658-**H**
Ethnicity: African-American/Black
Degree and Year: PhD 1981
Major Field: Clinical Psychology

MINK, Iris T.
Dept. of Psychiatry
760 Westwood Plaza
Los Angeles, CA 90024-1759
(310) 206-6082-**B**, (310) 476-2722-**H**, (310) 476-3989-**F**
irismink@ucla.edu
Ethnicity: Asian-American/Asian/Pacific Islander
Degree and Year: PhD 1971
Major Field: Developmental Psychology
Specialty: Mentally Retarded;Cross Cultural Processes;Family
Processes;Parent-Child Interaction

MINK, Oscar G.
University of Texas
Department of Education Administration
310 Education Building
Austin, TX 78712
(512) 837-9371-**B**, (512) 837-2060-**H**, (512) 835-4998-**F**
Ethnicity: American Indian/Alaska Native
Degree and Year: EdD 1961
Major Field: Counseling Psychology

MINO, Itsuko
Associate in Research
E.O. Rezschauer Institute
Harvard University
PO Box 380550
Cambridge, MA 02238-0550
(617) 242-1626-**B**, (617) 242-1626-**H**
minomiya@aol.rom
Ethnicity: Asian-American/Asian/Pacific Islander
Languages: Japanese
Degree and Year: EdD 1986
Major Field: Developmental Psychology
Specialty: Adult Development;Moral Development;Social
Psychology;Cognitive Development;Psychology of
Women;Suicide

MINTURN, Robin H.
360 W 62nd Street
Indianapolis, IN 46260-4716
(317) 259-4817-**B**
Ethnicity: Asian-American/Asian/Pacific Islander
Languages: Spanish
Degree and Year: PhD 1982
Major Field: Counseling Psychology
Specialty: Clinical Neuropsychology;Neuropsychology

MIO, Jeffery S.
CA State Polytechnic University, Pomona
Behavior Science Department
3801 West Temple Avenue
Pomona, CA 91768-2557
(909) 869-3899-**B**, (909) 597-1989-**H**, (509) 335-5043-**F**
jmio@csupomona.edu
Ethnicity: Asian-American/Asian/Pacific Islander
Degree and Year: PhD 1984
Major Field: Clinical Psychology
Specialty: Clinical Psychology;Cognitive Psychology;Cross Cultural
Processes;Family Therapy

MIRANDA, David J.
Rosewood Center
Rosewood Lane
Owings Mills, MD 21117
(410) 647-8840-**B**, (410) 255-1680-**H**
miranda@amdyne.net
Ethnicity: Hispanic/Latino
Languages: Portuguese, Spanish
Degree and Year: PhD 1991
Major Field: Clinical Psychology
Specialty: Attention Deficit Disorders;Adolescent Therapy;Mentally
    Retarded;Assessment/Diagnosis/Evaluation

MIRANDA, Jose P.
102 Canyon Rim Drive
Austin, TX 78746
1 800 792-9276-**B**, (512) 327-4968-**H**
Ethnicity: Hispanic/Latino
Languages: Spanish
Degree and Year: PhD 1995
Major Field: School Psychology
Specialty: Clinical Neuropsychology

MIRANDA, M.
Georgetown University Hospital
Department of Psychiatry
3800 Reservoir Road, NW
Washington, DC 20007-2113
(202) 687-8650-**B**, (301) 564-6676-**H**, (415) 206-8942-**F**
Ethnicity: Hispanic/Latino
Languages: Spanish
Degree and Year: PhD 1986
Major Field: Clinical Psychology
Specialty: Health Psychology;Depression;Clinical Research;Mental
    Health Services;Psychosomatic Disorders;Cognitive Behavioral
    Therapy

MIRANDA, Manuel R.
California State University, Los Angeles
Salazar Hall, Room C-120
5151 State University Avenue
Los Angeles, CA 90032
(323) 343-5337-**B**, (626) 793-1337-**H**, (323) 343-6410-**F**
mmiranda@calstatela.edu
Ethnicity: Hispanic/Latino
Languages: Spanish
Degree and Year: PhD 1971
Major Field: Gerontology
Specialty: Adult Development;Clinical Psychology;Ethnic
    Minorities;Epidemiology & Biometry;Gerontology/
    Geropsychology

MISRA, Rajendra K.
484 Miner Road
Highland Heights, OH 44143-1539
(216) 342-9868-**B**
Ethnicity: Asian-American/Asian/Pacific Islander
Languages: Hindi, Urdu, Bengali
Degree and Year: PhD 1968
Major Field: Personality Psychology
Specialty: Personality Disorders;Cross Cultural Processes;Community
    Psychology;Projective Techniques

MITCHELL, Horace
University of California, Irvine
405 Administration Building
Irvine, CA 92717
(714) 856-7253-**B**, (714) 725-2763-**F**
Ethnicity: African-American/Black
Degree and Year: PhD 1974
Major Field: Counseling Psychology
Specialty: Administration

MITCHELL, Howard E.
315 S. Camac Street
Philadelphia, PA 19107
(215) 735-1562-**B**, (215) 735-1562-**H**, (215) 735-1562-**F**
Ethnicity: African-American/Black
Languages: Italian
Degree and Year: PhD 1951
Major Field: Clinical Psychology
Specialty: Human Resources;Management & Organization;Cross
    Cultural Processes

MIURA, Irene T.
2225 Bunker Hill Dr
San Mateo, CA 94402-3832
(408) 924-3717-**B**, (415) 349-6954-**H**, (409) 924-3713-**F**
Ethnicity: Asian-American/Asian/Pacific Islander
Languages: Japanese
Degree and Year: PhD 1984
Major Field: Educational Psychology
Specialty: Child Development;Adolescent Development

MIYAHIRA, Sarah D.
5943 Kalanianaole Hwy
Honolulu, HI 96821-2309
(808) 566-1648-**B**, (808) 395-9151-**H**, (808) 944-7490-**F**
Ethnicity: Asian-American/Asian/Pacific Islander
Degree and Year: PhD 1976
Major Field: Counseling Psychology
Specialty: Ethnic Minorities;Human Resources;Management &
    Organization;Gender Issues

MIYAKE, Steven M.
300 Ala Moana Boulevard
Room #2322
Honolulu, HI 96850-0002
(808) 566-1657-**B**
Ethnicity: Asian-American/Asian/Pacific Islander
Degree and Year: PhD 1978
Major Field: Clinical Psychology
Specialty: Health Psychology;Behavior Therapy;Clinical
    Psychology;Biofeedback;Chronically Mentally Ill;Cognitive
    Behavioral Therapy

MIZOKAWA, Donald T.
University of Washington
College of Educational Psychology
322 Miller Hall, Rm. #DQ-12
Seattle, WA 98195
(206) 543-1846-**B**, (206) 543-8439-**F**
Ethnicity: Asian-American/Asian/Pacific Islander
Degree and Year: PhD 1974
Major Field: Educational Psychology

Specialty: Attribution Theory;Computer Applications and
  Programming;Cross Cultural Processes;Educational
  Psychology;Learning/Learning Theory

MIZWA, Martine M.
  Lac du Flambeau Family Resource Center
  Box 189
  La duc Flambeau, WI 54538
  (715) 588-9818-**B**, (906) 932-0454-**H**, (715) 588-3903-**F**
Ethnicity: American Indian/Alaska Native
Degree and Year: PhD 1993
Major Field: Clinical Psychology
Specialty: Clinical Psychology;Domestic Violence;Forensic Psychology

MOBLEY, Brenda D.
  Wright State University
  Ellis Hum Dev Inst. Sch. of Prof. Psychology
  9 N Edwin C. Moses Blvd.
  Dayton, OH 45407-2837
  (937) 775-4339-**B**, (937) 223-4601-**H**, (937) 775-4323-**F**
  brenda.mobley@wright.edu
Ethnicity: African-American/Black
Degree and Year: PhD 1973
Major Field: Clinical Psychology
Specialty: Psychotherapy;Sex/Marital Therapy;Psychopathology

MOCK, Matthew R.
  Berkeley Mental Health (FYC)
  John F. Kennedy Univesity
  Berkeley, CA 94705
  (510) 644-6617-**B**, (510) 848-9919-**H**, (510) 644-6021-**F**
Ethnicity: Asian-American/Asian/Pacific Islander
Degree and Year: PhD 1991
Major Field: Clinical Psychology
Specialty: Ethnic Minorities;Family Therapy;Cross Cultural
  Processes;Clinical Psychology;Behavior Therapy

MODIANO, Rachel
  710 Easton Avenue
  Somerset, NJ 08873
  (908) 828-4622-**B**, (908) 037-6641-**H**, (908) 828-0255-**F**
Ethnicity: Hispanic/Latino
Languages: Spanish
Degree and Year: PsyD 1986
Major Field: School Psychology
Specialty: Child Abuse;Forensic Psychology;Clinical Psychology;Child
  Development;Child Therapy

MODY, Zarin R.
  350 Bleecker Street, #4T
  New York, NY 10014
  (212) 243-2734-**H**
Ethnicity: Asian-American/Asian/Pacific Islander
Degree and Year: PsyD 1988
Major Field: School Psychology
Specialty: Child Therapy;HIV/AIDS;Family
  Therapy;Infancy;Psychotherapy

MOGRO, Ana Klatt
  5913 Vallejo Street
  Emeryville, CA 94608-2111
  (510) 784-4568-**B**, 510 482-2268-**H**
Ethnicity: Hispanic/Latino
Degree and Year: PhD 1988
Major Field: Clinical Psychology
Specialty: Psychotherapy

MOIDEEN, Yasmine
  Pilot City Mental Health Center
  1313 Penn Avenue North
  Minneaoplis, MN 55411
  (612) 348-4631-**B**, (612) 348-4773-**F**
  yasmine.moideen@colhennepin.mn
Ethnicity: Asian-American/Asian/Pacific Islander
Languages: Spanish
Degree and Year: PhD 1995
Major Field: Clinical Child Psychology
Specialty: Clinical Child Psychology;Ethnic Minorities;Marriage &
  Family;Family Therapy;Parent-Child Interaction

MOLDEN, Sabrina
  421 Hilliard Drive
  Fayetteville, NC 28311
  (919) 483-5171-**B**, (919) 488-8043-**H**
Ethnicity: African-American/Black
Degree and Year: PhD 1981
Major Field: Clinical Psychology
Specialty: Psychotherapy;Clinical Child Psychology

MONDOL, Merlyn D.
  4931 Indian Trail
  Saginaw, MI 48603-5575
Ethnicity: Asian-American/Asian/Pacific Islander
Degree and Year: PhD 1973
Major Field: Educational Psychology

MONDRAGON, Nathan J.
  SHL Aspen Tree
  PO Box 1347
  709 Grand Avenue
  Laramie, WY 82072
  (307) 721-5888-**B**, (307) 721-9480-**H**, (307) 721-2135-**F**
  nathanm@aspentree.com
Ethnicity: Hispanic/Latino
Degree and Year: PhD 1993
Major Field: Industrial/Organizational Psy.
Specialty: Industrial/Organizational Psychology;Management &
  Organization;Selection & Placement;Human
  Resources;Quantitative/Mathematical,
  Psychometrics;Organizational Development

MONGUIO, Ines
  1280 S Victoria Avenue
  Suite #260
  Ventura, CA 93003
  (805) 655-7919-**B**, (805) 647-9838-**H**, (805) 650-7485-**F**
Ethnicity: Hispanic/Latino
Languages: Spanish
Degree and Year: PhD 1989
Major Field: Clinical Psychology
Specialty: Clinical Neuropsychology;Affective Disorders;Cognitive
  Behavioral Therapy;Hypnosis/Hypnotherapy;Medical
  Psychology

MONSERRAT, Laura
  Monserrat Psychological Services, P.C.
  510 E 86 Street
  Apartment #18-E
  New York, NY 10028-7506

(212) 410-6500-**B**, (212) 628-7692-**H**, (212) 410-0101-**F**
Ethnicity: Hispanic/Latino
Degree and Year: PhD 1984
Major Field: Clinical Psychology
Specialty: Forensic Psychology;Psychotherapy

MONTALVO, Roberto E.
Alameda County Guidance Clinic
2200 Fairmont Drive
Fremont, CA 94536
(510) 667-7719-**B**, (510) 796-3034-**H**, (510) 667-3005-**F**
bcmontalvo@aol.com
Ethnicity: Hispanic/Latino
Languages: Spanish
Degree and Year: PhD 1980
Major Field: Clinical Psychology
Specialty: Adolescent Therapy;Clinical Psychology;Cognitive
    Behavioral Therapy;Crisis Intervention & Therapy;Personality
    Measurement

MONTEIRO, Kenneth P.
San Francisco State University
1600 Holloway Avenue
San Francisco, CA 94132
(415) 338-3459-**B**, (415) 338-0937-**F**
monteiro@sfsu
Ethnicity: African-American/Black
Languages: French
Degree and Year: PhD 1982
Major Field: Cognitive Psychology
Specialty: Social Cognition;Cultural & Social Processes;Lesbian & Gay
    Issuues

MONTEIRO, Rita C.
6971 Caminito Perico
San Diego, CA 92119-2425
(619) 552-8585-**B**, (619) 697-6648-**H**, (619) 552-4336-**F**
Ethnicity: African-American/Black
Degree and Year: PhD 1985
Major Field: Clinical Psychology
Specialty: Alcoholism & Alcohol Abuse

MONTEMAYOR, Raymond
Ohio State University
Department of Psychology
Columbus, OH 43210
(614) 292-3059-**B**, (614) 421-0285-**H**, (614) 292-4537-**F**
Ethnicity: Hispanic/Latino
Degree and Year: PhD 1974
Major Field: Developmental Psychology
Specialty: Adolescent Development;Developmental Psychology;Family
    Processes;Parent-Child Interaction;Social Development

MONTES, Francisco
1 Normandy Circle #A
Colorado Springs, CO 80906-3033
(719) 473-7444-**B**, (719) 578-0069-**H**, (719) 473-7892-**F**
ammontes@aol.com
Ethnicity: Hispanic/Latino
Languages: Spanish
Degree and Year: PhD 1974 MA 1973
Major Field: Developmental Psychology
Specialty: Applied Behavior Analysis;Behavior Therapy;Cognitive
    Behavioral Therapy

MONTESI, Alexandra Saba
2123 N Rodney Drive
Suite #304
Los Angeles, CA 90027
(213) 341-1994-**B**, (213) 878-5526-**H**, (213) 650-2493-**F**
Ethnicity: Hispanic/Latino
Languages: Italian, Portuguese, Spanish
Degree and Year: PhD 1982
Major Field: Clinical Psychology
Specialty: Assessment/Diagnosis/Evaluation;Clinical
    Neuropsychology;Clinical Psychology;Counseling
    Psychology;Industrial/Organizational
    Psychology;Gerontology/Geropsychology

MONTGOMERY, Robert L.
University of Missouri
Psychology Department
Rolla, MO 65401
Ethnicity: American Indian/Alaska Native
Degree and Year: PhD 1968
Major Field: Social Psychology
Specialty: Interpersonal Processes & Relations

MONTIJO, Jorge A.
Banco Cooperativo Plaza #1106
Ponce de Leon 623
San Juan, PR 00917
(787) 763-2660-**B**, (787) 754-2923-**H**, (787) 754-5918-**F**
jmontijo@hotmail.com
Ethnicity: Hispanic/Latino
Languages: Spanish
Degree and Year: PhD 1974
Major Field: Clinical Psychology
Specialty: Clinical Neuropsychology;Psychotherapy;Health
    Psychology;Assessment/Diagnosis/Evaluation;Political
    Psychology;Forensic Psychology

MONTOYA, E. Carolina
944 NW 106th Avenue Circle
Miami, FL 33172
(305) 221-4288-**B**
Ethnicity: Hispanic/Latino
Languages: Spanish
Degree and Year: PhD 1986
Major Field: Clinical Psychology
Specialty: Clinical Psychology

MOODY, Helaine L.
1806 S. Vine Street
Urbana, IL 61801
(217) 367-9020-**H**
Ethnicity: African-American/Black
Degree and Year: PhD 1957
Major Field: Clinical Psychology

MOON, Tae-Hyun
5674 Stoneridge Drive
Suite #217
Pleasanton, CA 94588
(510) 833-0731-**B**
Ethnicity: Asian-American/Asian/Pacific Islander
Degree and Year: PhD 1984
Major Field: Clinical Psychology
Specialty: Marriage & Family;Ethnic Minorities;Affective Disorders

MOORE, C. L.
Pediatric & Family Psychology Center
261 North Ruth Street, #111
St. Paul, MN 55119-4337
(651) 771-4766-**B**, (651) 834-0364-**H**, (651) 771-4784-**F**
Ethnicity: African-American/Black
Degree and Year: PhD 1973
Major Field: Health Psychology
Specialty: HIV/AIDS;Marriage & Family;Child & Pediatric
    Psychology;Parent-Child Interaction;Administration;Managed
    Care

MOORE, Carolyn D.
1503 Canterford Court
Virginia Beach, VA 23464-6756
(804) 495-8066-**B**
Ethnicity: African-American/Black
Degree and Year: PhD 1982
Major Field: Clinical Psychology
Specialty: Psychotherapy

MOORE, Cleo H.
1030 W Allens Lane
Philadelphia, PA 19119-3315
(215) 242-8753-**B**
Ethnicity: African-American/Black
Degree and Year: EdD 1962
Major Field: School Psychology
Specialty: Preschool & Day Care Issues

MOORE, Helen B.
49 Flanagan Dr
Framingham, MA 01701-3714
(508) 879-5006-**B**, (508) 879-5006-**H**, (508) 877-6368-**F**
Ethnicity: African-American/Black
Degree and Year: PhD 1977
Major Field: Educational Psychology
Specialty: Consulting Psychology;Counseling Psychology;Cross
    Cultural Processes;Group Psychotherapy;Organizational
    Development

MOORE, Sandra
234 E. Fern Ave., #204
Redlands, CA 92373
(909) 794-2161-**B**, (909) 798-2416-**H**
Ethnicity: African-American/Black
Degree and Year: PhD 1988
Major Field: Community Psychology
Specialty: Social Psychology;Social Behavior;Ethnic Minorities;Gender
    Issues;Social Cognition

MOORMAN-LEWIS, Deborah A.
5509 Silver Hill Road
Forestville, MD 20747-2049
Ethnicity: African-American/Black
Degree and Year: PhD 1983
Major Field: Clinical Psychology
Specialty: Medical Psychology

MORALES-BARRETO, Gisela
74 Meadowbrook Road
Newton, MA 02459
(617) 534-2610-**B**, (617) 332-1448-**H**, (617) 534-4688-**F**
Ethnicity: Hispanic/Latino
Languages: Spanish
Degree and Year: EdD 1990

Major Field: Counseling Psychology
Specialty: Counseling Psychology;Administration;Cross Cultural
    Processes;Consulting Psychology;Continuing Education

MORALES, Cynthia T.
25551 Baker Place
Stevenson Ranch, CA 91381-1509
(213) 825-6109-**B**
Ethnicity: Hispanic/Latino
Degree and Year: PhD 1986
Major Field: Counseling Psychology
Specialty: Crisis Intervention & Therapy;Case Management

MORALES, Eduardo S.
355 Buena Vista E #612W
San Francisco, CA 94117
(415) 252-1655-**B**, (415) 255-0633-**H**, (415) 255-0553-**F**
dremorales@aol.com
Ethnicity: Hispanic/Latino
Languages: Spanish
Degree and Year: PhD 1976 BS 1972
Major Field: Counseling Psychology
Specialty: Lesbian & Gay Issuues;Prevention;Drug Abuse;HIV/
    AIDS;Metacognition;Cross Cultural Processes

MORALES, Elias
P.O. Box 1254
Orlando, FL 32802-1254
(1800) 272-7252-**B**, (407) 658-4627-**H**
Ethnicity: Hispanic/Latino
Languages: Spanish
Degree and Year: MA 1981
Major Field: General Psy./Methods & Systems
Specialty: Clinical Psychology;Clinical Neuropsychology;Employee
    Assistance Programs;Ethnic Minorities;Crisis Intervention &
    Therapy

MORALES, Pamilla V.
Texas A&M University
704 Harrington
Department of EPSY
College Station, TX 77843-4225
(409) 845-9277-**B**, (409) 845-9277-**H**, (409) 862-1256-**F**
meepam@acs.tamu.edu
Ethnicity: Hispanic/Latino
Languages: Spanish
Degree and Year: PhD 1993
Major Field: Counseling Psychology
Specialty: Assessment/Diagnosis/Evaluation;Death & Dying;HIV/
    AIDS;Clinical Neuropsychology;Ethnic Minorities;Medical
    Psychology

MORA, Ralph
8607 North Boulevard
Fort Pierce, FL 34951
(561) 778-2798-**B**, (561) 778-1105-**F**
110651.1332@compuserve.com
Ethnicity: Hispanic/Latino
Languages: Spanish
Degree and Year: PhD 1983
Major Field: Clinical Psychology
Specialty: Forensic Psychology;Drug Abuse;Clinical Child
    Psychology;HIV/AIDS;Marriage & Family

MORDKA, Irwin
9464 E Calle Bolivar
Tucsan, AZ 85715
(520) 296-9092-**B**
gracunningham@worldnet.att.net
Ethnicity: Hispanic/Latino
Languages: Spanish
Degree and Year: PhD 1964
Major Field: Industrial/Organizational Psy.
Specialty: Industrial/Organizational Psychology;Organizational
   Development;Human Resources;Attitudes &
   Opinions;Management & Organization

MORGAN, Cynthia L.
CSU, Stanislaus
Department of Psychology
801 W Monte Vista
Turlock, CA 95380
(209) 667-3386-**B**
Ethnicity: African-American/Black
Degree and Year: PhD 1974
Major Field: Experimental Psychology
Specialty: Vision;Learning/Learning Theory;Cognitive Psychology

MORI, DeAnna L.
Boston VAMC
150 S Huntington Avenue
Boston, MA 02130-4820
(617) 232-9500-**B**
Ethnicity: Asian-American/Asian/Pacific Islander
Degree and Year: PhD 1986
Major Field: Clinical Psychology

MORI, Lisa T.
California State University
   @ Fullerton
Department of Psychology
Fullerton, CA 92634
(714) 773-2149-**B**
Ethnicity: Asian-American/Asian/Pacific Islander
Degree and Year: PhD 1987
Major Field: Clinical Psychology
Specialty: Child & Pediatric Psychology;Clinical Child
   Psychology;Ethnic Minorities

MORISHIGE, Howard H.
Seattle University
Counseling Center
Mcgoldrick Building
Seattle, WA 98122
(206) 296-6090-**B**, (206) 296-6087-**F**
morishig@seattleu.edu
Ethnicity: Asian-American/Asian/Pacific Islander
Degree and Year: PhD 1971
Major Field: Clinical Psychology
Specialty: Clinical Psychology;Counseling
   Psychology;Psychotherapy;Cross Cultural Processes;Training
   & Development

MORISHIMA, James K.
University of Washington
406A Miller Hall
Box 353600
Seattle, WA 98195-3600
(206) 685-1499-**B**, (206) 524-9242-**H**, (206) 543-8439-**F**

morisim@u.washington.edu
Ethnicity: Asian-American/Asian/Pacific Islander
Degree and Year: PhD 1967
Major Field: Social Psychology
Specialty: Survey Theory & Methodology;Cultural & Social
   Processes;Ethnic Minorities;Cross Cultural
   Processes;Computer Applications and Programming;Language
   Process

MORITA, Denise N.
Guthrie Medical Group, P.C.
2517 Vestal Parkway East
Vestal, NY 13850
(607) 798-1452-**B**, (607) 798-9527-**H**
DM9527@aol
Ethnicity: Asian-American/Asian/Pacific Islander
Degree and Year: PhD 1991
Major Field: Clinical Psychology
Specialty: Affective Disorders;Cognitive Behavioral Therapy;Parent
   Education;Clinical Child Psychology;Adolescent
   Therapy;Attention Deficit Disorders

MORITSUGU, John
Pacific Lutheran University
Department of Psychology
5232 Erskine Way, SW
Seattle, WA 98136
(206) 535-7650-**B**, (206) 937-1874-**H**, (206) 535-8305-**F**
moritsjn@plu.edu
Ethnicity: Asian-American/Asian/Pacific Islander
Degree and Year: PhD 1977
Major Field: Clinical Psychology
Specialty: Clinical Psychology;Community Psychology;Ethnic
   Minorities;Prevention;Stress

MORONES, Pete A.
University of Portland
5000 North Willamette Boulevard
Portland, OR 97203
(503) 283-7134-**B**, (503) 283-7199-**F**
morones@up.edu
Ethnicity: Hispanic/Latino
Languages: Spanish
Degree and Year: PhD 1994
Major Field: Clinical Psychology
Specialty: Individual Psychotherapy;Affective Disorders

MOROTE, Gloria
424 S Washington St
Alexandria, VA 22314-3630
(703) 683-2695-**B**, (703) 765-4424-**H**
Ethnicity: Hispanic/Latino
Languages: Spanish
Degree and Year: PhD 1985
Major Field: Clinical Child Psychology
Specialty: Clinical Neuropsychology;Clinical Child
   Neuropsychology;Assessment/Diagnosis/Evaluation;Cross
   Cultural Processes;Forensic Psychology

MORRIS, Dolores O.
290 Riverside Drive
New York, NY 10025-5277
(212) 222-1060-**H**, (212) 22 1060-**F**

domorris@worldnet.att.nete
Ethnicity: African-American/Black
Degree and Year: PhD 1974
Major Field: Clinical Psychology
Specialty: Psychoanalysis;Professional Issues in Psychology;Marriage
& Family;Psychotherapy;School Psychology;Special
Education

MORRIS, Edward F.
George Fox University
Graduate School of Clinical Psychology
Newberg, OR 97132
(503) 5554-2763-**B**, (503) 538-8535-**H**
Ethnicity: African-American/Black
Degree and Year: PhD 1984
Major Field: Clinical Psychology
Specialty: Administration;Clinical Child Psychology;Cross Cultural
Processes;Assessment/Diagnosis/Evaluation;Community
Psychology;Ethnic Minorities

MORRIS, Joseph R.
Western Michigan University
Department of Counselor Education and
Counseling Psychology
3102 Sangren Hall
Kalamazoo, MI 49008-5195
(616) 387-5112-**B**
morris@wmich.edu
Ethnicity: African-American/Black
Degree and Year: PhD 1975
Major Field: Counseling Psychology
Specialty: Counseling Psychology;Group Processes;Cultural & Social
Processes;Assessment/Diagnosis/Evaluation

MORSE, Roberta N.
1741 N 28th Street
Richmond, VA 23223-5317
(804) 643-6218-**B**
Ethnicity: African-American/Black
Degree and Year: PhD 1974
Major Field: Clinical Psychology
Specialty: Consulting Psychology

MORTIMER, Joan R.
10 Hopewell Trail
Chagrin Falls, OH 44022-2543
Ethnicity: Hispanic/Latino
Degree and Year: PhD 1971
Major Field: unknown
Specialty: Child Therapy;Depression

MOSLEY-HOWARD, Gerri S.
(203) McGuffey Hall
Oxford, OH 45056
(513) 529-6626-**B**, (513) 529-7270-**F**
mosleygs@muohio.edu
Ethnicity: African-American/Black
Degree and Year: PhD 1984
Major Field: Educational Psychology
Specialty: Educational Psychology;School Counseling;Cultural & Social
Processes;Gender Issues

MOSS, Ramona J.
Sapphire Bay W. D.31
St. Thomas, VI 00802

(340) 775-1103-**B**, (341) 775-1103-**H**, (340) 775-1103-**F**
Ethnicity: African-American/Black, Hispanic/Latino
Languages: Spanish
Degree and Year: PhD 1991
Major Field: Clinical Psychology
Specialty: Assessment/Diagnosis/Evaluation;Family
Processes;Personality Measurement;Clinical
Psychology;Individual Psychotherapy;School Psychology

MO, Suchoon
University of Southern Colorado
Department of Psychology
Pueblo, CO 81001
(719) 549-2700-**B**, (719) 547-3705-**H**, (719) 549-2705-**F**
Ethnicity: Asian-American/Asian/Pacific Islander
Languages: Korean
Degree and Year: PhD 1968
Major Field: Experimental Psychology
Specialty: Schizophrenia;Psychopathology;Psychoses;Sensory &
Perceptual Processes;Experimental Psychology

MOTES, Patricia S.
14 Hillpine Court
Columbia, SC 29212
(808) 734-7320-**B**, (803) 781-3248-**H**, (803) 734-0791-**F**
Ethnicity: African-American/Black
Degree and Year: PhD 1986
Major Field: Clinical Psychology
Specialty: Clinical Child Psychology;Clinical Psychology;Community
Psychology

MOUZON, Richard R.
Po Box 91250
Atlanta, GA 30364-1250
(404) 505-9416-**B**, (404) 349-4520-**H**
Ethnicity: African-American/Black
Degree and Year: PhD 1985
Major Field: Clinical Psychology
Specialty: Psychotherapy

MOYNIHAN, Kelly L.
417 1st Avenue, SE
Irvine Bldg., Suite #107
Cedar Rapids, IA 52401-1317
(319) 366-6329-**B**
Ethnicity: American Indian/Alaska Native
Degree and Year: MA 1984
Major Field: Counseling Psychology
Specialty: Psychotherapy;Community Mental Health

MOY, Samuel
970 Farmington Avenue
West Hartford, CT 06107-2126
(203) 561-6710-**B**
Ethnicity: Asian-American/Asian/Pacific Islander
Degree and Year: PhD 1987
Major Field: Clinical Psychology
Specialty: Community Mental Health

MUGA, Joe
California Department of Corrections
Pleasant Valley State Prison
PO Box 8500

Coalinga, CA 93210
  (209) 935-4900-**B**, (650) 355-2974-**H**, (209) 935-4961-**F**
Ethnicity: Hispanic/Latino
Degree and Year: PhD 1989
Major Field: Clinical Psychology
Specialty: Forensic Psychology;Correctional Psychology;Crime &
        Criminal Behavior;Clinical Psychology;Psychology & Law

MUIR-MALCOLM, Joan A.
  University of Miami
  Center for Family Studies
  1425 NW 10th Avenue,
  Third Floor
  Miami, FL 33136
  (305) 243-4592-**B**, (305) 418-4878-**H**, (305) 243-5577-**F**
  jmalcolm@mednet.med.miami.edu
Ethnicity: African-American/Black
Degree and Year: PhD 1995
Major Field: Clinical Psychology

MUIU, Charles
  PO Box 6747
  Omaha, NE 68106-0747
  (913) 357-6483-**B**
Ethnicity: African-American/Black
Degree and Year: PhD 1986
Major Field: Developmental Psychology
Specialty: Adolescent Development

MUJICA, Ernesto
  20 West 86th Street
  Suite 1C
  New York, NY 10024
  (212) 721-0369-**B**, (212) 721-0384-**H**
Ethnicity: Hispanic/Latino
Languages: Spanish
Degree and Year: PhD 1991
Major Field: Clinical Psychology
Specialty: Individual Psychotherapy;Group
        Psychotherapy;Psychoanalysis;Psychotherapy

MUKHERJEE, Subhash C.
  P.O. Box 514
  North Andover, MA 01845
  (978) 352-21-**B**, (978) 688-01-**H**
Ethnicity: Asian-American/Asian/Pacific Islander
Languages: Hindi, Urdu, Bengali
Degree and Year: PhD 1971
Major Field: General Psy./Methods & Systems
Specialty: Clinical Psychology;Assessment/Diagnosis/
        Evaluation;Affective Disorders;Administration;Mental Health
        Services

MULLER, Terry P.
  2161 Whippoorwill Road
  Charlottesville, VA 22901
  (703) 943-6637-**B**, (804) 293-4163-**H**
Ethnicity: American Indian/Alaska Native
Degree and Year: PhD 1987
Major Field: Clinical Psychology
Specialty: Neuropsychology

MUNFORD, Paul R.
  4921 St. Thomas Drive
  Fairoaks, CA 95628-5312
  (213) 733-8218-**B**, (916) 967-1853-**H**

Ethnicity: African-American/Black
Degree and Year: PhD 1971
Major Field: Clinical Psychology
Specialty: Medical Psychology

MUNOZ, Daniel G
  University Of California
  Counseling and Psychological Services
  Revelle Col, B-021
  La Jolla, CA 92037
  (619) 534-1579-**B**
Ethnicity: Hispanic/Latino
Degree and Year: PhD 1971
Major Field: Clinical Psychology
Specialty: Psychotherapy;Forensic Psychology

MUNOZ, John A.
  800 Riverside Drive
  Apartment # 2 J
  New York, NY 10032-7406
  (212) 787-6780-**B**
Ethnicity: Hispanic/Latino
Languages: Spanish
Degree and Year: PhD 1973
Major Field: Clinical Psychology
Specialty: Cross Cultural Processes;Psychoanalysis;Child
        Abuse;Projective Techniques;Mental Health Services

MUNOZ, Leticia S.
  River Valley Counseling Center, Inc.
  303 Beech Street
  Holyoke, MA 01040
  (413) 534-3361-**B**, (413) 586-4263-**H**, (413) 534-7158-**F**
Ethnicity: Hispanic/Latino
Languages: Spanish
Degree and Year: PsyD 1990
Major Field: Clinical Psychology
Specialty: Cognitive Behavioral Therapy;Eating Disorders;Affective
        Disorders;Stress

MUNOZ, Luis A.
  408 Casa Loma Court
  San Jose, CA 95129-1027
  (408) 244-0860-**B**
  lamunoe@aol.com
Ethnicity: Hispanic/Latino
Degree and Year: PhD 1975
Major Field: Clinical Psychology
Specialty: Clinical Psychology;School Psychology

MUNOZ, Marisol
  Marin County Mental Health Center
  250 Bon Air Road
  Greenbrae, CA 94904
  (415) 499-6787-**B**
Ethnicity: Hispanic/Latino
Languages: Spanish
Degree and Year: PhD 1991
Major Field: Clinical Psychology
Specialty: Clinical Psychology;Community Psychology;Personality
        Psychology

MUNOZ, Nina R.
  5199 E Pacific Coast Highway
  Suite #602

Long Beach, CA 90804
(310) 434-6597-**B**, (310) 434-6626-**H**
Ethnicity: Hispanic/Latino
Degree and Year: PhD 1989
Major Field: Clinical Psychology
Specialty: Clinical Psychology;Child Abuse;Depression;Health
  Psychology;Stress

MUNOZ, Ricardo F.
University of California, San Francisco
Department of Psychiatry
Suite #7M
San Francisco, CA 94110
(415) 206-5214-**B**, (415) 206-8942-**F**
munoz@itsa.ucsf.edu
Ethnicity: Hispanic/Latino
Languages: Spanish
Degree and Year: PhD 1977
Major Field: Clinical Psychology
Specialty: Prevention;Depression;Cognitive Behavioral
  Therapy;Community Psychology;Research & Training

MURADIAN, Mark G.
135 Juniper Drive
Avon, CT 06001-3472
(203) 224-2647-**B**
Ethnicity: Asian-American/Asian/Pacific Islander
Degree and Year: DPA 1984
Major Field: unknown

MURAKAMI, Janice
92 Adams Street
Burlington, VT 05489
(802) 863-6114-**B**, (802) 899-3558-**H**
Ethnicity: Asian-American/Asian/Pacific Islander
Degree and Year: PhD 1987
Major Field: Clinical Psychology
Specialty: Psychotherapy;Adolescent Therapy;Stress;Affective
  Disorders

MURAKAMI, Sharon
46-369 H-11 Haiku Road
Kaneohe, HI 96744
(808) 956-2247-**B**, (808) 235-5262-**H**
Ethnicity: Asian-American/Asian/Pacific Islander
Degree and Year: PhD 1983
Major Field: Developmental Psychology
Specialty: Adolescent Development;Adolescent Therapy;Human
  Development & Family Studies;Learning Disabilities;Parent
  Education

MURAKAWA, Fay
Saint John's Child and Family
  Developmental Center
1339 20th Street
Santa Monica, CA 90404
(310) 829-8688-**B**, (310) 829-8455-**F**
Ethnicity: Asian-American/Asian/Pacific Islander
Degree and Year: PhD 1986
Major Field: Clinical Psychology
Specialty: Assessment/Diagnosis/Evaluation;Training &
  Development;Ethnic Minorities;Mental Disorders;Hospital
  Care

MURFREE, JR., Joshua W.
408-B Leafmore Road
Rome, GA 30165-3800
(404) 295-6600-**B**
Ethnicity: African-American/Black
Degree and Year: PhD 1987
Major Field: Counseling Psychology
Specialty: Psychotherapy

MURILLO, Nathan
1577 N Via Norte
Palm Springs, CA 92262-4281
(818) 886-7913-**B**
Ethnicity: Hispanic/Latino
Languages: Spanish
Degree and Year: PhD 1965
Major Field: Clinical Psychology
Specialty: Individual Psychotherapy;Group Psychotherapy;Cross
  Cultural Processes;Training & Development;Ethnic Minorities

MURRAY, James L.
San Jacinto Community College
8060 Spencer Highway
Pasenda, TX 77501
(281) 476-1501-**B**, (409) 744-4791-**H**
lmrra@sjcd.central.cc.tx.us
Ethnicity: African-American/Black
Degree and Year: EdD 1998
Major Field: General Psy./Methods & Systems
Specialty: Administration;Mental Health Services;Stress;Crime &
  Criminal Behavior;Statistics

MUSGROVE, Barbara J.
1603 Rhode Island Avenue, N.E.
Suite 100 B
Washington, DC 20018
(202) 529-3637-**B**, (301) 630-1922-**H**
Ethnicity: African-American/Black
Degree and Year: PhD 1974
Major Field: Social Psychology
Specialty: Clinical Psychology;Drug Abuse;Attention Deficit
  Disorders;Employee Assistance Programs;Alcoholism &
  Alcohol Abuse

MUSSENDEN, Gerald
317 Cactus Road
Seffner, FL 33584
(813) 681-5958-**B**, (813) 685-5040-**H**
Ethnicity: Hispanic/Latino
Languages: Spanish
Degree and Year: PhD 1974
Major Field: Clinical Psychology
Specialty: Assessment/Diagnosis/Evaluation;Forensic
  Psychology;Individual Psychotherapy;Projective
  Techniques;Rehabilitation

MYERS, Ernest R.
University of the District of Columbia
4200 Connecticut Avenue, NW
Building 44
Suite 200
Washington, DC 20008
(202) 274-6447-**B**, (202) 882-8124-**H**, (202) 274-5003-**F**
Ethnicity: African-American/Black
Languages: French

Degree and Year: PhD 1976 MSW 1964
Major Field: Community Psychology
Specialty: Ethnic Minorities;Human Relations;Industrial/Organizational
 Psychology;Training & Development;Counseling Psychology

MYERS, Hector F.
 University of California, Los Angeles
 Department of Psychology
 Box 951563
 Los Angeles, CA 90095-1563
 (310) 825-1813-**B**, (310) 204-1644-**H**, (310) 206-5895-**F**
 myers@psych.ucla.edu
Ethnicity: African-American/Black
Languages: Spanish
Degree and Year: PhD 1974
Major Field: Clinical Psychology
Specialty: Stress;Ethnic Minorities;Cardiovascular Processes;Health
 Psychology;HIV/AIDS;Psychopathology

MYERS, Linda J.
 5800 Sunbury Road
 Gahanna, OH 43230-1152
 (614) 292-3447-**B**
Ethnicity: African-American/Black
Degree and Year: PhD 1975
Major Field: Clinical Psychology
Specialty: Interpersonal Processes & Relations;Health
 Psychology;Social Problems;Cross Cultural Processes;Cultural
 & Social Processes

NABORS, Nina A.
 Central Michigan University
 Sloan 104 Psychology Department
 Mt. Pleasant, MI 48859
 (517) 774-6490-**B**, (517) 779-8185-**H**
 nina.nabors@mich.edu
Ethnicity: African-American/Black
Degree and Year: PhD 1994
Major Field: Clinical Psychology
Specialty: Clinical Neuropsychology;Rehabilitation;Ethnic
 Minorities;Psychology of Women

NADAL-VAZQUEZ, Vilma Y.
 Montgomery County Public Schools
 Rocking Horse Road Center
 4910 Macon Road
 Rockville, MD 20852
 (301) 230-0670-**B**, (202) 363-3609-**H**, (202) 636-0665-**F**
 bonafe@aol.com
Ethnicity: Hispanic/Latino
Languages: French, Spanish
Degree and Year: PhD 1994
Major Field: Counseling Psychology
Specialty: Counseling Psychology;School Counseling;Adolescent
 Therapy;Cross Cultural Processes;Individual
 Psychotherapy;Group Psychotherapy

NAGAMOTO, Alan
 University of California @ Los Angeles
 4223 Math Science Building
 405 Hilgard Avenue
 Los Angeles, CA 90024-8313
 (310)825-0768-**B**, 310280-3287-**H**
Ethnicity: Asian-American/Asian/Pacific Islander

Degree and Year: PhD 1980
Major Field: Clinical Psychology
Specialty: Psychotherapy

NAGATA, Donna K.
 University of Michigan
 Department of Psychology
 525 East University
 Ann Arbor, MI 48109-1109
 (734) 647-3886-**B**, (734) 662-7627-**H**, (734) 764-3520-**F**
 nagata@umich
Ethnicity: Asian-American/Asian/Pacific Islander
Degree and Year: PhD 1981
Major Field: Clinical Psychology
Specialty: Ethnic Minorities;Clinical Child Psychology

NAGAYAMA HALL, Gordon C.
 Kent State University
 Department of Psychology
 Kent, OH 44242-0001
 (216) 672-2253-**B**, (216) 678-0401-**H**, (216) 672-3786-**F**
Ethnicity: Asian-American/Asian/Pacific Islander
Degree and Year: PhD 1982
Major Field: Clinical Psychology
Specialty: Aggression;Crime & Criminal Behavior;Assessment/
 Diagnosis/Evaluation;Sexual Behavior;Forensic Psychology

NAGY, Vivian T.
 Kaiser Permanente
 3516 Woodcliff Road
 Pasadema, CA 91188
 (626) 564-3742-**B**, (626) 564-3447-**F**
 vivian.t.nagy@kp.org
Ethnicity: Asian-American/Asian/Pacific Islander
Degree and Year: PhD 1974
Major Field: Social Psychology
Specialty: Program Evaluation;Organizational Development;Health
 Psychology;Research Design & Methodology;Survey Theory
 & Methodology

NAIDOO, Josephine C.
 Wilfrid Laurier University
 Psychology Department
 Waterloo, Ontario, N2L3C5
 CANADA
 (519) 884-1970-**B**, (519) 884-6060-**H**, (519) 746-7605-**F**
Ethnicity: Asian-American/Asian/Pacific Islander
Degree and Year: PhD 1966
Major Field: Social Psychology
Specialty: Cross Cultural Processes;Ethnic Minorities;Psychology of
 Women;Adolescent Development;Community Psychology

NAKAGAWA, Janice Y.
 1409 28th Street
 Suite 100
 Sacramento, CA 95820
 (916) 452-3756-**B**, (925) 228-9177-**H**, (916) 452-3757-**F**
 S13151@aol.com
Ethnicity: Asian-American/Asian/Pacific Islander
Degree and Year: PhD 1980
Major Field: Clinical Psychology
Specialty: Forensic Psychology;Correctional Psychology

NAKAMURA, Charles Y.
Department of Psychology
University of California
Los Angeles, CA 90024-1563
(310) 825-2305-**B**, (310) 826-5893-**H**
Ethnicity: Asian-American/Asian/Pacific Islander
Degree and Year: PhD 1956
Major Field: Clinical Psychology
Specialty: Child Development;Psychology of Women;Training &
    Development;Psychotherapy;Developmental Psychology

NAKAMURA, Linda K
Glen Roberts Child Study Center
1530 East Colorado Street
Glendale, CA 91205
(818) 244-0222-**B**, (310) 212-9727-**H**, (818) 243-5413-**F** k.net
Ethnicity: Asian-American/Asian/Pacific Islander
Degree and Year: Psy 1994 MA 1989
Major Field: Clinical Psychology
Specialty: Child Therapy;Clinical Psychology;Clinical Child
    Psychology;Marriage & Family

NARVAEZ, Darcia F.
University of Minnesota
150 Peik Hall
159 Pillsbury Drive
Minneapolis, MN 55455
617/626-7306-**B**, 617./624-8277-**F**
narvaez@ttc.umn.edu
Ethnicity: Hispanic/Latino
Languages: French, Spanish
Degree and Year: PhD 1993
Major Field: Educational Psychology
Specialty: Moral Development;Cognitive Development;Cultural &
    Social Processes;Values & Moral Behavior;Educational
    Psychology;Social Development

NATALICIO, Luiz
1113 Whitaker Lane
El Paso, TX 79902-2126
(915) 532-4621-**B**, (915) 545-2410-**H**
Ethnicity: Hispanic/Latino
Languages: Portuguese, Spanish
Degree and Year: PhD 1967
Major Field: Educational Psychology
Specialty: Clinical Psychology;Applied Behavior Analysis;Forensic
    Psychology;Learning/Learning Theory;Philosophy of Science

NATANI, Kirmach
Bi-State Neurometric Services
University Club Tower, Suite 800
1034 Southg Brentwood Boulevard
St. Louis, MO 631117
(314) 741-8900-**B**, (314) 426-1875-**H**, (618) 465-4790-**F**
Ethnicity: American Indian/Alaska Native, European/White
Degree and Year: PhD 1977 MSc 1970
Major Field: Neurosciences
Specialty: Clinical Research;Electrophysical Psychology;Clinical Child
    Neuropsychology;Cognitive Behavioral Therapy;Clinical
    Neuropsychology;Attention Deficit Disorders

NAVARRO FOLEY, Gloria L.
3509 Woodrow Street
Austin, TX 78705-1733

(512) 499-8071-**B**
Ethnicity: Asian-American/Asian/Pacific Islander
Degree and Year: PhD 1984
Major Field: School Psychology

NAVAS-ROBLETO, Jose J.
PO Box 41242
Santurce, PR 00940-1242
(787) 725-6500-**B**, (787) 791-2661-**H**
Ethnicity: Hispanic/Latino
Degree and Year: PhD 1984
Major Field: Clinical Psychology
Specialty: Rational-Emotive Therapy;Cognitive Behavioral Therapy

NAVEDO, Christella N.
Adm Beneficios
Puerto Rico Telephone Co
Praderas, DF-9
Valle Verde III
Bayamon, PR 00961
(787) 273-8076-**B**, (787) 795-0903-**H**, (787) 793-4494-**F**
Ethnicity: Hispanic/Latino
Languages: Spanish
Degree and Year: PhD
Major Field: Industrial/Organizational Psy.
Specialty: Assessment/Diagnosis/Evaluation;Industrial/Organizational
    Psychology;Research & Training;Performance
    Evaluation;Computer Applications and Programming

NAYAK, Madhabika B.
Department of Psychiatry
Faculty of Medicine
Kuwait University
PO Box 24923
Safat,
KUWAIT
965 533-0467-**B**, 965 488 5388-**H**, 965 533 8904-**F**
mnayak@hsc.kuniv.edu.kw
Ethnicity: Asian-American/Asian/Pacific Islander
Languages: Hindi, Urdu
Degree and Year: PhD 1994
Major Field: Clinical Psychology

NAZARIO, JR., Andres
Gainesville Family Institute
1031 NW 6th Street
Suite #C-2
Gainesville, FL 32601
(352) 376-5543-**B**, (352) 331-9891-**H**, (352) 376-2042-**F**
afno9650@afn.org
Ethnicity: Hispanic/Latino
Languages: Spanish
Degree and Year: PhD 1983 MS 1977
Major Field: Counseling Psychology
Specialty: Family Therapy;Marriage & Family;Lesbian & Gay
    Issuues;HIV/AIDS;Training & Development;Disadvantaged

NEAL-BARNETT, Angela M.
Kent State University
Department of Psychology
Kent, OH 44242-0001
(330) 672-2266-**B**, (330) 633-5990-**H**, (330) 672-3786-**F**
aneal@phoenix.kent.edu
Ethnicity: African-American/Black
Degree and Year: PhD 1988 MA 1985

Major Field: Clinical Psychology
Specialty: Clinical Child Psychology;Affective Disorders;Child
Development;Ethnic Minorities;Clinical Research;Mental
Health Services

NELSON-GOEDERT, Carolyn Y
20363 NW 32 Place
Miami, FL 33056-1857
305 354-8047-**B**, 305 623-8903-**H**
futrpsych@aol.com
Ethnicity: African-American/Black
Degree and Year:
Major Field: School Psychology

NELSON-LEGALL, Sharon A.
University of Pittsburgh
829 Lrdc Bldg
Univ Of Pittsburgh
Pittsburgh, PA 15260
(412) 624-7481-**B**, (412) 731-1559-**H**, (412) 624-9149-**F**
Ethnicity: African-American/Black
Languages: French
Degree and Year: PhD 1978
Major Field: Developmental Psychology
Specialty: Child Development;Interpersonal Processes &
Relations;Motivation;Social Cognition;Ethnic Minorities

NEMOTO, Tooru
University of California
@ San Francisco
Institute for Health Policy Studies
1388 Sutter Street - 11th Floor
San Francisco, CA 94109
(415) 476-5935-**B**, (415) 346-1794-**H**, (415) 476-0705-**F**
Ethnicity: Asian-American/Asian/Pacific Islander
Languages: Japanese
Degree and Year: PhD 1988
Major Field: Community Psychology
Specialty: Cultural & Social Processes;Drug Abuse;Ethnic
Minorities;HIV/AIDS;Research Design & Methodology;Policy
Analysis

NESBITT, Eric B.
Park Ridge Mental Health Center
1581 Long Pond Road
Rochester, NY 14626
(716) 723-7750-**B**, (716) 334-8358-**H**, (716) 723-7048-**F**
en@prhs.ima-net.com
Ethnicity: African-American/Black
Degree and Year: PhD 1977
Major Field: Clinical Psychology
Specialty: Child Therapy;Adolescent Therapy;Attention Deficit
Disorders;Conduct Disorders;Parent Education;Clinical Child
Psychology

NETTER, Beatriz E. C.
4180 La Jolla Village Drive
Suite #530
La Jolla, CA 92037
(619) 552-8912-**B**, (619) 546-8704-**H**
Ethnicity: Hispanic/Latino
Languages: Portuguese
Degree and Year: PhD 1990

Major Field: Clinical Psychology
Specialty: Psychotherapy;Projective Techniques;Cross Cultural
Processes;Child Therapy;Clinical Psychology

NETTER, Roberto
9510 Easter Way
San Diego, CA 92121
(619) 552-8911-**B**
Ethnicity: Hispanic/Latino
Languages: French, Portuguese, Spanish
Degree and Year: PhD 1989
Major Field: Clinical Psychology
Specialty: Cross Cultural Processes;Clinical Child Psychology;Forensic
Psychology;Psychotherapy

NETTLES, Arie L.
University of Michigan
School of Education
610 E. University, 1360-B
Ann Arbor, MI 48109-1259
(313) 763-6123-**B**, (313) 761-1821-**H**, (313) 763-1368-**F**
Ethnicity: African-American/Black
Degree and Year: PhD 1987
Major Field: Clinical Psychology
Specialty: Assessment/Diagnosis/Evaluation;School
Psychology;Preschool & Day Care Issues;Intelligence;Cross
Cultural Processes

NEWBURGH, Tracey LS
175 Brooks Avenue
Arlington, MA 02474
(508) 793-3363-**B**, (781) 641-3631-**H**
tnewburgh@holycross.edu
Ethnicity: African-American/Black, American Indian/Alaska Native
Degree and Year: PhD 1995
Major Field: Counseling Psychology

NEZU, Arthur M.
Allegheny University
of the Health Sciences
Department of Clinical & Health Psych.
Broad & Vine
Philadelphia, PA 19102-1192
(215) 762-4829-**B**, (215) 751-2769-**H**, (215) 762-8625-**F**
ne2ua@auhs.edu
Ethnicity: Asian-American/Asian/Pacific Islander
Degree and Year: PhD 1979
Major Field: Clinical Psychology
Specialty: Behavior Therapy;Cognitive Behavioral Therapy;Health
Psychology;Clinical Psychology;Clinical Research;Mentally
Retarded

NG, James T.
PO Box 1424
Monterey Park, CA 91754-8424
(818) 240-1000-**B**, (213) 670-9229-**H**
LeeFC@aol.com
Ethnicity: Asian-American/Asian/Pacific Islander
Languages: Chinese
Degree and Year: PhD 1981
Major Field: unknown
Specialty: Counseling Psychology;Ethnic Minorities;Organizational
Development;Applied Behavior Analysis;Training &
Development

NG, Pak C.
6316 Willow Glen Road
Midlothian, VA 23112
(804) 274-4228-**B**, (804) 744-0459-**H**
Ethnicity: Asian-American/Asian/Pacific Islander
Languages: Chinese
Degree and Year: PhD 1989
Major Field: Social Psychology
Specialty: Attitudes & Opinions

NGUYEN, Dao Q.
Two Clark Drive
San Mateo, CA 94401
(408) 874-7732-**B**, (408) 224-6072-**H**
dnguyen@jfku.edu
Ethnicity: Asian-American/Asian/Pacific Islander
Languages: French, Vietnamese
Degree and Year: PhD 1995 MIBA 1984
Major Field: Clinical Psychology
Specialty: Cross Cultural Processes;Clinical Psychology;Ethnic
Minorities

NHAN, Nguyen
4600 Oxford Street
Garrett Park, MD 20896-0174
(703) 777-3485-**B**
Ethnicity: Asian-American/Asian/Pacific Islander
Languages: Vietnamese
Degree and Year: PhD 1963
Major Field: Social Psychology
Specialty: Program Evaluation;Attitudes & Opinions

NICHOLSON, Liston O.
P.O. Box 255
West Brentwood, NY 11717-0255
(516) 789-8562-**B**
Ethnicity: African-American/Black
Degree and Year: PhD 1964
Major Field: Clinical Psychology

NICKERSON, Kim J.
American Psychological Association
Minority Fellowship Program
750 First Street, NE
Washington, DC 20002-4242
(202) 336-5981-**B**, (301) 937-3511-**H**, (202) 336-6012-**F**
knickerson@apa.org
Ethnicity: African-American/Black
Degree and Year: PhD 1992
Major Field: Community Psychology
Specialty: Ethnic Minorities;Social Problems;Mental Health
Services;Cultural & Social Processes;Community
Psychology;Research & Training

NICKS, T. Leon
U.S. Public Health Services
John F. Kennedy Federal Building
Region 1, Room #1826
Boston, MA 02203
(617) 525-1463-**B**, (508) 429-2028-**H**, (617) 565-4027-**F**
Ethnicity: African-American/Black

Languages: Spanish
Degree and Year: PhD 1960
Major Field: Clinical Psychology
Specialty: Administration;Community Mental Health;Ethnic
Minorities;Child & Pediatric Psychology

NIEMANN, Yolanda F
University of Houston
Psychology Department
Houston, TX 77204-5341
(713) 743-8524-**B**, 713 869-4551-**H**, 713 743-8588-**F**
yfniemann@uh.edu
Ethnicity: Hispanic/Latino
Languages: Spanish
Degree and Year: PhD 1992 MGd 1989
Major Field: Social Psychology
Specialty: Ethnic Minorities;Cross Cultural Processes;Social
Cognition;Group Processes;Cultural & Social Processes

NIETO-CARDOSO, Ezequiel
Hacienda del Jacal 1303
Mansiones del Valle
Queretaro 264, 76185
MEXICO
42-160208-**B**, 42-167898-**H**, 42-160208-**F**
ezequiel@ciateq.mx
Ethnicity: Hispanic/Latino
Languages: French, Spanish
Degree and Year: PhD 1975
Major Field: Counseling Psychology
Specialty: Clinical Psychology;Psychotherapy

NIEVES-GRAFALS, Sara
1400 Twentieth Street, NW
Suite #103
Washington, DC 20036
(202) 543-1247-**B**
Ethnicity: Hispanic/Latino
Languages: Portuguese, Spanish
Degree and Year: PhD 1980
Major Field: Clinical Psychology
Specialty: Psychotherapy;Assessment/Diagnosis/Evaluation;Cross
Cultural Processes;Clinical Psychology;Depression

NIEVES, Luis R.
Contemporary Psychology Institute
156 Tamarack Circle
Skillman, NJ 08558-2021
(609) 924-8010-**B**, (609) 921-6034-**H**
Ethnicity: Hispanic/Latino
Degree and Year: PsyD 1976
Major Field: Clinical Psychology
Specialty: Sex/Marital Therapy

NIHIRA, Kazuo
1750 Stone Canyon Road
Los Angeles, CA 90077
(310) 825-0204-**B**, (310) 472-9480-**H**, (310) 825-9875-**F**
Ethnicity: Asian-American/Asian/Pacific Islander
Languages: Japanese
Degree and Year: PhD 1965
Major Field: Quan/Math & Psychometrics/Stat
Specialty: Developmental Psychology;Cross Cultural Processes;Family
Processes;Measurement;Special Education

NINONUEVO, Fred
1518 East Lake Street, Suite 200
Minneapolis, MN 55407
(612) 724-3443-**B**, (612) 729-9713-**F**
frednino@msus1.msus.edu
Ethnicity: Asian-American/Asian/Pacific Islander
Degree and Year: PhD 1989
Major Field: Clinical Psychology
Specialty: Assessment/Diagnosis/Evaluation;Ethnic
   Minorities;Alcoholism & Alcohol Abuse;Program Evaluation

NISHI-STRATTNER, Linda
7420 SW Hunziker
Suite C
Tigard, OR 97223-8242
(503) 620-0157-**B**
Ethnicity: Asian-American/Asian/Pacific Islander
Degree and Year: PhD 1987
Major Field: Clinical Psychology
Specialty: Adolescent Therapy;Child Therapy;Family Therapy

NISHIO, Kazumi
8383 W Dry Creek Road
Healdsburg, CA 95448-9718
(707) 433-5954-**B**
Ethnicity: Asian-American/Asian/Pacific Islander
Degree and Year: PhD 1982
Major Field: Clinical Psychology
Specialty: Psychotherapy

NIWA, John S.
4860 86th Avenue, SE
Mercer Island, WA 98040-4606
(206) 544-4121-**B**
Ethnicity: Asian-American/Asian/Pacific Islander
Degree and Year: MA 1958
Major Field: unknown
Specialty: Human Factors

NIX-EARLY, Vivian
517 Roumfort Road
Philidelphia, PA 19119
(215) 436-3416-**B**, (215) 247-6821-**H**
Ethnicity: African-American/Black
Languages: Spanish
Degree and Year: PhD 1978
Major Field: Clinical Psychology
Specialty: Clinical Psychology;Individual
   Psychotherapy;Leadership;Training &
   Development;Psychotherapy

NOEL, Winifred
1677 Colusa Avenue
Davis, CA 95616
(916) 752-0871-**B**, (916) 758-1048-**H**
Ethnicity: African-American/Black
Degree and Year: EdD 1976
Major Field: Counseling Psychology
Specialty: Adult Development;Biofeedback;Personality
   Disorders;Administration

NOGALES, Ana
Nogales Psychological Counseling, Inc.
3550 Wilshire Boulevard

Suite #670
Los Angeles, CA 90010
(213) 413-7777-**B**, (213) 384-7660-**H**, (213) 384-2084-**F**
Ethnicity: Hispanic/Latino
Languages: Spanish
Degree and Year: PhD 1982
Major Field: Clinical Psychology
Specialty: Clinical Psychology;Cross Cultural Processes;Mass Media
   Communication;Forensic Psychology;Cognitive Psychology

NOLAN, JR., Benjamin C.
PO Box 2605
Middletown, CT 06457
(203) 347-2032-**B**, (203) 347-2032-**H**
Ethnicity: African-American/Black
Degree and Year: PhD 1980
Major Field: Clinical Psychology
Specialty: Clinical Child Psychology;Clinical Child
   Neuropsychology;Learning Disabilities;Assessment/Diagnosis/
   Evaluation;Community Mental Health

NOLAN, Beverly D.
886 Hillcrest Road
Ridgewood, NJ 07450-1131
Ethnicity: African-American/Black
Degree and Year: PhD 1983
Major Field: Counseling Psychology
Specialty: Psychotherapy

NOLLEY, David A.
1702 Peony Lane
San Jose, CA 95124
(408) 266-4939-**B**, (408) 266-4939-**H**, (408) 996-0294-**F**
danolley@aol.com
Ethnicity: American Indian/Alaska Native
Degree and Year: PhD 1974
Major Field: Neurosciences
Specialty: Applied Behavior Analysis;Mentally Retarded;Physiological
   Psychology;Sexual Behavior;Training & Development

NORMAN-JACKSON, Jacquelyn
87-49 Chevy Chase Street
Jamaica, NY 11432-2443
(718) 454-6264-**B**
Ethnicity: African-American/Black
Degree and Year: PhD 1976
Major Field: School Psychology

NORMAN, William H.
Butler Hospital
345 Blackstone Blvd.
Providence, RI 02906
(401) 455-6352-**B**
Ethnicity: African-American/Black
Degree and Year: PhD 1975
Major Field: Clinical Psychology
Specialty: Affective Disorders;Cognitive Behavioral
   Therapy;Assessment/Diagnosis/Evaluation;Clinical
   Research;Group Psychotherapy

NORONHA, Greta A.
604 N Pegram Street
Alexandria, VA 22304-2728
Ethnicity: Asian-American/Asian/Pacific Islander

Degree and Year: PhD 1976
Major Field: Clinical Psychology
Specialty: Drug Abuse

NORTON, A. Evangeline
1129 Towanda Terrace
Cincinnati, OH 45216
(513) 556-0648-**B**, (513) 242-2492-**H**, (513) 556-2302-**F**
Ethnicity: African-American/Black
Degree and Year: PhD 1961
Major Field: Clinical Psychology
Specialty: Clinical Psychology;Cross Cultural
Processes;Depression;Ethnic Minorities;Feminist Therapy

NOWATARI, Masahiro
Tamagawa University
6-1-1 Tamagawa Gakuen
Machida-Shi 194-860,
JAPAN
+042 739 8463-**B**, +427 739 8858-**F**
nowatari@eng.tamajawa.ac.jp
Ethnicity: Asian-American/Asian/Pacific Islander
Languages: Japanese
Degree and Year: PhD 1993
Major Field: Industrial/Organizational Psy.
Specialty: Social Psychology;Work Performance;Management &
Organization;Performance Evaluation;Organizational
Development;Group Processes

NUNEZ, Narina N
University of Wyoming
Department of Psychology
Box 3415
Laramie, WY 83071
(301) 766-6718-**B**, 307 766-2926-**F**
narina@uwyo.edu
Ethnicity: Hispanic/Latino
Degree and Year: PhD 1987 MS 1984
Major Field: Developmental Psychology
Specialty: Psychology & Law;Child Abuse;Developmental Psychology

NUTTALL, Ena V.
Northeastern University
Bouve Graduate School
203 Mugar Life Building
Boston, MA 02115
(617) 373-3297-**B**, (617) 969-6116-**H**, (617) 373-4701-**F**
evazquez-nuttall@nunnet.neu.ed
Ethnicity: Hispanic/Latino
Languages: Spanish
Degree and Year: EdD 1968
Major Field: School Psychology
Specialty: Cross Cultural Processes;Child Therapy;School
Psychology;Assessment/Diagnosis/Evaluation;School
Counseling;Counseling Psychology

NZEWI, Esther N.
California Institute of Integral Studies
9 Peter Yorke Way
San Francisco, CA 94132

(415) 674-5500-**B**, (415) 584-1256-**H**, (415) 674-5555-**F**
Ethnicity: African-American/Black
Degree and Year: PhD 1978
Major Field: Clinical Psychology
Specialty: Clinical Psychology;Cultural & Social Processes;Ethnic
Minorities;Cross Cultural Processes;Death & Dying

O'BRIEN, B. Marco
3284 North Hackett Avenue
Milwaukee, WI 53211
(414) 963-9810-**B**, (414) 963-4797-**H**
obrienm@milwaukee.tec.wi
Ethnicity: Hispanic/Latino
Languages: Spanish
Degree and Year: PhD 1982
Major Field: Educational Psychology
Specialty: Psychometrics;Cross Cultural Processes;Educational
Research;Program Evaluation;Educational Psychology;School
Psychology

O'NEILL-DEPUMARADA, Celeste
Azucena 6 Santa Maria
Rio Piedras, PR 00927
(809) 764-0000-**B**, (809) 758-3667-**H**
Ethnicity: Hispanic/Latino
Degree and Year: MA 1959
Major Field: Social Psychology
Specialty: Cross Cultural Processes

OANA, Leilani K.
15712 Mapleview Circle
Dallas, TX 75248-4225
(972)225-9780-**B**, 214 458-9695-**H**
Ethnicity: Asian-American/Asian/Pacific Islander
Languages: Japanese
Degree and Year: PhD 1984
Major Field: Clinical Psychology
Specialty: Gerontology/Geropsychology;Clinical
Psychology;Assessment/Diagnosis/Evaluation

OCASIO-GARCIA, Ketty
253 Chile Street
Cadiz Cond. 17-B
San Juan, PR 00917-2109
(809) 753-8112-**H**, (809) 782-4334-**F**
Ethnicity: Hispanic/Latino
Languages: Spanish
Degree and Year: PhD 1985
Major Field: Industrial/Organizational Psy.
Specialty: Industrial/Organizational Psychology;Professional Issues in
Psychology;Interpersonal Processes &
Relations;Organizational Development;Training &
Development;Stress

ODA, Ethel Aiko
University of Hawaii at Manoa
509 University Avenue
Suite #402
Honolulu, HI 96826
(808) 956-7501-**B**, (808) 956-3814-**F**
oda@hawaii.edu
Ethnicity: Asian-American/Asian/Pacific Islander
Degree and Year: PhD 1969
Major Field: Counseling Psychology

Specialty: Rehabilitation;Cross Cultural Processes;Ethnic
Minorities;Psychology of Women;Training & Development

OH, Jungyeol L.
California Department of Correction
14901 South Central Avenue
Chino, CA 91708
(909) 597-1821-**B**, (818) 790-7881-**H**, (818) 790-3061-**F**
Ethnicity: Asian-American/Asian/Pacific Islander
Degree and Year: PhD 1994
Major Field: Clinical Psychology
Specialty: Clinical Child Psychology;Ethnic Minorities;Problem
Solving;Assessment/Diagnosis/Evaluation;Forensic
Psychology;Parent Education

OHWAKI, Sonoko
Sonoma Developmental Center
P.O. Box 936
Eldridge, CA 95431-0936
(707) 938-6625-**B**
Ethnicity: Asian-American/Asian/Pacific Islander
Degree and Year: PhD 1959
Major Field: Developmental Psychology

OHYE, Bonnie Y.
10 Mt. Vernon Street
Marbelhead, MA 01945
(617) 979-7025-**B**, (617) 639-1634-**H**
Ethnicity: Asian-American/Asian/Pacific Islander
Degree and Year: PhD 1980
Major Field: Clinical Psychology
Specialty: Child & Pediatric Psychology

OKA, Evelyn R.
451 Erickson Hall
Mich State Univ
East Lansing, MI 48824-1034
(5173)55-6683-**B**, (517) 351-9543-**H**, (517) 353-6393-**F**
Ethnicity: Asian-American/Asian/Pacific Islander
Degree and Year: PhD 1984
Major Field: Developmental Psychology
Specialty: Cognitive Development;Educational
Psychology;Motivation;Parent-Child Interaction;School
Psychology

OKAGAKI, Lynn
Purdue University
Child Development and
Family Studies
West Lafayette, IN 47907-1267
(317) 494-2960-**B**
Ethnicity: Asian-American/Asian/Pacific Islander
Degree and Year: PhD 1984
Major Field: Developmental Psychology
Specialty: Cognitive Development;Educational Research;Ethnic
Minorities

OKAZAKI, Sumie
University of Wisconsin, Madison
Department of Psychology
1202 West Johnson Street
Madison, WI 53706
(608) 262-0389-**B**, (608) 829-0467-**H**, (608) 262-4029-**F**
sakazaki@facstaff.wisc.edu
Ethnicity: Asian-American/Asian/Pacific Islander

Languages: Japanese
Degree and Year: PhD 1994
Major Field: Clinical Psychology

OKIYAMA, Stephen L.
University of California
Veitch Student Center - Counseling
Riverside, CA 92521
(906) 787-5531-**B**, (909) 823-7546-**H**, (909) 787-2447-**F**
Ethnicity: Asian-American/Asian/Pacific Islander
Degree and Year: PhD 1989
Major Field: Clinical Psychology
Specialty: Individual Psychotherapy;Interpersonal Processes &
Relations;Clinical Psychology;Group Psychotherapy

OKONJI, Jacques A.
Prospect Pyschoeducational Service
International-PPSi
PO Box 6003
Colorado Springs, CO 80934-3212
(719) 577-3212-**B**, (719) 650-3600-**H**, (719) 591-2691-**F**
caddyking1@aol.com
Ethnicity: African-American/Black
Degree and Year: PhD 1994
Major Field: Educational Psychology
Specialty: Rehabilitation;Cross Cultural Processes;Educational
Psychology;Drug Abuse;Forensic Psychology;Training &
Development

OKORODUDU, Corahann
Rowan University
Psychology Department
Glassboro, NJ 08028-1701
(609) 256-4500-**B**, (609) 848-4961-**H**, (609) 848-0142-**F**
okorodudu@rowan.edu
Ethnicity: African-American/Black
Degree and Year: PhD 1966
Major Field: Developmental Psychology
Specialty: Motivation;Cross Cultural Processes;Human Development &
Family Studies;Cognitive Development;Ethnic
Minorities;Gender Issues

OLGUIN, Arthur
Santa Barbara City College
Psychology Department
721 Cliff Drive
Santa Barbara, CA 93109
(805) 965-0581-**B**, (805) 681-0541-**H**
olguin@earthlink.net
Ethnicity: Hispanic/Latino
Degree and Year: PhD 1991
Major Field: Social Psychology
Specialty: Program Evaluation;Job Satisfaction;Social
Psychology;Family Therapy;Industrial/Organizational
Psychology

OLIVAS, Romeo A.
194 Highland Court
Harrisonburg, VA 22801-2810
(703) 433-1261-**B**
Ethnicity: Hispanic/Latino
Degree and Year: PhD 1968
Major Field: Developmental Psychology

OLIVERO, Gerald
  Pan Am Building
  521 Fifth Avenue
  Suite #1700
  New York, NY 10175-0001
  (212) 316-2800-**B**
Ethnicity: Hispanic/Latino
Degree and Year: PhD 1973
Major Field: Industrial/Organizational Psy.
Specialty: Organizational Development

OLMEDO, Esteban L.
  California School of Professional
  Professional Psychology
  100 S Fremont Avenue
  Alhambra, CA 91803-4737
  (818) 284-2777-**B**, (818) 810-4224-**H**, (818) 284-0550-**F**
Ethnicity: Hispanic/Latino
Languages: Spanish
Degree and Year: PhD 1972
Major Field: Experimental Psychology
Specialty: Quantitative/Mathematical, Psychometrics;Cross Cultural
      Processes;Administration

OLMO, Manuel C.
  P.O. Box 2930
  Bayamon, PR 00960
  (787) 780-0775-**B**, (787) 740-1461-**H**, (787) 780-0775-**F**
Ethnicity: Hispanic/Latino
Languages: Spanish
Degree and Year: PhD 1978
Major Field: Clinical Psychology
Specialty: Attention Deficit Disorders;Child Abuse;Forensic
      Psychology;Psychometrics

OMIZO, Michael M.
  University of Hawaii at Manoa
  1776 University Avenue
  Honolulu, HI 96822
  (808) 956-4338-**B**, (808) 956-3814-**F**
  omizo@hawaii.edu
Ethnicity: Asian-American/Asian/Pacific Islander
Languages: Japanese
Degree and Year: PhD 1978
Major Field: Counseling Psychology
Specialty: Child Therapy;Counseling Psychology;Ethnic
      Minorities;Homelessness & Homeless Populations;School
      Counseling

OMOTO, Allen M.
  University of Kansas
  Department of Psychology
  426 Fraser Hall
  Lawrence, KS 66045
  (785) 864-9835-**B**, (785) 843-4909-**H**, (785) 864-5696-**F**
  omoto@ukans.edu
Ethnicity: Asian-American/Asian/Pacific Islander
Degree and Year: PhD 1989
Major Field: Social Psychology
Specialty: HIV/AIDS;Interpersonal Processes & Relations;Lesbian &
      Gay Issuues;Social Cognition;Social Problems

ONG, Eddie N.
  405 91st Street #4
  Daly City, CA 94015-1955

(415) 668-5960-**B**
Ethnicity: Asian-American/Asian/Pacific Islander
Degree and Year: PhD 1984
Major Field: Clinical Psychology

ONIZUKA, Richard K.
  Kaiser Permente
  5257 S Wadsworth
  Littleton, CO 80123-2228
  (303) 972-5366-**B**, (303) 646-0311-**H**, (303) 972-5017-**F**
Ethnicity: Asian-American/Asian/Pacific Islander
Degree and Year: PhD 1986
Major Field: Clinical Psychology
Specialty: Administration;Adolescent Therapy;Cross Cultural
      Processes;Managed Care;Ethnic Minorities

ONODA, Lawrence
  21243 Ventura Boulevard
  Woodland Hills, CA 91364
  (818) 704-9918-**B**, (805) 492-1641-**H**, (818) 704-1362-**F**
Ethnicity: Asian-American/Asian/Pacific Islander
Degree and Year: PhD 1974
Major Field: Counseling Psychology
Specialty: Clinical Psychology;Cognitive Behavioral Therapy;Family
      Therapy;Assessment/Diagnosis/Evaluation

OOMMEN THOMAS, Susy
  Kennedy Krieger Institute
  Johns Hopkins University
   School of Medicine
  707 North Broadway
  Baltimore, MD 21205
  (410) 674-4335-**H**
  susydn@gateway.net
Ethnicity: Asian-American/Asian/Pacific Islander
Languages: Spanish, Malayalan
Degree and Year: PhD 1996
Major Field: Clinical Psychology
Specialty: Child Abuse;Community Mental Health;Instructional
      Methods;Child Therapy;Cross Cultural
      Processes;Neuropsychology

ORABONA, Elaine
  U.S. Air Force
  501 Fisher Street
  Keesler Medical Center SGOH
  Biloxi, MS 39534
  (228) 377-6216-**B**, (228) 396-9798-**H**, (228) 377-6336-**F**
  majorabona@aol.com
Ethnicity: Hispanic/Latino
Degree and Year: PhD 1988 DOD 1996
Major Field: Psychopharmacology
Specialty: Continuing Education;Gender Issues;Medical
      Psychology;Ethnic Minorities;Group
      Psychotherapy;Psychopharmacology

ORTEGA, Richard J.
  18101 Marksman Circle
  Apartment #303
  Olney, MD 20832-1471
  (410) 795-2100-**B**, (301) 570-4450-**H**
Ethnicity: Hispanic/Latino
Degree and Year: PhD 1983

Major Field: Clinical Psychology
Specialty: Chronically Mentally Ill;Schizophrenia;Individual
Psychotherapy;Medical Psychology;Death & Dying

ORTEGA, Robert M.
The University of Michigan
School of Social Work
1080 South University   #2796
Ann Arbor, MI 48109-1106
(734) 763-6576-**B**, (734) 668-2924-**H**, (734) 763-3372-**F**
rmortega@umich.edu
Ethnicity: Hispanic/Latino
Languages: Spanish
Degree and Year: PhD 1991
Major Field: Social Psychology
Specialty: Child Abuse;Military Psychology;Social Psychology;Ethnic
Minorities;Interpersonal Processes & Relations

ORTIZ, Berta S.
119 San Vicente Blvd.
Suite #205
Beverly Hills, CA 90211
(310) 475-8317-**B**, (310) 475-8317-**H**
Ethnicity: Hispanic/Latino
Languages: Spanish
Degree and Year: PhD 1982
Major Field: Counseling Psychology
Specialty: Health Psychology;Assessment/Diagnosis/
Evaluation;Psychotherapy;Employee Assistance
Programs;Consulting Psychology

ORTIZ, Vilma
University of California
@ Los Angeles
Department of Sociology
Los Angeles, CA 90024
(310) 206-5218-**B**, (310) 206-1784-**F**
Ethnicity: Hispanic/Latino
Languages: Spanish
Degree and Year: PhD 1981
Major Field: unknown
Specialty: Ethnic Minorities

OSATO, Sheryl
West Los Angeles VAMC
Psychology Service (B116B)
11301 Wilshire Blvd.
Los Angeles, CA 90073
(310) 268-3336-**B**, (818) 783-6486-**H**, (310) 268-4725-**F**
sosato@ucla.edu
Ethnicity: Asian-American/Asian/Pacific Islander
Degree and Year: PhD 1986
Major Field: Clinical Psychology
Specialty: Gerontology/Geropsychology;Neuropsychology;Alzheimer's
Disease;Research & Training;Chronically Mentally Ill

OSHODI, John
The Oshodi Foundation
17325 NW 27 Avenue
Suite 209
Miami, Fl 33056
(305)/623-5979-**B**, 305/623-9414-**F**
jos5930458@aol.com
Ethnicity: African-American/Black

Degree and Year: PhD 1991
Major Field: Clinical Psychology
Specialty: Motivation;Forensic Psychology;Research &
Training;Cultural & Social Processes

OSORNO, Wendell A.
14035 E Progress Court
Aurora, CO 80015-1128
(303) 351-1635-**B**
Ethnicity: Asian-American/Asian/Pacific Islander, Hispanic/Latino
Degree and Year: PhD 1972
Major Field: Counseling Psychology

OTANI, Akira
University of Maryland
Shoemaker Bldg., Counseling Center
College Park, MD 20742-0001
(301) 314-7662-**B**, (301) 890-8546-**H**, (301) 314-9206-**F**
aotani@wam.umd.edu
Ethnicity: Asian-American/Asian/Pacific Islander
Degree and Year: EdD 1985
Major Field: Counseling Psychology
Specialty: Psychotherapy

OTERO, Rafael F.
5425 Plaza Drive
Texarkana, TX 75503
(903) 838-3711-**B**, (903) 832-2456-**H**, (903) 838-8879-**F**
tero@txk.net
Ethnicity: Hispanic/Latino
Languages: Spanish
Degree and Year: PhD 1982
Major Field: Clinical Psychology
Specialty: Pain & Pain Management;Clinical
Neuropsychology;Assessment/Diagnosis/Evaluation;Child
Therapy;Psychotherapy

OUTLAW, Patricia A.
Outlaw & Associates
2300 North Calvert Street
Suite 219
Baltimore, MD 21218-2547
(410) 235-4539-**B**, (410) 235-7108-**H**, (410) 235-6856-**F**
Ethnicity: African-American/Black
Degree and Year: PhD 1977 MA 1971
Major Field: Clinical Psychology
Specialty: Clinical Child Neuropsychology;HIV/
AIDS;Ethology;Psychotherapy;Pastoral Psychology

OU, Young-Shi
5563 Shepherdess Court
Columbia, MD 21045-2423
(301) 997-1560-**B**
Ethnicity: Asian-American/Asian/Pacific Islander
Degree and Year: PhD 1977
Major Field: Developmental Psychology

OVIDE, Christopher R.
2400 West Villard Avenue
Milwaukee, WI 53209
(414) 527-8450-**B**, (414) 321-1690-**H**, (414) 527-8046-**F**
covide@post.its.mcw.edu
Ethnicity: Hispanic/Latino
Degree and Year: EdD 1978
Major Field: Counseling Psychology

Specialty: Assessment/Diagnosis/Evaluation;Psychotherapy;Health
Psychology;Medical Psychology;Gerontology/
Geropsychology

OWENS-LANE, Jan
Hamden Medical Center
295 Washington Avenue
Suite 2
Hamden, CT 06518
(203)288-9666-**B**, 203/288-0344-**F**
jan.owens.lane@snet.net
Ethnicity: African-American/Black
Degree and Year: PhD 1980 MSW 1973
Major Field: Clinical Psychology
Specialty: Management & Organization;Rehabilitation;Cognitive
Behavioral Therapy;Sex/Marital Therapy;Problem
Solving;Stress

OWYANG, Walter
Canada College
Department of Psychology
4200 Farm Hill Boulevard
Redwood City, CA 94061
(650) 306-3464-**B**
wmoyang@pacbell.net
Ethnicity: Asian-American/Asian/Pacific Islander
Languages: Chinese
Degree and Year: PhD 1970
Major Field: Counseling Psychology
Specialty: Cognitive Behavioral Therapy;Community Mental
Health;Cross Cultural Processes;Forensic
Psychology;Psychometrics

OZAKI, Mona M.
5812 SE 22nd Avenue
Portland, OR 97202
(503) 256-3040-**B**, (503) 233-5639-**H**, (503) 256-9601-**F**
Ethnicity: Asian-American/Asian/Pacific Islander
Degree and Year: PhD 1985
Major Field: Clinical Psychology
Specialty: Child Abuse;Clinical Child Psychology;Community Mental
Health;Preschool & Day Care Issues

OZOA, Claudette
373 Partridge Street
Albany, NY 12208-2916
(518) 453-9220-**B**
Ethnicity: Asian-American/Asian/Pacific Islander, Hispanic/Latino
Degree and Year: PhD 1987
Major Field: Clinical Psychology
Specialty: Medical Psychology;Psychotherapy

OZUZU, Sam
3901 Elmcrest Drive
Pensacola, FL 32504
(904) 444-2364-**B**, (904) 484-8052-**H**
Ethnicity: African-American/Black
Degree and Year: PhD 1982
Major Field: unknown
Specialty: Applied Behavior Analysis;Experimental Analysis of
Behavior;Special Education

PACHECO, Angel E.
CE #649
10451 NW 28th Street
Suite #101

Miami, FL 33172-2100
(809) 685-7424-**B**, (809) 682-1091-**H**, (809) 685-7424-**F**
Ethnicity: Hispanic/Latino
Languages: Spanish
Degree and Year: PhD 1976
Major Field: Clinical Psychology
Specialty: Applied Behavior Analysis;Cognitive Behavioral
Therapy;Individual Psychotherapy;Sex/Marital
Therapy;Family Therapy

PAIGE, Roger
1230 N Doquesne
Joplin, MO 64801
(417) 782-1443-**B**, (417) 624-5194-**H**
Ethnicity: American Indian/Alaska Native
Degree and Year: PhD 1978
Major Field: Clinical Psychology
Specialty: Psychotherapy;Psychometrics;Neuropsychology;Employee
Assistance Programs;Biofeedback

PALOMARES, Ronald S.
Texas Woman's University
Department of Psychology and Philosophy
PO Box 425470
Dento, TX 76204
(940) 898-2303-**B**, (940) 898-2301-**F**
f_palomares@twu.edu
Ethnicity: Hispanic/Latino
Degree and Year: PhD 1992
Major Field: School Psychology
Specialty: Assessment/Diagnosis/Evaluation;Educational
Psychology;Psychopathology;Cross Cultural Processes

PANCIERA, Lawrence A.
Northern Pines Unified Services
P.O. Box 518
Cumberland, WI 54829-0518
(818) 841-1508-**B**
Ethnicity: Hispanic/Latino
Degree and Year: PhD 1974
Major Field: Clinical Psychology
Specialty: Forensic Psychology

PANG, Dawn
Central Oahu Family Guidance Center
860 Fourth Street
Pearl City, HI 96782
(808) 453-5900-**B**
Ethnicity: Asian-American/Asian/Pacific Islander
Degree and Year: PhD 1986
Major Field: Clinical Psychology
Specialty: Special Education;Clinical Child Psychology;Family
Therapy;Parent-Child Interaction;Community Mental
Health;Chronically Mentally Ill

PANG, Mark G.
Hudspeth Regional Cener
Highway 475 South
PO Box 127-B
Whitfield, MS 39193
(601) 664-6373-**B**, (601) 898-0841-**H**, (601) 354-6945-**F**
psych@hrc.state.ms.us

Ethnicity: Asian-American/Asian/Pacific Islander, Hispanic/Latino
Degree and Year: Phd 1989
Major Field: Industrial/Organizational Psy.
Specialty: Industrial/Organizational Psychology;Performance
　　　Evaluation;Research Design & Methodology;Management &
　　　Organization;Mentally Retarded;Organizational Development

PANIAGUA, Freddy A.
　　University of Texas
　　Department of Psychiatry
　　Medical Branch
　　Galveston, TX 77550
　　(409) 772-2419-**B**, (409) 986-6926-**H**, (407) 772-2885-**F**
　　fpaniagua@psypo.med.utm.edu
Ethnicity: Hispanic/Latino
Languages: Spanish
Degree and Year: PhD 1981
Major Field: Clinical Child Psychology
Specialty: Developmental Psychology;Applied Behavior
　　　Analysis;Behavior Therapy

PARASNIS, Ila
　　National Technical Institute
　　　for Deaf
　　1 Lomb Memorial Drive
　　Rochester, NY 14623-5603
　　(716) 475-6708-**B**
Ethnicity: Asian-American/Asian/Pacific Islander
Degree and Year: PhD 1980
Major Field: Experimental Psychology

PARASURAMAN, Raja
　　The Catholic University of America
　　Department of Psychology
　　Washington, DC 20064-0001
　　(202) 319-5825-**B**, (301) 365-6981-**H**
　　parasuraman@csu.deu
Ethnicity: Asian-American/Asian/Pacific Islander
Degree and Year: PhD 1976
Major Field: Experimental Psychology

PARDO, Ruben C.
　　2225 19th St
　　Sacramento, CA 95818-1621
　　(916) 322-8641-**B**, (818) 365-4605-**H**, (916) 322-0922-**F**
Ethnicity: Hispanic/Latino
Languages: Spanish
Degree and Year: PhD 1979
Major Field: unknown
Specialty: Vocational Psychology;Rehabilitation;Psychology &
　　　Law;Cross Cultural Processes;Consulting Psychology

PAREDES, JR., Frank C.
　　717 W Ashby
　　San Antonio, TX 78212
　　(210) 733-7373-**B**, (210) 733-7398-**F**
　　fcparede@texas.net
Ethnicity: Hispanic/Latino
Languages: Spanish
Degree and Year: PhD 1982
Major Field: Clinical Psychology
Specialty: Psychotherapy;Personality
　　　Disorders;Psychoanalysis;Psychology & Law;Ethnic
　　　Minorities

PARHAM, Patricia A.
　　2553 Lands End Dr.
　　Carrollton, Tx 75006
　　(972) 405-5182-**B**, (972) 418-1957-**H**, (972) 418-6077-**F**
　　parhament@webcombo.net
Ethnicity: African-American/Black
Degree and Year: PhD 1980
Major Field: unknown
Specialty: Program Evaluation;Organizational Development

PARHAM, Thomas A.
　　University of California
　　Assistant Vice-Chancellor
　　Counseling and Health Services
　　202 Student Services I
　　Irvine, CA 92697
　　(949) 824-4642-**B**, (949) 824-6586-**F**
　　taparham@uci.edu
Ethnicity: African-American/Black
Degree and Year: PhD 1982　MAEd 1978
Major Field: Counseling Psychology
Specialty: Cross Cultural Processes;Counseling Psychology;Ethnic
　　　Minorities

PARHAM, William D.
　　University of California, Los Angeles
　　Student Psychological Services
　　4223 Math Sciences Building
　　Los Angeles, CA 90024
　　(310) 825-0768-**B**, (310) 285-1475-**H**, (310) 206-7365-**F**
　　wparham@sps.saonet.ucla.net
Ethnicity: African-American/Black
Degree and Year: PhD 1981　ABPP 1992
Major Field: Counseling Psychology
Specialty: Individual Psychotherapy;Sports Psychology;Ethnic
　　　Minorities

PARK, Eyoungsoo
　　1244 Starlite Lane
　　Yuba City, CA 95991-6725
　　(916) 673-4049-**B**
Ethnicity: Asian-American/Asian/Pacific Islander
Degree and Year: PhD 1971
Major Field: Clinical Psychology
Specialty: Clinical Psychology;Community Psychology

PARKS, Carlton
　　Californai School of Professional Psychology
　　　Los Angeles
　　1000 South Fremon Avenue
　　Alhambra, CA 91803-1360
　　(626) 284-2777-**B**, (626) 284-0550-**F**
　　cparks@mail.cspp.edu
Ethnicity: African-American/Black
Degree and Year: PhD 1986
Major Field: Developmental Psychology
Specialty: Clinical Child Psychology;Developmental
　　　Psychology;Gender Issues;Lesbian & Gay Issuues;Sexual
　　　Behavior

PARKS, Fayth M.
　　University of South Carolina
　　Counseling & Human Development Ctr.
　　900 Assembly Street

Room 212
Columbia, SC 29208
(803) 777-5223-**B**, (803) 926-5985-**H**, (803) 777-5433-**F**
fparks@studaff.sa.sc.edu
Ethnicity: African-American/Black
Degree and Year: PhD 1996
Major Field: Counseling Psychology
Specialty: Ethnic Minorities;Curriculum Development/Evaluation;Drug
    Abuse;Counseling Psychology;Cultural & Social
    Processes;Family Processes

PARKS, Gregory S.
PO box 260
East Hampton, NY 11937
(202) 724-3121-**B**, 202 986-5329-**H**
Ethnicity: African-American/Black
Degree and Year:
Major Field: Clinical Psychology

PARLADE, Rafael J.
123 Live Oak Avenue
Daytona Beach, FL 32114-3440
(904) 255-1244-**B**, (904) 767-7764-**H**
Ethnicity: Hispanic/Latino
Degree and Year: PhD 1982
Major Field: Clinical Psychology
Specialty: Cognitive Behavioral Therapy;Family Therapy

PARSON, Erwin R.
PO Box 62
Perry Point, MD 21903-0062
Ethnicity: African-American/Black, Hispanic/Latino
Degree and Year: PhD 1977
Major Field: Clinical Psychology
Specialty: Psychotherapy

PASAMONTE, Ana M.
817 Myrna Drive
Hempstead, NY 11552
(718) 263-1919-**B**
Ethnicity: Hispanic/Latino
Languages: Spanish
Degree and Year: MA 1986
Major Field: Social Psychology
Specialty: School Psychology;Special Education

PASTER, Vera S.
30 Jordan Road
Hastings-on-Hudson, NY 10706
(212) 534-0516-**B**, (914) 478-1168-**H**
Ethnicity: African-American/Black
Degree and Year: PhD 1962
Major Field: Clinical Psychology
Specialty: Psychotherapy;Family Therapy;Feminist Therapy;Cross
    Cultural Processes;Prevention

PATEL, Sanjiv A.
Richard Hall Community Mental
    Health Center
500 North Bridge Street & Vogt Drive
Bridgewater, NJ 08807
(908) 253-3146-**B**, (732) 821-2005-**H**, (908) 704-1790-**F**
Ethnicity: Asian-American/Asian/Pacific Islander

Languages: Hindi, Gujarati
Degree and Year: PsyD 1995 MA 1990
Major Field: Clinical Psychology
Specialty: Clinical Psychology;Family Therapy;Cultural & Social
    Processes;Child Therapy;Individual Psychotherapy;Child
    Abuse

PATRICE, David
21 Wolden Square
Apartment #733
Cambridge, MA 02140
(617) 635-9635-**B**, (617) 547-1782-**H**, (637) 635-9692-**F**
Ethnicity: African-American/Black
Degree and Year: MA 1984
Major Field: School Psychology
Specialty: Cognitive Behavioral Therapy;Educational
    Psychology;Ethnic Minorities;Juvenile Delinquency;School
    Counseling

PATRICK, Carol L.
1037 W Market Street
Lima, OH 45805-2729
(419) 222-5077-**B**
Ethnicity: Hispanic/Latino
Degree and Year: PhD 1985
Major Field: Clinical Psychology
Specialty: Clinical Psychology

PATTERSON, Drayton R.
1836 East 219th Place
Sauk Village, IL 60411
(708) 758-7376-**H**
Ethnicity: African-American/Black
Degree and Year: PhD 1992
Major Field: School Psychology
Specialty: School Psychology;Forensic Psychology;Sports
    Psychology;Stress;General Psychology;Industrial/
    Organizational Psychology

PATTERSON, Mayin Lau
3510 North St. Mary's
Suite #200
San Antonio, TX 78212
(210) 733-8857-**B**, (210) 732-8574-**H**
mayla@stic.net
Ethnicity: Asian-American/Asian/Pacific Islander
Languages: Chinese
Degree and Year: MA 1966
Major Field: Clinical Psychology
Specialty: Clinical Psychology;Clinical Child Psychology;Drug
    Abuse;Gerontology/Geropsychology;Marriage & Family

PATTON, Kenneth
6333 Sagebrush Way
Sacramento, CA 95842
(916) 973-7480-**B**, (916) 332-1700-**H**
Ethnicity: African-American/Black
Degree and Year: PhD 1975
Major Field: Clinical Child Psychology
Specialty: Adolescent Therapy;Attention Deficit Disorders;Child
    Therapy;Family Therapy;Hypnosis/Hypnotherapy

PAYTON, Carolyn R.
3428 Quebec Street, N.W.
Washington, DC 20016

(202) 806-6870-**B**, (202) 966-4247-**H**
Ethnicity: African-American/Black
Degree and Year: EdD 1961
Major Field: Counseling Psychology
Specialty: Client-Centered Therapy;Counseling Psychology;Individual
   Psychotherapy;Lesbian & Gay Issuues

PEART-NEWKIRK, Natalia J.
   Columbia Associates in Psychiatry
   11402 Sunflower Lane
   Fairfax, VA 22030
   (703) 841-1317-**B**, (703) 293-9028-**H**
Ethnicity: African-American/Black, Hispanic/Latino
Degree and Year: PhD 1994
Major Field: Clinical Psychology
Specialty: Clinical Child Psychology;Learning Disabilities;Clinical
   Psychology;Parent-Child Interaction

PEAVYHOUSE, Betty M.
   1114 Sunset Road
   Wheaton, IL 60187-6120
   (708) 665-9590-**H**
Ethnicity: African-American/Black
Degree and Year: PsyD 19
Major Field: Clinical Psychology
Specialty: Assessment/Diagnosis/Evaluation;Clinical
   Psychology;Family Therapy;Group Psychotherapy

PEDEMONTE, Monica
   Biscayne Institute
   2785 NE 183 Street
   Miami, FL 33160
   (305) 932-8994-**B**, (954) 792-8808-**H**, (305) 932-9362-**F**
   bri@gate.net
Ethnicity: Hispanic/Latino
Languages: Spanish
Degree and Year: PhD 1985
Major Field: Health Psychology
Specialty: Clinical Psychology;Assessment/Diagnosis/
   Evaluation;HIV AIDS

PELAEZ, Carmen
   408-A Elizabeth Street
   Fort Lee, NJ 07024
   (201) 617-9651-**B**, (201) 461-2864-**H**
Ethnicity: Hispanic/Latino
Languages: Spanish
Degree and Year: PsyD 1981
Major Field: Clinical Psychology
Specialty: Psychoanalysis;Child Therapy;Preschool & Day Care
   Issues;Child Development;Parent-Child Interaction

PENISTON, Eugene G.
   S. Rayburn Memorial Veteran Center
   1201 East 9th Street
   Bonham, TX 75090
   (903) 583-6240-**B**, (903) 893-0906-**H**
Ethnicity: African-American/Black
Languages: German
Degree and Year: EdD 1972
Major Field: Clinical Psychology
Specialty: Clinical Psychology;Alcoholism & Alcohol
   Abuse;Biofeedback;Behavior Therapy;Psychoimmunology

PENN, Nolan E.
   University of California @ San Diego

School of Medicine
Psychiatry Department
9500 Gilman Drive
La Jolla, CA 92093-0603
(619) 534-0603-**B**, (619) 459-3829-**H**, (619) 459-3829-**F**
npenn@san.rr.com
Ethnicity: African-American/Black
Degree and Year: PhD 1958
Major Field: Clinical Psychology
Specialty: Experimental Psychology

PEOPLES, Kathleen
   Gallaudet University
   800 Florida Ave., N.E.
   Washington, DC 20002
   (202) 651-5260-**B**, (301) 206-5433-**H**, (202) 651-5745-**F**
Ethnicity: African-American/Black
Languages: American Sign Language
Degree and Year: PhD 1982
Major Field: Clinical Psychology
Specialty: Clinical Psychology;Individual Psychotherapy;Moral
   Development;Psychoanalysis

PEOPLES, Napoleon L.
   VA Commonwealth University
   PO Box 842525
   Richmond, VA 23227-4727
   (804) 828-3964-**B**, (804) 828-4488-**F**
   npeoples@saturn.vcu.edu
Ethnicity: African-American/Black
Degree and Year: PhD 1977
Major Field: Counseling Psychology
Specialty: Sex/Marital Therapy;Ethnic Minorities;Stress;Counseling
   Psychology

PERALTA, Carmelina
   4 Huntington Road
   Huntington, NY 11743-1703
   (516) 271-3319-**B**
Ethnicity: Hispanic/Latino
Languages: Spanish
Degree and Year: PhD 1989
Major Field: Clinical Psychology
Specialty: School Psychology

PEREIRA, Glona M.
   Aon Consulting
   2000 Bering Drive
   Suite 900
   Houston, TX 77057
   (713) 954-7416-**B**, (713) 954-7400-**F**
   gloria_pereira@aoncons.com
Ethnicity: Hispanic/Latino
Languages: Spanish
Degree and Year: PhD 1994
Major Field: Industrial/Organizational Psy.
Specialty: Selection & Placement;Work Performance

PEREZ EBRAHIMI, Concepcion
   3967 Sedgwick Avenue, 20A
   Bronx, NY 10463
   (718) 549-3033-**H**, (781) 549-3033-**F**
Ethnicity: Hispanic/Latino
Languages: Spanish
Degree and Year: MA 1988

Major Field: Clinical Psychology
Specialty: Administration;Case Management;Developmental
    Psychology;Adolescent Development;Clinical
    Psychology;Parent Education

PEREZ-ARCE, Patricia
    Substance Abuse Services
    Ward 93
    San Francisco General Hospital
    1001 Potrero Avenue
    San Francisco, CA 94110
    (415) 206-3949-**B**, (707) 935-7209-**H**, (415) 206-6875-**F**
Ethnicity: Hispanic/Latino
Languages: French, Spanish
Degree and Year: PhD 1985
Major Field: Clinical Psychology
Specialty: Neuropsychology;Drug Abuse

PEREZ-RAMOS, Juan
    Universidade de Sao Paulo
    Instituto de Psicologia
    Rua Pelagio Lobo, #107
    71-Sao Paulo
    05009-020 SP   71-,
    BRAZIL
    (110) 38621087-**B**, (110 38621087-**H**, (11) 38621087-**F**
    juanidi1@usp.br
Ethnicity: Hispanic/Latino
Languages: Portuguese, Spanish
Degree and Year: PhD 1967
Major Field: Industrial/Organizational Psy.

PEREZ, Carlos A.
    RD 6 Box 6
    East Stroudsburg, PA 18301
    (201) 319-3836-**B**, (201) 795-5270-**H**
Ethnicity: Hispanic/Latino
Languages: Portuguese, Spanish
Degree and Year: EdD 1979
Major Field: Counseling Psychology
Specialty: Counseling Psychology;Clinical Psychology

PEREZ, Cecilia M.
    135 Lincoln Avenue
    Elizabeth, NJ 07208
    (908) 352-7474-**B**, (908) 353-2958-**H**, (908) 965-3227-**F**
Ethnicity: Hispanic/Latino
Languages: Italian, Portuguese, Spanish
Degree and Year: MA 1978
Major Field: Counseling Psychology
Specialty: Crisis Intervention & Therapy;Child Abuse;Assessment/
    Diagnosis/Evaluation;Consulting Psychology;Counseling
    Psychology

PEREZ, Fred M.
    1717 N Bayshore Drive
    Suite #1756
    Miami, FL 33132-1158
    (305) 577-8333-**B**, (305) 577-4946-**H**, (305) 577-0068-**F**
Ethnicity: Hispanic/Latino
Languages: Spanish
Degree and Year: PhD 1979
Major Field: Developmental Psychology

Specialty: Psycholinguistic;Learning Disabilities

PEREZ, Juan C.
    Long Beach Memorial
    Rehabilitation Hospital
    2801 Atlantic Boulevard
    Long Beach, CA 90807
    (562) 933-9033-**B**, (562) 987-4332-**H**, (562) 434-6213-**F**
Ethnicity: Hispanic/Latino
Languages: Spanish
Degree and Year: PsyD
Major Field: Clinical Psychology
Specialty: Neuropsychology;Health Psychology;Rehabilitation

PEREZ, Ruperto M.
    University of Georgia
    Counseling and Testing Center
    Clark Howell Mall
    Athens, GA 30602-3333
    (706) 542-3183-**B**, (706) 369-3091-**H**, (706) 542-3915-**F**
    rperez@arches.uga.edu
Ethnicity: Asian-American/Asian/Pacific Islander
Degree and Year: PhD 1993 MA 1985
Major Field: Counseling Psychology
Specialty: Counseling Psychology;Lesbian & Gay Issuues;Ethnic
    Minorities;Gender Issues

PERILLA, Julia L.
    Georgia State University
    Department of Psychology
    University Plaza
    Atlanta, GA 30303
    (404) 651-2955-**B**, (404) 634-8079-**H**, (404) 651-1391-**F**
    jperilla@gsu.edu
Ethnicity: Hispanic/Latino
Languages: Spanish
Degree and Year: PhD 1995
Major Field: Clinical Psychology
Specialty: Domestic Violence;Psychology of Women;Feminist
    Therapy;Ethnic Minorities;Community Psychology

PERNELL, Eugene
    5031 Park Lake Rd
    East Lansing, MI 48823-3835
    (517) 332-0811-**B**, (517) 332-7479-**H**
Ethnicity: African-American/Black
Degree and Year: PhD 1971
Major Field: unknown
Specialty: Conduct Disorders

PERRY, Cereta E.
    1645 North Portal Drive, NW
    Washington, DC 20012
    (202) 722-6043-**B**
Ethnicity: African-American/Black
Degree and Year: PhD 1969
Major Field: unknown
Specialty: Family Therapy

PERRY, Jeanell
    South Beach Psychiatric Hospital
    25 Flatbush Avenue
    Adolescent Day Program
    Brooklyn, NY 11217
    (718) 858-4002-**B**, (732) 264-8257-**H**

Ethnicity: African-American/Black
Degree and Year: Phd 1984
Major Field: Clinical Child Psychology
Specialty: Adolescent Therapy;Ethnic Minorities;Special
      Education;Clinical Child
      Psychology;Psychotherapy;Assessment/Diagnosis/Evaluation

PETERS, James S.
   P.O. Box 431
   Storrs, CT 06268
   (203) 487-0823-**B**, (203) 487-0823-**H**
Ethnicity: African-American/Black
Degree and Year: PhD 1955
Major Field: Counseling Psychology
Specialty: Clinical Psychology;Counseling Psychology;Social
      Psychology

PETERS, Sheila
   4811 Fairmede, CT
   Nashville, TN 37218-1601
   speters@dubois.fisk.edu
   (615) 299-9568-**H** (615) 329-8535-**W**

PETTIGREW, Dorothy C.
   305 Moody, Ste #160
   Galveston, TX 77550-
   (409) 765-5070-**B**, (409) 763-6306-**F**
Ethnicity: African-American/Black
Languages: Spanish
Degree and Year: PsyD 1981
Major Field: Clinical Psychology
Specialty: Adolescent Therapy;Clinical Child Psychology;Cultural &
      Social Processes;Family Therapy;Projective Techniques

PFLAUM, John H.
   2266 N Prospect
   Room #200
   Milwaukee, WI 53202
   (414) 289-0559-**B**, (414) 962-7421-**H**
Ethnicity: Hispanic/Latino
Languages: Spanish
Degree and Year: PhD 1972
Major Field: Developmental Psychology
Specialty: Clinical Psychology;Gerontology/
      Geropsychology;Assessment/Diagnosis/
      Evaluation;Depression;Alzheimer's Disease

PHELPS, C. K.
   3437 Quincy Avenue
   Kansas City, MO 64128-2346
   (816) 861-0831-**H**
Ethnicity: African-American/Black
Degree and Year: PhD 1952
Major Field: Clinical Psychology

PHELPS, Rosemary E.
   240 Pebble Creek Drive
   Athens, GA 30605
   (706) 542-1812-**B**, (706) 353-6591-**H**
Ethnicity: African-American/Black
Degree and Year: PhD 1986
Major Field: Counseling Psychology
Specialty: Counseling Psychology;Cultural & Social Processes;Ethnic
      Minorities;Psychopathology;Psychotherapy

PHILLIPS, Campbell C.
   Kare Services Limited
   13 Havelock Street
   St. Clair
   Port-Of-Spain,
   TRINIDAD
   (868) 622-7581-**B**, (808) 524-1920-**H**, (868) 622-7581-**F**
   kares@tsttnet.tt
Ethnicity: African-American/Black
Degree and Year: PhD 1984 MA 1981
Major Field: Clinical Psychology
Specialty: Family Therapy;Sex/Marital Therapy;Employee Assistance
      Programs;Clinical Psychology;Individual
      Psychotherapy;Assessment/Diagnosis/Evaluation

PHILP, Frederick W.
   United States Air Force
   Education Services
   PO Box 105
   Sheppard Air Force Base
   Wichita Falls, TX 26311
   (904) 676-4838-**B**, (940) 855-7699-**H**, (940) 676-7714-**F**
Ethnicity: African-American/Black
Languages: French
Degree and Year: EdD 1979
Major Field: Counseling Psychology
Specialty: Adult Development;Group
      Processes;Administration;Training & Development;Family
      Processes

PICO, Daima
   Comprehensive Pain and Rehabilitation
      Center at South Shore Hospital
   600 Alton Road
   Miama Beach, FL 33139
   (305) 532-7246-**B**, (305) 221-2514-**H**
Ethnicity: Hispanic/Latino
Languages: Spanish
Degree and Year: PsyD 1994
Major Field: Clinical Psychology
Specialty: Pain & Pain Management;Cognitive Behavioral
      Therapy;Individual Psychotherapy;Rehabilitation;Affective
      Disorders;Clinical Neuropsychology

PIERCE, William D.
   Private Practice & Psychological and
      Human Resources Consultants
   361 Upper Terrace
   San Francisco, CA 94117
   (415) 771-3938-**B**, (415) 771-3938-**H**, (415) 777-5663-**F**
Ethnicity: African-American/Black
Degree and Year: PhD 1967
Major Field: Clinical Psychology
Specialty: Forensic Psychology;Community Mental Health;Mental
      Health Services;Psychopathology;Psychotherapy;Group
      Processes

PIERCY, Patricia A.
   211 N. Whitfield Street
   Suite #470
   Pittsburgg, PA 15206
   (412) 661-5970-**B**, (724) 444-1016-**H**, (412) 661-5924-**F**
Ethnicity: African-American/Black

Degree and Year: PhD 1976
Major Field: Clinical Psychology
Specialty: Adolescent Therapy;Child Abuse;Child Therapy

PINCHEIRA, Juan A.
201 Penn Center Blvd.
Pittsburgh, PA 15235-5435
(412) 824-8992-**B**
Ethnicity: Hispanic/Latino
Degree and Year: PhD 1976
Major Field: Clinical Psychology

PINDER-AMAKER, Stephanie L.
Seton Hall University
400 South Orange Avenue
South Orange, NJ 07079
(973) 275-2852-**B**, (973) 275-9075-**H**
Ethnicity: African-American/Black
Degree and Year: PhD 1988
Major Field: Clinical Psychology
Specialty: Clinical Psychology;Individual Psychotherapy;Health Psychology;Ethnic Minorities

PINDERHUGHES, Ellen B.
Vanderbilt University
Dept. of Psychology & Human Dev.
Box 512 Peabody College
Nashville, TN 37202-0512
(615) 322-8141-**B**, (615) 646-2837-**H**
pinderee@trvax.vanderbilt.edu
Ethnicity: African-American/Black
Degree and Year: PhD 1986
Major Field: Clinical Psychology
Specialty: Developmental Psychology;Human Development & Family Studies

PINDERHUGHES, Victoria A.
536 West 111th Street
Suite #45
New York, NY 10025
(212) 932-6620-**B**, (212) 662-2760-**H**
Ethnicity: African-American/Black
Degree and Year: PhD 1987
Major Field: Clinical Psychology
Specialty: Clinical Child Psychology;Assessment/Diagnosis/Evaluation;Giftedness;Child & Pediatric Psychology;Individual Psychotherapy

PINE, Charles J.
Upland Veterans Center
10B-RC 0637Psychology Science
Upland, CA 91786
(909) 890-0797-**B**
Ethnicity: American Indian/Alaska Native
Degree and Year: PhD 1979
Major Field: Clinical Psychology
Specialty: Ethnic Minorities;Alcoholism & Alcohol Abuse;Drug Abuse;Stress;Sports Psychology

PINTO, Alcides
113 Legion Avenue
Annapolis, MD 21401-4002
(410) 729-6319-**B**, (410) 267-9008-**H**, (410) 729-6800-**F**
chcpsych@juno.com

Ethnicity: Hispanic/Latino
Languages: Spanish
Degree and Year: PhD 1963
Major Field: Clinical Psychology
Specialty: Family Therapy;Assessment/Diagnosis/Evaluation;Ethnic Minorities;Mentally Retarded

PIRHEKAYATY-SORIANO, Tahereh
Institute for Multicultural Counseling
and Educational Services Center
3550 Wilshire Boulevard
Suite 410
Los Angeles, CA 90010
(213) 381-1250-**B**, (213) 665-0544-**H**, (213) 383-4803-**F**
tarapirimces@msn.com
Ethnicity: Asian-American/Asian/Pacific Islander, European/White
Languages: Farsi
Degree and Year: PhD 1985
Major Field: Clinical Psychology
Specialty: Clinical Psychology;Depression;Cross Cultural Processes;Parent-Child Interaction

PITA, Marcia E.
Hillsborogh County Schools
1107 West Coral Street
Tampa, FL 33602
(813) 273-7158-**B**, (813) 221-4035-**H**, (813) 221-4035-**F**
apita2prodigy.net
Ethnicity: Hispanic/Latino
Languages: Spanish
Degree and Year: PhD 1994
Major Field: Clinical Psychology
Specialty: School Psychology;Clinical Child Psychology;Ethnic Minorities;Clinical Psychology

PIZANO-THOMEN, Margarita
60 West 13th Street
Apartment #9F
New York, NY 10011-7919
(212) 675-2674-**B**
Ethnicity: Hispanic/Latino
Degree and Year: PsyD 1988
Major Field: Clinical Psychology
Specialty: Family Therapy

PLAZAS, Carlos A.
5655 N Drake
Chicago, IL 60659
(312) 878-8756-**B**, (312) 478-8138-**H**
Ethnicity: Hispanic/Latino
Languages: Spanish
Degree and Year: PhD 1972
Major Field: Clinical Psychology
Specialty: Alcoholism & Alcohol Abuse;Clinical Psychology;Community Mental Health;Drug Abuse;School Psychology

POAL, Pilar
Southhampton Psychiatric Associates
Suite A-200 Southhampton Office Park
928 Jaymer Road
Southhampton, PA 18966
(215) 355-2011-**B**, (610) 964-9528-**H**

Ethnicity: Hispanic/Latino
Languages: Spanish
Degree and Year: PhD 1989
Major Field: Clinical Psychology
Specialty: Rehabilitation;Brain Damage;Clinical
　　　　Psychology;Psychotherapy

POLITE, Craig K.
　One Battery Park Place
　27th Floor
　P.O. Box 19
　New York, NY 10004-1412
Ethnicity: African-American/Black
Degree and Year: PhD 1972
Major Field: Clinical Psychology
Specialty: Organizational Development

POLITE, Kenneth
　173 N Marengo
　# 407
　Pasadena, CA 91101-4522
　708 866-7661-**B**
Ethnicity: African-American/Black
Degree and Year: PhD 1983
Major Field: Clinical Psychology
Specialty: Clinical Psychology;Individual Psychotherapy;Child &
　　　　Pediatric Psychology;Ethnic Minorities;Cognitive Behavioral
　　　　Therapy

POMPA, Janiece L.
　546 Chipeta Wy #2249
　Salt Lake City, UT 84108-1241
　(801) 585-7555-**B**, (801) 582-4110-**H**, (801) 585-5845-**F**
　pompa_j@gse.utah.edu
Ethnicity: Hispanic/Latino
Degree and Year: PhD 1983
Major Field: Clinical Psychology
Specialty: Clinical Neuropsychology;Psychotherapy;Brain
　　　　Damage;Lesbian & Gay Issuues;Attention Deficit Disorders

PONS, Michael B.
　Health and Human Services Group
　25108 Marguerite Parkway
　Suite B/42
　Mission Viejo, CA 92692
　(949) 859-7460-**B**, (949) 768-3351-**H**, (949) 768-1667-**F**
　hhsg@ix.netcom.com
Ethnicity: Hispanic/Latino
Languages: Spanish
Degree and Year: PhD 1996 MA 1982
Major Field: Physiological Psychology
Specialty: Medical Psychology;Assessment/Diagnosis/
　　　　Evaluation;Biofeedback;Clinical Neuropsychology;Forensic
　　　　Psychology;Psychophysiology

PONTON, Marcel O.
　300 North Lake Avenue
　Suite 111-A
　Pasadena, CA 91101
　(626) 449-2484-**B**, (626) 798-9606-**H**, (626) 449-1107-**F**
　moponton@ucla.edu
Ethnicity: Hispanic/Latino
Languages: Spanish
Degree and Year: PhD 1989
Major Field: Clinical Psychology

Specialty: Neuropsychology;Rehabilitation;Central Nervous
　　　　System;Intelligence;Assessment/Diagnosis/Evaluation;Clinical
　　　　Child Neuropsychology

POON, Leonard W.
　University of Georgia
　Gerontology Center
　100 Candler Hall
　Athens, GA 30609
Ethnicity: Asian-American/Asian/Pacific Islander
Degree and Year: PhD 1972
Major Field: Experimental Psychology
Specialty: Memory

POPE-DAVIS, Donald B.
　University of Notre Dame
　Department of Psychology
　118 Haggar Hall
　Notre Dame, IN 46556
　(219) 631-7675-**B**, (219) 631-8883-**F**
Ethnicity: African-American/Black
Degree and Year: PhD 1989
Major Field: Counseling Psychology
Specialty: Counseling Psychology;Cross Cultural Processes;Cultural &
　　　　Social Processes;Ethnic Minorities;Individual Difference

POPE-TARRENCE, Jacqueline R.
　Western Kentucky University
　Tate Page Hall - 273
　Bowling Green, KY 42101
　(502) 745-2695-**B**, (502) 842-0710-**H**, (502) 745-6934-**F**
　jacqueline.pope-tarrence@wku.e
Ethnicity: African-American/Black
Degree and Year: PhD 1991
Major Field: Social Psychology
Specialty: Psychology & Law;Crime & Criminal Behavior;Cultural &
　　　　Social Processes;Attribution Theory;Social
　　　　Psychology;Experimental Psychology

POPE, Mark
　University of Missouri, St. Louis
　Division of Counseling
　8001 Natural Bridge Road
　St. Louis, MO 63121-4499
　(314) 516-7121-**B**, (314) 454-9300-**H**, (314) 516-5784-**F**
　pope@jinx.umsl.edu
Ethnicity: American Indian/Alaska Native
Degree and Year: EdD 1988
Major Field: Counseling Psychology
Specialty: Vocational Psychology;Lesbian & Gay
　　　　Issuues;Psychometrics;Cross Cultural Processes;HIV/
　　　　AIDS;Drug Abuse

PORCHE-BURKE, Lisa M.
　Phillips Graduate Institute
　5445 Balboa Boulevard
　Encino, CA 91316-1509
　(818) 386-5950-**B**
　lpburkel@aol.com
Ethnicity: African-American/Black
Languages: Spanish
Degree and Year: PhD 1983 MA 1981
Major Field: Counseling Psychology
Specialty: Social Psychology;Ethnic
　　　　Minorities;Leadership;Management & Organization

PORGES, Carlos R.
  NBHC, Inc.
  1555 Howell Branch Road
  Suite C-210
  Winter Park, FL 32789
  (407) 760-0007-**B**, (407) 882-3126-**H**, (407) 740-8360-**F**
  76511.2230@compuserve.com
Ethnicity: Hispanic/Latino
Languages: Spanish
Degree and Year: PsyD 1991
Major Field: Clinical Psychology
Specialty: Neuropsychology;Curriculum Development/
      Evaluation;Rehabilitation;Cross Cultural Processes

PORTER, Julia
  5328 29th St Nw
  Washington, DC 20015-1332
  (703) 247-4100-**B**, (202) 364-1382-**H**
Ethnicity: African-American/Black
Degree and Year: PhD 1987
Major Field: Clinical Psychology
Specialty: Adolescent Therapy

POSNER, Carmen A.
  4201 N Oak Park Avenue
  Chicago, IL 60634
  (312) 794-5500-**B**, (312) 794-3975-**F**
Ethnicity: Hispanic/Latino
Languages: Spanish
Degree and Year: PhD 1969
Major Field: Clinical Psychology
Specialty: Child & Pediatric Psychology

POSTON, II, Walker S.
  6019 Claridge
  Houston, TX 77096-5824
  (713) 795-7458-**B**, 713 496-6138-**H**, 713 798-4888-**F**
  walker@bcm.tmc.edu
Ethnicity: African-American/Black
Degree and Year: PhdD 1990
Major Field: Counseling Psychology
Specialty: Medical Psychology;Health Psychology;Eating
      Disorders;Clinical Research;Epidemiology & Biometry

POWELL, Lois
  12269 Carroll Mill Road
  Ellicott City, MD 21042
  (410) 531-2805-**B**, (301) 596-9114-**H**
Ethnicity: African-American/Black
Degree and Year: PhD 1972
Major Field: Clinical Psychology
Specialty: Individual Psychotherapy;Psychometrics;Experimental
      Psychology;Personality Measurement;Hypnosis/
      Hypnotherapy

POWERS, Keiko I.
  227 Green Healt Place
  Thousand Oaks, CA 91361-1109
  (213) 825-9057-**B**
Ethnicity: Asian-American/Asian/Pacific Islander
Degree and Year: PhD 1990
Major Field: unknown
Specialty: Psychometrics

PRADERAS, Kim
  4110 Guadalupe
  Austin, TX 78751-4296
  (512) 371-6654-**B**, (512) 458-4515-**H**, (512) 371-6849-**F**
Ethnicity: Hispanic/Latino
Languages: Spanish
Degree and Year: PhD 1987
Major Field: Clinical Psychology
Specialty: Assessment/Diagnosis/Evaluation;Psychotherapy;Hospital
      Care

PRADO, Haydee
  8550 W Flagler St
  # 105
  Miami, FL 33144-2037
  (305) 551-5787-**B**, (305) 406-2115-**H**, (305) 551-5786-**F**
Ethnicity: Hispanic/Latino
Languages: Spanish
Degree and Year: PsyD 1983
Major Field: Clinical Psychology
Specialty: Clinical Psychology;Psychotherapy;School
      Psychology;Learning Disabilities;Assessment/Diagnosis/
      Evaluation;Clinical Child Psychology

PRADO, William M.
  Consulting Psychologist
  59 Cimarron Valley Circle
  Little Rock, AR 72212
  (501) 371-9360-**B**
Ethnicity: Hispanic/Latino
Languages: Spanish
Degree and Year: PhD 1958
Major Field: Clinical Psychology
Specialty: Clinical Psychology;Alcoholism & Alcohol Abuse;Consulting
      Psychology;Intelligence

PRELOW, Hazel M.
  Arizona State University
  Program for Prevention Research
  PO Box 871108
  Tempe, AZ 85287
  (602) 727-6155-**B**, (602) 994-9749-**H**, (602) 965-5430-**F**
  hazel.prelow@asu.edu
Ethnicity: African-American/Black
Degree and Year: PhD
Major Field: Clinical Psychology
Specialty: Clinical Child Psychology;Community
      Psychology;Prevention;Cross Cultural Processes;Ethnic
      Minorities;School Psychology

PRENDES-LINTEL, Maria L.
  Lincoln Medical Education Foundation
  Behavioral Health Center
  4600 Valley Road, Suite 200
  Lincoln, NE 68510
  (402) 483-1116-**B**, (402) 483-4593-**H**, (402) 483-6543-**F**
  mprendeslintel@lmef.org
Ethnicity: Hispanic/Latino
Languages: Spanish
Degree and Year: PhD 1996 MSW 1977
Major Field: Counseling Psychology
Specialty: Counseling Psychology;Stress;Ethnic Minorities;Cross
      Cultural Processes;Health Psychology;General Psychology

PRICE, Alicia A.

1508 San Ignacio
Suite 100
Coral Gables, FL 33146
(305) 771-5653-**B**, (305) 271-5046-**H**, (305) 595-6015-**F**
Ethnicity: Hispanic/Latino
Degree and Year: PhD 1995
Major Field: Clinical Psychology
Specialty: Clinical Psychology;Stress;Health Psychology;Hypnosis/
Hypnotherapy

PRICE, Gregory E.
13738 Lynhurst Drive
Woodbridge, VA 22193-4351
(703) 643-2341-**B**, (703) 590-6821-**H**
Ethnicity: African-American/Black
Languages: Spanish
Degree and Year: PhD 1976
Major Field: Personality Psychology
Specialty: Correctional Psychology;HIV/AIDS;Individual
Psychotherapy;Personality;Ethnic Minorities

PRICE, Linda A.
3557 Faraday Lane
Virginia Beach, VA 23452
(804) 683-9057-**B**, (804) 498-3649-**H**
Ethnicity: African-American/Black
Degree and Year: EdD 1980
Major Field: Educational Psychology
Specialty: Developmental Psychology

PRIETO, Addys
1601 Palm Avenue
Suite 300
Pembroke Pines, FL 33026
(954) 432-9911-**B**, (954) 436-1103-**H**, (954) 436-1193-**F**
Ethnicity: Hispanic/Latino
Languages: Spanish
Degree and Year: PsyD 1994
Major Field: Clinical Psychology
Specialty: Assessment/Diagnosis/Evaluation;Gerontology/
Geropsychology;Clinical Psychology;Individual
Psychotherapy

PRIETO, Susan L.
Purdue University
CAPS
1826 Psyc
Room 1120
West Lafayette, IN 47907-1826
(765) 494-6995-**B**, (765) 496-3004-**F**
slprieto@psych.purdue.edu
Ethnicity: Hispanic/Latino
Languages: Spanish
Degree and Year: PhD 1990
Major Field: Counseling Psychology
Specialty: Affective Disorders;Cross Cultural
Processes;Depression;Personality Theory;Psychopathology

PRUITT, JR., Joseph H.
Human Development Associates, Inc.
7250 Franklin Avenue #1115
Los Angeles, CA 90046
(213) 874-6966-**B**, (213) 874-5895-**H**, (213) 874-1419-**F**
Ethnicity: African-American/Black

Degree and Year: PhD

Major Field: unknown

PRUTSMAN, Thomas D.
12 Rockwell Drive
Troy, PA 16947
(717) 297-2740-**H**
Ethnicity: American Indian/Alaska Native
Degree and Year: PhD 1961
Major Field: Clinical Psychology
Specialty: Neuropsychology;Consulting Psychology;Learning
Disabilities;Continuing Education

PUENTE, Antonio E.
University of North Carolina @ Wilmington
@ Wilmington
Department of Psychology
Wilmington, NC 28403
(910) 256-3365-**B**, (910) 962-3812-**H**, (910) 962-7010-**F**
Puente@uncwil.edu
Ethnicity: Hispanic/Latino
Languages: Spanish
Degree and Year: PhD 1978
Major Field: Physiological Psychology
Specialty: Clinical Neuropsychology;Brain Damage;Neurological
Disorders;Psychosomatic Disorders;Ethnic Minorities

PUERTAS, Lorenzo
781 Comanche Ln
Franklin Lakes, NJ 07417-2903
(201) 881-6183-**B**, (201) 847-1054-**H**
Ethnicity: Hispanic/Latino
Languages: Italian, Spanish
Degree and Year: PsyD 1982
Major Field: School Psychology
Specialty: School Psychology;Alcoholism & Alcohol Abuse;Mentally
Retarded;Cognitive Behavioral Therapy;Cultural & Social
Processes

PUGH, Roderick W.
Loyola University, Chicato
Professor of Emeritus
5201 South Cornell Avenue
Suite #25-C
Chicago, IL 60615
(312) 332-0536-**B**, (773) 288-5488-**H**
72752.47.compuserve.com
Ethnicity: African-American/Black
Degree and Year: PhD 1949
Major Field: Clinical Psychology
Specialty: Cognitive Behavioral Therapy;Individual
Psychotherapy;Stress;Cross Cultural Processes;Applied
Behavior Analysis;Managed Care

PUIG, Ange
Puig Associates
1060 Kings Highway N.
Suite #314
Cherry Hill, NJ 08034
(609) 482-7744-**B**, (609) 482-7744-**H**, (609) 779-2705-**F**
wtgm66a@prodigy.com
Ethnicity: Hispanic/Latino
Degree and Year: PhD 1991
Major Field: Counseling Psychology
Specialty: Psychotherapy;Sex/Marital Therapy;Crisis Intervention &
Therapy;Managed Care;Psychology & Law;Mental Health

Services

PUIG, Hector
Teachers Association Building
Teachers Bldg, Ste 402
452 Ponce De Leon
Hato Rey, PR 00918-3490
(787) 767-6722-**B**, (809) 758-9560-**H**, (809) 753-0334-**F**
Ethnicity: Hispanic/Latino
Degree and Year: PhD 1960
Major Field: Industrial/Organizational Psy.
Specialty: Industrial/Organizational Psychology;Management & Organization;Human Resources;Consulting Psychology;Selection & Placement

PULLIAM, Barbara A.
81 Irving Place
Suite #1B
New York, NY 10003-2209
(212) 777-8019-**B**, (201) 509-7335-**H**, (201) 509-7335-**F**
Ethnicity: African-American/Black
Degree and Year: PhD 1979
Major Field: Clinical Psychology
Specialty: Family Therapy;Gender Issues;Group Psychotherapy;HIV/AIDS;Psychoanalysis

PULLIUM, Rita M.
Elon College
222 9 CB
Elon College, NC 27244-2020
(919) 584-2186-**B**, (919) 587-6992-**H**
Ethnicity: Asian-American/Asian/Pacific Islander
Languages: Chinese
Degree and Year: PhD 1980
Major Field: Social Psychology
Specialty: Social Psychology;Social Cognition;Social Problems;Cross Cultural Processes;Industrial/Organizational Psychology

PUROCHIT, Arjun P.
Beechgrove Regional Children's Center
283 Inverness Cr
Kingston, ON K7M6P3
CANADA
(613) 546-4094-**B**, (613) 548-8810-**H**
Ethnicity: Asian-American/Asian/Pacific Islander
Degree and Year: PhD 1965
Major Field: Clinical Psychology

QUIJANO, Walter Y.
2040 North Loop 336, West
Suite #322
Conroe, TX 77304
(409) 539-2226-**B**, (409) 273-3192-**H**, (409) 539-6308-**F**
Ethnicity: Asian-American/Asian/Pacific Islander
Languages: Filipino
Degree and Year: PhD 1975
Major Field: Clinical Psychology

QUINN, Lisa
22 Rose Avenue
Chico, CA 95928-9617
(415) 444-2549-**B**
Ethnicity: American Indian/Alaska Native
Degree and Year: PhD 1990
Major Field: Clinical Psychology

QUINTANA, Stephen M.
University of Wisconsin
Department of Counseling Psychology
1000 Bascom Mall
Madison, WI 53706
(608) 262-6987-**B**, (608) 238-4211-**H**, (608) 265-3347-**F**
quintana@mail.seomadison.wes.e
Ethnicity: Hispanic/Latino
Degree and Year: PhD 1989
Major Field: Counseling Psychology
Specialty: Ethnic Minorities;Adolescent Development;Psychotherapy;Counseling Psychology

RAINWATER, III, Avie J.
Behavioral Health Group
PO Box 5596
Florence, SC 29502-5596
(843) 667-4949-**B**, (843) 667-3349-**F**
drajr3@aol.com
Ethnicity: American Indian/Alaska Native
Degree and Year: PhD 1989
Major Field: Clinical Psychology
Specialty: Affective Disorders;Biofeedback;Interpersonal Processes & Relations;Medical Psychology;Pain & Pain Management

RAJARAM, Suparna
Department of Psychology
SUNY at Stony Brook
Stony Brook, NY 11794-2500
(516)632-7841-**B**, 516/632-7876-**F**
srajaram@psych1.psy.sunysb.edu
Ethnicity: Asian-American/Asian/Pacific Islander
Languages: Hindi, Kannada
Degree and Year: PhD 1991
Major Field: Cognitive Psychology
Specialty: Memory

RAMASWAMI, Sundar
123 Old Belden Hill Road
Suite #9
Norwalk, CT 06850
(203) 358-8500-**B**, (203) 846-3969-**H**
Ethnicity: Asian-American/Asian/Pacific Islander
Degree and Year: PhD 1984
Major Field: Educational Psychology
Specialty: Clinical Psychology;Counseling Psychology;Community Psychology;Psychopharmacology;Personality Psychology

RAMBO, Lewis M.
26 Taft Avenue
Lexington, MA 02173
(617) 498-5216-**B**, (617) 862-6284-**H**, (617) 498-7228-**F**
Ethnicity: African-American/Black
Languages: Spanish
Degree and Year: PhD 1971
Major Field: Industrial/Organizational Psy.
Specialty: Management & Organization;Labor & Management Relations;Industrial/Organizational Psychology

RAMIREZ-CANCEL, Carlos M.
PO Box 426
Mayaguez, PR 00681
(787) 833-5880-**B**, (787) 833-5583-**H**

Ethnicity: Hispanic/Latino
Languages: French, Italian, Spanish
Degree and Year: PhD 1975
Major Field: Counseling Psychology
Specialty: Counseling Psychology;Developmental
Psychology;Educational Psychology;Clinical Psychology

RAMIREZ, David E.
Swarthmore College
Psychological Services
500 College Avenue
Swarthmore, PA 19081-1397
(610) 328-8059-B, (610) 328-1997-H, (610) 328-8673-F
dramire1@swarthmore.edu
Ethnicity: Hispanic/Latino
Languages: Spanish
Degree and Year: PhD 1986
Major Field: Counseling Psychology
Specialty: Psychotherapy;Psychoanalysis

RAMIREZ, John/Juan
Washington State University
Counseling Services
Pullman, WA 99164-4130
(509) 335-4511-B, (509) 335-2924-F
ramirezi@mail.wsu.edu
Ethnicity: Hispanic/Latino
Languages: Spanish
Degree and Year: PhD 1978
Major Field: Counseling Psychology
Specialty: Counseling Psychology;Depression;Ethnic
Minorities;Cognitive Behavioral Therapy;Behavior Therapy

RAMIREZ, Sylvia Z.
University of Texas at Austin
Department of Educational Psychology
Sanchez Building 504
Austin, TX 78712-1296
(512) 471-6466-B, (512) 832-5544-H
sramirez@utexas.edu
Ethnicity: Hispanic/Latino
Languages: Spanish
Degree and Year: PhD 1988
Major Field: School Psychology
Specialty: Consulting Psychology;Ethnic Minorities;Mentally
Retarded;Cross Cultural Processes

RAMOS-GRENIER, Julia
85 West Mountain Road
Collinsville, CT 06022-1523
860 693-9599-B, 860 693-6191-H, 860 693-9123-F
gca@nai.net
Ethnicity: Hispanic/Latino
Languages: Spanish
Degree and Year: PhD 1977
Major Field: Clinical Psychology
Specialty: Clinical Child Neuropsychology;Clinical Psychology;Ethnic
Minorities;Clinical Neuropsychology;Forensic
Psychology;Assessment/Diagnosis/Evaluation

RAMOS, Arnaldo J.
New York University
1 Washington Square Village   #4-0
New York, NY 10012
(718) 579-5156-B, (212) 477-3157-H

ajr2@is3.nyu.edu
Ethnicity: Hispanic/Latino
Languages: Spanish
Degree and Year: EdD 1987
Major Field: Clinical Child Psychology
Specialty: Ethnic Minorities;Cross Cultural Processes;Individual
Psychotherapy;Family Therapy;Adolescent Therapy

RAMSEUR, Howard P.
Massachusetts Institute of Technology
Medical Department
25 Carrleson Street, E23-361
Cambridge, MA 02139
(617)253-2916-B, 617/576-2416-H, 617/253-0162-F
hpram2@aol.com
Ethnicity: African-American/Black
Degree and Year: PhD 1975
Major Field: Personality Psychology
Specialty: Clinical Psychology;Organizational Development

RANDHAWA, Bikkar S.
University of Saskatchewan
Department of Educational Psychology
and Special Education
Saskatoon , SK, S7N 0X1
CANADA
(306) 966-7661-B, (306) 249-0049-H, (306) 966-7719-F
randhawa@sask.usask.ca
Ethnicity: Asian-American/Asian/Pacific Islander
Languages: Hindi, Urdu, Punjabi
Degree and Year: Phd 1969
Major Field: Quan/Math & Psychometrics/Stat
Specialty: Educational Psychology;Educational Research;Program
Evaluation;Research Design & Methodology;Statistics

RANGOONWALA, Rafique
43211 Babcock Avenue
Hemet, CA 92544-1706
(714) 927-4016-B
Ethnicity: Asian-American/Asian/Pacific Islander
Degree and Year: PhD 1981
Major Field: Counseling Psychology
Specialty: Clinical Neuropsychology;Psychotherapy

RATTENBURY, Francie R.
720 Lake Street
Suite #201
Oak Park, IL 60301
(708) 386-7953-B, (708) 386-7953-H
Ethnicity: Asian-American/Asian/Pacific Islander
Degree and Year: PhD 1985
Major Field: Clinical Psychology
Specialty: Psychotherapy;Adolescent Therapy;Research &
Training;Psychopathology;Clinical Psychology

RAVAL, Bina D.
11216 5 Springs Road
Lutherville, MD 21093-3525
Ethnicity: Asian-American/Asian/Pacific Islander
Degree and Year: PhD 19
Major Field: Counseling Psychology
Specialty: Psychotherapy

RAY, Arun B.
4815 Country Walk Lane
Sylvania, OH 43560-2958

(419) 537-9195-**B**, (419) 841-6395-**H**
Ethnicity: Asian-American/Asian/Pacific Islander
Languages: Bengali
Degree and Year: PhD 1967
Major Field: Clinical Psychology
Specialty: Behavior Therapy;Alcoholism & Alcohol
   Abuse;Depression;Family Therapy;Sexual Dysfunction

RAY, Jacqueline W.
107 Commodore Drive
Staten Island, NY 10309
(718) 262-2191-**B**, (718) 966-8952-**H**
Ethnicity: African-American/Black
Degree and Year: PhD 1975
Major Field: Community Psychology
Specialty: Administration;Interpersonal Processes & Relations;Training
   & Development;Psychology of Women;Leadership

RAY, Vivian D.
1070 West Allens Lane
Philadelphia, PA 19119
(215) 242-9422-**B**, (215) 242-9422-**H**
Ethnicity: African-American/Black
Degree and Year: PhD 1980
Major Field: unknown
Specialty: School Psychology;Assessment/Diagnosis/
   Evaluation;Preschool & Day Care Issues

REAMS, Bennie P
5253 Angeles Vista Boulevard
Los Angeles, CA 90043-1613
(213) 298-0083-**B**, 213 291-2923-**H**
Ethnicity: African-American/Black
Degree and Year: EdD 1980
Major Field: Counseling Psychology
Specialty: Marriage & Family;Learning Disabilities;School
   Psychology;Ethnic Minorities;School Counseling

REANDEAU, Sharon L
PO Box 1061
Fall Creek, OR 97438-0061
(503) 344-6929-**B**, (541) 747-2567-**H**
Ethnicity: American Indian/Alaska Native
Degree and Year: PhD 1989
Major Field: Counseling Psychology
Specialty: Psychotherapy

REAVES, Andrew L
University of Alabama
Department of Psychology
Box 870348
Tuscaloosa, AL 35487-0348
(205) 348-6619-**B**, (205) 752-2645-**H**, (205) 348-8648-**F**
areaves@gp.as.ua.edu
Ethnicity: African-American/Black
Degree and Year: PhD 1992
Major Field: Social Psychology
Specialty: Aggression;Cultural & Social Processes;Homicide;Human
   Ecology;Social Cognition;Social Psychology

REAVES, Juanita Y.
1526 Gallatin Place, NE
Washington, DC 20017
(202) 373-7521-**B**, (202) 529-6542-**H**, (202) 373-5427-**F**
Ethnicity: African-American/Black
Degree and Year: PhD 1981

Major Field: Developmental Psychology
Specialty: Administration;Developmental Psychology;Ethnic
   Minorities;Human Resources;Curriculum Development/
   Evaluation

REDD-BARNES, Renee A.
10209 64th Street
Kenosha, WI 53142-7829
(312) 996-8960-**B**
Ethnicity: African-American/Black
Degree and Year: PhD 1989
Major Field: Counseling Psychology
Specialty: Psychotherapy

REED, III, Jesse A.
11200 Westheimer
Suite #1050
Houston, TX 77042
(713) 783-7894-**B**, (713) 867-3447-**H**, (713) 783-6345-**F**
Ethnicity: African-American/Black
Degree and Year: PhD 1981
Major Field: Clinical Psychology
Specialty: Forensic Psychology;Individual Psychotherapy;Cultural &
   Social Processes;Family Therapy;Group Processes

REED, James D.
2114 Tecumseh River Drive
Lansing, MI 48906
(517) 377-0397-**B**, (517) 323-4009-**H**, (517) 377-0393-**F**
Ethnicity: African-American/Black
Degree and Year: PhD 1982
Major Field: Counseling Psychology
Specialty: Administration;Clinical Psychology;Community Mental
   Health;Mental Health Services;Military Psychology

REEVES, Alan
St. Louis County Government
Health Department
212 North 62nd Street
East St. Louis, IL 62203
(314) 854-6771-**B**, (618) 854-6773-**F**
Ethnicity: African-American/Black
Languages: American Sign Language
Degree and Year: PhD 1982
Major Field: School Psychology
Specialty: Clinical Child Psychology;Clinical Psychology;Group
   Psychotherapy;Eating Disorders;Projective Techniques

REID, Pamela T
University of Michigan
Instit. for Research on Gender & Women
460 West Hall
Ann Arbor, MI 48109-1092
734/764-9537-**B**, 313/577-6079-**H**, 212 642-1940-**F**
pamreid@umich.edu
Ethnicity: African-American/Black
Degree and Year: PhD 1975
Major Field: Developmental Psychology

REILLY, Patrick M.
422 45th Avenue
San Francisco, CA 94121
(415) 476-1129-**B**, (415) 752-7206-**H**, (415) 476-4275-**F**
reilly.patrick_m@sanfranscisco
Ethnicity: African-American/Black
Degree and Year: PhD 1989 MSW 1979

Major Field: Counseling Psychology
Specialty: Research & Training;Cognitive Behavioral
    Therapy;Aggression;Domestic Violence;Alcoholism & Alcohol
    Abuse;Drug Abuse

REISINGER, Curtis W.
  Hackensack University Medical Center
  Department of Psychiatry
  60 Second Street, Suite 122
  Hackensack, NJ 07601
  (201) 996-3443-**B**, (201) 996-3602-**F**
  creisinger@humed.com
Ethnicity: American Indian/Alaska Native
Degree and Year: PhD 1979
Major Field: Clinical Psychology
Specialty: Administration;Managed Care;Clinical Psychology

REISINGER, Mercedes C.
  2114 East Fort Union Boulevard
  Salt Lake City, UT 84121-3142
  (801) 942-9807-**B**, (801) 943-5101-**H**
Ethnicity: Hispanic/Latino
Degree and Year: PhD 1981
Major Field: Clinical Psychology
Specialty: Forensic Psychology

REY-CASSERLY, Celiane M.
  Children's Hospital
  Fejan 8
  300 Longwood Avenue
  Boston, MA 02115
  (617) 355-6708-**B**, (617) 729-4639-**H**, (617) 730-0457-**F**
  casserly@1.tch.harvard.edu
Ethnicity: Hispanic/Latino
Languages: French, Spanish
Degree and Year: PhD 1982
Major Field: Clinical Psychology
Specialty: Clinical Child Neuropsychology;Clinical
    Neuropsychology;Clinical Psychology;Clinical Child
    Psychology

REYES-MAYER, Erwin
  345 Ocean Dr, #601
  Miami Beach, FL 33139-6916
  (212) 678-3154-**B**, (212) 366-4921-**H**
Ethnicity: Hispanic/Latino
Languages: Spanish
Degree and Year: PhD 1981
Major Field: Counseling Psychology
Specialty: Educational Psychology;Counseling Psychology;Cultural &
    Social Processes;Curriculum Development/Evaluation;Group
    Processes

REYES, Carla J.
  Utah State University
  Department of Psychology
  2810 Old Main Hall
  Logan, UT 84322-2810
  (535) 797-1487-**B**, (4350 787-8949-**H**, (435) 797-1448-**F**
  carla@fs1.ed.usu.edu
Ethnicity: Hispanic/Latino
Languages: Spanish
Degree and Year: PhD 1996

Major Field: Clinical Child Psychology
Specialty: Child Abuse;Ethnic Minorities;Family Therapy;Clinical
    Child Psychology;Prevention;Clinical Research

REYNA, Valerie F.
  University of Arizona
  6060 E Calle Ojos Verdes
  Tucson, AZ 85750
  (520) 626-7377-**B**
  vreyna@u.arizona.edu
Ethnicity: Hispanic/Latino
Degree and Year: PhD 1981
Major Field: Cognitive Psychology
Specialty: Decision & Choice Behavior;Cognitive
    Development;Developmental Psychobiology;Cognitive
    Psychology;Experimental Psychology;Human Development &
    Family Studies

REZA, Ernesto M.
  5159 N Mt. View Avenue
  San Bernadino, CA 92407
  (909) 880-5745-**B**, (909) 882-8142-**H**, (909) 880-5994-**F**
Ethnicity: Hispanic/Latino
Languages: Spanish
Degree and Year: PhD 1992
Major Field: Industrial/Organizational Psy.

REZENTES, III, William C.
  3221 Allan Place
  Honolulu, HI 96817-5234
  (808) 734-0218W-**B**, s-**F**
Ethnicity: Hispanic/Latino
Degree and Year: PhD 1988
Major Field: Clinical Psychology
Specialty: Employee Assistance Programs

RHEE, Susan B.
  3605 Buckthorn Lane
  Downers Grove, IL 60515
  (708) 858-2800-**B**, (708) 969-6409-**H**, (708) 858-9399-**F**
Ethnicity: Asian-American/Asian/Pacific Islander
Languages: Korean
Degree and Year: EdD 1993
Major Field: Counseling Psychology
Specialty: Counseling Psychology;Vocational Psychology;Mental
    Health Services;School Psychology

RIBERA-GONZALEZ, Julio C.
  UPR Station
  PO Box 22724
  San Juan, PR 00931
  (787) 758-7575-**B**, (787) 743-4435-**H**
  ribera@prtc.net
Ethnicity: Hispanic/Latino
Languages: Spanish
Degree and Year: PhD 1984 MA 1978
Major Field: Counseling Psychology
Specialty: Assessment/Diagnosis/Evaluation;Counseling
    Psychology;Epidemiology & Biometry;Individual
    Psychotherapy;Marriage & Family

RICE, Donadrian
  West Georgia College
  Department of Psychology

Carrollton, GA 30118
Ethnicity: African-American/Black
Degree and Year: PhD 1977
Major Field: unknown

RICHARD, Harriette W.
330 Hembree Grove Terrace
Roswell, GA 30076
(706) 864-2745-**B**, (770) 619-0128-**H**, (770) 619-9567-**F**
rich1599@aol.com
Ethnicity: African-American/Black
Degree and Year: PhD 1982
Major Field: Developmental Psychology
Specialty: Stress;Child Development;Parent-Child Interaction;Ethnic Minorities;Gender Issues

RICHARDS, Henry J.
1600 S. Springwood Drive
Silver Spring, MD 20910
(410) 799-3400-**B**, (301) 589-6242-**H**, (410) 799-0004-**F**
Ethnicity: African-American/Black
Degree and Year: PhD 1987
Major Field: Clinical Psychology
Specialty: Drug Abuse;Alcoholism & Alcohol Abuse;Forensic Psychology;Crime & Criminal Behavior;Program Evaluation

RICHARDSON, E. Strong-Legs
Kiyan Indian Consultant Group
Wakpala Shungmanitu Indian Lodge
6404 Wolf Run Court
Fairfax Station, VA 22039-1519
(703) 764-2152-**B**, 703 764-2152-**H**
Ethnicity: American Indian/Alaska Native
Languages: German, Lakota
Degree and Year: PhD 1951 MEd 1949
Major Field: Clinical Psychology
Specialty: Clinical Psychology;Sex/Marital Therapy;Alcoholism & Alcohol Abuse;Family Therapy;Stress;Special Education

RICHARDSON, Frederick
17809 Harvest Avenue
Cerritos, CA 90701-3745
(213) 865-1928-**B**
Ethnicity: African-American/Black
Degree and Year: PhD 1972
Major Field: Clinical Psychology
Specialty: Psychotherapy

RIDDLE, P. Elayne
20708 Riptide Square
Sterling, VA 20165
(703)421-1711-**H**
Ethnicity: African-American/Black
Degree and Year: PhD 1978 MSW 1972
Major Field: Counseling Psychology
Specialty: Counseling Psychology;Client-Centered Therapy;Mental Health Services;Human Resources;Interpersonal Processes & Relations

RIDLEY, Charles R.
Indiana University
Department of Counseling and Educational Psychology
Bloomington, IN 47405
(812) 856-8340-**B**, (812) 856-8440-**F**
Ethnicity: African-American/Black
Degree and Year: PhD 1978
Major Field: Counseling Psychology
Specialty: Cross Cultural Processes;Counseling Psychology;Consulting Psychology;Religious Psychology;Selection & Placement

RIGRISH, Diana
Cincinnati VAMC Psychology Service
ML116B
3200 Vine Street
Cincinnati, OH 45220
(513) 475-6236-**B**, (5130 475-6379-**F**
Ethnicity: Asian-American/Asian/Pacific Islander
Languages: Chinese
Degree and Year: PhD 1988
Major Field: Clinical Psychology
Specialty: Clinical Neuropsychology

RIGUAL-LYNCH, Lourdes
#41 West 96 Street
Apartment #3A
New York, NY 10025
(212) 360-6353-**B**, (212) 663-9369-**H**
Ethnicity: Hispanic/Latino
Languages: Spanish
Degree and Year: PhD 1979
Major Field: Clinical Psychology
Specialty: Child & Pediatric Psychology;Homelessness & Homeless Populations;Learning Disabilities;Parent Education;Psychotherapy

RIVAS-VAZQUEZ, Ana A.
1385 Coral Way
Suite #402
Miami, FL 33145
(305) 858-3085-**B**, (305) 666-8117-**H**, (305) 856-8087-**F**
Ethnicity: Hispanic/Latino
Languages: Spanish
Degree and Year: PhD 1969
Major Field: Clinical Psychology
Specialty: Clinical Child Psychology;Clinical Psychology;Family Therapy;Forensic Psychology;Individual Psychotherapy

RIVERA-LOPEZ, Hector
Central County Mental Health Center
Child and Adolescent Services
1026 Oak Grove Road
Suite 11
Concord, CA 94518
(510) 604-6244-**B**, (510) 669-1940-**H**, (510) 646-5102-**F**
hlopez@pacbell.net
Ethnicity: Hispanic/Latino
Languages: Spanish
Degree and Year: PhD 1984 MS 1972
Major Field: Clinical Psychology
Specialty: Alcoholism & Alcohol Abuse;Clinical Psychology;Cross Cultural Processes;Family Therapy;Community Mental Health;Ethnic Minorities

RIVERA-MEDINA, Eduardo J.
361 San Genaro Street
Rio Piedras, PR 00926
(809) 755-1632-**H**
Ethnicity: Hispanic/Latino
Languages: Spanish
Degree and Year: PhD 1971

Specialty: Educational Psychology;Community Psychology;Consulting
Psychology;Gerontology/Geropsychology;Gender Issues

RIVERA-MOLINA, Elba
Cond. Midtown
Suite #413
Munoz Rivera 421
Hato Rey, PR 00918
(803) 758-5850-**B**, (803) 760-5796-**H**, (803) 754-4924-**F**
Ethnicity: Hispanic/Latino
Languages: Spanish
Degree and Year: PhD 1981 MA 1997
Major Field: Clinical Psychology
Specialty: Clinical Psychology;Intelligence;Group
Psychotherapy;Psychotherapy;Motivation

RIVERA-SINCLAIR, Elsa A.
116 Fleetwood Terrace
Silver Spring, MD 20910
(202) 373-6549-**B**, (301) 588-1468-**H**
Ethnicity: Hispanic/Latino
Degree and Year: PhD 1988
Major Field: Counseling Psychology
Specialty: Neuropsychology;Cultural & Social Processes;Clinical
Psychology;Death & Dying

RIVERA, Beatriz D.
University Station
P.O. Box 22724
San Juan, PR 00931-2724
(809) 763-4199-**B**, (809) 743-4435-**H**
Ethnicity: Hispanic/Latino
Languages: Spanish
Degree and Year: PhD 1982
Major Field: Counseling Psychology
Specialty: Psychotherapy;Rehabilitation;Mental Disorders;Measurement

RIVERA, Carmen J.
Sunset Park Mental Health Center
514 49th Street
Brooklyn, NY 11220
(718) 437-5218-**B**, (718) 871-2166-**H**
Ethnicity: Hispanic/Latino
Languages: Spanish
Degree and Year: PhD 1985
Major Field: Clinical Psychology
Specialty: Cross Cultural Processes;Affective Disorders;Ethnic
Minorities;Mental Health
Services;Psychoanalysis;Psychotherapy

RIVERA, Enrique
13731 Ishnala Circle
West Palm Beach, FL 33414
(407) 793-7678-**B**, (407) 798-2706-**H**
Ethnicity: Hispanic/Latino
Languages: Spanish
Degree and Year: PhD 1978
Major Field: Clinical Psychology
Specialty: Pain & Pain Management;Clinical Psychology;Cognitive
Behavioral Therapy;Cognitive Psychology;Biofeedback

RIVERA, Jo Ann M.
2157 Tomlinson Avenue

Bronx, NY 10461-1201
(718) 829-0652-**B**
Ethnicity: Hispanic/Latino
Degree and Year: PhD 1979
Major Field: Clinical Psychology
Specialty: Chronically Mentally Ill;Individual Psychotherapy;Sex/
Marital Therapy;Family Therapy;Psychoses;Cross Cultural
Processes

RIVERA, Miquela
2741 Indian School Road, NE
Albuguerque, NM 87106
(505) 255-8682-**B**, (505) 293-7328-**H**, (505) 255-2890-**F**
Ethnicity: Hispanic/Latino
Languages: Spanish
Degree and Year: PhD 1981
Major Field: Clinical Psychology
Specialty: Employee Assistance Programs;Management &
Organization;Psychotherapy;Assessment/Diagnosis/
Evaluation;Community Psychology

RIVERA, Nelson E.
Village for Families of Children, Inc.
1680 Albany Avenue
Hartford, CT 06105
(860) 297-0550-**B**, (203) 244-9447-**H**, (860) 231-8449-**F**
drrivera@aol.com
Ethnicity: Hispanic/Latino
Languages: Spanish
Degree and Year: PhD 1990
Major Field: Clinical Psychology
Specialty: Assessment/Diagnosis/Evaluation;Ethnic Minorities;Child &
Pediatric Psychology;Individual Psychotherapy;Family
Therapy

RIVERO, Estela M.
29 Loudon Parkway
Loudonville, NY 12211
(518) 442-5800-**B**, (518) 465-0772-**H**, (518) 442-5444-**F**
Ethnicity: Hispanic/Latino
Languages: Spanish
Degree and Year: PhD 1982
Major Field: Clinical Psychology
Specialty: Management & Organization;Ethnic
Minorities;Psychotherapy;Community Mental Health

RIVERS, Marie D.
3508 N Marengo Avenue
Altadena, CA 91001-4044
(313) 681-3323-**B**
Ethnicity: African-American/Black, American Indian/Alaska Native
Degree and Year: PhD 1959
Major Field: Developmental Psychology
Specialty: Psychotherapy;Gerontology/Geropsychology;Social
Development;Cultural & Social Processes;Family
Therapy;Parent Education

RIVERS, Miriam W.
630 River Gate Road
Chesapeake, VA 23322-3488
mwrivers@aol.cm
(757) 482-0617-**B**
Ethnicity: African-American/Black
Degree and Year: PhD 1966
Major Field: Counseling Psychology

Specialty: Clinical Psychology;Counseling Psychology;School
    Psychology

ROBERTIN, Hector
Hawaii Pacific University
41-549 Indaole Street
Waimanalo, HI 96795
(808) 383-2308-**B**, (808) 259-8740-**H**, (808) 259-8740-**F**
webmaster@rican.com
Ethnicity: Hispanic/Latino
Languages: French, Spanish, Thai,Vietnamese
Degree and Year: Phd 1979
Major Field: Neurosciences
Specialty: General Psychology;Hypnosis/Hypnotherapy;Educational
    Research

ROBERTS, Albert
1304 Woodside Parkway
Silver Spring, MD 20910
(202) 806-6805-**B**, (301) 588-8883-**H**, (202) 806-4873-**F**
Ethnicity: African-American/Black
Degree and Year: PhD 1971
Major Field: Developmental Psychology
Specialty: Social Development;Adolescent Development;Personality
    Measurement;Educational Psychology;Ethnic Minorities

ROBERTS, Harrell B.
Associates for Psychotherapy
604 Green Valley Road
Suite 408
Greensboro, NC 27408
(336) 854-4450-**B**, (336) 656-4944-**H**
Ethnicity: African-American/Black
Degree and Year: PhD 1983
Major Field: Personality Psychology
Specialty: Adolescent Therapy;Ethnic Minorities;Consulting
    Psychology;Clinical Psychology;Individual
    Psychotherapy;Feminist Therapy

ROBERTSON, John F.
Psychological and Consulting Services
285 Genesee Street
Utica, NY 13501
(315) 798-8066-**B**, 315 735-3551-**H**, 315 798-8736-**F**
nbac@borg.com
Ethnicity: African-American/Black
Degree and Year: PhD 1984
Major Field: Counseling Psychology
Specialty: Alcoholism & Alcohol Abuse;Family Therapy;Group
    Psychotherapy;Drug Abuse;Individual Psychotherapy;Ethnic
    Minorities

ROBERTS, Terrence J.
711 E Walnut, Suite 207
Pasadena, CA 91101
(818) 440-9754-**B**, (818) 440-9754-**H**
Ethnicity: African-American/Black
Degree and Year: PhD 1976
Major Field: Educational Psychology
Specialty: Adolescent Therapy;Marriage & Family;Stress;Human
    Relations;Family Therapy

ROBEY, Dale L.
1512 N. Willow

Broken Arrow, OK 74012-9147
217 932-2242-**B**, 217 923-3794-**H**
Ethnicity: American Indian/Alaska Native
Degree and Year: EdD 1963
Major Field: unknown

ROBINSON, Gregory F.
The University of Akron
Counseling, Testing, and Career Center
163 Simmons Hall
Akron, OH 44325-4303
(330) 972-7082-**B**, (330) 867-4261-**H**, (330) 972-5679-**F**
gfr@uakron.edu
Ethnicity: African-American/Black
Degree and Year: PhD 1991
Major Field: Counseling Psychology
Specialty: Counseling Psychology;Training & Development;Vocational
    Psychology;Cultural & Social Processes

ROBINSON, Jane A.
A Counseling Place
3011 Grand Boulevard
Suite 1710
Detroit, MI 48202-3013
(313) 875-4433-**B**, (313) 865-4129-**H**, 313 875-3993-**F**
Ethnicity: African-American/Black
Degree and Year: PhD 1978
Major Field: Clinical Psychology
Specialty: Individual Psychotherapy;School Psychology

ROBINSON, John D
Howard University
College of Medicine
6735 13th Place, NW
Washington, DC 20012
(202) 865-6611-**B**, 202 722-5211-**H**, 202 865-6212-**F**
jdrobinson@aol.com
Ethnicity: African-American/Black
Languages: German, Spanish
Degree and Year: EdD 1972 MPH 1981
Major Field: Counseling Psychology
Specialty: Medical Psychology;Lesbian & Gay
    Issuues;Administration;Professional Issues in
    Psychology;Psychopathology;Psychosomatic Disorders

ROBINSON, W. LaVome
DePaul University
Department of Psychology
2219 North Kenmore
Chicago, IL 60614-3054
(312) 362-582-**B**, (312) 348-0920-**H**, (312) 362-8279-**F**
Ethnicity: African-American/Black
Degree and Year: PhD 1980
Major Field: Clinical Psychology
Specialty: HIV/AIDS;Prevention;Community Psychology;Health
    Psychology;Adolescent Development

RODRIGUEZ, Carlos J.
Po Box 7671
Pueblo, CO 81007-0671
(719) 584-4760-**B**, (719) 543-3919-**H**
Ethnicity: Hispanic/Latino
Degree and Year: PhD 1981
Major Field: Counseling Psychology

Specialty: Community Mental Health

RODRIGUEZ, Carmen G.
467 State Street
Brooklyn, NY 11217-1802
(212) 304-5250-**B**, (212) 305-7024-**F**
Cr14@columbia.edu
Ethnicity: Hispanic/Latino
Languages: Spanish
Degree and Year: PhD 1985
Major Field: Counseling Psychology
Specialty: Psychobiology;Parent-Child Interaction;Preschool & Day
Care Issues;Child Abuse;Administration

RODRIGUEZ, David A.
170 Crescent Street
Woodbridge, NJ 11120
(718) 248-6366-**B**
Ethnicity: Hispanic/Latino
Languages: Spanish
Degree and Year: PhD 1987
Major Field: Industrial/Organizational Psy.
Specialty: Industrial/Organizational Psychology;Human Resources;Job
Satisfaction;Organizational Development;Motivation

RODRIGUEZ, Ester R.
Arizona State University
723 West 17th Place
Tempe, AZ 85281
(602) 965-4316-**B**, (602) 966-0396-**H**, (602) 965-0212-**F**
aterr@asuvm.inre.asu.edu
Ethnicity: Hispanic/Latino
Languages: Spanish
Degree and Year: PhD 1994
Major Field: Counseling Psychology
Specialty: Ethnic Minorities;Counseling Psychology;Psychology of
Women;Family Therapy;Gender Issues

RODRIGUEZ, Lavinia
144 Whitaker Road
Lutz, FL 33549
(813)-949-4143-**B**, (813) 949-4143-**H**
Ethnicity: Hispanic/Latino
Languages: Spanish
Degree and Year: PhD 1981
Major Field: Clinical Psychology
Specialty: Eating Disorders;Cognitive Behavioral Therapy

RODRIGUEZ, Luis J.
1424 Ortega Ave
Coral Gables, FL 33134-2252
(305) 552-2399-**B**, (305) 444-3197-**H**
Ethnicity: Hispanic/Latino
Degree and Year: PhD 1990
Major Field: unknown
Specialty: Employee Assistance Programs;Drug Abuse

RODRIGUEZ, Manuel D.
Youthrack, Inc.
10184 West Belleview Avenue
Suite #300
Littleton, CO 80127
(303) 904-0998-**B**, (303) 680-1757-**H**, (303) 904-1798-**F**
ytdrrodriguez@plinet.com
Ethnicity: Hispanic/Latino
Languages: Spanish

Degree and Year: PhD 1989
Major Field: Clinical Psychology
Specialty: Clinical Psychology;Consulting Psychology;Managed
Care;Conduct Disorders;Juvenile Delinquency;Management &
Organization

RODRIGUEZ, Maria A.
Hunter College, 1004-EB
695 Park Avenue
New York, NY 10021
(212) 772-5754-**B**
Ethnicity: Hispanic/Latino
Degree and Year: PhD 1986
Major Field: Counseling Psychology

RODRIGUEZ, Ramon O.
VA Medical Center
Psychology Service (116B)
One Veterans Plaza
San Juan, PR 00927-5800.
(787) 758-7575-**B**, (787) 782-9472-**H**, (787) 766-6192-**F**
Ethnicity: Hispanic/Latino
Languages: Spanish
Degree and Year: PsyD 1983
Major Field: Clinical Psychology
Specialty: Behavior Therapy;Health Psychology;Gerontology/
Geropsychology

RODRIGUEZ, Richard A.
University of California, Berkeley
Counseling & Psychological Services
2222 Bancroft Way
The Tang Center
Berkeley, CA 94720
(510) 642-9494-**B**, (415) 252-7895-**H**, (510) 642-2368-**F**
rrodriguez@uhs.berkeley.edu
Ethnicity: Hispanic/Latino
Languages: Spanish
Degree and Year: PhD 1991
Major Field: Counseling Psychology
Specialty: Cross Cultural Processes;Lesbian & Gay Issuues;Ethnic
Minorities;HIV/AIDS;Child Abuse;Group Psychotherapy

RODRIGUEZ, Rogelio E.
523 S Lombard
Oak Park, IL 60304
(312) 666-6500-**B**, (708) 848-5462-**H**
Ethnicity: Hispanic/Latino
Languages: Spanish
Degree and Year: PhD 1986
Major Field: Clinical Psychology
Specialty: Clinical Psychology;Affective Disorders;Ethnic
Minorities;Psychotherapy;Assessment/Diagnosis/Evaluation

RODRIGUEZ, Wilfredo
1014 Carpenter Street
Philadelphia, PA 19147-3704
(215) 581-3806-**B**, (215) 625-8441-**H**
Ethnicity: Hispanic/Latino
Degree and Year: PhD 1990
Major Field: Clinical Psychology
Specialty: Clinical Neuropsychology

ROEHLKE, Helen J.
University of Missouri
Counseling Center

119 Parker Hall
Columbia, MO 65211
(573) 882-6601-**B**, (573) 446-0232-**H**, (573) 884-4936-**F**
Ethnicity: Hispanic/Latino
Languages: Spanish
Degree and Year: EdD 1965
Major Field: Counseling Psychology
Specialty: Counseling Psychology;Psychotherapy;Individual
Psychotherapy;Feminist Therapy;Training &
Development;Lesbian & Gay Issuues

ROGERS, Melvin L.
313 Crest Park Road
Philidelphia, PA 19119
(215) 247-9001-**B**, (215) 248-3588-**H**, (215) 247-9030-**F**
Ethnicity: African-American/Black
Languages: Spanish
Degree and Year: PhD 1977
Major Field: Clinical Psychology
Specialty: Clinical Psychology;Family Therapy;Group
Psychotherapy;Individual Psychotherapy;Marriage &
Family;Continuing Education

ROGLER, Lloyd H.
Fordham University
441 East Fordham Road
Faculty Memorial Hall 417
Bronx, NY 10458
(718)817-4087-**B**, 718/817-5779-**F**
rogler@murray.fordham.edu
Ethnicity: Hispanic/Latino
Languages: Spanish
Degree and Year: PhD 1957
Major Field: Community Psychology
Specialty: Interpersonal Processes & Relations;Mental
Disorders;Philosophy of Science;Medical Psychology;Mental
Health Services;Social Behavior

ROHILA, Pritam K.
831 Lancaster Drive, NE
Suite #214
Salem, OR 97301-2930
(503) 362-4635-**B**, (503) 393-8305-**H**, (503) 362-7297-**F**
rohila_phd@hotmail.com
Ethnicity: Asian-American/Asian/Pacific Islander
Languages: Hindi, Urdu, Punjabi
Degree and Year: PhD 1969
Major Field: Counseling Psychology
Specialty: Neurological Disorders;Medical Psychology;Attention
Deficit Disorders;Depression;Assessment/Diagnosis/
Evaluation;Psychotherapy

ROIG, Miguel
31 Lincoln Ave
Rumson, NJ 07760-2050
(718) 390-4513-**B**, (908) 758-1347-**H**
Ethnicity: Hispanic/Latino
Languages: Spanish
Degree and Year: PhD 1989
Major Field: Cognitive Psychology
Specialty: Cognitive Psychology;Experimental Psychology;General
Psychology;Information Processing;Memory

ROJAS, Rebecca S

Antioch University
13274 Fiji Way
Marina del Rey, CA 90292
(310) 578-1080-**B**, 310 827-6672-**H**, 310 822-4824-**F**
Ethnicity: American Indian/Alaska Native, Hispanic/Latino
Degree and Year: PhD 1995 MA 1982
Major Field: Counseling Psychology
Specialty: Crisis Intervention & Therapy;Gender Issues;Personality
Measurement;Cross Cultural Processes;Ethnic
Minorities;Child Development

ROLLOCK, David
Purdue University
Department of Psychological Sciences
1364 Psychological Sciences Building
Room 1162
West Lafayette, IN 47907-1364
(765) 494-6996-**B**, (317) 873-5734-**H**, (765) 496-2670-**F**
rollock@psyc.purdue.edu
Ethnicity: African-American/Black
Degree and Year: PhD 1989
Major Field: Clinical Psychology
Specialty: Individual Difference

ROLL, Samuel
University of New Mexico
Psychology Department
Albuquerque, NM 87131
(505) 277-4121-**B**, (505) 243-2635-**H**, (505) 277-1394-**F**
rollnroll@aol.com
Ethnicity: Hispanic/Latino
Languages: Spanish
Degree and Year: PhD 1968
Major Field: Clinical Psychology
Specialty: Psychotherapy;Psychoanalysis;Cross Cultural
Processes;Projective Techniques;Forensic Psychology

ROMAN, Hugo
Calderon De La Barca
W3-52 Urb Hucares
San Juan, PR 00926
(787) 721-5645-**B**, (787) 292-1659-**H**
Ethnicity: Hispanic/Latino
Languages: Spanish
Degree and Year: PhD 1992
Major Field: Clinical Psychology
Specialty: Assessment/Diagnosis/Evaluation;Attention Deficit
Disorders;Child Abuse;Clinical Psychology;School Psychology

ROMERO, Arturo
1904 Pepperdale Dr
Rowland Heights, CA 91748-3252
(805) 940-3537-**B**, (909) 595-0234-**H**
Ethnicity: Hispanic/Latino
Languages: Spanish
Degree and Year: PhD 1982
Major Field: Developmental Psychology
Specialty: Crisis Intervention & Therapy;Mental Health
Services;Psychotherapy

ROMERO, Augusto
16705 Dawn Haven Rd
Hacienda Hghts, CA 91745-5614
(626) 571-1838-**B**, (626) 369-6577-**H**, (626) 571-8349-**F**

drromero@ic.netcom
Ethnicity: Hispanic/Latino
Languages: Spanish
Degree and Year: PhD 1991
Major Field: Clinical Psychology
Specialty: Assessment/Diagnosis/Evaluation;Clinical
Neuropsychology;Family Therapy;Group
Psychotherapy;Individual Psychotherapy

ROMERO, Jose
654 Water Street
Apartment #2B
New York, NY 10002-8215
(718) 782-2200-**B**, (212) 962-0549-**H**
Ethnicity: Hispanic/Latino
Languages: Spanish
Degree and Year: PhD 1982
Major Field: Clinical Psychology
Specialty: Psychosomatic Disorders;Gerontology/Geropsychology

ROMERO, Regina E.
Psychological and Educational
Associates Inc.
6929 Georgia Avenue, NW
Washington, DC 20012
(202) 726-6062-**B**, (202) 882-6913-**H**, (202) 726-0032-**F**
Ethnicity: African-American/Black
Degree and Year: PhD 1983
Major Field: Clinical Psychology
Specialty: Psychotherapy;Depression;Management &
Organization;Alcoholism & Alcohol Abuse;Training &
Development

ROMEY, Carol M.
University Station
Recinto Sur #315 Ofc 2a
San Juan, PR 00901
(787) 725-4572-**B**, (787) 767-6448-**H**, (809) 721-4391-**F**
Ethnicity: Hispanic/Latino
Languages: Spanish
Degree and Year: PhD 1981
Major Field: Clinical Psychology
Specialty: Assessment/Diagnosis/Evaluation;Crime & Criminal
Behavior;Family Therapy;Forensic Psychology;Professional
Issues in Psychology

ROMNEY, Patricia
Hampshire College
64 Carriage Ln
Amherst, MA 01002-3303
(413) 256-0490-**B**, (413) 253-9349-**H**, (413) 549-0707-**F**
Ethnicity: African-American/Black
Languages: Spanish
Degree and Year: PhD 1980
Major Field: Clinical Psychology
Specialty: Eating Disorders;Clinical Psychology;Family Therapy;Ethnic
Minorities;Psychology of Women

ROOT, Maria P. P.
2457 26th Avenue East
Seattle, WA 98112-2612
(206) 324-1480-**B**, (206) 324-1480-**H**
Ethnicity: Asian-American/Asian/Pacific Islander
Degree and Year: PhD 1983
Major Field: Clinical Psychology

Specialty: Cross Cultural Processes;Eating Disorders;Family
Therapy;Feminist Therapy;Psychosomatic Disorders

ROQUE, Sylvia A.
900 North Lake Shore Drive
#1508
Chicago, IL 60611
(312) 943-8852-**B**, (312) 943-4450-**F**
Ethnicity: Asian-American/Asian/Pacific Islander
Languages: Tagalog
Degree and Year: PhD 1973
Major Field: Clinical Psychology
Specialty: Assessment/Diagnosis/Evaluation;Depression;Projective
Techniques;Clinical Child Psychology;Mental Health
Services;Special Education

ROSADO, John W.
Freehold Psychology Group
149 West Main
Freehold, NJ 07728
(723) 780-9898-**B**, (723) 389-2788-**H**
Ethnicity: Hispanic/Latino
Languages: Spanish
Degree and Year: PhD 1982
Major Field: School Psychology
Specialty: Marriage & Family;Parent-Child
Interaction;Personality;School Psychology;Special Education

ROSALES, Israel B.
1559 Sacramento Street
San Francisco, CA 94109
(415) 753-7783-**B**, (415) 922-8477-**H**, (415) 753-7767-**F**
Ethnicity: Hispanic/Latino
Languages: Spanish
Degree and Year: PhD 1990
Major Field: Clinical Psychology
Specialty: Child Abuse;Adolescent Therapy;Family Therapy;Juvenile
Delinquency;Religious Psychology

ROSARIO, Margaret
The City College of Graduate School
City University of New York
Psychology Department
138th Street & Convent Avenue
New York, NY 10031
(212) 650-5420-**B**, (201) 866-1432-**H**, (212) 650-5659-**F**
Ethnicity: Hispanic/Latino
Languages: Spanish
Degree and Year: PhD 1985
Major Field: Community Psychology
Specialty: HIV/AIDS;Health Psychology;Adolescent
Development;Sexual Behavior;Stress

ROSENQUIST, Henry S.
9971 Quail Boulevard
Apartment #1109
Austin, TX 78758-5792
Ethnicity: Asian-American/Asian/Pacific Islander
Degree and Year: PhD 1964
Major Field: Experimental Psychology
Specialty: Motor Performance

ROSIN, Susana A.

P.O. Box 20671
Houston, TX 77225
(713) 523-0000-**B**, (713) 523-0006-**F**
Ethnicity: Hispanic/Latino
Languages: Spanish
Degree and Year: PhD 1984
Major Field: Clinical Child Psychology
Specialty: Eating Disorders;Child & Pediatric Psychology;Projective
Techniques;Family Therapy;Intelligence

ROSSELLO, Jeannette
Edificio Midtown Ofic
Ave Munoz Rivera 421
Office #206
Hato Rey, PR 00919
Ethnicity: Hispanic/Latino
Degree and Year: PhD 1980
Major Field: Clinical Psychology
Specialty: Psychotherapy

ROSS, Sandra I.
34 Crest Drive
White Plains, NY 10607
(914) 592-8270-**H**
Ethnicity: African-American/Black
Degree and Year: PhD 1988
Major Field: Clinical Psychology
Specialty: Attention Deficit Disorders;Conduct Disorders;Ethnic
Minorities;Death & Dying;Educational
Psychology;Assessment/Diagnosis/Evaluation

ROUCE, Sandra
1615 Calumet
Houston, TX 77004
(713) 520-0985-**B**, (713) 988-2676-**H**, (713) 529-1738-**F**
Ethnicity: African-American/Black
Degree and Year: PhD 1975
Major Field: Clinical Psychology
Specialty: Child Abuse;Clinical Child Psychology;Clinical
Psychology;Psychopathology;Assessment/Diagnosis/
Evaluation

ROUNTREE, Yvonne B.
160 Cabrini Blvd.
Suite #101
New York, NY 10033-1145
(212) 928-3394-**B**
Ethnicity: African-American/Black
Degree and Year: PhD 1981
Major Field: Clinical Psychology
Specialty: Psychotherapy

ROY, Swati
2960 Juanita Place
Fullerton, CA 92635
(562) 651-3328-**B**
Ethnicity: Asian-American/Asian/Pacific Islander
Languages: Bengali
Degree and Year: PhD 1987
Major Field: Clinical Psychology
Specialty: Gerontology/Geropsychology;Chronically Mentally
Ill;Schizophrenia;Psychopathology;Research & Training

RUBIO, Charles T.

2127 Executive Park Drive
Opelika, AL 36801-6041
Ethnicity: Hispanic/Latino
Degree and Year: PhD 1975
Major Field: Clinical Psychology
Specialty: Psychotherapy

RUFFINS, Stephen A.
Long Island University: CW Post
Psychology Dept/Doctoral Program
Brookville, NY 11548-
(516) 299-4277-**B**, 212 684-3552-**H**, 516 299-2738-**F**
sruffins@titan.liunet.edu
Ethnicity: African-American/Black
Degree and Year: PhD 1988
Major Field: Clinical Psychology
Specialty: Psychotherapy

RUIZ, Fernando
P.O. Box 337
Downey, CA 902411
(213) 589-1902-**B**, (213) 589-1805-**F**
Ethnicity: Hispanic/Latino
Languages: Spanish
Degree and Year: PhD 1981
Major Field: Clinical Psychology
Specialty: Cognitive Psychology;Child Abuse;Domestic
Violence;Psychosomatic Disorders;Forensic Psychology

RUIZ, Nicholas J.
Winona State University
1650 97th Street, East
Inver Grove Heights, MN 55077
(507) 285-7136-**B**, (612) 451-7794-**H**
Ethnicity: Hispanic/Latino
Degree and Year: PhD 1991
Major Field: Counseling Psychology
Specialty: Counseling Psychology;Cognitive Behavioral Therapy;Job
Satisfaction;Adult Development;Crisis Intervention &
Therapy;Cross Cultural Processes

RUIZ, Sonia I.
2220 SW 25th Street
Miami, FL 33133
(305) 637-2585-**B**, (305) 858-6098-**H**
Ethnicity: Hispanic/Latino
Languages: Spanish
Degree and Year: PsyD 19
Major Field: Clinical Psychology

RUSSELL, David M.
780 Farmington Avenue
West Hartford, CT 06119
(203) 231-9191-**B**, (203) 285-0525-**H**
Ethnicity: African-American/Black
Degree and Year: PhD 1982
Major Field: Clinical Psychology
Specialty: Psychotherapy;Clinical Research;Emotion;Memory

RUTH, Richard
11303 Amherst Avenue
Suite #1
Wheaton, MD 20902
(301) 933-3072-**B**

Ethnicity: Hispanic/Latino
Languages: Spanish
Degree and Year: PhD 1986
Major Field: Clinical Psychology
Specialty: Cross Cultural Processes;Ethnic Minorities;HIV/
AIDS;Psychoanalysis;Assessment/Diagnosis/Evaluation

RYAN, Loye M.
1707 SE 154th Avenue
Vancouver, WA 98684-9009
(503) 224-1223-B, (206) 253-3900-H
Ethnicity: American Indian/Alaska Native
Degree and Year: EdD 1976
Major Field: Counseling Psychology

RYAN, Robert A.
Clinical Mental Health
1707 SE 154th Avenue
Vancouver, WA 98683
(503) 681-1453-B, (360) 253-3900-H, (360) 253-3900-F
runrr@aol.com
Ethnicity: American Indian/Alaska Native
Degree and Year: EdD 1973
Major Field: Counseling Psychology
Specialty: Alcoholism & Alcohol Abuse;Ethnic Minorities;Counseling
Psychology;Adolescent Therapy;Drug Abuse

SACASA, Rafael E.
9034 Westheimer
235
Houston, TX 77063
(713) 789-7560-B, (713) 975-0348-H
Ethnicity: Hispanic/Latino
Languages: German
Degree and Year: PhD 1993
Major Field: Clinical Psychology
Specialty: Behavior Therapy;Clinical Psychology;Medical
Psychology;Biofeedback;Cognitive Behavioral Therapy;Pain &
Pain Management

SADLER, Mark S.
4520 S. Harvard
Suite #200
Tulsa, OK 74135
(918) 743-3224-B
Ethnicity: American Indian/Alaska Native
Degree and Year: PhD 1982
Major Field: Counseling Psychology
Specialty: Adolescent Therapy;Child Therapy;Family Therapy;Group
Psychotherapy;Individual Psychotherapy

SAENZ, Javier
2787 E 4510 South
Salt Lake City, UT 84117-4658
(801) 262-8416-B, (801) 277-3436-H
Ethnicity: Hispanic/Latino
Languages: Spanish
Degree and Year: PhD 1965
Major Field: Community Psychology

SAENZ, Karol K.
2787 E 4510 S
Salt Lake City, UT 84117-4658

(801) 272-4010-B, (801) 277-3436-H
Ethnicity: Hispanic/Latino
Degree and Year: PhD 1982
Major Field: Counseling Psychology
Specialty: Chronically Mentally Ill;Cross Cultural Processes;Marriage
& Family;Group Processes

SAITO, Gloria C.
4232 Wilshire Blvd.
Oakland, CA 94602
(510) 642-9494-B, (510) 482-3959-H
Ethnicity: Asian-American/Asian/Pacific Islander
Languages: Japanese
Degree and Year: PhD 1983
Major Field: Clinical Psychology
Specialty: Clinical Child Psychology;Community Psychology;Cross
Cultural Processes;Family Therapy;Psychotherapy

SAKAMOTO, Katsuyuki
California School
of Professional Psychology
1005 Atlantic Avenue
Alameda, CA 94501
(510) 521-4964-B, (510) 523-4738-H, (510) 521-5121-F
kats@clas.org
Ethnicity: Asian-American/Asian/Pacific Islander
Degree and Year: PhD 1971
Major Field: Experimental Psychology
Specialty: Administration;Attitudes & Opinions;Ethnic
Minorities;Experimental Psychology;General Psychology

SAKATA, Robert T.
502 Bayberry Drive
Chapelhill, NC 27514-9123
(919) 966-3351-B, (919) 929-4443-H
Ethnicity: Asian-American/Asian/Pacific Islander
Degree and Year: PhD 1970
Major Field: Counseling Psychology
Specialty: Brain Damage;Rehabilitation;Research Design &
Methodology;Counseling Psychology;Medical
Psychology;Educational Psychology

SAKURAI, Mariko
22 King Street
Newton, MA 02166-1204
(508) 588-2425-B
Ethnicity: Asian-American/Asian/Pacific Islander
Degree and Year: PhD 1990
Major Field: Clinical Psychology
Specialty: Child Therapy;Group Psychotherapy

SALAIS, A. Joseph
938 Dewing Avenue
Suite 3
LaFayette, CA 94549
(925) 942-7110-B, (925) 671-0667-H, (925) 284-1919-F
lps@ix.netcom.com
Ethnicity: Hispanic/Latino
Degree and Year: PhD 1987
Major Field: Clinical Psychology
Specialty: Clinical Psychology;Organizational
Development;Assessment/Diagnosis/Evaluation

SALAS, Eduardo

Naval Air Warfare Center
12350 Research Parkway
Orlando, FL 32024
(407) 380-4651-**B**, (407) 646-7238-**H**, (407) 380-4110-**F**
eduardo_salas@ntsc.navy.mil
Ethnicity: Hispanic/Latino
Languages: Spanish
Degree and Year: PhD 1984 MS 1980
Major Field: Industrial/Organizational Psy.
Specialty: Industrial/Organizational Psychology;Group Processes;Work
   Performance;Human Factors;Training & Development;Military
   Psychology

SALAS, Jesus A.
   Center for Integrative Psychotherapy
   2151 South Cedar Crest Boulevard
   Suite 211D
   Allentown, PA 18103
   (610) 432-5066-**B**, (610) 398-7043-**H**, (610) 432-0973-**F**
   jasalas@compuserve.com
Ethnicity: Hispanic/Latino
Languages: Spanish
Degree and Year: MA 1986
Major Field: Clinical Psychology
Specialty: Cognitive Behavioral Therapy;Health
   Psychology;Biofeedback;Stress

SALDANA, Delia H.
   University of Texas
   Health Sciences Center
   Department of Psychiarty
   7703 Floyd Curl Drive
   San Antonio, TX 78284-7792
   (210) 531-8352-**B**, (210) 531-8169-**F**
   saldana@uthscsa.dcci.com
Ethnicity: Hispanic/Latino
Languages: Spanish
Degree and Year: PhD 1988
Major Field: Clinical Psychology
Specialty: Chronically Mentally Ill;Community Mental Health;Cross
   Cultural Processes;Ethnic Minorities;Mental Health Services

SALEEM, Rakhshanda
   2921 21st Street
   Boulder, CO 80304-2747
   (970) 491-6877-**B**, (970) 491-1032-**F**
   saleem@lamar.colostate.edu
Ethnicity: Asian-American/Asian/Pacific Islander
Languages: Hindi, Urdu
Degree and Year:
Major Field: Counseling Psychology

SALGADO DE SNYDER, V. Nelly S.
   Mexican Institute of Psychiatry
   Calzada Mexico - Xochimilco #101
   Delegacion Tlalpan
   Mexico, D.F., 14370
   Mexico
   0115256552811-**B**, 0115273 117914-**H**, 0115273 117914-**F**
   salgadvn@imp.edu.mx
Ethnicity: Hispanic/Latino
Languages: Spanish
Degree and Year: PhD 1986
Major Field: Social Psychology

Specialty: Social Problems;Gender Issues;Stress;Cultural & Social
   Processes

SALGANICOFF, Matilde
   556 North 23rd Street
   Philidelphia, PA 19130
   (215) 751-0396-**B**
Ethnicity: Hispanic/Latino
Languages: Spanish
Degree and Year: EdD 1978
Major Field: Clinical Psychology
Specialty: Adult Development;Family Therapy;Feminist
   Therapy;Psychology of Women

SALONE, Lavorial
   Metropolitan State University
   Student Counseling Services
   730 Hennepin Avenue
   Minneapolis, MN 55403-1897
   (612) 373-2710-**B**, (612) 623-7997-**H**, (612) 341-7399-**F**
   salone@msus1.msus.edu
Ethnicity: African-American/Black, Asian-American/Asian/Pacific
Islander
Degree and Year: PhD 1995 MA 1983
Major Field: Counseling Psychology
Specialty: Developmental Psychology;Ethnic Minorities;Industrial/
   Organizational Psychology;Disadvantaged;Group
   Processes;Psychotherapy

SALTER, Beatrice R.
   Park Heights
   1421 East Duval Street
   Philadelphia, PA 19138-1101
   (215) 438-5454-**B**
Ethnicity: African-American/Black
Degree and Year: PhD 1982
Major Field: Clinical Psychology
Specialty: Psychotherapy

SALTER, Dianne S.
   7600 Stenton Avenue
   Suite 4-D
   Philadelphia, PA 19118
   (215) 247-9001-**B**, (215) 248-3588-**H**, (215) 247-9030-**F**
Ethnicity: African-American/Black
Degree and Year: PhD 1977 JD 1987
Major Field: Clinical Psychology

SALWAY, Milton R.
   28609 Vista Madera
   Rancho Palos Verdes, CA 90275
   (310) 547-2848-**B**, (310) 547-2848-**H**
Ethnicity: Asian-American/Asian/Pacific Islander
Degree and Year: PhD 1980
Major Field: Clinical Psychology
Specialty: Industrial/Organizational Psychology;Alcoholism & Alcohol
   Abuse;Managed Care;Training & Development;Employee
   Assistance Programs

SAMAAN, Makram K.
   2933 Cottage Way
   Sacramento, CA 95825-1842
   (916) 972-0800-**B**

Ethnicity: African-American/Black
Degree and Year: PhD 1970
Major Field: Clinical Psychology

SAMANIEGO, Sandra
  43-A Garrison Avenue
  Jersey City, NJ 07306
  (212) 439-3365-**B**, (201) 656-5008-**H**, (212) 861-4400-**F**
Ethnicity: Hispanic/Latino
Languages: Spanish
Degree and Year: PhD 1980
Major Field: Clinical Psychology
Specialty: Clinical Psychology;Individual Psychotherapy;Group
    Psychotherapy;Psychometrics;Cross Cultural Processes

SAMANO, Italo A.
  P.O. Box 4138
  Berghein, TX 78004-4138
  (210) 530-1100-**B**, (210) 336-3099-**H**
Ethnicity: Hispanic/Latino
Degree and Year: PhD 1987
Major Field: Clinical Psychology

SAMFORD, Judith A.
  47-328 Mawaena Street
  Apartment C
  Kaneohe, HI 96744-4700
  (808) 236-8335-**B**, (808) 239-7090-**H**, (808) 247-7335-**F**
  samfor@hgea.org
Ethnicity: American Indian/Alaska Native
Degree and Year: PhD 1981
Major Field: Clinical Psychology
Specialty: Hypnosis/
    Hypnotherapy;Psychoses;Administration;Chronically
    Mentally Ill

SAMPSON, Myrtle B.
  4608 Splitrail Court
  Greensboro, NC 27406-9059
  (919) 272-1237-**B**, (336) 697-1220-**H**
Ethnicity: African-American/Black
Degree and Year: PhD 1980 EdD 1976
Major Field: Counseling Psychology
Specialty: Audition;Educational Psychology;Personality;Cognitive
    Behavioral Therapy;Individual Psychotherapy;Social
    Psychology

SAMUELS, Robert M.
  65 Chiswick Road
  Cranston, RI 02905-3710
  (203) 243-2929-**B**
Ethnicity: African-American/Black
Degree and Year: PhD 1987
Major Field: Clinical Psychology
Specialty: Family Therapy

SAMUEL, Valerie J.
  Massachusetts General Hospital
  Harvard Medical School
  WACC 725, AOHD Study
  15 Parkman Street
  Boston, MA 02114
  (617)724-1531-**B**, 617/497-2253-**H**, 617/724-1540-**F**
  samuel@helix.mgh.harvard.edu
Ethnicity: African-American/Black
Degree and Year: PhD 1988

Major Field: Clinical Child Psychology
Specialty: Psychopathology;Psychotherapy;Parent-Child
    Interaction;Research & Training;Juvenile Delinquency

SAN LUIS, Roberto R.
  Pierce Wood Memorial Hospital
  Mental Health, G
  5847 SE Highway 31
  Arcadia, FL 34266-9627
  (941) 494-3323-**B**, (941) 494-6995-**H**, (941) 494-4273-**F**
Ethnicity: Asian-American/Asian/Pacific Islander
Languages: Filipino
Degree and Year: PhD 1968
Major Field: Clinical Psychology
Specialty: Gerontology/Geropsychology;Mental Health
    Services;Neuropsychology;Alzheimer's Disease;Behavior
    Therapy

SAN MIGUEL, Christopher L.
  VA Medical Center
  Department of Psychology
  2300 Ramsey
  Fayetteville, NC 28301-3856
  (512) 590-0938-**B**
Ethnicity: Hispanic/Latino
Degree and Year: PhD 1976
Major Field: Clinical Psychology
Specialty: Psychotherapy

SANCHEZ-CASO, Luis M.
  Calle Central #659
  Miramar
  Apartment #7
  San Juan, PR 00907-3407
  (783)-0123-**B**, 723-4909-**H**
Ethnicity: Hispanic/Latino
Languages: Spanish
Degree and Year: PhD 1992
Major Field: Clinical Psychology

SANCHEZ-HUCLES, Janis V.
  Old Dominion University
  Psychology Dept.
  Norfolk, VA 23529
  (757) 683-4439-**B**, (757) 481-9989-**H**, (757) 683-5087-**F**
  JSH100F@viper.mgb.odu.edu
Ethnicity: African-American/Black
Degree and Year: PhD 1980
Major Field: Clinical Psychology
Specialty: Psychotherapy

SANCHEZ-TORRENTO, Eugenio
  1226 Lisbon Street
  Coral Gables, FL 33134
  (305) 444-2690-**B**, (305) 444-2690-**H**
Ethnicity: Hispanic/Latino
Languages: Portuguese, Spanish
Degree and Year: PhD 1976
Major Field: Clinical Psychology
Specialty: Adolescent Therapy;Alcoholism & Alcohol Abuse;Clinical
    Child Psychology;Drug Abuse;Family Therapy

SANCHEZ, David M.
  1802 Nuevo Road

Henderson, NV 89014
(702) 454-1140-**B**, (702) 451-0500-**H**, (702) 454-1140-**F**
Ethnicity: Hispanic/Latino
Degree and Year: MA 1973
Major Field: General Psy./Methods & Systems
Specialty: Statistics

SANCHEZ, Debra A.
1002 North Benton Avenue
Helene, MT 59601
(406) 449-7753-**B**, (406) 449-3940-**H**
Ethnicity: Hispanic/Latino
Degree and Year: PhD 1987
Major Field: Clinical Psychology
Specialty: Adolescent Therapy;Cognitive Behavioral
Therapy;Assessment/Diagnosis/
Evaluation;Psychopathology;Psychopathology

SANCHEZ, H.G.
P.O. Box 14631
San Luis Obispo, CA 93406
(805) 547-7900-**B**
Ethnicity: Hispanic/Latino
Languages: Spanish
Degree and Year: PhD 1986
Major Field: Clinical Psychology
Specialty: Mental Health Services;Correctional Psychology;Crisis
Intervention & Therapy;Forensic Psychology;Chronically
Mentally Ill

SANCHEZ, Juan
Florida International University
Department of Psychology
University Park
Miami, FL 33199
(305) 348-3387-**B**, (305) 348-3879-**F**
sanchezj@fiu.edu
Ethnicity: Hispanic/Latino
Languages: Spanish
Degree and Year: PhD 1989
Major Field: Industrial/Organizational Psy.
Specialty: Human Relations;Human Resources;Industrial/Organizational
Psychology;Labor & Management Relations;Job Satisfaction

SANCHEZ, Victor C.
P.O. Box 3353
South Pasadena, CA 91031-6353
(818) 798-8682-**B**
Ethnicity: Hispanic/Latino
Degree and Year: PhD 1978
Major Field: Clinical Psychology

SANCHEZ, William
Northeastern University
203 Lake Hall
Boston, MA 02115
(617) 373-2404-**B**, (617) 969-5651-**H**, (617) 373-4595-**F**
Ethnicity: Hispanic/Latino
Languages: Spanish
Degree and Year: PhD 1978
Major Field: Clinical Psychology
Specialty: Child & Pediatric Psychology;Ethnic Minorities;Mentally
Retarded;Assessment/Diagnosis/Evaluation;Rehabilitation

SANCHO, Ana M.
Hutchinson & Associates
222 West Gregory Boulevard
Suite 100
Kansas City, MO 64114
(816) 361-0664-**B**, (913) 789-7723-**H**, (816) 361-0677-**F**
sanchosama@aol.com
Ethnicity: Hispanic/Latino
Languages: Spanish
Degree and Year: PhD 1994
Major Field: Counseling Psychology
Specialty: Psychotherapy;Cross Cultural Processes;Interpersonal
Processes & Relations;Assessment/Diagnosis/
Evaluation;Training & Development;Gender Issues

SANDERS-THOMPSON, Vetta L.
University of Missouri, St. Louis
9900 Martingale Road
St. Louis, MO 63137
(314) 516-5409-**B**, (314) 868-6833-**H**, (314) 516-5392-**F**
sv/sand@ums/vma.ums.edu
Ethnicity: African-American/Black
Degree and Year: PhD 1988
Major Field: Clinical Psychology
Specialty: Ethnic Minorities;Child Therapy;Clinical Child
Psychology;Community Mental Health

SANDERS, Betty M.
Lockheed-Martin
10814 Oak Hollow Drive
Houston, TX 77024
(281) 483-0047-**B**, (713) 984-9191-**H**, (281) 244-5193-**F**
betty.sanders1@jsc.nasa.gov
Ethnicity: African-American/Black
Degree and Year: PhD 1984
Major Field: Industrial/Organizational Psy.
Specialty: Leadership;Management & Organization;Engineering
Psychology;Administration;Organizational
Development;Human Factors

SANDERS, Daniel W.
130 Strecker Drive
Tallmadge, OH 44278
(330) 633-1206-**B**, (330) 630-2121-**H**, (330) 633-1364-**F**
dansanders@neo.rr.com
Ethnicity: African-American/Black
Degree and Year: PhD 1984
Major Field: Counseling Psychology
Specialty: Sex/Marital Therapy;Assessment/Diagnosis/
Evaluation;Ethnic Minorities;Vocational Psychology;Religious
Psychology

SANDERS, Gilbert O.
Alaska Native Medical Center
Psychiatry Department
4320 Diplomacy Drive
Suite 200
Anchorage, AK 99508
(907) 729-2500-**B**, (907) 729-2525-**F**
gsanders@akanmc.alaska.ihs.gov
Ethnicity: American Indian/Alaska Native
Languages: Spanish
Degree and Year: EdD 1974
Major Field: Counseling Psychology
Specialty: Drug Abuse;Biofeedback;Marriage & Family

SANDOVAL, Jonathan
  University of California
  Division of Education
  One Shields Avenue
  Davis, CA 95616
  (916) 752-3198-**B**, (916) 752-5411-**F**
  jhsandoval@ucdavis.edu
  Ethnicity: Hispanic/Latino
  Languages: German, Spanish
  Degree and Year: PhD 1969
  Major Field: School Psychology
  Specialty: School Psychology;Prevention;Measurement;Individual
    Difference;Crisis Intervention & Therapy

SANER-YIU, Li-Chia
  4, Place Des Alpes
  Geneva, 1201
  SWITZERLAND
  011 412906 1720-**B**, 41 22 7381737-**F**
  saneryiu@csend.org
  Ethnicity: Asian-American/Asian/Pacific Islander
  Degree and Year: EdD 1978
  Major Field: Industrial/Organizational Psy.
  Specialty: Organizational Development;Management &
    Organization;Leadership;Counseling Psychology;Training &
    Development;Cross Cultural Processes

SANTIAGO-NEGRON, Salvador
  Caribbean Center for Advanced Studies
  PO Box 9023711
  San Juan, PR 00902-3711
  (787) 725-6500-**B**, (78763-0095-**H**, (787) 721-7187-**F**
  Ethnicity: Hispanic/Latino
  Degree and Year: PhD 1993 MPH 1982
  Major Field: School Psychology
  Specialty: Learning Disabilities

SANTIAGO, Lydia V.
  Kaiser Medical Group Oakland
  280 West MacArthur Boulevard
  Oakland, CA 94611
  (510) 596-1459-**B**, (501) 233-8297-**H**
  Ethnicity: Hispanic/Latino
  Degree and Year: PhD 1991
  Major Field: Clinical Child Psychology
  Specialty: Medical Psychology;Neurological Disorders;Ethnic
    Minorities

SANTINI-HERNANDEZ, Ernesto
  Winston Churchill #128
  Suite 150
  San Juan, PR 00926
  (787) 725-4572-**B**, (787) 754-6983-**H**, (787) 725-4572-**F**
  Ethnicity: Hispanic/Latino
  Languages: Spanish
  Degree and Year: PhD 1991
  Major Field: Clinical Psychology
  Specialty: Forensic Psychology;Clinical Psychology;Assessment/
    Diagnosis/Evaluation

SANTOS DE BARONA, Maryann
  Arizona State University
  Division of Psychology in Education
  Box 870611

Tempe, AZ 85287-0611
  (602) 965-3384-**B**, (602) 820-7774-**H**, (602) 965-0300-**F**
  Ethnicity: Hispanic/Latino
  Degree and Year: PhD 1981
  Major Field: School Psychology
  Specialty: Assessment/Diagnosis/Evaluation;Preschool & Day Care
    Issues;Special Education;Ethnic Minorities;Preschool & Day
    Care Issues

SANUA, Victor D.
  St. Johns University
  2416 Quentin Road
  Brooklyn, NY 11229
  (718) 990-6368-**B**, (718) 339-0337-**H**, (718) 990-6705-**F**
  sanuan@stjohns.edu
  Ethnicity: Hispanic/Latino
  Languages: French, Italian, Spanish
  Degree and Year: PhD 1956
  Major Field: Clinical Psychology
  Specialty: Autism;Clinical Psychology;Cross Cultural Processes;Ethnic
    Minorities;Schizophrenia

SAPP, Marty
  Dept. of Educational Psychology
  2400 E. Hartford Avenue
  Milwaukee, WI 53211
  (414) 229-6347-**H**, (414) 229-4939-**F**
  sapp@uwm.edu
  Ethnicity: African-American/Black
  Languages: Spanish, Swahili
  Degree and Year: EdD 1988
  Major Field: Counseling Psychology
  Specialty: Counseling Psychology;Hypnosis/
    Hypnotherapy;Quantitative/Mathematical,
    Psychometrics;Stress;Rational-Emotive Therapy

SARAF, Komal C.
  1430 Riverside Drive
  Trenton, NJ 08618
  (908) 521-0030-**B**, (609) 394-8238-**H**
  Ethnicity: Asian-American/Asian/Pacific Islander
  Languages: Hindi, Urdu, Punjabi,Gujrati
  Degree and Year: PhD 1980
  Major Field: Clinical Psychology
  Specialty: Assessment/Diagnosis/Evaluation;Cross Cultural
    Processes;Mental Health Services;Juvenile
    Delinquency;Cognitive Behavioral Therapy

SARMIENTO, Robert F.
  1202 Rosemeadow Drive
  Houston, TX 77094-2920
  (713) 465-2456-**B**
  Ethnicity: Hispanic/Latino
  Degree and Year: PhD 1973
  Major Field: Clinical Psychology
  Specialty: Rational-Emotive Therapy

SASAO, Toshiaki
  International Christian University
  10-2, Osawa 3-Chome
  Mitaka-Shi
  Tokyo 181-8585,
  JAPAN
  +81-422-33-3188-**B**, +81-433-34-3578-**H**, +81-422-34-6982-**F**

sasao@icu.ac.jp
Ethnicity: Asian-American/Asian/Pacific Islander
Languages: Japanese
Degree and Year: PhD 1988
Major Field: Community Psychology
Specialty: Cross Cultural Processes;Drug Abuse;Cultural & Social
Processes;Alcoholism & Alcohol Abuse;Ethnic
Minorities;Community Psychology

SASSCER-BURGOS, Julie
1135 Ingate Road
Baltimore, MD 21227
(410) 792-4022-**B**, (410) 242-1719-**H**, (410) 792-0439-**F**
Ethnicity: Hispanic/Latino
Languages: French, Spanish
Degree and Year: PsyD 1988
Major Field: Clinical Psychology
Specialty: Forensic Psychology;Group Psychotherapy;Family
Therapy;Child Therapy

SATO, Susan D.
Medical College Of Georgia
1940 Cottonwood Dr
Aiken, SC 29803-5783
(404) 721-2161-**B**, (803) 648-2466-**H**
Ethnicity: Asian-American/Asian/Pacific Islander
Degree and Year: PhD 1984
Major Field: Clinical Psychology
Specialty: Medical Psychology

SAUCEDO, Carlos
14030 Saddle Ridge Road
Sylmar, CA 91342-1063
(818) 362-5454-**B**
Ethnicity: Hispanic/Latino
Languages: Spanish
Degree and Year: PhD 1980
Major Field: Clinical Psychology
Specialty: Clinical Psychology;Clinical Neuropsychology;Clinical Child
Neuropsychology

SAUCEDO, Carlos
10324 Balboa Blvd.
Suite #200
Granada Hills, CA 91344
(818) 362-5454-**B**
Ethnicity: Hispanic/Latino
Languages: Spanish
Degree and Year: PhD 1980
Major Field: Clinical Psychology
Specialty: Clinical Psychology;Clinical Neuropsychology;Clinical Child
Neuropsychology

SAUL, Tuck T.
627 Whilehaven Court
Westerville, OH 43081-3772
(614) 451-0176-**B**, (614) 794-1755-**H**, (614) 451-8138-**F**
Ethnicity: Asian-American/Asian/Pacific Islander
Degree and Year: PhD 1980
Major Field: Counseling Psychology
Specialty: Psychotherapy

SAUNDERS, Walter C.

Springdale Professional Center
3110 Provo Court
Suite #A
San Jose, CA 95127-1034
(408) 272-4321-**B**, (408) 259-1126-**H**
Ethnicity: Hispanic/Latino
Languages: Spanish
Degree and Year: PhD 1974
Major Field: Clinical Psychology
Specialty: Family Therapy;Alcoholism & Alcohol Abuse;Hypnosis/
Hypnotherapy;Group Psychotherapy

SAVAGE, JR., James E.
Institute for Life Enrichment
7852 16th Street, NW
Washington, DC 20012
(202) 291-5008-**B**, (202) 882-2996-**H**, (202) 291-2080-**F**
Ethnicity: African-American/Black
Languages: German
Degree and Year: PhD 1971
Major Field: Clinical Psychology
Specialty: Individual Psychotherapy;Assessment/Diagnosis/
Evaluation;Employee Assistance Programs

SAX, Kenji W.
University of Cincinnati
231 Bethesda Avenue (ML559)
Cincinnati, OH 45229-2827
(513) 558-4902-**B**, (513) 321-2571-**H**, (513) 558-4805-**F**
saxkw@email.uc.edu
Ethnicity: Asian-American/Asian/Pacific Islander
Degree and Year: PhD 1995 MS 1992
Major Field: Experimental Psychology
Specialty: Brain Functions;Cognitive
Psychology;Neuropsychology;Psychopathology;Neurophysiology

SAYAMA, Mike K.
2612 Peter Street
#A
Honolulu, HI 96816-2014
808 942-7171-**B**
Ethnicity: Asian-American/Asian/Pacific Islander
Degree and Year: PhD 1982
Major Field: Clinical Psychology

SCHACHT, Thomas E.
614 W Locust Street
Johnson City, TN 37604
(615) 929-6305-**B**, (615) 929-1076-**H**, (615) 461-7033-**F**
Ethnicity: Hispanic/Latino
Degree and Year: PsyD 1980
Major Field: Clinical Psychology
Specialty: Clinical Psychology;Psychotherapy;Psychology &
Law;Forensic Psychology;Research & Training

SCHENQUERMAN, Berta N.
243 Moraga
San Francisco, CA 94122
(415) 564-3415-**B**, (415) 564-3415-**H**
Ethnicity: Hispanic/Latino
Languages: Spanish
Degree and Year: PhD 1980
Major Field: Clinical Psychology
Specialty: Assessment/Diagnosis/Evaluation;Clinical Psychology;Ethnic

Minorities;Family Therapy;Medical Psychology

SCHLESINGER, Laura Ann
30 Lomo Avenue
Suite 300
Kahului, HI 96732
(808) 871-7502-**B**, (808) 874-0854-**H**, (808) 871-9726-**F**
Ethnicity: Asian-American/Asian/Pacific Islander
Degree and Year: MA 1978
Major Field: Clinical Psychology
Specialty: Alcoholism & Alcohol Abuse;Family Therapy

SCHLESINGER, Susana J.
16284 Prince Drive
South Holland, IL 60473
(708) 210-133-**B**, (773) 238-7637-**H**, (708) 331-8670-**F**
Ethnicity: Hispanic/Latino
Languages: Spanish
Degree and Year: PhD 1983 MTM 1980
Major Field: Counseling Psychology

SCHMAJUK, Nestor
Northwestern University
Department of Psychology
Evanston, IL 60208
(708) 491-5517-**B**, (708) 491-7859-**F**
Ethnicity: Hispanic/Latino
Languages: Spanish
Degree and Year: PhD 1986
Major Field: Neurosciences
Specialty: Experimental Psychology;Learning/Learning
    Theory;Psychophysiology;Psychopathology;Brain Functions

SCHREIER, Raquel L.
2410 E. Hammond Lake Drive
Bloomfield Hills, MI 48302
(313) 334-3444-**B**, (313) 338-0273-**H**
Ethnicity: Hispanic/Latino
Languages: Spanish
Degree and Year: PhD 1971
Major Field: Clinical Psychology
Specialty: Behavior Therapy;Clinical Neuropsychology;Cognitive
    Behavioral Therapy;Ethnic Minorities;Medical Psychology

SCHROFF, Kamal
43 Winchester Drive
East Windsor, NJ 08520-2608
(609) 443-5009-**B**, (609) 443-5009-**H**
Ethnicity: Asian-American/Asian/Pacific Islander
Languages: Hindi, Marathi
Degree and Year: PhD 1974
Major Field: Clinical Psychology
Specialty: Assessment/Diagnosis/Evaluation;Mentally Retarded;Cross
    Cultural Processes;Developmental
    Psychology;Psychotherapy;Personality

SCOTT-JONES, Diane
Boston College
Department of Psychology
Mcguinn Hall 435
140 Commonwealth Avenue
Chestnut Hill, MA 02467
(617) 552-3972-**B**, (617) 552-0523-**F**
diane.scott-jones.1@bc.edu
Ethnicity: African-American/Black
Degree and Year: PhD 1979

Major Field: Developmental Psychology
Specialty: Adolescent Development;Cultural & Social Processes;Ethnic
    Minorities;Developmental Psychobiology;Policy Analysis

SCOTT, Linda D.
35 Riverbank Road
Northampton, MA 01060
(413) 545-2337-**B**, (413) 584-5764-**H**, (413) 545-9602-**F**
becklin@uhs.umass.edu
Ethnicity: African-American/Black
Degree and Year: PhD 1986
Major Field: Clinical Psychology
Specialty: Psychotherapy;Ethnic Minorities;Feminist Therapy

SCOTT, Merilla M.
17415 Raymer Street
Northridge, CA 91325-3449
(818) 993-7196-**B**
Ethnicity: African-American/Black
Degree and Year: PhD 1988
Major Field: Clinical Psychology
Specialty: Child Therapy;Crisis Intervention & Therapy

SEARCY, Mary L.
600 Ridgewell Way
Silver Spring, MD 20902
(202) 806-6974-**B**, (301) 622-9381-**H**
Ethnicity: African-American/Black
Degree and Year: PhD 1980
Major Field: Clinical Psychology
Specialty: Individual Psychotherapy;Marriage & Family;Child &
    Pediatric Psychology;Assessment/Diagnosis/Evaluation;Ethnic
    Minorities

SEDA, Gilbert
Naval Medical Center Portsmouth
3006 Acres Road
Portsmouth, VA 22703
(757) 314-6738-**B**, (757) 483-1022-**H**
gseda@med.navy.mi
Ethnicity: Hispanic/Latino
Degree and Year: PhD 1992
Major Field: Clinical Psychology
Specialty: Psychopharmacology

SEDO, Manuel A.
9 Ingleside Road
Natick, MA 01760-1415
(617) 635-9635-**B**, (508) 655-6970-**H**
Ethnicity: Hispanic/Latino
Languages: French, Italian, Spanish, Catalan
Degree and Year: PhD 1987
Major Field: Counseling Psychology
Specialty: Cognitive Development;Learning
    Disabilities;Neuropsychology;Child Development;Individual
    Psychotherapy

SEITZ, Kathleen
508 Southlawn
East Lansing, MI 48823-3138
(517) 332-5612-**B**
Ethnicity: Asian-American/Asian/Pacific Islander
Degree and Year: PhD 1986
Major Field: unknown

Specialty: Family Therapy

SELGAS, James W.
1400 Quail Hollow Road
Harrisburg, PA 17112
(717) 780-2519-**B**, (717) 545-6090-**H**
Ethnicity: Hispanic/Latino, European/White
Degree and Year: EdD 1970
Major Field: Counseling Psychology
Specialty: Behavior Therapy;Cognitive Behavioral Therapy;School Psychology;Sports Psychology

SELLARDS, Robert
705 Octavia St
New Orleans, LA 70115-3155
(504) 897-2892-**B**, (504) 897-2892-**H**
Ethnicity: American Indian/Alaska Native
Degree and Year: PhD 1981
Major Field: Counseling Psychology

SEN, Tapas K.
29 Arden Road
Mountain Lakes, NJ 07046-1513
(973) 625-2779-**B**, (973) 625-2779-**H**
ssits@att.net
Ethnicity: Asian-American/Asian/Pacific Islander
Languages: Hindi, Bengali
Degree and Year: PhD 1963
Major Field: unknown
Specialty: Human Factors;Psychometrics;Organizational Development;Industrial/Organizational Psychology

SERAFICA, Felicisima C.
Ohio State University
Department of Psychology
214 Townshend Hall
1885 Neil Avenue
Columbus, OH 43210-1222
(614) 292-0483-**B**, (614) 267-8545-**H**
serafica.1@osu.edu
Ethnicity: Asian-American/Asian/Pacific Islander
Languages: Spanish, Tagalog
Degree and Year: PhD 1973
Major Field: Clinical Psychology
Specialty: Clinical Child Psychology;Developmental Psychology

SERRANO-GARCIA, Irma
University of Puerto Rico
PO Box 23174
San Juan, PR 00931-3174
(787) 764-74670-**B**, (787) 789-2188-**H**, (787) 758-4213-**F**
Ethnicity: Hispanic/Latino
Languages: Spanish
Degree and Year: PhD 1978 PDoc 1985
Major Field: Community Psychology
Specialty: Community Psychology;HIV/AIDS

SEYMOUR, Guy O.
872 East Confederate Avenue, S.E.
Atlanta, GA 30316
(404) 624-9624-**B**
guy0@ix.netcom.com
Ethnicity: African-American/Black
Degree and Year: PhD 1971
Major Field: unknown

Specialty: Professional Issues in Psychology;Cultural & Social Processes

SHAHANI-DENNING, Comila
102 Hofstra Univ
906 Huntington
Hempstead, NY 11550-1090
(516) 292-6242-**B**, (516) 333-2362-**H**, (516) 463-6010-**F**
Ethnicity: Asian-American/Asian/Pacific Islander
Languages: Hindi
Degree and Year: PhD 1988
Major Field: Industrial/Organizational Psy.
Specialty: Stress;Industrial/Organizational Psychology;Gender Issues

SHAH, Vasantkumar B.
90 McGuire Street
Metuchen, NJ 08840
(732) 549-0032-**H**, (732) 549-0032-**F**
Ethnicity: Asian-American/Asian/Pacific Islander
Languages: Hindi
Degree and Year: PhD 1964
Major Field: Clinical Psychology
Specialty: Developmental Psychology;Child Development;Clinical Psychology;Administration;Mental Disorders

SHAPIRO, Ester R.
150 Otis Street
West Newton, MA 02165
(617) 287-6360-**B**, (617) 964-0997-**H**
Ethnicity: Hispanic/Latino
Degree and Year: PhD 1979
Major Field: Clinical Psychology
Specialty: Human Development & Family Studies

SHARMA, Greesh C.
699 West Trenton Avenue
Morrisville, PA 19067
(215) 295-3099-**B**, (215) 493-2006-**H**, (215) 493-2006-**F**
Ethnicity: Asian-American/Asian/Pacific Islander
Languages: Hindi, Urdu, Brijbhasha
Degree and Year: PhD 1978
Major Field: Clinical Psychology
Specialty: Cognitive Behavioral Therapy;Clinical Psychology;Depression;Family Therapy;Drug Abuse

SHARMA, Satanand
Inglewood Medical
and Mental Health Services
2421 Nalin Drive
Bel Air, CA 90077
(310) 671-0555-**B**, (310) 476-9214-**H**, (310) 674-5292-**F**
Ethnicity: Asian-American/Asian/Pacific Islander
Languages: Fijian
Degree and Year: PhD 1973
Major Field: Psychopharmacology
Specialty: Drug Abuse;Drug Abuse

SHARMA, Vijai P.
2150 North Ocoee St.
Cleveland, TN 37311
(423) 476-1933-**B**, (423) 479-5747-**H**, (423) 476-1933-**F**
Ethnicity: Asian-American/Asian/Pacific Islander
Languages: Hindi
Degree and Year: PhD 1977
Major Field: Clinical Psychology
Specialty: Adolescent Therapy;Clinical Child Psychology;Clinical

Psychology;Health Psychology;Cognitive Behavioral Therapy

SHARP, Jude C.
1947 Divisadero Street
Suite 2
San Francisco, CA 94115
(415) 922-9013-**B**, (510) 841-7154-**H**, (510) 549-0475-**F**
judesharp@aol.com
Ethnicity: African-American/Black
Degree and Year: PhD 1987 MA 1981
Major Field: Clinical Psychology
Specialty: Cognitive Behavioral Therapy;Depression;Affective
        Disorders;Cross Cultural Processes;Employee Assistance
        Programs;Group Processes

SHAW, Paula
4829 16th St NW
Washington, DC 20011-4332
(202) 726-7700-**B**, (202) 723-3667-**H**, (202) 726-7717-**F**
Ethnicity: African-American/Black
Degree and Year: PhD 1977
Major Field: Clinical Psychology
Specialty: Mental Health Services;Cognitive Behavioral
        Therapy;Alcoholism & Alcohol Abuse;Marriage &
        Family;Managed Care

SHAW, Terry G.
P.O. Box 470
McAlester, OK 74502
(918) 423-1267-**B**, (918) 426-6780-**H**
Ethnicity: American Indian/Alaska Native
Degree and Year: PhD 1976
Major Field: Neurosciences
Specialty: Clinical Neuropsychology;Neuropsychology;Neurological
        Disorders;Brain Damage;Alzheimer's Disease

SHEA-MARTINEZ, Herminia E.
2134 Main Street, Suite 250
Huntinton Beach, CA 92648
(714) 847-4415-**B**, (714) 969-6621-**F**
Ethnicity: Hispanic/Latino
Languages: Spanish
Degree and Year: PhD 1988
Major Field: Clinical Psychology
Specialty: Child Therapy;Ethnic Minorities;Psychology of
        Women;Cognitive Behavioral Therapy;Family Therapy;Stress

SHELL, Juanita
Health and Hospital Corporation
Bellevue Hospital Center
27th Street adn First Avenue
Bronx, NY 10452
(718) 861-4509-**B**, (718) 681-7562-**H**
Ethnicity: African-American/Black
Degree and Year: PhD 1977 Cert 1991
Major Field: Clinical Psychology
Specialty: Clinical Child Psychology;Psychoanalysis;Forensic
        Psychology;Assessment/Diagnosis/Evaluation;Autism

SHEN, John
850 Columbia Road #204
Westlake, OH 44145
(440) 871-0950-**B**, (440) 871-4640-**F**
Ethnicity: Asian-American/Asian/Pacific Islander
Languages: Chinese
Degree and Year: PhD 1972

Major Field: Clinical Psychology
Specialty: Pain & Pain Management;Sexual Dysfunction

SHIMA, Fred M.
11421 Albata
Los Angeles, CA 90049-3403
Ethnicity: Asian-American/Asian/Pacific Islander
Degree and Year: PhD 1968
Major Field: unknown
Specialty: History & Systems of Psychology;Memory

SHIMIZU, Annette A.
Straub Clinic & Hosp Inc.
888 S King Street
Honolulu, HI 96813
(808) 522-4521-**B**
Ethnicity: Asian-American/Asian/Pacific Islander
Degree and Year: PhD 1976
Major Field: Clinical Psychology

SHIMODA, Kim C.
Children's National Medical Center
Department of Hematology/Oncology
111 Michigan Avenue, NW
Washington, DC 20010
(202) 884-2806-**B**, (202) 884-2976-**F**
kshimoda@cnmc.org
Ethnicity: Asian-American/Asian/Pacific Islander
Degree and Year: PhD 1993
Major Field: Clinical Child Psychology
Specialty: Child & Pediatric Psychology;Pain & Pain
        Management;Behavior Therapy;Clinical Child
        Neuropsychology

SHING, Marn-Ling
Center for Child Development
TALPEH Municipal Teachers College
1 AI Kuo West Road
Taipei 100   419,
TAIWAN
Ethnicity: Asian-American/Asian/Pacific Islander
Degree and Year: PhD 1987
Major Field: Developmental Psychology

SHIPP, Pamela L.
1414 N. Novada Avenue
Colorado Springs, CO 80907
(719) 475-8038-**B**, (719) 632-3063-**F**
Ethnicity: African-American/Black
Degree and Year: PhD 1985
Major Field: Counseling Psychology
Specialty: Cross Cultural Processes;Adolescent
        Therapy;Leadership;Marriage & Family;Group
        Psychotherapy

SHIRAKAWA, Patti
1481 S King Street
Suite #528
Honolulu, HI 96814-2601
(808) 944-9940-**B**
Ethnicity: Asian-American/Asian/Pacific Islander
Degree and Year: PhD 1982
Major Field: Clinical Psychology
Specialty: Family Therapy

SHIRES, Michael R.
Community Hospital of Lancaster
1012 Beech Street
Reading, PA 19605
(717) 239-4241-**B**, (717) 394-7072-**F**
michael.shires@chol.org
Ethnicity: Asian-American/Asian/Pacific Islander
Degree and Year: MA 1982
Major Field: Counseling Psychology
Specialty: Humanistic Psychology;Health Psychology;Adolescent
    Therapy

SHOHET, Jacqueline M.
10571 La Dona Drive
Garden Grove, CA 92640-1616
(714) 537-9193-**H**, (714) 537-4031-**F**
Ethnicity: American Indian/Alaska Native
Degree and Year: PhD 1959
Major Field: Developmental Psychology
Specialty: Developmental Psychology;Neurological Disorders

SHON, Elizbabeth
745 Marengo Avenue
Pasadena, CA 91106
(323) 256-8203-**H**
Ethnicity: Asian-American/Asian/Pacific Islander
Degree and Year: PhD 1988
Major Field: Clinical Psychology
Specialty: Clinical Psychology;Psychotherapy;Ethnic
    Minorities;Affective Disorders;Eating Disorders

SHOPSHIRE, Michael S.
University of California, San Francisco
74 New Montgomery Street
Suite 440
San Francisco, CA 94105
(415) 597-9278-**B**, (707) 575-0732-**H**, (415) 597-9277-**F**
mshopshire@aol.com
Ethnicity: Asian-American/Asian/Pacific Islander
Degree and Year: Ph' 1993
Major Field: Clinical Psychology
Specialty: Drug Abuse;Clinical Research

SHROFF, Kamal
43 Winchester Drive
East Windsor, NJ 08520-2608
(609) 443-5009-**B**, (609) 443-5009-**H**
Ethnicity: Asian-American/Asian/Pacific Islander
Languages: Hindi
Degree and Year: PhD 1974
Major Field: Clinical Psychology
Specialty: Assessment/Diagnosis/Evaluation;Developmental
    Psychology;Mentally Retarded;Psychotherapy;Cross Cultural
    Processes

SHUFFER, JR., Jacob M.
45136 N Roden Avenue
Lancaster, CA 93535-2668
Ethnicity: Hispanic/Latino
Degree and Year: MA 1979
Major Field: unknown
Specialty: Correctional Psychology

SHUM, Hilda B.
22232 Belleau Ct
Calabasas, CA 91302-5876
(510) 596-1476-**B**, (818) 225-7226-**H**
Ethnicity: Asian-American/Asian/Pacific Islander
Degree and Year: PhD 1985
Major Field: Clinical Psychology
Specialty: Child & Pediatric Psychology;Clinical Child
    Psychology;Adolescent Therapy;Cognitive Behavioral
    Therapy;Parent-Child Interaction

SHUM, Hilda B.
22232 Belleau Ct
Calabasas, CA 91302-5876
(510) 596-1476-**B**, (818) 225-7226-**H**
Ethnicity: Asian-American/Asian/Pacific Islander
Degree and Year: PhD 1985
Major Field: Clinical Psychology
Specialty: Child & Pediatric Psychology;Clinical Child
    Psychology;Adolescent Therapy;Cognitive Behavioral
    Therapy;Parent-Child Interaction

SIKES, Melvin P.
8703 Point West Drive
Austin, TX 78759-7336
(512) 345-2045-**B**
Ethnicity: African-American/Black
Degree and Year: PhD 1950
Major Field: Clinical Psychology
Specialty: Group Psychotherapy

SIKKA, Anjoo
University of Houston - Downtown
One Main Street
Houston, TX 77002
(713) 221-8156-**B**, (713) 880-2524-**H**, (713) 226-5234-**F**
sikka@uh.dt.edu
Ethnicity: Asian-American/Asian/Pacific Islander
Languages: Hindi
Degree and Year: PhD 1991
Major Field: Educational Psychology
Specialty: Educational Psychology;Ethnic Minorities;Adolescent
    Development;Creativity;Attitudes & Opinions;Assessment/
    Diagnosis/Evaluation

SILLING, S. Marc
The University of Akron
Coordinator of Testing
Psychologist (OH #3261)
Akron, OH 44325-4303
(330) 972-7085-**B**, (330) 633-3465-**H**, (330) 972-5679-**F**
msilling@akron.edu
Ethnicity: American Indian/Alaska Native
Degree and Year: PhD 1981
Major Field: Counseling Psychology
Specialty: Alcoholism & Alcohol Abuse;Assessment/Diagnosis/
    Evaluation;Computer Applications and Programming

SILVA, Santiago
University of Texas, Pan American
1201 West University Drive
STUS. Room 618
Edinburg, TX 78539
(956) 381-2585-**B**, (956) 664-1428-**H**, (956) 316-7015-**F**

Ethnicity: Hispanic/Latino
Languages: Spanish
Degree and Year: PhD 1991
Major Field: Counseling Psychology
Specialty: HIV/AIDS;Marriage & Family;Lesbian & Gay Issuues

SIMMS PUIG, Jan
Puig Associates, P.A.
1060 Kings Highway North
Suite 314
Cherry Hill, NJ 08034
(609) 482-7755-**B**, (609) 983-4132-**H**, (609) 779-2705-**F**
wtmg66a@prodigy.com
Ethnicity: African-American/Black
Degree and Year: EdD 1976
Major Field: School Psychology
Specialty: Family Therapy;Special Education

SIMPSON, Adelaide W.
4110 Hillcrest Road
Richmond, VA 23225
(804) 273-1760-**B**, (804) 233-2098-**H**
asimp1007@aol.com
Ethnicity: African-American/Black
Degree and Year: PhD 1983
Major Field: Clinical Psychology
Specialty: Psychotherapy;Clinical Child Psychology;Ethnic
Minorities;Stress;Affective Disorders

SIMS-PATTERSON, Sandra
Spelman College
Psychology Department
P.O. Box 353
Atlanta, GA 30314-0353
(404) 222-8350-**B**, (404) 691-8350-**H**
Ethnicity: African-American/Black
Degree and Year: PhD 19
Major Field: Developmental Psychology

SINGG, Sangeeta
3318 Grandview
San Angelo, TX 76904
(915) 942-2208-**B**, (915) 944-0273-**H**
Ethnicity: Asian-American/Asian/Pacific Islander
Languages: Hindi, Urdu, Punjabi
Degree and Year: PhD 1981
Major Field: Educational Psychology
Specialty: Counseling Psychology;Group Psychotherapy;Individual
Psychotherapy;Family Therapy;Psychopathology

SINGH, Darshan
10763 Elmcrest Drive
Clive, IA 50325-6657
(515) 242-7714-**B**, (515) 225-8254-**H**, (515) 223-8993-**F**
gnoodine@ins.net
Ethnicity: Asian-American/Asian/Pacific Islander
Languages: Hindi, Urdu, Punjabi
Degree and Year: EdD 1986
Major Field: School Psychology
Specialty: Cross Cultural Processes;Educational Psychology;Ethnic
Minorities;School Psychology;Child Development;Counseling
Psychology

SINGH, Nirbhay N.
Medical College of Virginia
P.O. Box 489
Richmond, VA 23075-0489
(804) 786-4393-**B**
Ethnicity: Asian-American/Asian/Pacific Islander
Degree and Year: PhD 1979
Major Field: Psychopharmacology

SINGH, R. K. Janmeha
1172 Moccasin Court
Clayton, CA 94517-1245
(510) 825-1793-**B**, (510) 947-3867-**H**
Ethnicity: Asian-American/Asian/Pacific Islander
Languages: Hindi, Urdu, Punjabi
Degree and Year: PhD 1965
Major Field: Clinical Psychology

SINGH, Ramadhar
National University of Singapore
Dept Of Psychol & Soc Wrk
10 Kent Ridge Crescent
Singapore 392,
SINGAPORE
(011) 65874350-**B**, (011) 65872931-**H**
swksingh@leonis.nus.edu.sg
Ethnicity: Asian-American/Asian/Pacific Islander
Languages: Hindi
Degree and Year: PhD 1973
Major Field: Social Psychology
Specialty: Industrial/Organizational Psychology;Personality
Psychology;Developmental Psychology

SINGH, Silvija S.
6533 Darlington Road
Pittsburgh, PA 15217-1839
(412) 422-7227-**B**, (412) 421-3715-**H**
Ethnicity: Asian-American/Asian/Pacific Islander
Languages: French
Degree and Year: PhD 1987
Major Field: Clinical Psychology
Specialty: Creativity;Ethnic Minorities;Psychology of Women;Sex/
Marital Therapy;Group Psychotherapy

SINGLETON, Edward G.
Mayatech Corporation
8737 Colesville Road
Sixth Floor
Silver Spring, MD 20910
(301) 587-1600-**B**, (410) 744-0963-**H**, (410) 744-4604-**F**
edward@mayatech.com
Ethnicity: African-American/Black
Degree and Year: PhD 1985 MA 1982
Major Field: Personality Psychology
Specialty: Drug Abuse;Alcoholism & Alcohol Abuse;Assessment/
Diagnosis/Evaluation;Research Design & Methodology;Training &
Development;Research & Training

SINHA, Birendra
University of Alberta
Department of Psychology
8 Whitemud Place
Edmonton, AB T6H5X4
CANADA

Ethnicity: Asian-American/Asian/Pacific Islander
Degree and Year: PhD 1966
Major Field: unknown
Specialty: **Biofeedback**
SINHA, Sachchida
Rajasthan University
E-42, Sector-13
Malaviya Nagar
Jaipur ,Rajasthan, 302017
INDIA
00910141-552644-**H**, 0091-141-41763-**F**
Ethnicity: Asian-American/Asian/Pacific Islander
Languages: Hindi
Degree and Year: PhD 1964
Major Field: Environmental Psychology
Specialty: Behavior Genetics;Clinical Neuropsychology;Experimental
Psychology;Human Ecology;Neuropsychology;Neurosciences

SISON, Cecile E.
VA Hudson Valley Health Care System
Route 9A
PO Box 100
Montrose, NY 10548
(914) 737-4400-**B**, (914) 739-9416-**H**, (914) 734-7002-**F**
sison.cecile@montrose.va.gov
Ethnicity: Asian-American/Asian/Pacific Islander
Languages: Filipino
Degree and Year: PhD 1991
Major Field: Clinical Psychology
Specialty: Gerontology/
Geropsychology;Schizophrenia;Emotion;Clinical Research

SITHARTHAN, Thiagarajan
7 Roselea Way
nsw, 2118 040-,
AUSTRALIA
02-5167412-**B**, 02-8713981-**H**
Ethnicity: Asian-American/Asian/Pacific Islander
Languages: Tamil
Degree and Year: MPs 1985
Major Field: Clinical Psychology
Specialty: Alcoholism & Alcohol Abuse;Behavior Therapy;Clinical
Psychology;Cognitive Behavioral Therapy;Health Psychology

SLAUGHTER-DEFOE, Diana T.
University of Pennsylvania
3700 Walnut Street
Graduate School of Education
Human Develop. & Social Policy Program
Philadelphia, PA 19104-6216
(215) 573-3947-**B**, (212) 563-2151-**H**, (212) 898-4399-**F**
dianad@gsu.upenn.edu
Ethnicity: African-American/Black
Degree and Year: PhD 1968
Major Field: Developmental Psychology
Specialty: Child Development;Disadvantaged;Parent Education;Parent-
Child Interaction;Human Development & Family Studies

SLOAN, R. Lloyd
Howard University
Psychology Department

525 Bryant Street, NW
Washington, DC 20001-2326
(202) 636-6805-**B**
Ethnicity: Hispanic/Latino
Degree and Year: PhD 1972
Major Field: Social Psychology
Specialty: Attitudes & Opinions;Interpersonal Processes & Relations

SMEDLEY, Joseph W.
The Consulting Services Group, International
1464 North Central Avenue
Indianapolis, IN 46202
(317) 278-4586-**B**, (317) 630-4973-**H**, (317) 238-9676-**F**
jl_smedley@msn.com
Ethnicity: African-American/Black
Degree and Year: PhD 1983
Major Field: Industrial/Organizational Psy.
Specialty: Training & Development;Organizational
Development;Industrial/Organizational Psychology;Cultural & Social
Processes;Management & Organization;Cross Cultural Processes

SMITH, JR., Theodore R.
Psychological Assessment and
    Treatment Center
5038 San Juan Avenue
Jacksonville, FL 32210
(904) 384-1036-**B**, (904) 384-1036-**F**
Ethnicity: African-American/Black
Degree and Year: PsyD 1982
Major Field: Clinical Psychology
Specialty: Clinical Psychology;Cognitive Psychology;Hypnosis/
    Hypnotherapy;Gerontology/Geropsychology;Clinical
    Neuropsychology;Stress

SMITH, Althea
57 Cameron Avenue
Somerville, MA 02144-2430
(617) 876-9257-**B**
Ethnicity: African-American/Black
Degree and Year: PhD 1978
Major Field: Social Psychology
Specialty: Psychology of Women

SMITH, Alvin E.
422 Pacific Street
Brooklyn, NY 11217
(718) 221-7376-**B**, (718) 855-6082-**H**
Ethnicity: African-American/Black
Degree and Year: PhD 1984
Major Field: Clinical Psychology
Specialty: Adolescent Therapy;Community Mental Health;Group
    Psychotherapy;Family Therapy;Homelessness & Homeless
    Populations

SMITH, Benjamin
3504 Sequoia Avenue
Baltimore, MD 21215-7211
(301) 367-7541-**B**
Ethnicity: African-American/Black
Degree and Year: PhD 1951
Major Field: Educational Psychology
Specialty: Educational Research

SMITH, Carol Y.
C.Y. Smith & Associates, Inc., D.B.A. The
Samuel Center for Psychology Services
4465 North Oakland Avenue
Shorewood, WI 53211
(414) 962-9351-**B**, (414) 354-4972-**H**, (414) 354-3621-**F**
drcymith@compuserve.com
Ethnicity: African-American/Black
Languages: Spanish
Degree and Year: PhD 1984
Major Field: Clinical Psychology

SMITH, Charles E.
1320 W Locust Avenue
Lompoc, CA 93436-7503
Ethnicity: African-American/Black
Degree and Year: PhD 1985
Major Field: Clinical Psychology

SMITH, Cherryl R.
1721 Irving St. NW
Washington, DC 20010
(301) 699-3744-**B**, (202) 265-9895-**H**
Ethnicity: African-American/Black
Degree and Year: PhD 1978
Major Field: Clinical Psychology
Specialty: Adolescent Therapy;Attention Deficit
Disorders;Assessment/Diagnosis/Evaluation;Child
Therapy;Clinical Child Psychology

SMITH, Iola R.
11216 Green Dragon Court
Hobbits Glen
Columbia, MD 21044-1025
Ethnicity: African-American/Black
Degree and Year: PhD 1966
Major Field: Educational Psychology

SMITH, Michael C.
Smith & Cemerihs
210 West 22nd Street
Suite 119
Oak Brook, IL 60523
(630) 574-9084-**B**, (630) 834-9338-**H**, (630) 782-6069-**F**
Ethnicity: Asian-American/Asian/Pacific Islander
Degree and Year: PhD 1992
Major Field: Clinical Psychology
Specialty: Clinical Child Psychology;Forensic Psychology;Medical
Psychology;Cognitive Behavioral Therapy;Marriage &
Family;Cross Cultural Processes

SMITH, Teresa D.
2008 Kanawha Blvd., East
Charleston, WV 25311-2204
(304) 344-0349-**B**
Ethnicity: Asian-American/Asian/Pacific Islander
Degree and Year: PhD 1974
Major Field: Clinical Psychology
Specialty: Biofeedback

SMITH, Walanda W.
Children's Rehabilitative Services

124 West Thomas Road
Phoenix, AZ 85013
(602) 406-4098-**B**, (602) 406-7166-**F**
Ethnicity: African-American/Black
Degree and Year: PhD 1996 MA 1983
Major Field: Clinical Psychology
Specialty: Clinical Psychology;Mentally Retarded;Child & Pediatric
Psychology

SMITH, William
235 West Macarthur Blvd.
Suite #401
Oakland, CA 94611
(510) 653-6456-**B**, (510) 653-6456-**F**
Ethnicity: African-American/Black
Degree and Year: PhD 1979
Major Field: Clinical Psychology
Specialty: Child Therapy;Forensic
Psychology;Psychotherapy;Projective Techniques

SMITH, William F.
1401 12th Avenue, South
St. Petersberg, FL 33705-2309
Ethnicity: African-American/Black
Degree and Year: PhD 1979
Major Field: Clinical Psychology
Specialty: Clinical Psychology

SNOWDEN, Lonnie R.
1090 Warfield Avenue
Oakland, CA 94610-1612
(510) 642-1252-**B**, 510 452-2125-**H**, (510) 643-6126-**F**
Ethnicity: African-American/Black
Degree and Year: PhD 1975
Major Field: Clinical Psychology

SOBRINO, James F.
231 W 20th Street
New York, NY 10011
(212) 795-0860-**B**, (212) 929-6042-**H**
Ethnicity: Hispanic/Latino
Languages: Spanish
Degree and Year: PhD 1965
Major Field: Clinical Psychology
Specialty: Individual Psychotherapy;Group
Psychotherapy;Community Mental
Health;Administration;Sex/Marital Therapy

SODOWSKY, Gargi R.
University of Nebraska
Dept. of Educational Psychology
118 Bancroft Hall
Lincoln, NE 68588-0345
(402) 472-2245-**B**, (402) 489-2017-**H**
Ethnicity: Asian-American/Asian/Pacific Islander
Languages: French, Hindi, Bengali,Marathi
Degree and Year: PhD 1988
Major Field: Counseling Psychology
Specialty: Ethnic Minorities;Cross Cultural Processes;Gender
Issues;Measurement;Personality Measurement

SOFTAS, Basilia C.
University Northern Colorado

Division of Professional Psychology
Counseling Psychology
McKee Hall 248
Greeley, CO 80639-0001
(970) 351-1631-**B**
Ethnicity: Hispanic/Latino
Degree and Year: PhD 1984
Major Field: unknown
Specialty: Family Therapy

SOLER, Robin E
1310 Carriage Place Court
Decatur, GA 30033
(404) 298-1980-**H**
robinsoler@um.cc.umich.edu
Ethnicity: Hispanic/Latino
Degree and Year: PhD 1994
Major Field: Developmental Psychology
Specialty: Ethnic Minorities;Stress;Human Development & Family
Studies

SOLOMON, Sondra E.
University of Vermont
Department of Psychology
John Dewey Hall
Burlington, VT 05401
(802) 656-3034-**B**, (802) 893-9978-**H**, (802) 656-8783-**F**
sondrasolomon@uvm.edu
Ethnicity: African-American/Black
Degree and Year: PhD 1994
Major Field: Clinical Psychology
Specialty: Clinical Psychology;Cultural & Social Processes

SOMERVILLE, Addison W.
California State University
Department of Psychology
6000 J. Street
Sacramento, CA 95819-6007
(916) 383-7145-**B**, (916) 383-8366-**H**, (916) 388-0826-**F**
awsomer101@aol.com
Ethnicity: African-American/Black, American Indian/Alaska Native
Degree and Year: PhD 1963
Major Field: Developmental Psychology
Specialty: Developmental Psychology;Ethnic Minorities;Parent-Child
Interaction;Psychopathology;Psychotherapy;Sex/Marital
Therapy

SOMJEE, Lubna
Yale-School of Medicine
Yale Psychiatric Institute
184 Liberty Street
New Haven, CT 06520
(203) 737-2762-**B**, (203) 772-3673-**H**, (203) 785-7855-**F**
lsomjee@aol.com
Ethnicity: Asian-American/Asian/Pacific Islander
Languages: Urdu
Degree and Year: PhD 1999
Major Field: Clinical Psychology
Specialty: Clinical Psychology

SOMODEVILLA, S. A.
8500 Stemmons Freeway
Suite #6025, LB 47

Dallas, TX 75247
(214) 905-4308-**B**, (214) 343-4035-**H**
Ethnicity: Hispanic/Latino
Languages: Spanish
Degree and Year: PhD 1971
Major Field: Clinical Psychology
Specialty: Assessment/Diagnosis/Evaluation;Clinical
Psychology;Industrial/Organizational
Psychology;Psychotherapy;Stress

SOMWARU, Jwalla P.
Minneapolis Department
of Education
550 Cedar Street
St. Paul, MN 55101-2233
Ethnicity: Asian-American/Asian/Pacific Islander
Degree and Year: EdD 1967
Major Field: unknown
Specialty: Clinical Psychology

SONNEBORN, Dean R.
3535 Old Mountainview Drive
Lafayette, CA 94549-4918
(415) 284-5838-**B**
Ethnicity: Hispanic/Latino
Degree and Year: MA 1979
Major Field: unknown
Specialty: Community Mental Health

SORIANO, Fernando I.
8522 Neva Avenue
San Diego, CA 92123
619 594-3640-**B**, (619) 569-8900-**H**, 619 495-7704-**F**
fsoriano@sunstroke.sdsu.edu
Ethnicity: Hispanic/Latino
Languages: Spanish
Degree and Year: PhD 1987
Major Field: Social Psychology
Specialty: Social Behavior;Aggression;Family Processes;Crime &
Criminal Behavior;Social Behavior

SORIANO, Marcel
California State University, Los Angeles
5151 State University Drive
KHC1065
Los Angeles, CA 90032-4226
(213) 343-4255-**B**, (909) 483-2415-**H**, (213) 343-4252-**F**
msorian@calstatela.edu
Ethnicity: Hispanic/Latino
Languages: Spanish
Degree and Year: PhD 1984
Major Field: Counseling Psychology
Specialty: Counseling Psychology;Special Education

SOSA, Juan N.
715 E Idaho
Las Cruces, NM 88001
(505) 523-0482-**B**, (505) 522-8154-**H**
Ethnicity: Hispanic/Latino
Languages: Spanish
Degree and Year: PhD 1974
Major Field: Clinical Psychology

SOTO, Elaine
17 Revolutionary Road

Cortlandt Manor, NY 10567
(212) 679-9442-**B**
delsoto@bestweb.net
Ethnicity: Hispanic/Latino
Languages: Spanish
Degree and Year: PhD 1979 EdM 1973
Major Field: Clinical Psychology

SOTO, George M.
106 Kenilworth Street
Philadelphia, PA 19147-3410
(215) 925-7828-**H**
Ethnicity: Hispanic/Latino
Degree and Year: MA/M 1982
Major Field: Counseling Psychology

SOTO, Tomas A.
3301 North Seeley Street
Chicago, IL 60618
(773) 404-9084-**B**, (312) 633-3002-**F**
tsoto567@aol.com
Ethnicity: Hispanic/Latino
Languages: Spanish
Degree and Year: PhD 1991
Major Field: Clinical Psychology
Specialty: Lesbian & Gay Issuues;HIV/AIDS;Program
Evaluation;Individual Psychotherapy;Drug Abuse

SOUTHERLAND, Deborah L.
Dayton Correctional Institution
4104 Germantown Street
Dayton, OH 45408
(937) 263-0060-**B**, (937) 263-6721-**F**
Ethnicity: African-American/Black
Degree and Year: PhD 1987
Major Field: Clinical Psychology
Specialty: Assessment/Diagnosis/Evaluation;Forensic
Psychology;Clinical Psychology;Adult Development

SOZA, Anthony M.
8618 Sepulveda Blvd
330
Los Angeles, CA 90045-4005
(310) 338-1301-**B**
Ethnicity: Hispanic/Latino
Degree and Year: PhD 1992
Major Field: Clinical Psychology
Specialty: Family Therapy;Adolescent Therapy;Social Skills;Parent-
Child Interaction;Individual Psychotherapy

SPEIGHT, Suzette L.
Loyola University Chicago
1041 Ridge Road
Wilmette, IL 60091
(847) 853-3348-**B**, (847) 853-3375-**F**
sspeigh@luc.edu
Ethnicity: African-American/Black
Degree and Year: PhD 1990
Major Field: Counseling Psychology
Specialty: Ethnic Minorities;Training & Development;Cultural & Social
Processes;Prevention

SPENCER, Margaret B.
University of Pennsylvania
Graduate School of Education
3700 Walnut Street

Philadelphia, PA 19104-6216
(215) 898-1945-**B**, (215) 573-3893-**F**
marges@gse.upenn.edu
Ethnicity: African-American/Black
Degree and Year: PhD 1976
Major Field: Developmental Psychology
Specialty: Human Development & Family Studies;Adolescent
Development;Cultural & Social Processes;Child
Development;Ethnic Minorities;Developmental Psychology

SPIDELL HELMS, Dorothy J.
New Center Community Mental Health Center
2051 West Grand Boulevard
Detroit, MI 48208
(313) 961-3200-**B**, (313) 869-2703-**H**
dolary@aol.com
Ethnicity: African-American/Black
Degree and Year: MA 1992
Major Field: Clinical Psychology
Specialty: Clinical Psychology;Domestic Violence;HIV/
AIDS;Chronically Mentally Ill;Forensic Psychology;Individual
Psychotherapy

SPIVEY, Philop B.
140 Riverside Drive
Suite 1A
New York, NY 10024
(212) 873-4803-**B**, (212) 664-8803-**F**
Ethnicity: African-American/Black
Degree and Year: PhD 1984
Major Field: Clinical Psychology
Specialty: Alcoholism & Alcohol Abuse;Ethnic Minorities;HIV/
AIDS;Drug Abuse;Lesbian & Gay Issuues

SPRAINGS, Violet E.
89 Moraga Way
Orinda, CA 94563-3543
(510) 253-1906-**B**, (510) 254-4621-**H**, (510) 253-1595-**F**
Ethnicity: African-American/Black
Degree and Year: PhD 1982
Major Field: Educational Psychology
Specialty: Assessment/Diagnosis/
Evaluation;Neuropsychology;Intelligence;Juvenile
Delinquency;Learning Disabilities

SPROUSE, Agnes A.
289 Bilmar Place
Englewood, NJ 07631
(718) 681-6538-**B**, (201) 816-1306-**H**
Ethnicity: African-American/Black
Degree and Year: PhD 1988
Major Field: School Psychology
Specialty: Assessment/Diagnosis/Evaluation;Developmental
Psychology;Learning/Learning Theory;Rational-Emotive
Therapy

SRINIVASAN, Sampurna
Comprehensive Care Center
201 Mechanic Street
Lexington, KY 40507-1004
(606)233-0444-**B**, 606/224-8411-**H**, 606/281-2114-**F**
Ethnicity: Asian-American/Asian/Pacific Islander
Languages: Hindi, Tamil
Degree and Year: PhD 1978
Major Field: Clinical Psychology

Specialty: Assessment/Diagnosis/Evaluation;Clinical
Psychology;Community Mental Health;Chronically Mentally
Ill;Cognitive Behavioral Therapy;Depression

SRIVASTVA, Suresh
Case Western Reserve University
Dept. of Organizational Behavior
Sears Library Building
Cleveland, OH 44106
(216) 368-2128-**B**, (216) 932-0737-**H**
Ethnicity: Asian-American/Asian/Pacific Islander
Degree and Year: PhD 1960
Major Field: unknown
Specialty: Organizational Development

ST. LEGER, Sidney C.
Substance Abuse Treatment Prog.
Bobby E. Wright Comp.
Community Mental Health
9 South Kedzte Avenue
Chicago, IL 60612
(312) 722-7900-**B**, (312) 487-8541-**H**, (312) 722-0644-**F**
Ethnicity: African-American/Black
Degree and Year: PhD 1993
Major Field: Clinical Psychology
Specialty: Individual Psychotherapy;Alcoholism & Alcohol
Abuse;Drug Abuse;Assessment/Diagnosis/Evaluation;Mental
Health Services

STALLWORTH, Lisa M.
University of Massachusetts
Department of Psychology
Tobin Hall
Amherst, MA 01003
(413) 545-0049-**B**, (413) 545-0996-**F**
stallworth@psychumass.edu
Ethnicity: African-American/Black
Degree and Year: PhD 1975
Major Field: Social Psychology
Specialty: Group Processes;Social Cognition;Experimental
Psychology;Social Psychology;Psycholinguistic

STARKS-WILLIAMS, Mary L.
1301 Joliet
Detroit, MI 48207-2833
(313) 393-9603-**H**
Ethnicity: African-American/Black
Degree and Year: PhD 1974
Major Field: School Psychology
Specialty: School Psychology;Educational Psychology

STASSON, Mark F.
Virginia Commonwealth University
Department of Psychology
808 West Franklin Street
Box 842018
Richmond, VA 23284-2018
(804) 828-6330-**B**, *804) 754-3445-**H**
Ethnicity: Hispanic/Latino
Degree and Year: PhD 1989 MA 1987
Major Field: Social Psychology
Specialty: Social Psychology;Group Processes;Attitudes &
Opinions;Quantitative/Mathematical, Psychometrics

STEELE, Marilyn
Consulting and Clinical Services
1220 S. Sierra Bonita Avenue
Los Angeles, CA 90019
(323) 936-0343-**B**, (323) 936-0343-**H**
dr_mls@earthlink.net
Ethnicity: African-American/Black
Degree and Year: PhD 1986
Major Field: Clinical Child Psychology
Specialty: Parent Education;Child Development;Program
Evaluation;Prevention;Research & Training;Cultural & Social
Processes

STEELE, Robert E.
University of Maryland
College of Behavioral & Social Sciences
2141 Tydings Hall
College Park, MD 20742-7200
(301) 405-0161-**B**
Ethnicity: African-American/Black
Degree and Year: PhD 1975
Major Field: Community Psychology
Specialty: Community Mental Health

STEPHENS, Dorothy W.
The Rehabilitation Center
3701 Bellemenda Avenue
Evansville, IN 47714-0161
(812) 479-1411-**B**
Ethnicity: Asian-American/Asian/Pacific Islander
Languages: Chinese
Degree and Year: PhD 1974
Major Field: Clinical Psychology
Specialty: Attention Deficit Disorders;Autism;Physically
Handicapped;Learning Disabilities

STERLING, Sharon E.
96 Chadbourne Road
Rochester, NY 14618-1136
(716) 723-7750-**B**
Ethnicity: Asian-American/Asian/Pacific Islander
Degree and Year: PhD 1986
Major Field: Clinical Psychology

STERN, Marilyn
SUNY Albany
Dept. of Counseling Psychology
Educ 220
1400 Washington Avenue
Albany, NY 12222-0100
(518) 442-5039-**B**, (518) 442-4953-**F**
ms127@cnsvax.albany.edu
Ethnicity: Hispanic/Latino
Degree and Year: PhD 1984
Major Field: Counseling Psychology
Specialty: Health Psychology

STEVENSON, JR., Edward E.
137 Putnam Avenue
Freeport, NY 11520-1151
(718) 262-2693-**B**, (516) 868-2583-**H**
Ethnicity: African-American/Black
Degree and Year: PhD 1974

Major Field: Clinical Psychology
Specialty: Clinical Child Psychology;Clinical Psychology;Community Mental Health;Stress;Training & Development

STEWART, Arleen R.
2595 Mission Suite 311
San Francisco, CA 94110
(415)-550-8400-**B**
Ethnicity: Hispanic/Latino
Languages: Spanish
Degree and Year: PhD 1973
Major Field: Clinical Psychology
Specialty: Individual Psychotherapy;Cross Cultural Processes;Ethnic Minorities;Organizational Development;Clinical Child Psychology;Community Psychology

STEWART, G. Keith
407 Arcadia Place
San Antonio, TX 78209-5920
Ethnicity: American Indian/Alaska Native
Degree and Year: EdD 1973
Major Field: Clinical Psychology

STEWART, Sunita M.
C/O Jones, Day
PO Box 660623
Dallas, TX 75266-0623
(852) 2819-2821-**B**, (852) 2810-6009-**H**, (852) 2855-9528-**F**
smstewar@hkucc.hku.hk
Ethnicity: Asian-American/Asian/Pacific Islander
Languages: Urdu
Degree and Year: PhD 1981
Major Field: Clinical Psychology
Specialty: Cross Cultural Processes;Adolescent Development;Depression;Child & Pediatric Psychology;Clinical Child Psychology;Health Psychology

STEWART, Vlenaetha
4015 Kimberly Woods Drive
Flint, MI 48504-1140
(313) 760-1022-**B**
Ethnicity: African-American/Black
Degree and Year: PhD 1983
Major Field: Clinical Psychology
Specialty: Special Education;Assessment/Diagnosis/Evaluation;Child & Pediatric Psychology;Psychotherapy;Sports Psychology

STOKES, Devon R.
St. Peter Hospital
Behavioral Science
Family Practice Resident
525 Lily Road, NE
Olympia, WA 98506-6905
(206) 493-7230-**B**, (360) 438-0686-**H**, (206) 493-4071-**F**
stokesd@psph.providence.org
Ethnicity: African-American/Black
Degree and Year: PhD 1983
Major Field: Clinical Psychology
Specialty: Medical Psychology;Training & Development;Family Therapy;Psychotherapy;Cross Cultural Processes

STONE, G. Vaughn
Wisconsin Department of Corrections
Seven Lincoln Avenue
Waupun, WI 53963
(920) 324-5577-**B**, (920) 324-3083-**H**

Ethnicity: American Indian/Alaska Native
Degree and Year: PhD 1970
Major Field: Counseling Psychology
Specialty: Clinical Psychology;Counseling Psychology;Pain & Pain Management;Correctional Psychology;Medical Psychology;Psychotherapy

STONE, Lynn J.
Unites States Air Force
PO Box 514
USAFA, CO 80840-0514
(719) 333-2987-**B**
Ethnicity: African-American/Black
Degree and Year: PhD 1994 MA 1991
Major Field: Quan/Math & Psychometrics/Stat
Specialty: Counseling Psychology;Program Evaluation;Psychometrics

STRICKLAND, Tony L
C.R. Drew University of Medicine &
Science, Biobehavioral Research Center
& Laboratory, Department of Psychiatry
1621 East 120th Street, Mail Point 19-B
Los Angeles, CA 90059
(213) 563-5915-**B**, (310) 673-3765-**F**
tstrick@ucla.edu
Ethnicity: African-American/Black
Degree and Year: PhD 1986
Major Field: Clinical Psychology
Specialty: Neuropsychology;Psychobiology;Drug Abuse;Psychopharmacology;Clinical Neuropsychology;Gerontology/Geropsychology

STRINGER, Anthony Y.
Emory University
Center for Rehabilitation Medicine
1441 Clifton Road, NE
Atlanta, GA 30088
(404) 712-5567-**B**, (404) 712-5668-**F**
astring@emory.edu
Ethnicity: African-American/Black
Degree and Year: PhD 1984
Major Field: Clinical Psychology
Specialty: Neuropsychology;Neurological Disorders;Clinical Neuropsychology;Brain Damage;Vocational Psychology

STROUD, Barbara
Los Angeles Child Guidance Clinic
3787 South Vermont Avenue
Los Angeles, CA 90007
(213) 766-2360-**B**, (213) 766-2350-**F**
Ethnicity: African-American/Black
Degree and Year: PhD 1992
Major Field: Clinical Child Psychology
Specialty: Special Education;Adolescent Therapy;Child Development;School Counseling;Group Psychotherapy;Child Therapy

SUAREZ-BALCAZAR, Yolanda
Loyola University Chicago
6525 North Sheridan
Chicago, IL 60626
ysuarez@wpo.luc.edu
Ethnicity: Hispanic/Latino
Languages: Spanish
Degree and Year: PhD 1987

Major Field: Community Psychology
Specialty: Community Psychology;Disadvantaged;Ethnic
Minorities;Program Evaluation;Social Change;Prevention

SUAREZ-CROWE, Yolanda
Jacksonville State University
Psychology Department
700 Pelham Road North
Jacksonville, AL 36265
(205) 782-5808-**B**, (205) 435-3337-**H**
Ethnicity: Hispanic/Latino
Languages: Spanish
Degree and Year: PhD 1975
Major Field: Clinical Psychology
Specialty: Behavior Therapy;Clinical
Research;Psychopathology;Applied Behavior
Analysis;Affective Disorders

SUAREZ, Alejandra
45th Street Clinic
1629 North 45th Street
Seattle, WA 98103
(206) 633-3350-**B**, (206) 525-3253-**H**, (206) 623-3113-**F**
aleja@u.washington.edu
Ethnicity: Hispanic/Latino
Languages: Spanish, Esperanto
Degree and Year: PhD 1986
Major Field: Clinical Psychology
Specialty: Adult Development;Mental Health Services;Ethnic
Minorities;Emotional Development

SUAREZ, Carlota
68 Montague
Brooklyn, NY 11201
(718) 951-5931-**B**
Ethnicity: Hispanic/Latino
Languages: Spanish
Degree and Year: PhD 1972
Major Field: Clinical Psychology
Specialty: Clinical Psychology;Clinical Child Psychology

SUAREZ, Enrique M.
1450 Madruga Avenue, Suite 205
Coral Gables, FL 33146
(305) 667-4101-**B**, (305) 661-7222-**F**
Ethnicity: Hispanic/Latino
Degree and Year: PhD 1974 MA 1973
Major Field: Experimental Psychology
Specialty: Psychotherapy;Industrial/Organizational Psychology;Clinical
Psychology

SUAREZ, Miguel G.
31 Woodland St #1-r
Hartford, CT 06105
(203) 278-9090-**B**, (203) 724-1103-**H**
Ethnicity: Hispanic/Latino
Degree and Year: PhD 1983
Major Field: unknown
Specialty: Neuropsychology;Rehabilitation

SUAREZ, Susan D.
The Sage Colleges
140 New Scotland Avenue

Albany, NY 12208
(518) 445-1746-**B**, (518) 283-4641-**H**
Ethnicity: Hispanic/Latino
Degree and Year: PhD 1982
Major Field: Comparative Psychology
Specialty: Comparative Psychology;Psychobiology;Physiological
Psychology;Experimental Psychology;Developmental
Psychology

SUDEVAN, Padmanbhan
University of Wisconsin
Department of Psychology
Stevens Point, WI 54481
(715) 346-3960-**B**, (715) 342-1921-**H**
psudevan@uwsp.edu
Ethnicity: Asian-American/Asian/Pacific Islander
Languages: French, Hindi, Malayalam, Tamil
Degree and Year: PhD 1981
Major Field: Cognitive Psychology
Specialty: Information Processing;Memory;Computer Applications and
Programming;Quantitative/Mathematical, Psychometrics

SUE, David
Western Washington University
Department of Psychology
Bellingham, WA 98225
(206) 650-3573-**B**, (206) 671-6033-**H**
Ethnicity: Asian-American/Asian/Pacific Islander
Degree and Year: PhD 1973
Major Field: Clinical Psychology
Specialty: Cross Cultural Processes;Counseling
Psychology;Psychotherapy;Group Psychotherapy;Mental
Disorders

SUE, Derald W.
California School of Professional Psych.
1005 Atlantic Avenue
Alameda, CA 94501-1148
(510) 523-2300-**B**
dsue@haywire.csuhayward.edu
Ethnicity: Asian-American/Asian/Pacific Islander
Degree and Year: PhD 1969
Major Field: Counseling Psychology
Specialty: Counseling Psychology;Cross Cultural Processes;Deviant
Behavior;Ethnic Minorities;Communication

SUE, Stanley
University of California
Department of Psychology
Davis, CA 95616
(530) 754-6173-**B**, (925) 932-0839-**H**, (530) 752-2087-**F**
ssue@ucdavis.edu
Ethnicity: Asian-American/Asian/Pacific Islander
Languages: Chinese
Degree and Year: PhD 1971
Major Field: Clinical Psychology
Specialty: Ethnic Minorities;Mental Health
Services;Psychotherapy;Community Psychology;Cultural &
Social Processes

SUGAI, Don P.
Lahey Clinic
41 Mall Road
Department of Psychiatry
Burlington, MA 01805

(781) 233-8925-**B**, (978) 456-3387-**H**, (781) 273-9235-**F**
don.p.sugai@lahey.hitchcock.og
Ethnicity: Asian-American/Asian/Pacific Islander
Degree and Year: PhD 1978
Major Field: Clinical Child Psychology
Specialty: Adolescent Therapy;Child Therapy;Assessment/Diagnosis/
Evaluation;Behavior Therapy

SUGAWARA, Hazuki M.
Nihon Keizai Shimbun, Inc.
1-9-5 Otemachi
Chiyoda-Ku
Tokyo,
JAPAN
81-3-5562-6540-**F**
vyv02471@niftyserve.org.jp
Ethnicity: Asian-American/Asian/Pacific Islander
Languages: Japanese
Degree and Year: PhD 1994
Major Field: Quan/Math & Psychometrics/Stat
Specialty: Quantitative/Mathematical, Psychometrics;Industrial/
Organizational Psychology

SUINN, Richard M.
Colorado State University
Department of Psychology
Fort Collins, CO 80523
(970) 491-1351-**B**, (970) 484-4829-**H**, (970) 491-6408-**F**
suin@lamar.colostate.edu
Ethnicity: Asian-American/Asian/Pacific Islander
Degree and Year: PhD 1959
Major Field: Clinical Psychology
Specialty: Behavior Therapy;Sports
Psychology;Administration;Counseling Psychology

SUNDARARAJAN, Louise Kuen-Wei L.
Rochester Psychiatric Center, New York
691 French Rd
Rochester, NY 14618-5244
(716) 473-3230-**B**, (716) 461-0995-**H**
louisela@frontiernet.net
Ethnicity: Asian-American/Asian/Pacific Islander
Languages: Chinese
Degree and Year: PhD 1980 EdD 1988
Major Field: Counseling Psychology
Specialty: Humanistic Psychology;Schizophrenia;Hypnosis/
Hypnotherapy;Family Therapy;Drug Abuse

SUNG, Yong H.
90 Marywood Trail
Wheaton, IL 60187
(708) 773-6633-**B**, (708) 462-7036-**H**, (708) 773-6949-**F**
Ethnicity: Asian-American/Asian/Pacific Islander
Languages: Korean
Degree and Year: PhD 1975
Major Field: Industrial/Organizational Psy.
Specialty: Management & Organization;Measurement;Decision &
Choice Behavior;Leadership

SUN, Irene L.
7132 Nimrod Dr
Huntington Bch, CA 92647-6222
(714) 770-0855-**B**, (714) 841-7437-**H**

trenesun@aol.com
Ethnicity: Asian-American/Asian/Pacific Islander
Languages: Chinese
Degree and Year: PsyD 1985
Major Field: School Psychology
Specialty: Clinical Child Psychology;Individual
Psychotherapy;Marriage & Family;Child Therapy;Parent-
Child Interaction

SUTTON, David
4305 Callahan Road
Big Spring, TX 79720
(915) 263-7361-**B**, (915) 264-0605-**H**, (915) 728-7834-**F**
Ethnicity: American Indian/Alaska Native
Languages: Spanish
Degree and Year: PhD 1982
Major Field: Counseling Psychology
Specialty: Counseling Psychology;Clinical Psychology;Alcoholism &
Alcohol Abuse;Drug Abuse;Group Psychotherapy

SUTTON, Sharon E.
University of Michigan
College of Architecture and
Urban Planning
Ann Arbor, MI 48109-2069
(313) 936-0201-**B**, (313) 426-2665-**H**, (313) 763-2322-**F**
Ethnicity: African-American/Black
Languages: Spanish
Degree and Year: PhD 1982
Major Field: Environmental Psychology
Specialty: Curriculum Development/Evaluation;Educational
Psychology;Environmental Psychology;Group Processes

SUZUKI, Lisa A.
New York University
239 Green Street - Fourth Floor
Department of Applied Psychology
New York, NY 10003
(212) 998-5575-**B**, (212) 254-2882-**H**, (212) 995-4358-**F**
lasl@is.nyu.edu
Ethnicity: Asian-American/Asian/Pacific Islander
Degree and Year: PhD 1992 MeD 1985
Major Field: Counseling Psychology
Specialty: Assessment/Diagnosis/Evaluation;Cross Cultural Processes

SWANEY, Gyda
Confederated Salish & Kootenai Tribes
Tribal Mental & Addiction Treatment
PO Box 427
St. Ignatius, MT 59865
(406) 745-4363-**B**, (406) 745-4363-**F**
Ethnicity: American Indian/Alaska Native
Degree and Year: PhD 1986
Major Field: Clinical Psychology
Specialty: Alcoholism & Alcohol Abuse;Eating Disorders;Crisis
Intervention & Therapy;Child Abuse;Ethnic Minorities

SWAN, June A.
7152 Breno Place
Alta Loma, CA 91701
(909) 944-4043-**H**
Ethnicity: Asian-American/Asian/Pacific Islander
Languages: Burmese
Degree and Year: PhD 1993

Major Field: Clinical Psychology
Specialty: Group Psychotherapy;Attention Deficit Disorders;Cognitive Behavioral Therapy;Child Therapy;Ethnic Minorities;Parent Education

SWANSTON, Melvon C.
764 South Drive
Baldwin, NY 11510
(718) 221-7607-**B**, (516) 481-3680-**H**
Ethnicity: African-American/Black
Degree and Year: PhD 1982
Major Field: Cognitive Psychology
Specialty: Clinical Psychology;Cognitive Behavioral Therapy;Cultural & Social Processes;Industrial/Organizational Psychology;Behavior Therapy

SY, Michael J.
Southdown
1335 St. John's Sideroad East
Ontario L4G 3G8,
CANADA
(416) 727-7214-**B**, (416) 853-1467-**H**
Ethnicity: Asian-American/Asian/Pacific Islander
Languages: Chinese, Filipino
Degree and Year: PhD 1980
Major Field: Clinical Psychology
Specialty: Alcoholism & Alcohol Abuse;Cardiovascular Processes;Clinical Neuropsychology;Counseling Psychology;Depression

SZAPOCZNIK, Jose
Center for Family Studies
1425 NW 10th Avenue
3rd Floor
Miami, FL 33136
(305) 548-4592-**B**, (305) 443-4408-**H**, (305) 547-5577-**F**
Ethnicity: Hispanic/Latino
Languages: Spanish
Degree and Year: PhD 1977 MS 1973
Major Field: Clinical Psychology
Specialty: Clinical Psychology;Drug Abuse;Ethnic Minorities;Family Therapy;HIV/AIDS

TABACHNIK, Samuel
2955 Shattuck Avenue
Suite #10
Berkeley, CA 94705
(510) 845-3525-**B**, (510) 845-3382-**F**
destz@aol.com
Ethnicity: Hispanic/Latino
Languages: Spanish
Degree and Year: PhD 1985
Major Field: Clinical Psychology
Specialty: Adolescent Therapy;Cross Cultural Processes;Managed Care;Family Therapy;Ethnic Minorities;Military Psychology

TAI, Chun-Nan
1F, 31 Lane 22, Hsien-Yan Rd
Wen-San District
Taipei, 419,
TAIWAN
(011) 886-6-23-**B**, (011) 886-6-23-**H**
Ethnicity: Asian-American/Asian/Pacific Islander

Languages: Chinese
Degree and Year: DMin 1989
Major Field: Counseling Psychology
Specialty: Marriage & Family;Religious Psychology;Consulting Psychology;Clinical Psychology;Educational Psychology

TAKAHASHI, Lorey K.
University of Michigan
Medical School
Department of Psychology
600 Highland Avenue
Madison, WI 53792
(608) 263-6063-**B**, (608) 833-0603-**H**, (608) 263-0265-**F**
Ethnicity: Asian-American/Asian/Pacific Islander
Degree and Year: PhD 1982
Major Field: Physiological Psychology
Specialty: Developmental Psychobiology;Hormones & Behavior;Neurosciences;Psychobiology;Stress

TAKAMINE, Sandra
P.O. Box M
Hakalau, HI 96710
(808) 933-4080-**B**, (808) 963-6762-**H**
Ethnicity: Asian-American/Asian/Pacific Islander
Languages: Japanese
Degree and Year: PhD 1979
Major Field: Clinical Psychology
Specialty: Assessment/Diagnosis/Evaluation;Clinical Child Neuropsychology;Behavior Therapy;Cognitive Behavioral Therapy;Crisis Intervention & Therapy

TAKANISHI, Ruby
Foundation for Child Development
145 East 32nd Street
14th Floor
New York, NY 10010
212/213-8337-**B**, 212/213-5897-**F**
Ethnicity: Asian-American/Asian/Pacific Islander
Degree and Year: PhD 1973 MA 1969
Major Field: Developmental Psychology
Specialty: Adolescent Development;Child Development;Preschool & Day Care Issues;Policy Analysis;Educational Research

TAKEMOTO-CHOCK, Naomi
1978 Komohana Ext.
Hilo, HI 96720
(808) 959-4948-**B**, (808) 959-4948-**H**, (808) 959-4948-**F**
Ethnicity: Asian-American/Asian/Pacific Islander
Degree and Year: PhD 1985
Major Field: Clinical Psychology
Specialty: Cognitive Behavioral Therapy;Ethnic Minorities;Clinical Psychology;Adolescent Therapy;Cross Cultural Processes

TAKUSHI, Ruby Y.
University of Washington
Department of Psychology
Box 351525
Seattle, WA 98108
(206) 616-5765-**B**, (206) 722-8386-**H**, (206) 685-1310-**F**
Ethnicity: Hispanic/Latino
Degree and Year: PhD 1990
Major Field: Clinical Psychology

Specialty: Clinical Psychology;Group Psychotherapy;Alcoholism &
Alcohol Abuse;Drug Abuse

TAMAYO, Federico M. V.
2983 B Gardner LP
Fort Meade, MD 20755-2011
(202) 576-1065-**B**
Ethnicity: Asian-American/Asian/Pacific Islander
Degree and Year: PhD 1975
Major Field: unknown

TAMAYO, Jose M.
JMT Psychological Services
446 S Quincy
Hinsdale, IL 60521-3952
(773) 535-8956-**B**, (630) 325-2381-**H**
Ethnicity: Hispanic/Latino
Languages: French, Spanish
Degree and Year: PhD 1985
Major Field: Educational Psychology
Specialty: School Psychology;Neuropsychology;Assessment/Diagnosis/
Evaluation;Special Education;School Counseling

TAMURA, Leonard J.
Asian/Pacific Development Center
1825 York Street
Denver, CO 80206
(303) 393-0304-**B**, (303) 933-3616-**H**
Ethnicity: Asian-American/Asian/Pacific Islander
Degree and Year: PhD 1991
Major Field: Clinical Psychology
Specialty: Ethnic Minorities;Cross Cultural Processes;Clinical
Psychology;Psychometrics;Religious Psychology

TANA, Joseph
Governors Hospital
227 Madison Street
New York, NY 10002
(718) 597-7467-**H**
Ethnicity: Asian-American/Asian/Pacific Islander
Languages: Chinese
Degree and Year: PhD 1993
Major Field: School Psychology
Specialty: School Psychology;Sleep Disorders;Psychometrics;Mental
Health Services

TANAKA-MATSUMI, Junko
127 Hofstra University
Department of Psychology
Monroe Hall, Room #034
Hempstead, NY 11550
(516) 463-5633-**B**, (516) 678-5695-**H**, (516) 463-6052-**F**
psyjtm@hofstra.edu
Ethnicity: Asian-American/Asian/Pacific Islander
Languages: Japanese
Degree and Year: PhD 1978
Major Field: Clinical Psychology
Specialty: Depression;Emotion;Applied Behavior Analysis;Behavior
Therapy;Cross Cultural Processes

TANAKA, Koji
Okayama University
1-17-1-104
Tsushima-kuwanoki

Okayama 700-0084,
JAPAN
086-251-7721-**B**, 086-256-0656-**H**, 086-256-0656-**F**
tanaka@cc.okyama-u.ac.jp
Ethnicity: Asian-American/Asian/Pacific Islander
Degree and Year: PhD 1987
Major Field: Social Psychology
Specialty: Health Psychology;Interpersonal Processes &
Relations;Social Psychology;Stress;Vocational Psychology

TANAKA, Yasumasa
Gakushuin University 1-5-1 Mejiro
Department of Political Science
Toshima-Ku,
JAPAN
(03)9 86-0221-**B**, (03)5 992-1006-**F**
Ethnicity: Asian-American/Asian/Pacific Islander
Degree and Year: PhD 1963
Major Field: Social Psychology
Specialty: Attitudes & Opinions;Communication

TAN, Gabriel
VA Medical Center
Psychology Service (116B)
2002 Holcombe Boulevard
Houston, TX 77030
(713) 794-7858-**B**, (713) 242-1698-**H**, (713) 794-7835-**F**
tan.gabriel@houston.va.gov
Ethnicity: Asian-American/Asian/Pacific Islander
Languages: Chinese
Degree and Year: PhD 1980
Major Field: Clinical Psychology
Specialty: Pain & Pain Management;Drug Abuse;Biofeedback;Clinical
Neuropsychology;Medical Psychology;Rehabilitation

TANG, Terry
35593 Gleason Lane
Fremont, CA 94536
(408) 432-8500-**B**, (510) 794-4923-**H**, (510) 794-4923-**F**
bkoon@sjm.infi.net
Ethnicity: Asian-American/Asian/Pacific Islander
Languages: Chinese
Degree and Year: PhD 1973
Major Field: Experimental Psychology
Specialty: Clinical Psychology;Developmental
Psychology;Experimental Psychology;Forensic
Psychology;Medical Psychology

TANG, Thomas L P
Middle Tennessee State University
Department of Management
PO Box 516
Murfreesboro, TN 37132
(617) 898-2005-**B**, (615) 791-9847-**H**, (615) 898-5308-**F**
ttang@mtsu.edu
Ethnicity: Asian-American/Asian/Pacific Islander
Languages: Chinese
Degree and Year: PhD 1981
Major Field: Industrial/Organizational Psy.
Specialty: Human Resources;Management & Organization;Job
Satisfaction;Leadership;Measurement

TAN, Josephine
Lakehead University
Psychology Department

955 Oliver Road
Thunder Bay
Ontario, P7B 5E1
CANADA
(807) 346-7751-**B**, (807) 346-7734-**F**
jtan@sky.lakeheadu.ca
Ethnicity: Asian-American/Asian/Pacific Islander
Languages: Chinese, Malay, Bahasa Kebangsaan
Degree and Year: PhD 1992 MA 1985
Major Field: Clinical Psychology
Specialty: Depression;Gender Issues;Domestic Violence;Clinical Psychology;Clinical Child Psychology

TAN, Rowena N.
University of Northern Iowa
334 Baker Hall
Cedar Falls, IA 50614-0505
(319)273-7286-**B**, 319/277-6672-**H**, 319/273-6188-**F**
rowena.tan@uni.edu
Ethnicity: Asian-American/Asian/Pacific Islander
Degree and Year: PhD 1996 BA 1996
Major Field: Counseling Psychology
Specialty: Counseling Psychology

TAN, Siang-Yang Y.
Fuller Graduate School of Psychology
180 North Oakland Avenue
Pasadena, CA 91101
(626) 584-5532-**B**, (626) 355-0933-**H**, (626) 584-9630-**F**
Ethnicity: Asian-American/Asian/Pacific Islander
Degree and Year: PhD 1980
Major Field: Clinical Psychology
Specialty: Cognitive Behavioral Therapy;Cross Cultural Processes;Health Psychology;Pain & Pain Management;Religious Psychology

TAPO, Linda J.
948 Lewis Pl
Shreveport, LA 71103-2638
(318) 531-3922-**B**, (-**H**
Ethnicity: African-American/Black
Degree and Year: PhD 1980
Major Field: Clinical Psychology
Specialty: Individual Psychotherapy;Assessment/Diagnosis/ Evaluation;Family Therapy;HIV/AIDS;Child Therapy

TATARA, Mikihachiro
18-15 Zigozen 1 Chome
Hatsuka-Ichi
Hiroshima 738,
197 - JAPAN
(082) 293-2500-**B**
Ethnicity: Asian-American/Asian/Pacific Islander
Degree and Year: PhD 1962
Major Field: Clinical Psychology
Specialty: Psychotherapy

TATE, Donald
Donald Tate, PhD, P.C.
14930 Faust Avenue
Detroit, MI 48223-2306
(313) 276-6759-**B**, (313) 877-8027-**H**, (313) 838-2518-**F**
duck-tate@aol.com
Ethnicity: African-American/Black
Degree and Year: PhD 1980

Major Field: Clinical Psychology
Specialty: Adult Development;Drug Abuse;Hypnosis/Hypnotherapy

TATSUGUCHI, Rosalie K.
3221 Waialae Ave, Ste 378
Honolulu, HI 96816-5845
(808) 735-1214-**B**, (808) 261-8312-**H**
Ethnicity: Asian-American/Asian/Pacific Islander
Degree and Year: PhD 1980
Major Field: Clinical Psychology
Specialty: Family Therapy;Learning Disabilities

TATUM, Beverly D.
Mount Holyoke College
32 Pioneer Knolls
Florence, MA 01062-3409
(413) 538-2086-**B**, (413) 586-0415-**H**, (413) 538-2327-**F**
Ethnicity: African-American/Black
Degree and Year: PhD 1984
Major Field: Clinical Psychology
Specialty: Adolescent Development;Ethnic Minorities;Human Development & Family Studies;Cross Cultural Processes

TAYLOR, Flor N.
Private Practice
324 Centre Street
South Orange, NJ 07079
(973) 761-5322-**B**, (973) 762-9396-**H**, (973) 762-2619-**F**
diagnosis@aol.com
Ethnicity: African-American/Black, American Indian/Alaska Native
Degree and Year: PhD 1994
Major Field: Counseling Psychology
Specialty: Group Processes;Organizational Development;Individual Psychotherapy

TAYLOR, Gary
P.O. Box 23
Buies Creek, NC 27506
(919) 893-1649-**B**, (919) 892-4712-**H**
Ethnicity: American Indian/Alaska Native
Degree and Year: PhD 1984
Major Field: School Psychology
Specialty: Assessment/Diagnosis/Evaluation;Community Mental Health;Child Therapy;Mentally Retarded;Personality Theory

TAYLOR, Palmeda D.
220 River Oak Cove
Nashville, TN 37214-4801
(615) 366-2789-**B**, 615 885-2282-**H**
Ethnicity: African-American/Black
Degree and Year: PhD 1981
Major Field: Clinical Psychology
Specialty: Chronically Mentally Ill;Group Psychotherapy;Individual Psychotherapy;Managed Care;Mental Health Services

TAYLOR, Peggy S.
42105 Manista Way
Murrieta, CA 92562-8235
(714) 676-3455-**B**, (714) 677-6868-**H**
Ethnicity: American Indian/Alaska Native
Degree and Year: PsyD 1983
Major Field: Clinical Psychology
Specialty: Affective Disorders;Cognitive Behavioral Therapy;Crisis Intervention & Therapy;Family Therapy;Psychopathology

TAYLOR, Stephen Q.
20 Kirsi Circle
Westford, MA 01886-2015
(508) 692-6407-**B**
Ethnicity: Hispanic/Latino
Degree and Year: PhD 1986
Major Field: Clinical Psychology
Specialty: Psychotherapy

TAZEAU, Yvette N.
2550 Samaritan Drive
Suite E
San Jose, CA 95124
(408) 977-7117-**B**, (408) 813-4871-**H**, (408) 358-9856-**F**
ytazeau@ix.netcom.com
Ethnicity: Hispanic/Latino
Languages: Spanish
Degree and Year: PhD 1995 MS 1993
Major Field: Clinical Psychology
Specialty: Clinical Neuropsychology;Gerontology/
Geropsychology;Ethnic Minorities;Assessment/Diagnosis/
Evaluation;Clinical Psychology;Industrial/Organizational
Psychology

TEITEL, Raquel S.
5610 Wisconsin Avenue
Suite #606
Bethesda, MD 20815-4417
(202) 362-1103-**B**
Ethnicity: Hispanic/Latino
Degree and Year: PhD 1973
Major Field: Clinical Psychology
Specialty: Psychotherapy

TEIXEIRA, Michael A.
328 Shepard Street
Suite #1
Lansing, MI 48912-2717
(517) 482-6106-**B**
Ethnicity: Hispanic/Latino
Degree and Year: PhD 1982
Major Field: Clinical Psychology
Specialty: Psychotherapy

TEJEDA, Manuel J.
Gettysburg College
Department of Management
North Washington Street
Gettysburg, PA 17325
(717) 337-6646-**B**, (717) 337-6488-**F**
mtejeda@gettsburg.edu
Ethnicity: Hispanic/Latino
Languages: Spanish
Degree and Year: PhD 1994 MsED 1989
Major Field: Industrial/Organizational Psy.
Specialty: Leadership;Quantitative/Mathematical,
Psychometrics;Clinical Research;Management &
Organization;Research Design & Methodology;Drug Abuse

TENG, Evelyn L.
Univ. of So. CA, School of Medicine
2025 Zonal Avenue
Los Angeles, CA 90033
(213) 226-7385-**B**, (213) 226-5869-**F**
eteng@hsc.usc.edu
Ethnicity: Asian-American/Asian/Pacific Islander
Languages: Chinese
Degree and Year: PhD 1963 MS 1960
Major Field: Neurosciences
Specialty: Adult Development;Alzheimer's Disease;Assessment/
Diagnosis/Evaluation;Clinical Neuropsychology;Cross Cultural
Processes

TENG, L. Neal
564 NE Ravenna Boulevard
Seattle, WA 98115
(206) 527-2266-**B**
Ethnicity: Asian-American/Asian/Pacific Islander
Languages: Chinese, German
Degree and Year: PhD 1982
Major Field: Clinical Psychology
Specialty: Assessment/Diagnosis/Evaluation;Cultural & Social
Processes;Pastoral Psychology;Sex/Marital Therapy;Vocational
Psychology

TEO, Thomas
York University
Department of Psychology
47000 Keele Street
Toronto, Ontario, M3J1P3
Canada
(416) 736-2100-**B**, (416) 736-5814-**F**
tteo@yorku.ca
Ethnicity: Asian-American/Asian/Pacific Islander
Languages: German
Degree and Year: PhD 1992 MsL 1986
Major Field: General Psy./Methods & Systems
Specialty: History & Systems of Psychology;Developmental
Psychology;Social Psychology;Philosophy of Science;Cultural
& Social Processes;Ethnic Minorities

THIMOTHEOSE, K. G.
3048 Brewster Court
West Bloomfield, MI 48322-2421
Ethnicity: Asian-American/Asian/Pacific Islander
Degree and Year: PhD 1975
Major Field: unknown
Specialty: Psychotherapy;Sexual Dysfunction;Clinical
Psychology;Family Therapy

THOMAS, JR., Charles B.
University of Michigan @ Flint
Department of Sociology
Flint, MI 48502
(313) 762-3340-**B**, (313) 230-0281-**H**, (313) 762-3687-**F**
Ethnicity: African-American/Black
Degree and Year: PhD 1976
Major Field: Social Psychology
Specialty: Values & Moral Behavior;Social Psychology;Ethnic
Minorities;Gender Issues;Research Design & Methodology

THOMAS, Anita J.
Northeastern Illinois University
Counselor Education
5500 North St. Louis Avenue
Chicago, IL 60625
(773) 794-2847-**B**, (847) 816-7950-**H**, (773) 794-6243-**F**
athomas7@niu.edu

Ethnicity: African-American/Black
Degree and Year: PhD 1995 MA 1992
Major Field: Counseling Psychology
Specialty: Marriage & Family;Ethnic Minorities;Child
    Therapy;Adolescent Therapy

THOMAS, Hilton T.
  3300 Waverly Hills Rd
  Lansing, MI 48917-4305
  (517) 321-5900-**B**, (517) 485-1546-**H**
Ethnicity: African-American/Black
Degree and Year: PhD 1982
Major Field: Clinical Psychology
Specialty: Family Therapy

THOMAS, Joseph E.
  16-W 731 89th Place
  Hinsdale, IL 60521
  (630) 357-1188-**B**, (630) 887-0425-**H**, (630) 887-1842-**F**
  piravom@aol.com
Ethnicity: Asian-American/Asian/Pacific Islander
Languages: Malayalam
Degree and Year: PhD 1969
Major Field: Health Psychology
Specialty: Attention Deficit Disorders;Biofeedback;Health
    Psychology;Hypnosis/Hypnotherapy;Pain & Pain
    Management;Psychotherapy

THOMAS, Thomas J.
  Bi Polar Inc
  PO Box 160220
  Austin, TX 78716-0220
  (512) 327-2656-**B**, (512) 327-5415-**H**, (512) 327-7516-**F**
  cherocreek@aol.com
Ethnicity: American Indian/Alaska Native
Languages: French
Degree and Year: PhD 1982
Major Field: Educational Psychology
Specialty: Consulting Psychology;Personality;Statistics;Quantitative/
    Mathematical, Psychometrics;Communication

THOMPSON, Chalmer E.
  Indiana University
  School of Education
  201 N. Rose Avenue, Rm 4024
  Bloomington, IN 47403
  (812) 856-8319-**B**, (812) 856-8440-**F**
  chathomp@indiana.edu
Ethnicity: African-American/Black
Degree and Year: PhD 1988
Major Field: Counseling Psychology
Specialty: Counseling Psychology;Cross Cultural Processes;Ethnic
    Minorities;Gender Issues;Personality

THOMPSON, Veronique L.
  Wright Institute
  2728 Durant Avenue
  Berkeley, CA 94703
  (510) 841-9230-**B**, (510) 763-2440-**H**, (510) 549-2591-**F**
  vthompson@wrightinsti.edu
Ethnicity: African-American/Black
Degree and Year: PhD 1989
Major Field: Clinical Psychology
Specialty: Family Therapy;Parent-Child Interaction;Ethnic

Minorities;Developmental Psychology;Community
Psychology

THORN, Isabel M.
  International Monetary Fund
  235 Midsummer Circle
  Gaithersburg, MD 20878
  (202) 623-7633-**B**, (301) 990-7619-**H**, (301) 258-7349-**F**
Ethnicity: Hispanic/Latino
Languages: American Sign Language, Spanish
Degree and Year: PhD 1980
Major Field: unknown
Specialty: Human Resources;Industrial/Organizational
    Psychology;Organizational Development;Management &
    Organization;Counseling Psychology

THORNTON, Dozier W.
  Michigan State University
  Department of Psychology
  Psychology Research Building
  East Lansing, MI 48824
  (517) 355-0300-**B**, (517) 332-2853-**H**, (517) 336-1171-**F**
Ethnicity: African-American/Black
Degree and Year: PhD 1966
Major Field: Clinical Psychology
Specialty: Cognitive Behavioral Therapy;Depression;Experimental
    Analysis of Behavior;Prevention;Sex/Marital Therapy

THORSON, Billie J.
  380 Bailey Plantation Drive
  Richmond Hill, GA 31324-3032
Ethnicity: American Indian/Alaska Native
Degree and Year: PhD 1986
Major Field: Clinical Psychology
Specialty: Clinical Child Psychology;Child Therapy;Assessment/
    Diagnosis/Evaluation;Parent-Child Interaction;Family Therapy

THURMAN, Pamela J.
  2319 Antelope
  Ft. Collins, CO 80535
  (303) 491-0251-**B**, (303) 491-0527-**F**
Ethnicity: American Indian/Alaska Native
Degree and Year: PhD 1990
Major Field: Clinical Psychology
Specialty: Cross Cultural Processes;Child Therapy;Alcoholism &
    Alcohol Abuse;Drug Abuse;Gender Issues

TIEN, Liang
  33309 First Way South
  Building A
  Suite #204
  Federal Way, WA 98003-6260
  (206) 874-0420-**B**, (206) 644-2491-**H**
Ethnicity: Asian-American/Asian/Pacific Islander
Languages: Chinese
Degree and Year: PhD 1985
Major Field: Clinical Psychology
Specialty: Clinical Psychology;Individual Psychotherapy;Marriage &
    Family;Cross Cultural Processes;Ethnic Minorities

TIGGLE, Ronald B.
  1058 Spring Valley Court
  Fort Washington, MD 20744
  (703) 274-5610-**B**, (301) 248-8029-**H**, (703) 274-857-**F**
Ethnicity: African-American/Black
Degree and Year: PhD 1983

Major Field: Social Psychology
Specialty: Attitudes & Opinions;Industrial/Organizational
Psychology;Health Psychology;Job Satisfaction;Gender Issues

TING-CHAU, Theodora
California School of
Professional Psychology
2170 Century Park East
Suite 605
Los Angeles, CA 90067-2213
Ethnicity: Asian-American/Asian/Pacific Islander
Degree and Year: PhD 1973
Major Field: Industrial/Organizational Psy.

TIRADO, John
531 E Roosevelt Road
Wheaton, IL 60187-5583
Ethnicity: Hispanic/Latino
Degree and Year: PhD 1975
Major Field: Clinical Psychology
Specialty: Psychotherapy

TIRADO, Linda Ann
16151 Wood Acres Road
Los Gatos, CA 95030-3037
(408) 399-1500-**B**, (408) 354-2238-**H**
Ethnicity: Hispanic/Latino
Languages: Spanish
Degree and Year: PhD 1981
Major Field: Clinical Psychology
Specialty: Family Therapy

TISCHER, Hans
11625 Bailey Mountain Trail
Midlothian, VA 23112-3062
Ethnicity: Hispanic/Latino
Degree and Year: MA 1968
Major Field: Clinical Psychology

TOBIAS, Manuel D.
3576 Third Avenue
San Diego, CA 92103-4909
(619) 295-2749-**B**
Ethnicity: Asian-American/Asian/Pacific Islander
Degree and Year: PhD 1980
Major Field: Clinical Psychology

TODD-MANCILLAS, William R.
1034 Cordelia Court
Chico, CA 95926-7142
Ethnicity: Hispanic/Latino
Degree and Year: PhD 1976
Major Field: Social Psychology
Specialty: Values & Moral Behavior

TOLDSON, Ivory L.
CPHC Community Mental Health Center
861 Main Street
Baton Rouge, LA 70802
(504) 383-3013-**B**, (504) 774-0109-**H**, (504) 383-0030-**F**
itoldson@premier.ent
Ethnicity: African-American/Black
Degree and Year: EdD 1971

Major Field: Counseling Psychology
Specialty: Attention Deficit Disorders;Cross Cultural Processes;Sexual
Behavior;Child Abuse;Personality Disorders;Structured
Outpatient Services

TOM, Agnes
1480 Chippewa Pathway
Riverwoods, IL 60015-1611
(708) 578-3761-**B**
Ethnicity: Asian-American/Asian/Pacific Islander
Degree and Year: PhD 1981
Major Field: Counseling Psychology
Specialty: Psychotherapy

TOMES, Henry
American Psychological Association
Public Interest Directorate
750 First Street, NE
Washington, DC 20002-4242
(202) 336-6050-**B**, (301) 951-0904-**H**, (202) 336-5723-**F**
ltomes@apa.org
Ethnicity: African-American/Black
Degree and Year: PhD 1963
Major Field: Clinical Psychology
Specialty: Clinical Psychology;Community Psychology

TOMLINSON-CLARKE, Saundra M.
Graduate School of Education
Department of Educational Psychology
New Brunswick, NJ 08903-5050
(732) 932-7946-**B**, (908) 246-3901-**H**
Ethnicity: African-American/Black
Degree and Year: PhD 1983
Major Field: Counseling Psychology
Specialty: Cross Cultural Processes;Ethnic Minorities;Cultural & Social
Processes

TOMS, Esther C.
P.O. Box 26087
Washington, DC 20001-0087
Ethnicity: African-American/Black
Degree and Year: PhD 1955
Major Field: Clinical Psychology
Specialty: Clinical Psychology

TOOMER, Jethro W.
Florida International University
Tamiami Trail, DM 201B
Miami, FL 33199
(305) 348-2089-**B**, (305) 255-8846-**H**, (305) 348-3205-**F**
Ethnicity: African-American/Black
Languages: French
Degree and Year: PhD 1973
Major Field: unknown
Specialty: Forensic Psychology;Assessment/Diagnosis/
Evaluation;Cross Cultural Processes

TOPOLSKI, James M.
6408 Lansdowne Avenue
St. Louis, MO 63109
(314) 644-7974-**B**, (314) 353-7026-**H**, (314) 644-8370-**F**
Ethnicity: Hispanic/Latino
Languages: Spanish
Degree and Year: PhD 1984

Major Field: General Psy./Methods & Systems
Specialty: Drug Abuse;Mental Health Services;Program
Evaluation;Industrial/Organizational Psychology;Quantitative/
Mathematical, Psychometrics

TORIGOE, Rodney Y.
VAMROC -116B
PO Box 50188
Honolulu, HI 96813
(808) 566-1495-**B**, (808) 373-9425-**H**, (808) 566-1817-**F**
Torigoe Rodney@honolulu.va.gov
Ethnicity: Asian-American/Asian/Pacific Islander
Languages: Hawaiian
Degree and Year: PhD 1976
Major Field: Clinical Psychology
Specialty: Sexual Dysfunction;Cross Cultural Processes;Ethnic
Minorities;Health Psychology;Pain & Pain Management

TORO-ALFONSO, Jose
Fundacion Sida
1200 16th Street Caparra Terrace
San Juan, PR 00921
(787) 782-9600-**B**, (787) 721-9171-**H**, (787) 782-1411-**F**
fndjoe@juno.com
Ethnicity: Hispanic/Latino
Languages: Spanish
Degree and Year: PhD 1990 MS 1988
Major Field: Clinical Psychology
Specialty: HIV/AIDS;Sexual Behavior;Sex/Marital Therapy;Family
Therapy

TORO, Carlos A.
A-5 Las Garzas
Tierralta
Guaynabo, PR 00926-9537
(809) 731-8056-**B**
Ethnicity: Hispanic/Latino
Degree and Year: PhD 1976
Major Field: Industrial/Organizational Psy.
Specialty: Management & Organization;Organizational Development

TORO, Haydee
Department of Children and Families
12664 NW 12th Court
Sunrise, FL 33323
(954) 467-4218-**B**, (954) 467-5949-**F**
Ethnicity: Hispanic/Latino
Languages: Spanish
Degree and Year: PhD 1988 MA 1988
Major Field: Developmental Psychology
Specialty: Behavior Therapy;Mentally Retarded;Parent
Education;Applied Behavior Analysis;Special Education

TORRES-SAENZ, Jorge
1915 NE 39th Street
Portland, OR 97212
(503) 667-0117-**B**, 503 667-0117-**H**
Ethnicity: Hispanic/Latino
Languages: Spanish
Degree and Year: PsyD 1993
Major Field: Clinical Psychology
Specialty: Community Mental Health;Family Therapy

TORRES, Mario A.
12 Linnaean St

Cambridge, MA 02138-1613
(617) 547-0931-**H**
Ethnicity: Hispanic/Latino
Languages: French, Spanish
Degree and Year: PhD 1988
Major Field: Clinical Psychology
Specialty: Assessment/Diagnosis/Evaluation;Psychopathology;Forensic
Psychology

TOSHIMA, Tamotsu
Chuo-3 Chome 8-11
Kure 737,
197 - JAPAN
Ethnicity: Asian-American/Asian/Pacific Islander
Degree and Year: PhD 1989
Major Field: Experimental Psychology
Specialty: Neuropsychology

TOSTADO, John F.
23432 Blue Bird Drive
Lake Forest, CA 92630
(909) 558-8615-**B**, (949) 837-8811-**H**, (909) 558-0171-**F**
jflora-tostado@ccmail.llu.edu
Ethnicity: Hispanic/Latino
Degree and Year: PhD 1974
Major Field: Clinical Psychology
Specialty: Clinical Psychology;Individual Psychotherapy;Family
Therapy;Assessment/Diagnosis/Evaluation;Adolescent
Therapy

TOWNS-MIRANDA, Luz
105 Payson Avenue
Suite #1
New York, NY 10034
(212) 942-2695-**B**, (212) 942-2695-**H**, (212) 942-2695-**F**
ltm_phd@aol.com
Ethnicity: Hispanic/Latino
Degree and Year: PhD 1985
Major Field: Clinical Psychology
Specialty: Clinical Child Psychology;Clinical Psychology;Child
Abuse;Psychology of Women;Gerontology/
Geropsychology;Psychoanalysis

TREADWELL, Marsha J.
1096 Tevlin Street
Albany, CA 94706
(510) 428-3356-**B**, (510) 524-4978-**H**
Ethnicity: African-American/Black
Degree and Year: PhD 1985
Major Field: Clinical Child Psychology
Specialty: Child & Pediatric Psychology;Clinical Child
Psychology;Hypnosis/Hypnotherapy;Psychotherapy;Human
Development & Family Studies

TRIMBLE, Joseph E.
Harvard University
Radcliffe Institute for Advanced Study
The Henry A. Murray Center
10 Garden Street
Cambridge MA 02138-3993
(617) 495-8140-**B**, (617) 496-3993-**F**
trimble@radcliffe.edu

Ethnicity: American Indian/Alaska Native
Degree and Year: PhD 1969

Major Field: Social Psychology
Specialty: Cultural & Social Processes;Ethnic Minorities;Drug
Abuse;Social Change;Research Design & Methodology

TRIPLETT, Sheila J.
Buchanan Counseling Center-Clarian, Inc.
1812 North Capitol Avenue
448 Wile Hall
Indianapolis, IN 46206
(317) 929-8613-**B**, (317) 929-5961-**F**
striplett@clarian.com
Ethnicity: African-American/Black
Degree and Year: PhD 1994
Major Field: Clinical Psychology
Specialty: Adolescent Development;Child Abuse;Ethnic
Minorities;Problem Solving;Interpersonal Processes &
Relations

TROTMAN, Frances K.
999 Teaneck Road
Teaneck, NJ 07666
(201) 833-2181-**B**, (201) 833-4326-**H**
Ethnicity: African-American/Black
Languages: French, Italian, Portuguese, Spanish
Degree and Year: PhD 1976
Major Field: Counseling Psychology

TROUTT, Bobbye V.
250 W 90th St #8k
New York, NY 10024-1141
(212) 362-1920-**B**, (212) 362-1920-**H**
Ethnicity: African-American/Black
Degree and Year: PhD 1980
Major Field: Clinical Psychology
Specialty: Psychotherapy

TRUE, Reiko Homma
5326 Silva Avenue
El Cerrito, CA 94530
(510) 233-2082-**H**, (510) 233-29977-**F**
rhtrue@aol.com
Ethnicity: Asian-American/Asian/Pacific Islander
Languages: Japanese
Degree and Year: PhD 1976
Major Field: Clinical Psychology
Specialty: Community Mental Health;Ethnic Minorities;Clinical
Psychology;Health Psychology;Management & Organization

TRUFANT, Carol A.
PO Box 8072
Berkeley, CA 94707-8072
(510) 746-1646-**H**
Ethnicity: African-American/Black
Languages: Italian
Degree and Year: PhD 1977 MA 1972
Major Field: Clinical Child Psychology
Specialty: Systems Analysis;Family Processes;Cultural & Social
Processes;Clinical Child Psychology;Social
Learning;Alzheimer's Disease

TSAI, Mavis
3245 Fairview Avenue, East
Suite #303
Seattle, WA 98102
(206) 323-8447-**B**, (206) 322-1067-**H**

Ethnicity: Asian-American/Asian/Pacific Islander
Languages: Chinese
Degree and Year: PhD 1982
Major Field: Clinical Psychology
Specialty: Psychotherapy;Psychology of Women;Ethnic
Minorities;Personality Disorders;Child Abuse

TSANG, Michael Hing- Pui
The Chinese University of Hong Kong
Department of Psychology
Shatin
New Territories,
Hong Kong
(852) 2609-6195-**B**, (852) 2994-1005-**H**, (852) 2603-5019-**F**
mhptsang@psy.cuhk.edu.hk
Ethnicity: Asian-American/Asian/Pacific Islander
Languages: Chinese
Degree and Year: Phd 1993 MS 1994
Major Field: Clinical Psychology
Specialty: Clinical Psychology;Counseling Psychology;Health
Psychology;Clinical Neuropsychology;Gerontology/
Geropsychology;Psychotherapy

TSUI, Alice M.
731 W Meseto Circle
Mesa, AZ 85210-7552
(602) 954-3273-**B**
Ethnicity: Asian-American/Asian/Pacific Islander
Degree and Year: PhD 1978
Major Field: Clinical Psychology
Specialty: Sex/Marital Therapy

TSUI, Ellen C.
85 Livingston Street
Brooklyn, NY 11201
(718) 694-0938-**H**
Ethnicity: Asian-American/Asian/Pacific Islander
Languages: Chinese
Degree and Year: PhD 1989
Major Field: Educational Psychology
Specialty: Applied Behavior Analysis

TSUJIMOTO, Richard N.
Pitzer College
Department of Psychology
Claremont, CA 91711
(909) 607-3779-**B**, (909) 625-4522-**H**, (909) 621-8521-**F**
richard_tsujimoto@pitzer.edu
Ethnicity: Asian-American/Asian/Pacific Islander
Degree and Year: PhD 1974
Major Field: Clinical Psychology
Specialty: Child Abuse;Decision & Choice Behavior;Ethnic
Minorities;Program Evaluation;Juvenile Delinquency;Mental
Health Services

TSUKAMOTO, Donna E.
44-114 Nanamoana Street
Kaneohe, HI 96744-2555
Ethnicity: Asian-American/Asian/Pacific Islander
Degree and Year: PsyD 1983
Major Field: Clinical Psychology
Specialty: Psychotherapy

TSUSHIMA, William T.
Straub Clinic
888 South King Street
Honolulu, HI 96813
(808) 522-4521-**B**, (808) 732-1155-**H**, (808) 522-3526-**F**
Ethnicity: Asian-American/Asian/Pacific Islander
Degree and Year: PhD 1967
Major Field: Clinical Psychology
Specialty: Neuropsychology;Medical Psychology;Biofeedback;Learning
Disabilities;Forensic Psychology

TUCKER, Dorothy M.
PO Box 62309
Los Angeles, CA 90062-9998
(213) 293-2646-**B**, (310) 559-1607-**H**, (213) 296-4752-**F**
drdotdot@earthlink.net
Ethnicity: African-American/Black
Degree and Year: PhD 1976 PhD 1972
Major Field: Clinical Psychology
Specialty: Child Abuse;Forensic Psychology;Consulting
Psychology;Ethnic Minorities;Organizational
Development;Family Therapy

TUCKER, James L.
Colorado Boys Ranch Foundation
28071 Highway 102
PO Box 681
La Junta, CO 81050-2424
(719) 384-5981-**B**, (719) 384-2617-**H**, (719) 384-2617-**F**
jltucker@iguana.ruralnet.net
Ethnicity: African-American/Black
Degree and Year: PhD 1978
Major Field: Clinical Child Psychology
Specialty: Clinical Child Psychology;Cognitive
Development;Autism;Child Development;Deviant
Behavior;Psychotherapy

TUCKER, Samuel J.
735 Peyton Road, SW
Atlanta, GA 30311
(404) 522-2916-**B**, (404) 755-4244-**H**, (404) 522-2916-**F**
Ethnicity: African-American/Black
Degree and Year: PhD 1969
Major Field: Counseling Psychology
Specialty: Clinical Psychology;Neuropsychology;Mentally
Retarded;Disadvantaged;Counseling Psychology

TUNG, May
1733 Scott St
San Francisco, CA 94115-3030
(415) 923-1028-**B**
Ethnicity: Asian-American/Asian/Pacific Islander
Languages: Chinese, Mandarin
Degree and Year: PhD 1979
Major Field: Clinical Psychology
Specialty: Clinical Psychology;Cross Cultural Processes;Individual
Psychotherapy;Cultural & Social
Processes;Neuroses;Assessment/Diagnosis/Evaluation

TURNBOUGH, P. Diane
University of Nevada @ Las Vegas
Psychology Department
4505 S. Maryland Parkway
Las Vegas, NV 89154

(702) 895-3328-**B**, (702) 798-7997-**H**
Ethnicity: American Indian/Alaska Native
Degree and Year: PhD 1972
Major Field: Clinical Psychology
Specialty: Affective Disorders;Clinical Psychology;Cognitive
Behavioral Therapy;Employee Assistance Programs;Gender
Issues

TURNER, Alvin L.
1701 Augustine Cut-Off, Suite 13
Suite 13
Wilimington, DE 19803
(302) 656-7224-**B**, (302) 762-6163-**H**, (302) 656-1220-**F**
Ethnicity: African-American/Black
Languages: French
Degree and Year: PhD 1980
Major Field: Counseling Psychology
Specialty: Adolescent Therapy;Family Therapy;Health
Psychology;Hypnosis/Hypnotherapy;Cross Cultural
Processes

TURNER, Castellano
95 Wood End Road
Newton Highland, MA 02161-1402
(617) 965-6636-**B**
Ethnicity: African-American/Black
Degree and Year: PhD 1966
Major Field: Clinical Psychology

TURNER, Darrell D.
University of Chicago Hospital
Department of Psychiatry
5841 S Maryland, Dept. #MC3077
Chicago, IL 60637
(312) 702-9725-**B**, (312) 702-6454-**F**
Ethnicity: Hispanic/Latino
Degree and Year: PhD 1989
Major Field: Clinical Psychology
Specialty: Psychotherapy;Medical Psychology

TURNER, Samuel M.
University of Maryland
Department of Psychology
College Park, MD 20742
(301) 405-0232-**B**, (803) 405-8154-**F**
turner@bss3.umd.edu
Ethnicity: African-American/Black
Degree and Year: PhD 1975
Major Field: Clinical Psychology
Specialty: Behavior Therapy;Neuroses;Ethnic Minorities;Clinical
Psychology;Mental Health Services;Clinical Research

TWE, Boikai S.
Sinclair Community College
Psychology Department
444 West Third Street
Dayton, OH 45406
(937) 512-2913-**B**, (937) 274-0906-**H**, (937) 512-5192-**F**
btwe@sinclair.edu
Ethnicity: African-American/Black
Degree and Year: EdD 1985
Major Field: Educational Psychology
Specialty: Community Psychology;Educational Psychology;General
Psychology;Cross Cultural Processes;Ethnic Minorities

UGWUEGBU, Denis C.
University of Ibadan
Psychology, Faculty of Social Science
Oyo Road
Ibadan, Oyo,
NIGERIA
011 022400-550-**B**, 011 022550-1985-**H**
Ethnicity: African-American/Black
Degree and Year: PhD 1973
Major Field: Social Psychology
Specialty: Attribution Theory

UNDERWOOD, Robert J.
73 Elk Street
San Francisco, CA 94131-2841
Ethnicity: African-American/Black
Degree and Year: PhD 1967
Major Field: Clinical Psychology

UNO, Elizabeth
823 33rd Ave
San Francisco, CA 94121-3429
(415) 751-7210-**B**
Ethnicity: Asian-American/Asian/Pacific Islander
Degree and Year: PhD 1979
Major Field: Clinical Psychology
Specialty: Child Therapy

UNSON, Delia C. O.
The Integral Psychology Center
1619 Monroe Street
Madison, WI 53711-2021
Ethnicity: Asian-American/Asian/Pacific Islander, Hispanic/Latino
Degree and Year: PhD 1986
Major Field: Counseling Psychology

UPADHYAYA, Shripati
Learning Disability Directorate
Bradford Community Health
4 Queens Road
Bradford, England, BD8 7BT
UNITED KINGDOM
02174-481161-**B**, 01977-683715-**H**, 01274-771106-**F**
Ethnicity: Asian-American/Asian/Pacific Islander
Languages: Hindi, Urdu, Gujrati
Degree and Year: PhD 1975
Major Field: Clinical Psychology
Specialty: Assessment/Diagnosis/Evaluation;Autism;Clinical
    Psychology;Cognitive Behavioral Therapy;Learning
    Disabilities;Mentally Retarded

URBINA, Susana P.
University of North Florida
1301 First Street, South
#1407
Jacksonville Beach, FL 32250
(904) 646-2808-**B**, (904) 246-4143-**H**, 904 646-2563-**F**
surbina@unf.edu
Ethnicity: Hispanic/Latino
Languages: French, German, Italian, Spanish
Degree and Year: PhD 1972
Major Field: Quan/Math & Psychometrics/Stat
Specialty: Assessment/Diagnosis/Evaluation;Quantitative/
    Mathematical, Psychometrics;Projective Techniques;Clinical
    Neuropsychology;Intelligence;History & Systems of
    Psychology

URQUIZA, Anthony J.
University of California, Davis Medical Ctr.
Pediatrics
2516 Stockton Boulevard
Sacramento, CA 95817
(916) 734-7608-**B**, (916) 456-2236-**F**
ajurquiza@ucdavis.edu
Ethnicity: Hispanic/Latino
Degree and Year: PhD 1988
Major Field: Clinical Child Psychology
Specialty: Child Abuse;Child & Pediatric Psychology;Child
    Therapy;Ethnic Minorities;Research Design & Methodology

UYEDA, Arthur A.
1500 Tanager Lane
Petaluma, CA 94954
(707) 763-8585-**H**
Ethnicity: Asian-American/Asian/Pacific Islander
Degree and Year: PhD 1960
Major Field: Comparative Psychology
Specialty: Neurophysiology;Physiological Psychology;Mentally
    Retarded;Behavior Therapy;Psychometrics

UZZELL, Barbara P.
Memorial Neurological Association
7777 SW Freeway
Suite 900
Houston, TX 77074
(713) 772-4600-**B**, (281) 997-6757-**H**, (281) 997-9422-**F**
bpuzzell@hal-pc.org
Ethnicity: American Indian/Alaska Native
Degree and Year: PhD 1970
Major Field: Clinical Psychology
Specialty: Neuropsychology;Clinical Neuropsychology;Neurological
    Disorders;Rehabilitation;Brain Functions

VADA, Alejo
5949 SW 41st Street
Miami, FL 33155-5203
(305) 947-5597-**B**
Ethnicity: Hispanic/Latino
Degree and Year: PhD 1977
Major Field: Counseling Psychology
Specialty: Forensic Psychology

VAID, Jyotsna
Texas A&M
Psychology Department
College Station, TX 77843-4235
(409) 845-2576-**B**, (409) 845-4727-**F**
jxv@psyc.tamu.edu
Ethnicity: Asian-American/Asian/Pacific Islander
Languages: French, Hindi
Degree and Year: PhD 1982
Major Field: Experimental Psychology
Specialty: Cognitive Psychology;Psycholinguistic;Psychology of
    Women

VAKHARIYA, Sobha
4102 Golf Ridge Drive East
Bloomfield Hills, MI 48302
(248) 538-0598-**H**
sobhav@aol.com
Ethnicity: Asian-American/Asian/Pacific Islander
Languages: Hindi
Degree and Year: PsyD 1999
Major Field: Clinical Psychology

VALDES, Luis F.
RHR International Company
1355 Peachtree Street
Suite 1400
Atlanta, GA 30309-3274
(404) 870-9160-**B**, (770) 414-8625-**H**, (404) 870-9164-**F**
lvaldes@rhrinternational.com
Ethnicity: Hispanic/Latino
Degree and Year: PhD 1984
Major Field: Counseling Psychology

VALDES, Maria
Dept. of Social Services
4500 East 7th Ave
Denver, CO 80220-5012
(303) 727-2938-**B**, (303) 355-5818-**H**
Ethnicity: Hispanic/Latino
Languages: Spanish
Degree and Year: PhD 1978
Major Field: Community Psychology

VALDES, Thusnelda M.
2003 Shadow Creek
Houston, TX 77017
(713) 743-5412-**B**, (713) 941-3812-**H**
Ethnicity: Hispanic/Latino
Languages: Spanish
Degree and Year: EdD 1979
Major Field: Counseling Psychology
Specialty: Ethnic Minorities;Assessment/Diagnosis/
Evaluation;Vocational Psychology;Stress;Training &
Development

VALDEZ, JR., Romulo
PO Box 5911
Manchester, NH 03108-5911
(603) 622-9262-**B**, (603) 472-4932-**H**
Ethnicity: Asian-American/Asian/Pacific Islander
Degree and Year: PhD 1984
Major Field: Counseling Psychology
Specialty: Adolescent Therapy;Child Therapy;Marriage &
Family;Psychotherapy;Drug Abuse

VALDEZ-MENCHACA, Marta C.
University of California
@ Santa Barbara
Graduate School of Education
Department of Education
Santa Barbara, CA 93106
Ethnicity: Hispanic/Latino
Degree and Year: PhD 1990
Major Field: Developmental Psychology

VALDEZ, Jesse N.
University of Denver
College of Education, AHB
24450 South Vine Street
Denver, CO 80208
(303) 871-2482-**B**, (303) 758-0143-**H**, (303) 871-4456-**F**
jevaldez@du.edu
Ethnicity: Hispanic/Latino
Languages: Spanish
Degree and Year: PhD 1985
Major Field: Counseling Psychology
Specialty: Psychotherapy;Alcoholism & Alcohol Abuse;Health
Psychology;Affective Disorders;Gender Issues;Counseling
Psychology

VALDIVIA, Lino
2140 W Chapman
Suite #123
Orange, CA 92680
(714) 978-9008-**B**, (714) 838-7334-**H**, (714) 978-2337-**F**
Ethnicity: Hispanic/Latino
Languages: Spanish, Quechua
Degree and Year: PsyD 1985
Major Field: Clinical Psychology
Specialty: Forensic Psychology;Neuropsychology

VALENCIA-LAVER, Debra
Cal Poly State University
Department of Psychology
and Human Development
San Luis Obispo, CA 93407
(805) 756-1603-**B**, (805) 772-5059-**H**, (805) 756-1134-**F**
dlvalenc@calpoly.edu
Ethnicity: Hispanic/Latino
Degree and Year: PhD 1992
Major Field: Cognitive Psychology
Specialty: Memory;Psycholinguistic;Gerontology/
Geropsychology;Information Processing;Language Process

VALENTINER, David P.
Northern Illinois University
Department of Psychology
Dekalb, IL 60115
(815) 753-786-**B**, (815) 758-1865-**H**, (815) 75308088-**F**
dvalentiner@niv.edu
Ethnicity: Asian-American/Asian/Pacific Islander
Degree and Year: PhD 1994
Major Field: Clinical Psychology
Specialty: Stress

VALLEY, John A.
37825 Lakeshore Blvd.
PO Box 5302
Willowick, OH 44094
(216) 946-5225-**B**, (216) 946-5225-**H**
Ethnicity: American Indian/Alaska Native
Languages: French, Latin
Degree and Year: MA 1975
Major Field: Counseling Psychology
Specialty: Counseling Psychology;Religious
Psychology;Depression;Psychotherapy;Sexual Behavior

VALTIERRA, Mary
2950 Vecino Drive
Sacramento, CA 95833-1703
(916) 564-8515-**B**

Ethnicity: Hispanic/Latino
Degree and Year: PhD 1989
Major Field: Clinical Psychology
Specialty: Clinical Psychology

VANCE, Ellen B.
1900 N. Northlake Way
Suite 127
Seattle, WA 98103
(206) 525-1382-**B**, (206) 527-2332-**H**
Ethnicity: Asian-American/Asian/Pacific Islander
Degree and Year: PhD 1975
Major Field: Clinical Psychology
Specialty: Marriage & Family;Family Therapy;Sex/Marital
Therapy;Cross Cultural Processes

VANCE, Marilyn M.
Euclid Guild Associates
25100 Euclid Avenue
Suite 212
Euclid, OH 44117-2620
(440) 975-0734-**B**, (440) 543-4693-**H**
Ethnicity: African-American/Black
Degree and Year: PhD 1980
Major Field: Clinical Psychology
Specialty: Family Therapy

VANDERHOST, Leonette
250 East 87th Street
New York, NY 10128
(212) 831-8063-**B**, (212) 831-8063-**H**
Ethnicity: African-American/Black
Degree and Year: PhD 1966
Major Field: Clinical Psychology
Specialty: Parent-Child Interaction;Affective Disorders;Individual
Psychotherapy;Adolescent Therapy;Family Therapy

VANDERPOOL, Andrea T.
7 Hathaway Court
Silver Spring, MD 20903
(301) 460-7112-**B**, (301) 460-6317-**H**
Ethnicity: African-American/Black
Degree and Year: PhD 1979
Major Field: Educational Psychology
Specialty: Child Therapy;Group Psychotherapy;Learning
Disabilities;Adolescent Therapy;Parent-Child
Interaction;Psychotherapy

VARGAS, Alice M.
University of New Mexico, CPH
UNM Carrie Tingley Hospital
Department of Pediatrics
1127 University Boulevard, NE
Albuquerque, NM 87102-1740
(505) 272-4244-**B**, (505) 856-1664-**H**
Ethnicity: American Indian/Alaska Native, Hispanic/Latino
Languages: Spanish
Degree and Year: PhD 1983
Major Field: Counseling Psychology
Specialty: Adolescent Therapy;Assessment/Diagnosis/Evaluation;Child
& Pediatric Psychology;Clinical Psychology;Ethnic Minorities

VARGAS, Luis A.

UNM Children's Psychiatric Hosp.
1001 Yale Blvd., NE
Albuquerque, NM 87131
(505) 843-2900-**B**, (505) 897-7634-**H**, (505) 843-0052-**F**
Ethnicity: Hispanic/Latino
Languages: Spanish
Degree and Year: PhD 1982
Major Field: Clinical Psychology
Specialty: Clinical Child Psychology;Cultural & Social Processes;Ethnic
Minorities;Family Therapy;Death & Dying

VARGAS, M. Angelica
New Life Counseling Counseling Center
817 East Southmore
Pasadena, TX 77502
(713) 475-0072-**B**, (713) 541-6232-**H**, (713) 541-6232-**F**
Ethnicity: Hispanic/Latino
Languages: Spanish
Degree and Year: MA 1993
Major Field: Clinical Psychology
Specialty: Affective Disorders;Alcoholism & Alcohol Abuse;Pain &
Pain Management;Psychotherapy;Stress;Depression

VARGAS, Manuel J.
1560 Happy Valley Road
Crown Point, IN 46307-9300
(219) 988-4580-**H**
Ethnicity: Hispanic/Latino
Languages: Spanish
Degree and Year: PhD 1952
Major Field: Clinical Psychology
Specialty: Individual Psychotherapy;Adolescent Therapy;Community
Mental Health;Group Psychotherapy;Hypnosis/
Hypnotherapy

VARKI, C. Paily
1010 Glen Road
Wallingford, PA 19086
(215) 525-9620-**B**, (215) 876-6901-**H**
Ethnicity: Asian-American/Asian/Pacific Islander
Languages: Malayalam
Degree and Year: PhD 1975
Major Field: Clinical Psychology
Specialty: Depression;Affective Disorders;Schizophrenia;Cognitive
Behavioral Therapy;Marriage & Family

VASQUEZ, Melba
Vasquez & Associates
2901 Bee Cave Road
PO Box N
Austin, TX 78746
(512) 329-8000-**B**, (512) 327-4218-**H**, (512) 329-8299-**F**
melvasquez@aol.com
Ethnicity: Hispanic/Latino
Languages: Spanish
Degree and Year: PhD 1978
Major Field: Counseling Psychology
Specialty: Depression;Ethnic Minorities;Feminist Therapy;Group
Psychotherapy;Psychotherapy

VASQUEZ, Michael B.
4400 Shandwick Drive
Apt 154
Sacramento, CA 95842-5713

Ethnicity: Hispanic/Latino
Degree and Year: PhD 1983
Major Field: Clinical Psychology

VAUGHAN, Elaine
University of California
Program in Social Ecol.
Irvine, CA 92717
(714) 856-7184-**B**
Ethnicity: African-American/Black
Degree and Year: PhD 1986
Major Field: Social Psychology
Specialty: Environmental Psychology

VAUGHANS, Kirkland C.
New Hope Guild: East New York
100 Pennsylvania Avenue
Brooklyn, NY 11207
(516) 643-0615-**B**, (516) 643-0615-**H**, (718) 485-4018-**F**
jicap66@aol.com
Ethnicity: African-American/Black
Degree and Year: PhD 1985 Cert 1996
Major Field: Clinical Psychology
Specialty: Adolescent Therapy;Child Therapy

VAZQUEZ, Carlos D.
2024 Becquer Street
El Senorial
San Juan, PR 00926
(809) 748-0056-**B**, (787) 761-5716-**H**, (809) 748-0056-**F**
Ethnicity: Hispanic/Latino
Languages: Spanish
Degree and Year: PhD 1974 MA 1957
Major Field: Clinical Psychology
Specialty: Group Processes;Group Psychotherapy;Interpersonal
Processes & Relations;Family Processes

VAZQUEZ, Cesar D.
Po Box 22776
San Juan, PR 00931-2776
(787) 764-000-**B**, (787) 751-5110-**H**, (787) 751-5110-**F**
cvazque@caribe.net
Ethnicity: Hispanic/Latino
Languages: Spanish
Degree and Year: PhD 1987
Major Field: Counseling Psychology
Specialty: Assessment/Diagnosis/Evaluation;Consulting
Psychology;Counseling Psychology;Cross Cultural
Processes;Adolescent Therapy

VAZQUEZ, Rosa
26 West 9th Street
Suite 1-C
New York, NY 10011
(212) 475-1787-**B**
Ethnicity: Hispanic/Latino
Languages: Spanish
Degree and Year: PhD 1989
Major Field: Clinical Psychology
Specialty: Child Therapy;Child Development;Infancy;Parent-Child
Interaction;Marriage & Family

VAZQUEZ-RUIZ, Francisco
2100 Antiuguia St. Apolo
Guaynabo, PR 00969
(809) 764-0000-**B**, (809) 790-4229-**H**, (809) 764-5238-**F**

Ethnicity: Hispanic/Latino
Languages: Spanish
Degree and Year: PhD 1976
Major Field: General Psy./Methods & Systems
Specialty: Child Abuse;Prevention;Professional Issues in
Psychology;Crisis Intervention & Therapy;Counseling
Psychology

VEGA, Jose G.
222 West B Street
Pueblo, CO 81003-3404
(719) 544-8520-**B**, (719) 564-5903-**H**
Ethnicity: Hispanic/Latino
Languages: Spanish
Degree and Year: PhD 1979
Major Field: Counseling Psychology
Specialty: Clinical Neuropsychology;Counseling Psychology;Mental
Health Services;Ethnic Minorities;Rehabilitation

VEGA, Star
California Behavioral Medical Group
8141 East 2nd Sreet
Suite 305
Downey, CA 90241
(310) 904-2771-**B**, (818) 541-1229-**H**, (310) 904-2773-**F**
kwikmind@aol.com
Ethnicity: Hispanic/Latino
Languages: Spanish
Degree and Year: PhD 1983
Major Field: Clinical Psychology
Specialty: Forensic Psychology;Clinical Neuropsychology;Cross
Cultural Processes;Employee Assistance Programs;Ethnic
Minorities

VEGEGA, Maria E.
4726 S 29th Street
Suite #A-2
Arlington, VA 22206-1333
(202) 366-5590-**B**
Ethnicity: Hispanic/Latino
Degree and Year: PhD 1980
Major Field: Social Psychology
Specialty: Attitudes & Opinions

VELASCO, Frank E.
7544 Trask Ave
Playa Del Rey, CA 90293-8043
(310) 574-1748-**B**, (310) 821-5602-**F**
Ethnicity: Hispanic/Latino
Languages: Spanish
Degree and Year: PhD 1984
Major Field: Clinical Psychology
Specialty: Child Abuse;Clinical Psychology;Family Therapy;Managed
Care;Rehabilitation

VELASQUEZ, John M.
University of the Incarnate Word
Department of Psychology
4301 Broadway
San Antonio, TX 78209
(210) 829-3960-**B**, (210) 590-0044-**H**, (210) 829-3880-**F**
velasqe@universe.uitwtx.edu
Ethnicity: Hispanic/Latino
Degree and Year: PhD 1995
Major Field: Clinical Psychology

Specialty: Clinical Psychology;Pain & Pain Management;Community
 Psychology;Ethnic Minorities;Hypnosis/
 Hypnotherapy;Program Evaluation

VELASQUEZ, Roberto J.
 SDSU-UCSD Joint PhD Program
 6363 Alvarado Court #103
 San Diego, CA 92120-4913
 (619) 594-6105-**B**, (619) 421-9170-**H**
 rvelasquez@sunstroke.sdsu.edu
Ethnicity: Hispanic/Latino
Languages: Spanish
Degree and Year: PhD 1986
Major Field: Clinical Psychology
Specialty: Assessment/Diagnosis/Evaluation;Counseling
 Psychology;Ethnic Minorities;Mental
 Disorders;Psychopathology

VELAYO, Richard S.
 Pace University
 130 Water Street, 4-A
 New York, NY 10005
 (212) 346-1506-**B**, (212) 825-1154-**H**, (212) 346-1618-**F**
 rvelayo@pace.edu
Ethnicity: Asian-American/Asian/Pacific Islander
Languages: Filipino
Degree and Year: PhD 1993 MA 1988
Major Field: Educational Psychology
Specialty: Educational Technology;Cognitive Psychology;Experimental
 Psychology;Computer Applications and
 Programming;Information Processing

VELEZ-DIAZ, Angel
 1559 San Remo Avenue
 Coral Gables, FL 33146-3008
 (305) 665-6445-**B**, (305) 856-6483-**H**
 avd@earthlink.net
Ethnicity: Hispanic/Latino
Languages: Portuguese, Spanish
Degree and Year: PhD 1970
Major Field: Clinical Psychology
Specialty: Clinical Psychology;Personality Measurement;Vocational
 Psychology;Mental Disorders;Clinical Neuropsychology

VELEZ, Maria T.
 University of Arizona
 Counseling and Testing Services
 Old Main, 200 West
 Tuson, AZ 85721
 (602) 621-7591-**B**, (602) 743-9760-**H**, (602) 621-8158-**F**
Ethnicity: Hispanic/Latino
Languages: Spanish
Degree and Year: PhD 1983
Major Field: Clinical Psychology
Specialty: Clinical Psychology;Human Relations;Human
 Resources;Ethnic Minorities

VERA, Elizabeth M.
 Loyola University Chicago
 1014 Ridge Road
 Wilmette, IL 60091
 (847) 853-3351-**B**, (773) 274-6483-**H**, (847) 853-3375-**F**
 evera@luc.edu
Ethnicity: Hispanic/Latino

Languages: Spanish
Degree and Year: PhD 1993 MA 1990
Major Field: Counseling Psychology
Specialty: Prevention;Counseling Psychology;Community
 Psychology;Ethnic Minorities

VERGHESE, Cherian
 12625 Laurie Dr
 Silver Spring, MD 20904-1504
 (202) 994-6550-**B**
Ethnicity: Asian-American/Asian/Pacific Islander
Degree and Year: PhD 1988
Major Field: Counseling Psychology
Specialty: Psychotherapy

VIALE-VAL, Graciela
 1641 Hinman, 3rd Flr
 Evanston, IL 60201-4509
 (312) 433-8552-**B**, (708) 864-9514-**H**
Ethnicity: Hispanic/Latino
Languages: Spanish
Degree and Year: PsyD 1981
Major Field: Clinical Psychology
Specialty: Suicide;Forensic Psychology;Juvenile
 Delinquency;Adolescent Therapy;Psychotherapy

VICENTE, Peter J.
 Riverhills Healthcare, Inc.
 111 Wellington Medicine Place
 Cincinnati, OH 45219
 (513) 241-2370-**B**, (513) 271-7099-**H**, (513) 241-6053-**F**
 pvicente@compuserve.com
Ethnicity: Hispanic/Latino
Languages: Spanish
Degree and Year: PhD 1975
Major Field: Counseling Psychology
Specialty: Pain & Pain Management;Rehabilitation;Medical
 Psychology;Behavior Therapy;Counseling
 Psychology;Medical Psychology

VIGIL, Patricia L.
 Colorado State University
 2012 Devonshire Drive
 Fort Collins, CO 80524
 (970) 491-5748-**B**, (970) 223-4713-**H**, (970) 491-5748-**F**
 pvigil@vines.colostate.edu
Ethnicity: Hispanic/Latino
Degree and Year: PhD 1988
Major Field: Counseling Psychology
Specialty: Ethnic Minorities;Counseling Psychology;Death &
 Dying;Cross Cultural Processes;Child Abuse;Feminist
 Therapy

VILLEGAS, Orlando L.
 3190 Kenicott
 Walled Lake, MI 48390-1676
 (313) 646-6990-**B**, 313 788-0286-**H**
Ethnicity: Hispanic/Latino
Degree and Year: MA 1978
Major Field: Educational Psychology
Specialty: Educational Research;Neuropsychology

VILLEJO, Ron E.
 20 South Clark Street
 Third Floor
 Chicago, IL 60603

(312) 201-0200-**B**, (847) 543-9412-**H**, (312) 201-1907-**F**
landville@aol.com
Ethnicity: Asian-American/Asian/Pacific Islander
Degree and Year: PhD 1993 BA 1981
Major Field: Clinical Child Psychology
Specialty: Clinical Psychology;Adolescent Development

VILLELA, Leopoldo F.
Leopoldo F. Vilvela, PhD, Inc.
2595 Mission Street
Suite #211
San Francisco, CA 94110
(415) 641-7169-**B**, (415) 695-9461-**H**, (425) 641-0307-**F**
lvpsyinc.@worldnet.ait.net
Ethnicity: Hispanic/Latino
Languages: Spanish
Degree and Year: PhD 1975
Major Field: Clinical Psychology
Specialty: Clinical Psychology;Community Psychology;Gerontology/
     Geropsychology;Clinical Child Psychology

VISWESVARAN, Chockalingam
Florida International University
Department of Psychology
University Park
Miami, FL 33199
(305) 348-4165-**B**, (305) 385-3408-**H**, (305) 348-3879-**F**
vish@fiu.edu
Ethnicity: Asian-American/Asian/Pacific Islander
Languages: Tamil
Degree and Year: PhD 1973
Major Field: Industrial/Organizational Psy.
Specialty: Performance
     Evaluation;Measurement;Psychometrics;Personality;Quantitative/
     Mathematical, Psychometrics;Labor & Management Relations

VONTRESS, Clemmont E.
2301 Naylor Road, S.E.
Washington, DC 20020
(202) 994-6856-**B**, (202) 584-1255-**H**
Ethnicity: African-American/Black
Languages: French
Degree and Year: PhD 1965
Major Field: unknown
Specialty: Cross Cultural Processes;Ethnic Minorities;HIV/
     AIDS;Lesbian & Gay Issuues;Stress

VRANIAK, Damian A.
W3177 Hamilton Road
Springbrook, WI 54875-9314
(715) 766-2029-**B**
maaingan@spacestar.net
Ethnicity: American Indian/Alaska Native
Degree and Year: PhD 1980
Major Field: Clinical Psychology
Specialty: Clinical Psychology;Clinical Child Psychology;Counseling
     Psychology;School Psychology;Cross Cultural Processes

WAGNER, Aureen Pinto
247 Park Avenue
Rochester, NY 14607
(716) 594-4770-**B**, (716) 594-5404-**H**, (716) 594-4207-**F**
aureen@eznet.net
Ethnicity: Asian-American/Asian/Pacific Islander

Languages: Hindi
Degree and Year: PhD 1989
Major Field: Clinical Child Psychology
Specialty: Adolescent Therapy;Affective Disorders;Clinical Child
     Psychology;Cognitive Behavioral Therapy;Behavior
     Therapy;Child Therapy

WAKEMAN, Richard J.
Ochsner Clinic
Department of Psychiatry
1514 Jefferson Highway
New Orleans, LA 70121
(504) 842-3845-**B**, (504) 899-0607-**H**, (504) 842-3236-**F**
Ethnicity: Asian-American/Asian/Pacific Islander
Degree and Year: PhD 1975
Major Field: Clinical Psychology
Specialty: Managed Care;Health Psychology;Neuropsychology;Pain &
     Pain Management;Sports Psychology

WALCOTT, Delores D.
Western Michigan University
2510 Faunee Student Services Building
Kalamazoo, MI 49008
(616) 387-1850-**B**, (616) 372-3037-**H**, (616) 387-1884-**F**
delores.walcott@umich.edu
Ethnicity: African-American/Black
Degree and Year: PsyD
Major Field: Clinical Psychology
Specialty: Juvenile Delinquency;Cross Cultural Processes;Sexual
     Physiology/Behavior;Assessment/Diagnosis/
     Evaluation;Research & Training;Forensic Psychology

WALIA, Kusum
Five Riverside Drive #411
Binghamton, NY 13905-4610
(518) 439-5396-**B**, (518) 439-2915-**H**
Ethnicity: Asian-American/Asian/Pacific Islander
Languages: Hindi, Punjabi
Degree and Year: PhD 1979
Major Field: School Psychology
Specialty: Assessment/Diagnosis/Evaluation;Cognitive Behavioral
     Therapy;Family Therapy;Psychotherapy;Stress

WALKER, L. Gorman
Dupree Counseling Services
10736 Jefferson Bulding #649
Culver City, CA 90230-4969
(310) 642-0841-**B**, (310) 642-5995-**F**
Ethnicity: African-American/Black, European/White
Degree and Year: PhD
Major Field: Clinical Psychology
Specialty: Employee Assistance Programs;Psychometrics;Assessment/
     Diagnosis/Evaluation;Cognitive Behavioral Therapy;Crisis
     Intervention & Therapy;Managed Care

WALKER, Lila K.
Morehouse College
1445 Monroe Drive #E-7
Atlanta, GA 30324
(770) 996-2224-**B**, (404) 892-4691-**H**, (770) 996-5469-**F**
Ethnicity: African-American/Black
Degree and Year: PhD 1991
Major Field: Clinical Psychology
Specialty: Neuropsychology;Clinical Neuropsychology;Assessment/
     Diagnosis/Evaluation

WALKER, Lola
  Lola Gorman Walker, PhD
  10736 Jefferson Boulevard #649
  Culver City, CA 90230
  (310) 642-0841-**B**, (310) 649-3651-**H**, (310) 642-5995-**F**
  Ethnicity: African-American/Black
  Degree and Year: PhD 1988 MA 1983
  Major Field: Clinical Psychology
  Specialty: Employee Assistance Programs;Ethnic Minorities;Marriage
      & Family;Crisis Intervention & Therapy;Forensic
      Psychology;Individual Psychotherapy

WALKER, O'Neal A.
  Federal Correctional Institutional
  Psychology Department
  501 Gary Hill Road
  Edgefield, SC 29824
  (803) 637-1500-**B**, (706) 863-5215-**H**, (706) 869-9059-**F**
  janeal2@aol.com
  Ethnicity: African-American/Black
  Degree and Year: PhD 1993 MS 1986
  Major Field: Clinical Psychology
  Specialty: Administration;Clinical Psychology;Ethnic
      Minorities;Alcoholism & Alcohol Abuse;Crime & Criminal
      Behavior;Crisis Intervention & Therapy

WALTON, Duncan E.
  Rutgers University
  Graduate School of Education
  10 Seminary Place
  New Brunswick, NJ 08903
  (908) 932-7297-**B**, (908) 756-6131-**H**, (908) 932-8206-**F**
  Ethnicity: African-American/Black
  Degree and Year: PhD 1956
  Major Field: Clinical Psychology
  Specialty: Counseling Psychology;Cross Cultural Processes;Ethnic
      Minorities;Psychotherapy

WANG, Alvin
  University of Central Florida
  Department of Psychology
  Orlando, FL 32816
  (407)823-2568-**B**, 407/539-3015-**H**
  awang@pegasus.cc.ucf.edu
  Ethnicity: Asian-American/Asian/Pacific Islander
  Degree and Year: PhD 1980
  Major Field: Experimental Psychology
  Specialty: Learning/Learning Theory;Memory

WANG, Edward S.
  46 Meadowbrook Rd
  Chestnut Hill, MA 02167-2933
  (617) 727-4923-**B**, (617) 734-2013-**H**
  Ethnicity: Asian-American/Asian/Pacific Islander
  Degree and Year: PsyD 1987
  Major Field: Clinical Psychology

WANG, James D.
  407 N Hebard Street
  Knoxville, IL 61448-1174
  (309) 289-2614-**B**
  Ethnicity: Asian-American/Asian/Pacific Islander
  Degree and Year: PhD 1941
  Major Field: Clinical Psychology
  Specialty: Group Psychotherapy;Family Therapy

WANG, Margaret C.
  Temple University
  933 Ritter Hall Annex
  Philidelphia, PA 19122
  (215) 204-3001-**B**, (215) 664-7176-**H**, (215) 204-5130-**F**
  Ethnicity: Asian-American/Asian/Pacific Islander
  Languages: Chinese
  Degree and Year: PhD 1968
  Major Field: Educational Psychology
  Specialty: Child Development;Educational Psychology;Learning
      Disabilities;Educational Research;Special Education

WANG, Paul H.
  15671 Sugarridge Court
  Chesterfield, MO 63017-5218
  Ethnicity: Asian-American/Asian/Pacific Islander
  Degree and Year: PhD 1983
  Major Field: Clinical Psychology
  Specialty: Cognitive Behavioral Therapy

WANG, Richard S.
  Number One Kimber Court
  East Northport, NY 11731-1355
  (516) 757-5014-**H**
  rsw39@juno.csm
  Ethnicity: Asian-American/Asian/Pacific Islander
  Degree and Year: MA 1969
  Major Field: Counseling Psychology

WANG, Wen-Hsiu
  National Hsinchu Teachers College
  No. 521, Nan-Ta Road
  Hsinchu,
  TAIWAN
  01188635213132-**B**, 01188635611529-**H**, 01188635611529-**F**
  wwant@cc.nhctc.edu.edu
  Ethnicity: Asian-American/Asian/Pacific Islander
  Degree and Year: EdD 1993
  Major Field: Counseling Psychology
  Specialty: Child Therapy;Client-Centered Therapy;Gender
      Issues;Group Processes;School Counseling;Training &
      Development

WANG, Youde
  Office of Education
  721 Fairfax Avenue
  Norfolk, VA 23507-2007
  (757) 446-8488-**B**, (508) 842-8738-**H**, (757) 446-8416-**F**
  yw@worf.evms.edu
  Ethnicity: Asian-American/Asian/Pacific Islander
  Languages: Chinese
  Degree and Year: PhD 1988
  Major Field: Health Psychology
  Specialty: Sports Psychology;Stress;Motor Performance;Statistics

WARD, Alan J.
  University of Illinois at Chicago
  Department of Psychiatry
  5415 North Sheridan Road
  Suite 4301
  Chicago, IL 60640
  (773) 996-8698-**B**, (773 271-4439-**H**, (773) 271-4439-**F**
  alanw28981@aol.com

Ethnicity: African-American/Black
Degree and Year: PhD 1965 AM 1960
Major Field: Clinical Psychology
Specialty: Clinical Child Psychology;Individual Psychotherapy;Family
　　　Processes

WARD, Connie M.
　Counseling Center
　Georgia State University
　106 Courtland
　Atlanta, GA 30303
　(404) 651-2211-**B**, (404) 651-1714-**F**
Ethnicity: African-American/Black
Degree and Year: PhD 1980
Major Field: Counseling Psychology
Specialty: Adult Development;Counseling Psychology;Cross Cultural
　　　Processes;Ethnic Minorities;Vocational Psychology

WARD, Lucretia M.
　University of Michigan
　Psychology Department
　525 East University Avenue
　Ann Arbor, MI 48109-1109
　(734) 764-0430-**B**, (734) 764-3520-**F**
　ward@umich.edu
Ethnicity: African-American/Black
Degree and Year: PhD 1995
Major Field: Developmental Psychology
Specialty: Adolescent Development;Gender Issues;Sexual
　　　Behavior;Child Development;Mass Media
　　　Communication;Ethnic Minorities

WASHINGTON, Anita C.
　33343 Ladoga Avenue
　Long Beach, CA 90808
　(310) 425-9825-**B**, (310) 421-2225-**H**, (310) 421-2225-**F**
Ethnicity: African-American/Black
Degree and Year: PhD 1969
Major Field: Clinical Psychology
Specialty: Clinical Psychology;Crisis Intervention & Therapy;Family
　　　Therapy;Depression;Drug Abuse

WASHINGTON, Dianna E.
　14547 Jaystone Drive
　Silver Spring, MD 20905
　(301) 384-9394-**B**, (301) 384-9441-**H**
Ethnicity: African-American/Black
Degree and Year: PhD 1982
Major Field: Clinical Psychology
Specialty: Affective Disorders;Assessment/Diagnosis/
　　　Evaluation;Depression;Stress;Family Therapy

WASHINGTON, Robert A.
　St. Francis Center
　5135 MacArthur Boulevard
　Washington, DC 20011
　(202) 363-8500-**B**, 202 291-2824-**H**, 202 363-4989-**F**
Ethnicity: African-American/Black
Degree and Year: PhD 1974
Major Field: Clinical Psychology
Specialty: Clinical Psychology;Death & Dying

WATANABE-MURAOKA, Agnes M.
　19-10-1010 Higashi-Cho
　ISOGO-K4

　Yokohama 197,
　JAPAN
　(011) 81-035-4-**B**, (011) 81-033-3-**H**
Ethnicity: Asian-American/Asian/Pacific Islander
Languages: Japanese
Degree and Year: PhD 1980
Major Field: Counseling Psychology
Specialty: Counseling Psychology;Vocational Psychology;School
　　　Counseling;Gerontology/Geropsychology

WATTS, Charlotte B.
　Henrico Area Mental Health
　 and Retardation Services
　10299 Woodman Road
　Richmond, VA 23060
　(804) 261-8500-**B**, (804) 739-7295-**H**, (804) 261-8480-**F**
　wat30@cohenrico.va.us
Ethnicity: African-American/Black
Degree and Year: PhD 1996 MS 1993
Major Field: Counseling Psychology
Specialty: Family Therapy;Counseling Psychology;Interpersonal
　　　Processes & Relations

WATTS, Roderick J.
　DePaul University
　Department of Psychology
　2219 North Kenmore Avenue
　Chicago, IL 60614-3504
　(312) 325-2016-**B**, (708) 524-4695-**H**, (312) 362-8279-**F**
Ethnicity: African-American/Black
Degree and Year: PhD 1984
Major Field: Community Psychology
Specialty: Community Psychology;Ethnic Minorities;Program
　　　Evaluation

WEBB, Wanda
　708 Madras Lane
　Charlotte, NC 28211
　(704) 892-2297-**B**, (704) 365-1791-**H**, (704) 365-9973-**F**
Ethnicity: African-American/Black
Degree and Year: PhD 1984
Major Field: Counseling Psychology
Specialty: Cognitive Behavioral Therapy;Child Abuse;Alcoholism &
　　　Alcohol Abuse;Psychotherapy;Depression;Marriage & Family

WEBSTER, E. Carol
　4330 West Broward Blvd.
　Suite I
　Plantation, FL 33317
　(305) 584-6746-**B**
Ethnicity: African-American/Black
Degree and Year: PhD 1978
Major Field: Clinical Psychology
Specialty: Clinical Psychology

WELLONS, Retha V.
　805 Red Leaf Court
　San Francisco, CA 94134-3157
　(415) 585-5919-**B**, (415) 585-5972-**F**
Ethnicity: African-American/Black
Degree and Year: PhD 1978
Major Field: Industrial/Organizational Psy.
Specialty: Leadership;Group Processes;Organizational
　　　Development;Industrial/Organizational Psychology;Survey
　　　Theory & Methodology

WELLS, Annie M.
919 Corley Drive, SE
Huntsville, AL 35802
(205) 851-5528-**B**, (205) 881-4753-**H**
Ethnicity: African-American/Black
Languages: German
Degree and Year: PhD 1970
Major Field: unknown
Specialty: Experimental Psychology;Counseling Psychology;Health
	Psychology;Clinical Psychology;Psychopharmacology

WEST, Gerald I.
San Francisco State University
Dean of Faculty Affairs
1600 Holloway
San Francisco, CA 94132
(415) 338-2204-**B**, (415) 338-3901-**F**
gwest@sfsu.edu
Ethnicity: African-American/Black
Degree and Year: PhD 1967
Major Field: Counseling Psychology
Specialty: Counseling Psychology;Administration;Consulting
	Psychology;Cross Cultural Processes;Family Therapy

WEST, James E.
P.O. Box 1867
Marion, IN 46952
(765) 674-3321-**B**, (765) 674-7165-**H**
Ethnicity: African-American/Black
Degree and Year: PhD 1981
Major Field: Counseling Psychology
Specialty: Counseling Psychology;Sex/Marital Therapy;HIV/
	AIDS;Stress

WESTON, Raymond E.
Memorial Sloan Kettering Cancer Center
1275 York Avenue
New York, NY 10021
(212) 583-3047-**B**, (718) 258-8642-**H**
Ethnicity: African-American/Black
Degree and Year: PhD 1977
Major Field: Clinical Psychology
Specialty: Clinical Psychology;Community Mental Health;Cognitive
	Behavioral Therapy;Ethnic Minorities;HIV/AIDS

WHANG, Patricia A.
Auburn University
4064 Haley Center
Auburn University, AL 36849
(334) 844-3056-**B**, (334) 844-3072-**F**
Ethnicity: Asian-American/Asian/Pacific Islander
Degree and Year: PhD 1991
Major Field: Educational Psychology
Specialty: Educational Psychology;Ingestive Behavior &
	Nutrition;Motivation

WHISENTON, Joffre T.
3283 Spreading Oak Drive, SW
Atlanta, GA 30311-2939
(404) 696-0340-**B**
Ethnicity: African-American/Black
Degree and Year: PhD 1968
Major Field: Educational Psychology

WHITAKER, Arthur L.
39 Emily Jeffers Road
Randolph, MA 02368-2849
(617) 986-6360-**H**
Ethnicity: African-American/Black
Languages: French
Degree and Year: PhD 1973
Major Field: Counseling Psychology
Specialty: Clinical Psychology;Pastoral Psychology;Marriage &
	Family;Mental Health Services;Counseling Psychology

WHITAKER, Sandra V.
Govenors State University
Psychology Department
University Park, IL 60466
(708) 534-4907-**B**, (708) 798-5720-**H**, (708) 534-8451-**F**
s-whitak@govst.edu
Ethnicity: Hispanic/Latino
Languages: Spanish
Degree and Year: PhD 1972
Major Field: Clinical Psychology
Specialty: Assessment/Diagnosis/Evaluation;Psychology of
	Women;School Psychology;Social Psychology;Ethnic
	Minorities

WHITEHEAD, Barry X.
The Youth Camps
1001 West Van Buren
Sixth Floor
Chicago, IL 60607
(312) 243-0533-**B**, (847) 758-0762-**H**
Ethnicity: African-American/Black
Degree and Year: EdD 1988 MeD 1976
Major Field: Counseling Psychology
Specialty: Counseling Psychology;Drug Abuse;Psychoses;Behavior
	Therapy;Family Therapy;Sex/Marital Therapy

WHITEHEAD, Jesse
15 Canterbury Ln
Tinton Falls, NJ 07724-2804
(908) 542-1170-**B**, (908) 542-5925-**H**
Ethnicity: African-American/Black
Degree and Year: PsyD 1983
Major Field: unknown
Specialty: Adolescent Therapy

WHITEHURST, JR., William H.
Brightwood Station
P.O. Box 55493
Washington, DC 20040-5493
Ethnicity: African-American/Black
Degree and Year: MA 1955
Major Field: Clinical Psychology
Specialty: Social Psychology

WHITE, Joseph L.
University of California, Irvine
School of Social Services
3151 Social Science Plaza
Irvine, CA 72697-5100
(949) 824-7137-**B**, (949) 559-7379-**H**, (949) 824-6057-**F**
jlwhite@uic.edu
Ethnicity: African-American/Black

Degree and Year: PhD 1961
Major Field: Clinical Psychology
Specialty: Adolescent Development;Adult Development;Client-
    Centered Therapy;Clinical Psychology;Counseling Psychology

WHITE, Voncile
    12 Inman Street
    Apartment #55
    Cambridge, MA 02139-2419
    (781) 283-2327-**B**, (617) 492-0532-**H**, (781) 28303720-**F**
    vwhite@wellesley.edu
Ethnicity: African-American/Black
Degree and Year: EdD 1985
Major Field: Counseling Psychology
Specialty: Counseling Psychology;Psychology of Women;Ethnic
    Minorities;Clinical Psychology;Adult Development

WHITTEN, Lisa A.
    SUNY College at Old Westbury
    PO Box 210
    Psychology Programs
    Old Westbury, NY 11568-0210
    (516) 876-3124-**B**, (21) 926-9425-**H**, (516) 876-3299-**F**
    lwhitt@aol.com
Ethnicity: African-American/Black
Degree and Year: PhD 1982 BA 1977
Major Field: Clinical Psychology
Specialty: Cultural & Social
    Processes;Depression;Psychotherapy;Curriculum
    Development/Evaluation;Marriage & Family;Ethnic Minorities

WIBBERLY, Kathy H.
    Virginia Department of Health
    1500 East Main Street
    Suite 27 Box 2448
    Richmond, VA 23219
    (804) 786-1211-**B**, (804) 346-3356-**H**, (804) 371-0116-**F**
    kwibberly@vdh.state.va.us
Ethnicity: Asian-American/Asian/Pacific Islander
Languages: Chinese
Degree and Year: PhD 1995
Major Field: Counseling Psychology
Specialty: Group Processes;Prevention;Program Evaluation;Marriage &
    Family;Community Psychology;Ethnic Minorities

WICKRAMASEKERA, Ian E.
    PO Box 5247
    Hercules, CA 94547
    510 245-7022-**B**
    iwickram@igc.apc.org
Ethnicity: Asian-American/Asian/Pacific Islander
Languages: Singhalese
Degree and Year: PhD 1969
Major Field: Clinical Psychology
Specialty: Psychophysiology;Psychosomatic
    Disorders;Biofeedback;Hypnosis/Hypnotherapy;Pain & Pain
    Management

WILKINSON, H. Sook
    708 Parleman Drive
    Bloomfield Hills, MI 48304
    (313) 649-0001-**B**, (313) 645-6719-**H**
Ethnicity: Asian-American/Asian/Pacific Islander
Languages: Korean
Degree and Year: PhD 1981

Major Field: Clinical Child Psychology
Specialty: Child Therapy;Cross Cultural Processes;Individual
    Psychotherapy;Psychology of Women;Psychotherapy

WILLIAMS-MARKUM, Deirdre
    Rice University Counseling Center
    6100 Main Street - MS #19
    Houston, TX 77005
    (713) 527-4867-**B**, (281) 554-3298-**F**
    jazzy@rice.edu
Ethnicity: African-American/Black
Degree and Year: PhD 1993
Major Field: Clinical Psychology
Specialty: Assessment/Diagnosis/Evaluation;Ethnic
    Minorities;Psychology of Women;Adolescent
    Therapy;Personality Disorders;Eating Disorders

WILLIAMS-PETERSEN, Janice
    Family Life Institute
    3661 W Oakland Parkway
    Suite #300
    Ft. Lauderdale, FL 33311-1145
Ethnicity: African-American/Black
Degree and Year: PhD 1984
Major Field: Clinical Psychology
Specialty: Clinical Psychology;Community Psychology

WILLIAMS, Carrolyn N.
    11 Beech Street
    East Orange, NJ 07018-3003
    (973) 674-3663-**H**
Ethnicity: African-American/Black
Degree and Year: PhD 1984 MS 1971
Major Field: Community Psychology
Specialty: Adolescent Development;Child Abuse;Parent-Child
    Interaction;Alcoholism&AlcoholAbuse;HIVAIDS;Research&Training

WILLIAMS, Daniel E.
    1837 Rangewood Court
    Plainfield, NJ 07060
    (201) 675-9200-**B**, (908) 754-0186-**H**, (201) 678-8432-**F**
Ethnicity: African-American/Black
Degree and Year: PhD 1968
Major Field: General Psy./Methods & Systems
Specialty: Clinical Psychology;Child Therapy;Marriage &
    Family;Psychometrics;Psychopathology

WILLIAMS, David R.
    University of Michigan
    Institute for Social Research
    PO Box 1248
    Ann Arbor, MI 48106-1248
    (734) 936-0649-**B**, (734) 572-7742-**H**, (734) 647-6972-**F**
    wildavid@umich.edu
Ethnicity: African-American/Black
Degree and Year: PhD 1986
Major Field: unknown
Specialty: Ethnic Minorities;Health Psychology;Mental
    Disorders;Mental Health Services;Religious Psychology

WILLIAMS, Eddie E.
    VA Medical Center
    Psychology Service (116B)
    3001 Greenbay Road
    North Chicago, IL 60064-3034
    (708) 688-1900-**B**, (708) 249-2317-**H**

Ethnicity: African-American/Black
Degree and Year: PhD 1975
Major Field: Counseling Psychology
Specialty: Cross Cultural Processes;Drug Abuse;Ethnic
        Minorities;Forensic Psychology;Psychology & Law

WILLIAMS, Estelle M.
  Los Angeles School District
  450 North Grand Avenue
  Los Angeles, CA 90012
  (310) 444-9913-**B**, (213) 295-0318-**H**
Ethnicity: African-American/Black
Degree and Year: MS 1958
Major Field: Educational Psychology

WILLIAMS, Everett B.
  Turrell Fund
  21 Van Vleck Street
  Montclair, NJ 07042-2358
  (973) 783.9358-**B**, (973) 744-4377-**H**, (973) 783-9283-**F**
  ebelvinw@turrellfund.com
Ethnicity: African-American/Black
Degree and Year: PhD 1962 MSB 1970
Major Field: Clinical Psychology
Specialty: Cognitive Psychology;Problem Solving;Thought
        Processes;Management & Organization;Prevention;Values &
        Moral Behavior

WILLIAMS, Indy J.
  10521 Mereworth Lane
  Oakton, VA 22124
  (703) 938-5105-**H**
Ethnicity: African-American/Black
Degree and Year: PhD 1984
Major Field: Clinical Psychology
Specialty: Employee Assistance Programs;Clinical
        Psychology;Assessment/Diagnosis/Evaluation;Adult
        Development

WILLIAMS, Karen P. W.
  1911 Huntington Drive, #B
  Duarte, CA 91010
  (909) 981-2938-**B**, (818) 303-0526-**H**
Ethnicity: African-American/Black
Degree and Year: PhD 1979
Major Field: Clinical Child Psychology
Specialty: Clinical Child Psychology;Depression;Managed
        Care;Stress;Psychology of Women

WILLIAMS, Mary Beth
  Trauma Recovery Education
  9 North Third Street
  Suite 100 #14
  Warrenton, VA 20186
  (540) 341-7339-**B**, (540) 347-3408-**H**, (540) 341-7339-**F**
  mbethwms@citizen.infi.net
Ethnicity: American Indian/Alaska Native
Languages: German
Degree and Year: PhD 1990
Major Field: Clinical Psychology

WILLIAMS, Medria L.
  429 Grace Avenue
  Inglewood, CA 90301
  (213) 912-3942-**B**, (310) 412-7701-**H**, (310) 394-5348-**F**
Ethnicity: African-American/Black

Degree and Year: PhD 1985
Major Field: Clinical Psychology
Specialty: Adolescent Therapy;Alcoholism & Alcohol Abuse;Eating
        Disorders;Group Processes;Ethnic Minorities

WILLIAMS, Michael A.
  Professional Psychological Service
  4130 Linden Avenue
  Suite 309
  Dayton, OH 45432-3034
  (513) 254-7301-**B**, (613) 837-3961-**H**, (513) 254-2117-**F**
Ethnicity: African-American/Black
Degree and Year: EdD 1980
Major Field: Clinical Child Psychology
Specialty: Adolescent Therapy;Assessment/Diagnosis/Evaluation;Child
        Therapy;Family Therapy

WILLIAMSON, Diane H.
  3227 East 31st Street #104
  Tulsa, OK 74105
  (918) 742-4566-**B**, (918) 745-0890-**F**
  dwmson@lbm.net
Ethnicity: American Indian/Alaska Native
Degree and Year: EdD 1971 MTA 1969
Major Field: Developmental Psychology
Specialty: Neuropsychology;Mentally Retarded;Learning
        Disabilities;Psychopharmacology;Physically
        Handicapped;Brain Damage

WILLIAMS, Phyllis J.
  6 Valley Forge Road
  New Castle, DE 19720-4212
  (201) 647-0180-**B**, 302 322-5396-**H**
Ethnicity: African-American/Black
Degree and Year: PhD 1979
Major Field: Clinical Psychology
Specialty: Alcoholism & Alcohol Abuse;Drug Abuse

WILLIAMS, Rebecca E.
  VA San Diego Healthcare System
  3350 LaJolla Village Drive
  San Diego, CA 92161
  (619) 640-4590-**B**, (619) 640-4583-**F**
Ethnicity: African-American/Black, Hispanic/Latino
Degree and Year: PhD 1996 MeD 1988
Major Field: Clinical Psychology
Specialty: Chronically Mentally Ill;Clinical Psychology;Structured
        Outpatient Services;Alcoholism & Alcohol Abuse;Training &
        Development;Rehabilitation

WILLIAMS, Steve
  American Society of Association Executives
  1575 I Street, NW
  Washington , DC 20005-1168
  (202) 626-ASAE-**B**, (202) 842-1109-**F**
  swilliams@asaenet.org
Ethnicity: African-American/Black
Degree and Year: PhD 1997 MS 1994
Major Field: Clinical Psychology
Specialty: Clinical Psychology;Psychopathology;Suicide;Survey
        Theory & Methodology;Cultural & Social Processes;Crisis
        Intervention & Therapy

WILLIAMS, Victoria F.
  5312 Montague Street #4
  Charlotte, NC 28205-7956

(704) 567-9213-**H**
Ethnicity: African-American/Black
Degree and Year: PsyD 1986
Major Field: Clinical Psychology
Specialty: Clinical Psychology;Individual
Psychotherapy;Psychotherapy;Assessment/Diagnosis/
Evaluation;Personality Disorders;Ethnic Minorities

WILLIAMS, Willie S.
20310 Chagrin Blvd.
Shaker Heights, OH 44122-4973
(216) 491-9405-**B**
Ethnicity: African-American/Black
Degree and Year: PhD 1970
Major Field: Counseling Psychology

WILLIS, Cynthia E.
University of Nebraska
Psychology Department
209 Burnett Hall
Lincoln, NE 68588-0308
(402) 472-3740-**B**, (402) 435-4299-**H**
Ethnicity: American Indian/Alaska Native
Degree and Year: PhD 1990
Major Field: Social Psychology
Specialty: Ethnic Minorities;Cultural & Social Processes;Social
Cognition;Social Behavior;Psychology & Law

WILLIS, Diane J.
University of Oklahoma Health Services Center
Child Study Center
1100 N.E. 13th Street
Oaklahoma City, OK 73117
(405) 271-5700-**B**, (405) 364-9091-**H**, (405) 271-8835-**F**
dwillis@ouhsc.edu
Ethnicity: American Indian/Alaska Native
Degree and Year: PhD 1970
Major Field: Clinical Child Psychology
Specialty: Administration;Child Abuse;Child & Pediatric
Psychology;Clinical Child Psychology;Training &
Development

WILSON, Jennifer
1570 Crescent Hills Drive
La Crescent, MN 55947-9650
(608) 785-8073-**B**
Ethnicity: American Indian/Alaska Native
Degree and Year: PhD 1983
Major Field: unknown
Specialty: Counseling Psychology

WILSON, Lloyd K.
14603 Green Oaks Woods
San Antonio, TX 78249-1435
(210) 601-0142-**B**, (210) 492-0803-**H**, (210) 691-1438-**F**
Ethnicity: American Indian/Alaska Native
Degree and Year: PhD 1984
Major Field: unknown
Specialty: Rehabilitation;Neuropsychology;Vocational
Psychology;Brain Damage;Assessment/Diagnosis/Evaluation

WILSON, Margaret
3209 N Military Road

Arlington, VA 22207-4157
(202) 373-7387-**B**
Ethnicity: African-American/Black
Degree and Year: PhD 1978
Major Field: Clinical Psychology
Specialty: Developmental Psychology

WILSON, Melvin N.
University of Virginia
Dept. of Psychology
102 Gilmer Hall
Charlottesville, VA 22903
(804) 982-4750-**B**, (804) 982-4766-**F**
Ethnicity: African-American/Black
Degree and Year: PhD 1977
Major Field: Clinical Psychology
Specialty: Community Mental Health;Ethnic Minorities;Family
Processes;Domestic Violence;Cross Cultural Processes

WILSON, Shirley B.
8825 Lanier Drive
Silver Spring, MD 20910-2306
(202) 865-4569-**B**, (301) 589-8425-**H**, (202) 865-4558-**F**
iamshirley@aol.com
Ethnicity: African-American/Black
Degree and Year: PhD 1973
Major Field: Developmental Psychology
Specialty: Clinical Child Psychology;Medical Psychology;Mental
Health Services;Psychotherapy;Mental Disorders;Learning
Disabilities

WILSON, Susan B.
Swope Parkway
Community Mental Health Center
3801 Blue Parkway
Kansas City, MO 64030
(816) 922-7645-**B**, (816) 761-8201-**H**, (816) 929-2636-**F**
Ethnicity: African-American/Black
Degree and Year: PhD 1985 MS 1981
Major Field: Clinical Psychology
Specialty: Ethnic Minorities;Administration;Attention Deficit
Disorders;Managed Care;Affective Disorders;Consulting
Psychology

WILSON, Woodrow
9361 SW 62nd Street
Miami, FL 33173
(305) 342-3425-**B**, (305) 595-3344-**H**, (305) 271-7744-**F**
pepwilson@aol.com
Ethnicity: African-American/Black
Degree and Year: PhD 1974
Major Field: Clinical Psychology
Specialty: Clinical Psychology;Ethnic Minorities;Parent
Education;Counseling Psychology;Medical
Psychology;Administration

WINDHAM, Thomas L.
University Corporation for
Atmospheric Research (UCAR)
2830 Iliff Street
Boulder, CO 80303
(303) 447-5028-**B**, (303) 499-2740-**H**, (303) 447-5024-**F**
twindham@ucar.edu
Ethnicity: African-American/Black, American Indian/Alaska Native

Degree and Year: PhD 1975
Major Field: Social Psychology
Specialty: Social Psychology;Personality Psychology;Community
Psychology

WINFREY, Angela D.
Pennsylvania Hospital
Hall Mercer - Room 6A
800 Spruce Street
Phildelphia, PA 19107
(215) 829-5711-**B**, (215) 748-4554-**H**, (215) 829-5282-**F**
winfread@dca.net
Ethnicity: African-American/Black
Degree and Year: PhD 1998 MA 1973
Major Field: Neurosciences
Specialty: Child
Development;Neuropsychology;Psychopharmacology;Child &
Pediatric Psychology;Neurological Disorders;Assessment/
Diagnosis/Evaluation

WINFREY, LaPearl L.
American School of Professional
Psychology - Virginia Campus
1400 Wilson Boulevard
Suite 110
Arlington, VA 22209
(703) 243-5300-**B**, (703) 243-8973-**F**
lapwinf@aol.com
Ethnicity: African-American/Black
Degree and Year: PhD 1988
Major Field: Clinical Psychology
Specialty: Cognitive Behavioral Therapy;Ethnic Minorities;Cross
Cultural Processes;Consulting Psychology;Psychotherapy

WINTER, Amal
21433 Broadway Road
Los Gatos, LA 95030
(408) 353-1786-**B**, (408) 353-5438-**F**
Ethnicity: Asian-American/Asian/Pacific Islander
Languages: Arabic
Degree and Year: PhD 1973
Major Field: Clinical Psychology
Specialty: Community Mental Health;Assessment/Diagnosis/
Evaluation;Ethnic Minorities;Family Therapy;Alcoholism &
Alcohol Abuse

WIN, U. Kyaw
24941 Mustang Drive
Laguna Hills, CA 92653-5730
(714) 432-5860-**B**
Ethnicity: Asian-American/Asian/Pacific Islander
Degree and Year: PhD 1971
Major Field: Counseling Psychology

WISNER, Roscoe W.
266 East Greenwich Avenue
Roosevelt, NY 11575
(516) 868-5715-**H**
Ethnicity: African-American/Black
Degree and Year: EdD 1963
Major Field: unknown
Specialty: Administration;Assessment/Diagnosis/
Evaluation;Professional Issues in Psychology;Counseling

Psychology

WITTER, Jeanette M.
1015 Spring Street
Suite 301
Silver Spring, MD 20910
(301) 587-1919-**B**, (301) 559-7740-**H**, (301) 587-2943-**F**
jmew@erols.com
Ethnicity: African-American/Black
Degree and Year: PhD 1986 MpLi 1985
Major Field: Clinical Psychology
Specialty: Clinical Psychology;Depression;Lesbian & Gay
Issuues;Individual Psychotherapy;Ethnic
Minorities;Psychology of Women

WONG-NGAN, Julia A.
5441 SW Macadam
Suite #102
Portland, OR 97201
(503) 242-0490-**B**, (503) 774-0938-**H**, (503) 222-5480-**F**
Ethnicity: Asian-American/Asian/Pacific Islander
Degree and Year: PhD 1985
Major Field: Clinical Psychology
Specialty: Neuropsychology;Pain & Pain Management;Gerontology/
Geropsychology

WONG-RIEGER, Durhane
University of Windsor
Department of Psychology
401 Sunset Avenue
Windsor, Ontario, N9B 3G4
CANADA
(519) 253-4232-**B**, (519) 256-9471-**H**, (519) 973-7021-**F**
Ethnicity: Asian-American/Asian/Pacific Islander
Languages: Chinese, French
Degree and Year: PhD 1981
Major Field: Social Psychology
Specialty: Program Evaluation;Organizational Development;Psychology
of Women;Consulting Psychology;HIV/AIDS

WONG, Deborah A.
1440 West Main Street
Tipp City, OH 45371-2804
(513) 339-8907-**B**
Ethnicity: Asian-American/Asian/Pacific Islander
Degree and Year: PhD 1985
Major Field: Clinical Psychology
Specialty: Psychotherapy

WONG, Dorothy L.
4747 Bellaire Road
Suite #354
Bellaire, TX 77401
(713) 668-8228-**B**, (713) 664-9744-**H**, (713) 668-8283-**F**
Ethnicity: Asian-American/Asian/Pacific Islander
Languages: Chinese
Degree and Year: PhD 1975
Major Field: Developmental Psychology
Specialty: Clinical Psychology;Assessment/Diagnosis/Evaluation;Child
Abuse;Forensic Psychology;Family Therapy

WONG, Florence C
St. John's University, New York
Department of Psychology
8000 Utopia Parkway
Jamaica, NY 11439

(718) 990-1553-**B**, 718 658-0514-**H**
wongf@sjuvm.stjohns.edu
Ethnicity: Asian-American/Asian/Pacific Islander
Languages: Spanish
Degree and Year:
Major Field: Clinical Child Psychology

WONG, Frankie Y.
Fenway Community Health Center
7 Haviland Street
Boston, MA 02115
(617) 267-4700-**B**, (617) 522-0714-**H**, (617) 536-8602-**F**
fwong@fchc.org
Ethnicity: Asian-American/Asian/Pacific Islander
Languages: Chinese
Degree and Year: PhD 1990
Major Field: Social Psychology
Specialty: Alcoholism & Alcohol Abuse;Community
    Psychology;Gender Issues;HIV/AIDS

WONG, Hermund
Association in Counseling
  Mediation Therapy
646 29th Avenue
Suite 101
San Francisco, CA 94121-2821
(415) 221-1637-**B**, (415) 221-1637-**H**
Ethnicity: Asian-American/Asian/Pacific Islander
Languages: Chinese
Degree and Year: MA 1968
Major Field: unknown
Specialty: Psychotherapy;Stress;Domestic Violence;Psychosomatic
    Disorders;Death & Dying;Alzheimer's Disease

WONG, Jane L.
University of Northern Iowa
Department of Psychology
Cedar Falls, IA 50614
(319) 273-2223-**B**, (319) 277-9642-**H**, (319) 273-6188-**F**
jane.wong@uni.edu
Ethnicity: Asian-American/Asian/Pacific Islander
Degree and Year: PhD 1988
Major Field: Clinical Psychology
Specialty: Neuropsychology;Assessment/Diagnosis/Evaluation;Clinical
    Neuropsychology;Clinical Psychology;Cognitive Behavioral
    Therapy

WONG, Jessie
Clark Institute of Psychiatry
Health System Res. Unit
250 College Street
Toronto
Ontario M5T 1R8,
CANADA
(416) 979-6877-**B**, (416) 495-1776-**F**
Ethnicity: Asian-American/Asian/Pacific Islander
Languages: Chinese
Degree and Year: MA 1977
Major Field: Experimental Psychology
Specialty: Statistics

WONG, Kit L.
96 Mason Drive

Princeton, NJ 08540-5408
(609) 921-6936-**H**, (609) 921-6936-**F**
Ethnicity: Asian-American/Asian/Pacific Islander
Languages: Chinese
Degree and Year: PhD 1976
Major Field: Clinical Psychology
Specialty: Psychoanalysis;Psychotherapy;Forensic
    Psychology;Personality Disorders;Cross Cultural Processes

WONG, Lily Y.S
National Institute of Education
PO Box 214144
Sacramento, CA 95821-0144
Ethnicity: Asian-American/Asian/Pacific Islander
Languages: Chinese
Degree and Year: PhD 1987
Major Field: Educational Psychology
Specialty: Adolescent Development;Attribution Theory;Child
    Development;Cognitive Development;Creativity

WONG, Lily H.
Southeast Asia Union College
273 Upper Serangoon Road
Singapore, 392,
SINGAPORE
011 65-285-7-**B**, 011 65-285-7-**H**
Wongly@Singnet.com.sg
Ethnicity: Asian-American/Asian/Pacific Islander
Degree and Year: EdD 1976
Major Field: Educational Psychology

WONG, Martin R.
1623 Colorado Drive
East Lansing, MI 48823
(616) 966-5600-**B**, (517) 337-2299-**H**
Ethnicity: Asian-American/Asian/Pacific Islander
Degree and Year: PhD 1969
Major Field: Counseling Psychology
Specialty: Rehabilitation;Educational Psychology

WONG, Philip S
New School for Social Research
Department of Psychology
65 Fifth Avenue
New York, NY 10003
(212) 229-5778-**B**, (212) 873-1215-**H**, (212) 989-0846-**F**
pswong@newschool.edu
Ethnicity: Asian-American/Asian/Pacific Islander
Languages: 03 Cantonese, 03 Mandarin
Degree and Year: PhD 1992
Major Field: Clinical Psychology
Specialty: Clinical Psychology;Psychotherapy;Cognitive
    Psychology;Psychoanalysis;Ethnic
    Minorities;Psychophysiology

WONG, Roderick
University of British Colombia
Department of Psychology
Vancouver, BC V6T1W5
CANADA
(604) 228-2719-**B**
Ethnicity: Asian-American/Asian/Pacific Islander
Degree and Year: PhD 1963

Major Field: unknown

WONG, Tony M.
   Biola University
   6 Woodside Lane
   Pittsford, NY 14534-2308
   (213) 903-4867-**B**
Ethnicity: Asian-American/Asian/Pacific Islander
Degree and Year: PhD 1982
Major Field: unknown
Specialty: Clinical Neuropsychology

WONG, Wilson
   2443 Harrods Pointe Trace
   Lexington, KY 40514-1407
   (201) 358-9296-**B**
Ethnicity: Asian-American/Asian/Pacific Islander
Degree and Year: PhD 1968
Major Field: unknown
Specialty: Industrial/Organizational Psychology

WOOD, JR., Nollie P.
   Baltimore City Health Department
   1221 East Oliver St
   Baltimore, MD 21202-5721
   (301) 396-9944-**B**
Ethnicity: African-American/Black
Degree and Year: PhD 1985
Major Field: Clinical Psychology
Specialty: Alcoholism & Alcohol Abuse

WOOD, Keith A.
   Emory University
   Department of Psychiatry
   80 Bulter Street, SE
   Atlanta, GA 30335
   (404) 589-4795-**B**
Ethnicity: African-American/Black
Degree and Year: PhD 1976
Major Field: Clinical Psychology
Specialty: Experimental Analysis of Behavior

WOODLAND, Calvin E.
   Bergen Community College
   400 Paramus Road
   Paramus, NJ 07652-1595
   (201) 447-7491-**B**, (201) 447-3730-**F**
Ethnicity: African-American/Black
Degree and Year: PsyD 1997 EdD 1975
Major Field: Clinical Psychology

WOODS, Delma M.
   1106 Woodhaven Drive
   Charleston, SC 29407-3739
   (803) 571-6800-**B**
Ethnicity: African-American/Black
Degree and Year: PhD 1987
Major Field: Clinical Psychology

WOO, Rose
   16 South Oakland Avenue
   Suite 214
   Pasadena, CA 91101
   (626) 568-3856-**H**
Ethnicity: Asian-American/Asian/Pacific Islander

Degree and Year: PhD 1991 PhD 1981
Major Field: Clinical Psychology
Specialty: Psychoanalysis;Infancy;Clinical Child Psychology;Eating
      Disorders

WOO, Tae O.
   135 Oak Knoll Circle
   Millersville, PA 17551
   (717) 872-3088-**B**, (717) 872-1677-**H**
Ethnicity: Asian-American/Asian/Pacific Islander
Languages: Korean
Degree and Year: PhD 1982
Major Field: Social Psychology
Specialty: Cultural & Social Processes;Gender Issues;Health
      Psychology;Interpersonal Processes & Relations;Personality
      Psychology

WOOTEN, William
   University of Central Florida
   Psychology Department
   Orlando, FL 32816-1390
   (407) 823-2552-**B**, (407) 365-9918-**H**, (407) 823-5862-**F**
   wwooten@pegasus.cc.ucf.edu
Ethnicity: African-American/Black
Degree and Year: PhD 1980
Major Field: Industrial/Organizational Psy.
Specialty: Selection & Placement;Training & Development;Work
      Performance;Performance Evaluation;Quantitative/
      Mathematical, Psychometrics;Psychometrics

WORD, James C.
   DC Department of Corrections
   Lorton, VA 22079
   (703) 643-6305-**B**, (202) 722-6181-**H**, (703) 643-0738-**F**
Ethnicity: African-American/Black
Languages: Spanish
Degree and Year: PhD 1974 JD 1983
Major Field: Clinical Psychology
Specialty: Correctional Psychology;Mental Health Services;Forensic
      Psychology

WORRELL, Frank C.
   Pennsylvania State University
   Educational School Psychology and
     Special Education
   227 Cedar Building
   University Park, PA 16802
   (814) 865-1881-**B**, (814) 466-6158-**H**, (814) 863-1002-**F**
   fcw3@psu.edu
Ethnicity: African-American/Black
Degree and Year: PhD 1994
Major Field: School Psychology
Specialty: Adolescent Development;Prevention;Giftedness;School
      Psychology

WRIGHT, Doris J.
   1924 Lexington Lane
   Manhattan, KY 66503-7549
   (785) 532-5541-**B**
   djwright@ksu.edu
Ethnicity: African-American/Black
Degree and Year: PhD 1982
Major Field: Counseling Psychology

Specialty: Ethnic Minorities;Gender Issues;Health
Psychology;Organizational Development;Counseling
Psychology

WRIGHT, Michael F.
2632 San Pablo, #a
Berkeley, CA 94702-2249
(415) 845-2045-**B**, (510) 848-6463-**H**
Ethnicity: African-American/Black
Degree and Year: PhD 1976
Major Field: Clinical Psychology
Specialty: Religious Psychology;Forensic Psychology;Assessment/
Diagnosis/Evaluation;Neuropsychology;Ethnic Minorities

WU, Jing-Jyi
Fulbright Foundation
1-A Chuan Chow St.
Taipei, TAIWAN
(01)1886223327400-**B**, (01)1886223325445-**F**
jjwu@saec.saec.ude.twy
Ethnicity: Asian-American/Asian/Pacific Islander
Degree and Year: PhD 1967
Major Field: Educational Psychology
Specialty: Creativity;Cross Cultural Processes

WU, Li-Chuan
Department of Educational Psychology
& Counseling
National Taiwan Normal University
Taipei,
TAIWAN
(02) 2395 2445-**B**, (02) 2535 1370-**H**, (02) 2535 1491-**F**
linsh@cc.ntu.edu.tw
Ethnicity: Asian-American/Asian/Pacific Islander
Languages: Chinese
Degree and Year: PhD 1994 MS 1985
Major Field: Counseling Psychology
Specialty: Interpersonal Processes & Relations;Individual
Psychotherapy;Counseling Psychology;Psychotherapy;Parent
Education;Rational-Emotive Therapy

WU, Sheila T.
Asian Pacific Counseling
and Treatment Ceners
520 South LaFayette Park Place
Third Floor
Los Angeles, CA 90057
(213) 252-2111-**B**, (213) 267-4535-**H**, (213) 252-2199-**F**
s.wu@juno.com
Ethnicity: Asian-American/Asian/Pacific Islander
Languages: Chinese
Degree and Year: PhD 1991 MA 1989
Major Field: Clinical Psychology
Specialty: Administration;Clinical Child Psychology;Family
Therapy;Child Abuse;Community Mental Health;Parent
Education

WU, Shi-Jiuan
The New England Home
for Little Wanderers
Everrett House
232 Centre Street
Dorchester, MA 02124
617 232-8610-**B**, 617 388-9124-**H**, 617 388-9124-**F**

fcchou@athena.mit.edu
Ethnicity: Asian-American/Asian/Pacific Islander
Languages: Chinese, 03 Mandarin
Degree and Year: PhD 1993
Major Field: Counseling Psychology
Specialty: Family Processes;Gerontology/Geropsychology;Marriage &
Family;Family Therapy;Human Development & Family
Studies;Ethnic Minorities

WYATT, Gail E.
University of California, LA
Neuropsychiatric Institute
760 Westwood Plaza
Los Angeles, CA 90095-8353
(310) 825-0193-**B**, (310) 206-9137-**F**
gwyatt@mednet.ucla.edu
Ethnicity: African-American/Black
Degree and Year: PhD 1973
Major Field: Clinical Psychology
Specialty: Sexual Behavior;Sexual Dysfunction;Child Abuse;Cultural &
Social Processes

WYCHE, SR., LaMonte G.
7426 Carroll Avenue
Takoma Park, MD 20912
(202) 806-7350-**B**, (301) 270-3958-**H**, (202) 806-7018-**F**
Ethnicity: African-American/Black
Degree and Year: PhD 1973
Major Field: School Psychology
Specialty: School Psychology;Disadvantaged;Learning
Disabilities;Child Therapy;Parent Education;Human
Resources

WYCHE, Karen F.
New York University
School of Social Work
One Washington Square North
New York, NY 10003-6654
(212) 998-5971-**B**, (212) 995-4172-**F**
kfw1@is5.nyu.edu
Ethnicity: African-American/Black
Degree and Year: PhD 1984
Major Field: Clinical Psychology
Specialty: Cultural & Social Processes;Gender Issues;Social
Development;Preschool & Day Care Issues

WYNNE, Michael
Compton College
1111 East Artesia Boulevard
Compton, CA 90221
(310) 900-1600-**B**, (818) 765-7542-**H**, (818) 982-9162-**F**
mw_ppweix.netcom.com
Ethnicity: African-American/Black
Degree and Year: PhD 1981 MPA 1981
Major Field: Clinical Psychology
Specialty: Ethnic Minorities;Developmental Psychology;Human
Development & Family Studies;Clinical Child
Psychology;Community Psychology

XU, Gang
Jefferson Medical College
Center for Research in Medical Education
1025 Walnut Street
Suite 119
Philadelphia, PA 19107

(215) 955-8907-**B**, (609) 795-9968-**H**, (215) 923-6937-**F**
Ethnicity: Asian-American/Asian/Pacific Islander
Degree and Year: PhD
Major Field: Cognitive Psychology
Specialty: Cognitive Psychology;Cross Cultural Processes;Social
Psychology;Experimental
Psychology;Psychometrics;Personality

YABUSAKI, Ann S.
555 Pierce Street
Suite #3
Albany, CA 94706
(510) 527-7688-**B**, (510) 524-4008-**H**, (510) 526-2521-**F**
Ethnicity: Asian-American/Asian/Pacific Islander
Degree and Year: PhD 1992
Major Field: Clinical Psychology
Specialty: Alcoholism & Alcohol Abuse;Ethnic Minorities;Cross
Cultural Processes;Family Therapy;Cultural & Social
Processes

YAMADA, Elaine M.
4511 Clifton Road
Baltimore, MD 21216-1646
Ethnicity: Asian-American/Asian/Pacific Islander
Degree and Year: PhD 1975
Major Field: Clinical Psychology
Specialty: Psychotherapy

YAMAGUCHI, Harry G.
1708 Arden Drive
Bloomington, IN 47401
(812) 855-2311-**B**, (812) 323-9670-**H**
Ethnicity: Asian-American/Asian/Pacific Islander
Languages: Japanese
Degree and Year: PhD 1949
Major Field: Experimental Psychology
Specialty: Community Mental Health;Child Development;Child
Therapy;Clinical Psychology;Cognitive Behavioral Therapy

YAMAGUCHI, Mitsue Y.
423 S Pacific Costal Highway
Suite #102
Redondo Beach, CA 90277
(310) 541-2174-**B**, (310) 540-5864-**H**, (310) 540-8904-**F**
Ethnicity: Asian-American/Asian/Pacific Islander
Degree and Year: PhD 1988
Major Field: Clinical Psychology
Specialty: Cognitive Behavioral Therapy;Affective Disorders;Cultural
& Social Processes;Health Psychology;Cross Cultural
Processes

YAMAMURA, Lorraine M.
3231 Ocean Park Boulevard
Suite 204
Santa Monica, CA 90405
(310) 392-5209-**B**
Ethnicity: Asian-American/Asian/Pacific Islander
Languages: Japanese
Degree and Year: PhD 1985
Major Field: unknown
Specialty: Psychotherapy;Emotional Development;Interpersonal
Processes & Relations;Depression;Ethnic Minorities;Marriage
& Family

YANAGIDA, Evelyn H.

Kapiolani Medical Center
1319 Punahow Street
Honolulu, HI 96826
(808) 983-8368-**B**, (808) 983-8629-**F**
eviey@kapiolani.org
Ethnicity: Asian-American/Asian/Pacific Islander
Degree and Year: PhD 1979
Major Field: Clinical Psychology
Specialty: Clinical Child Psychology;Child Therapy;Assessment/
Diagnosis/Evaluation;Learning Disabilities

YAN, Bernice
University of British Columbia
1350 West 7th Avenue
Vancouver, BC, V6H-3WS
CANADA
(604) 731-0630-**F**
bernice.yan@uba.ca
Ethnicity: Asian-American/Asian/Pacific Islander
Languages: Chinese
Degree and Year: PhD 1995 MsC 1973
Major Field: Educational Psychology
Specialty: Psychometrics;Developmental Psychology;Cognitive
Development;Mental Health Services;Psychotherapy

YANCEY, Angela L.
2301 Georgian Way,#32
Wheaton, MD 20902-1863
(202) 373-7461-**B**, (301) 933-5289-**H**, (202) 373-7578-**F**
Ethnicity: African-American/Black
Degree and Year: PhD 1988 MA 1982
Major Field: Clinical Psychology
Specialty: Clinical Psychology;Forensic
Psychology;Psychopathology;Administration;Mental Health
Services

YANG, Raymond K.
Colorado State University
Human Development & Family Studies
102 Gifford Building
Fort Collins, CO 80523-0001
(303) 491-5718-**B**, (303) 491-7975-**F**
Ethnicity: Asian-American/Asian/Pacific Islander
Degree and Year: PhD 1971
Major Field: Developmental Psychology
Specialty: Child Development;Family Processes

YAP, Kim O.
Northwest Region Educational Library
101 SW Main
Suite 500
Portland, OR 97204-3213
(503) 275-9587-**B**, (503) 524-0559-**H**, (503) 275-9489-**F**
Ethnicity: Asian-American/Asian/Pacific Islander
Languages: Chinese
Degree and Year: PhD 1973
Major Field: Educational Psychology
Specialty: Program Evaluation;Measurement;Policy
Analysis;Instructional Methods;Curriculum Development/
Evaluation

YASUTAKE, Joseph Y.
1731 Septembersong Court
San Jose, CA 95131-2754
(408) 923-2883-**B**

Ethnicity: Asian-American/Asian/Pacific Islander
Degree and Year: PhD 1974
Major Field: Industrial/Organizational Psy.

YEE, Albert H.
 Florida International University
 Educational and Pychological Department
 Miami, FL 33199
 (305) 348-2610-**B**, (305) 594-7142-**F**
Ethnicity: Asian-American/Asian/Pacific Islander
Degree and Year: EdD 1965
Major Field: Educational Psychology
Specialty: Cultural & Social Processes;Educational Psychology

YEE, Barbara W. K.
 University of Texas Medical Branch
  at Galveston
 Health Promotion and Gerontology
 School of Allied Health Science
 Galveston, TX 77555-1028
 (409) 772-3038-**B**, (409) 740-1648-**H**, (409) 772-3014-**F**
 byee@utmb.edu
Ethnicity: Asian-American/Asian/Pacific Islander
Degree and Year: PhD 1982
Major Field: Gerontology
Specialty: Adult Development;Ethnic Minorities;Health
  Psychology;Cross Cultural Processes;Cultural & Social
  Processes

YEE, Brian W.
 P.O. Box 2636
 Carefree, AZ 85377-2636
 (602) 264-6402-**B**
Ethnicity: Asian-American/Asian/Pacific Islander
Degree and Year: PhD 1975
Major Field: Clinical Psychology
Specialty: Psychotherapy;Forensic Psychology

YEE, Jane K.
 100 S Ellsworth Avenue
 Suite #802
 San Mateo, CA 94401
 (650) 343-7902-**B**, (650) 325-1288-**F**
Ethnicity: Asian-American/Asian/Pacific Islander
Languages: Chinese
Degree and Year: PhD 1985
Major Field: Clinical Psychology
Specialty: Adult Development;Depression;Individual
  Psychotherapy;Marriage & Family;Parent-Child Interaction

YEE, Jennie Hy
 4004 Oakmore Road
 Oakland, CA 94602-1835
 (510) 398-0981-**B**, (510) 530-5733-**H**
Ethnicity: Asian-American/Asian/Pacific Islander
Degree and Year: PhD 1983
Major Field: Clinical Psychology
Specialty: Community Mental Health

YEE, Randall W.
 1165 Brockman Lane
 Sonoma, CA 95476-7654
 (707) 578-4379-**B**
Ethnicity: Asian-American/Asian/Pacific Islander

Degree and Year: PhD 1978
Major Field: Clinical Psychology
Specialty: Clinical Neuropsychology;Psychotherapy

YEE, Tina T.
 Division of Mental Health and
  Substance Abuse (5th Floor)
 1380 Howard Street
 San Francisco, CA 94103
 (415) 255-3422-**B**, (415) 752-6499-**H**, (415) 255-3567-**F**
Ethnicity: Asian-American/Asian/Pacific Islander
Degree and Year: PhD 1979
Major Field: Clinical Psychology
Specialty: Community Mental Health;Cross Cultural
  Processes;Training & Development;Ethnic Minorities

YI, Kris Y.
 11777 San Vicente Boulevard #700
 Los Angeles, CA 90049
 (310) 820-1724-**B**, (909) 621-2030-**H**, (909) 624-5948-**F**
 kyi@pomona.edu
Ethnicity: Asian-American/Asian/Pacific Islander
Languages: Korean
Degree and Year: PhD 1989
Major Field: Clinical Psychology
Specialty: Psychotherapy;Ethnic Minorities;Eating Disorders

YING, Yu-Wen
 University of California
  @ Berkeley
 School of Social Welfare
 120 Haviland Hall
 Berkeley, CA 94720-7400 7400
 (510) 643-6672-**B**, (510) 652-2150-**H**, 510 643-6126-**F**
 ywying10@socrates.berkeley.edu
Ethnicity: Asian-American/Asian/Pacific Islander
Languages: Chinese, German, 03 Mandarin
Degree and Year: PhD 1982
Major Field: Clinical Psychology
Specialty: Cross Cultural Processes;Ethnic
  Minorities;Depression;Prevention;Cultural & Social
  Processes;Clinical Psychology

YNIGUEZ, Linda E.
 6503 Greenleaf Avenue
 Suite C
 Whittier, CA 90601-4138
 (562) 693-4697-**B**, (213) 936-5560-**H**, (562) 698-1447-**F**
 drlinders@shrinkrap.com
Ethnicity: Hispanic/Latino
Degree and Year: PhD 1988
Major Field: Clinical Psychology
Specialty: Psychotherapy;Medical Psychology;Personality
  Disorders;Cross Cultural Processes;Depression

YORK, Joan E. S.
 138 Sanhican Drive
 Trenton, NJ 08618-5026
 (609) 292-8543-**B**, (609) 396-4887-**H**, (609) 633-8584-**F**
 jesy@email.msn.com
Ethnicity: African-American/Black
Degree and Year: PhD 1989

Major Field: Counseling Psychology

Specialty: Counseling Psychology;Alcoholism & Alcohol Abuse;Drug Abuse;Ethnic Minorities;Individual Psychotherapy

YORK, Mary J.
9327 Woodley Avenue
North Hills, CA 91343
(818) 830-1901-**B**, (818) 892-7743-**H**
Ethnicity: American Indian/Alaska Native
Languages: French, Apache, Penobscot
Degree and Year: PhD 1989
Major Field: Counseling Psychology
Specialty: Cross Cultural Processes;Cultural & Social Processes;Ethnic Minorities;Eating Disorders;Psychology of Women

YOSHIMURA, G. Joji
1 Baker Street
2A
San Francisco, CA 94117-3042
(415) 299-4004-**B**, (415)487-9644-**H**
Ethnicity: Asian-American/Asian/Pacific Islander
Degree and Year: PhD 1985
Major Field: Clinical Psychology
Specialty: Child Therapy;Family Therapy;Cross Cultural Processes;Industrial/Organizational Psychology;Adolescent Therapy

YOSHIMURA, Kari K.
595 East Colorado Boulevard, Suite 628
Pasadena, CA 91101
(626) 432-8113-**B**, (626) 441-3991-**F**
Ethnicity: Asian-American/Asian/Pacific Islander
Degree and Year: PhD 1992
Major Field: Clinical Psychology
Specialty: Ethnic Minorities;Psychology of Women

YOUNG, David A.
Health Psychology Associates
4482 Barranca Pkwy, Ste 130
Irvine, CA 92604-4744
(714) 551-4272-**B**, (714) 731-3572-**H**, (949) 551-6406-**F**
dayimagine@earthlink.net
Ethnicity: Asian-American/Asian/Pacific Islander
Degree and Year: PhD 1982 MPH 1984
Major Field: Clinical Psychology
Specialty: Health Psychology;Biofeedback;Child & Pediatric Psychology;Attention Deficit Disorders;Managed Care

YOUNG, Kimberly S.
University of Pittsburgh
Department of Psychology
300 Campus Drive
Bradford, PA 16701
(814) 362-5092-**B**, (814) 362-4913-**H**, (814) 368-9560-**F**
ksy@netaddiction.com
Ethnicity: American Indian/Alaska Native
Degree and Year: PsyD 1994
Major Field: Clinical Psychology
Specialty: Training & Development;Consulting Psychology;Information Processing;Clinical Psychology;Computer Applications and Programming;Mass Media Communication

YU, Angelita M.
Jacqueline L. Navin, PhD and Associates
1208 Churchville Road
Suite 300
Bel Air, MD 21014
(410) 638-5422-**B**, (410) 879-6770-**H**
ayu@ndm.edu
Ethnicity: Asian-American/Asian/Pacific Islander
Degree and Year: PhD 1995
Major Field: Counseling Psychology
Specialty: Family Therapy;Marriage & Family;Cross Cultural Processes;Counseling Psychology;Sex/Marital Therapy;Eating Disorders

YUEN, Lenora L.
667 Lytton Avenue
Palo Alto, CA 94301
(415) 322-1688-**B**
Ethnicity: Asian-American/Asian/Pacific Islander
Degree and Year: PhD 1980
Major Field: Clinical Psychology
Specialty: Psychotherapy;Psychoanalysis;Work Performance;Marriage & Family;Psychopathology

YU, Howard K.
City College of San Francisco
50 Phean Avenue
San Francisco, CA 94112
(415) 561-1929-**B**, (415) 561-1861-**F**
hyu@ccsf.cc.ca.us
Ethnicity: Asian-American/Asian/Pacific Islander
Languages: Chinese
Degree and Year: PhD 1981
Major Field: Educational Psychology
Specialty: Educational Research

YUN, S.B.
2828 Churchill Drive
Columbus, OH 43221
(513) 642-1065-**B**, (614) 481-8296-**H**, (513) 644-8172-**F**
Ethnicity: Asian-American/Asian/Pacific Islander
Languages: Korean
Degree and Year: M.Ed 1970
Major Field: Counseling Psychology
Specialty: Forensic Psychology;Correctional Psychology;Psychometrics;Personality Disorders;Counseling Psychology

YU, Pamela
1301 Capital of Texas Highway South
Suite #A-240
Austin, TX 78746
(512) 327-2008-**B**, (512) 328-4308-**H**
Ethnicity: Asian-American/Asian/Pacific Islander
Degree and Year: PhD 1979
Major Field: Clinical Psychology
Specialty: Family Therapy;Child Therapy;Adolescent Therapy;Marriage & Family;Child Development

ZALDIVAR, Luis R.
Comprehensive Psychological and
 Psychiatric Services. P.A.
1050 NW 15th Street, Suite 209
Boca Ratton, FL 33486
(561) 392-4415-**B**, (567) 883-5710-**H**, (561) 395-9754-**F**

Ethnicity: Hispanic/Latino
Languages: Spanish
Degree and Year: PhD 1982
Major Field: Clinical Psychology
Specialty: Clinical Psychology;Individual Psychotherapy;Affective Disorders;Family Therapy;Adolescent Therapy;Assessment/ Diagnosis/Evaluation

ZAMUDIO, Anthony
California Medical Center
Family Practice Residency Program
1338 S. Hope Street
Los Andeles, CA 90015
(213) 651-6371-**B**, (213) 651-6371-**H**
Ethnicity: Hispanic/Latino
Languages: Spanish
Degree and Year: PhD 1987
Major Field: Clinical Psychology
Specialty: Affective Disorders;Community Mental Health;Health Psychology;Mental Disorders;Lesbian & Gay Issuues

ZANE, Nolan W.S
University of California
Graduate School of Education
Santa Barbara, CA 93106-9490
(805) 893-8564-**B**, (310) 470-7159-**H**, (805) 893-8055-**F**
zane@education.ucsb.edu
Ethnicity: Asian-American/Asian/Pacific Islander
Degree and Year: PhD 1987
Major Field: Clinical Psychology
Specialty: Ethnic Minorities;Cultural & Social Processes;Research Design & Methodology;Psychotherapy;Program Evaluation

ZARAGOZA, Maria S.
Kent State University
Department of Psychology
Kent, OH 44242
(216) 672-2018-**B**
mzarago@kentvm
Ethnicity: Hispanic/Latino
Degree and Year: PhD 1984
Major Field: Cognitive Psychology
Specialty: Memory;Forensic Psychology

ZAVALA-MARTINEZ, Iris
Calle Lopez Landron 1563, #5
Santurce, PR 00911-
(809) 721-3233-**B**, (809) 724-0322-**H**
Ethnicity: Hispanic/Latino
Degree and Year: PhD 1984
Major Field: Clinical Psychology
Specialty: Community Mental Health

ZAVALA, Albert
377 S Mathilda Avenue
Sunnyvale, CA 904086
(408) 742-1922-**B**, (408) 733-6653-**H**
Ethnicity: Hispanic/Latino
Languages: Spanish
Degree and Year: PhD 1966
Major Field: unknown
Specialty: Human Factors;Human Resources;Leadership;Accident Prevention/Safety;Ethnic Minorities

ZAYAS-BAZAN, Carmen
16969 NW 67th Avenue
Suite #201
Miami, FL 33015
(305) 556-6972-**B**, (305) 596-6989-**H**, (305) 556-4929-**F**
Ethnicity: Hispanic/Latino
Languages: Spanish
Degree and Year: PsyD 1983
Major Field: Clinical Psychology
Specialty: Cognitive Behavioral Therapy;Hypnosis/ Hypnotherapy;Lesbian & Gay Issuues;Family Therapy

ZAYAS, Luis H.
Fordham University
Graduate School of Social Services
Tarrytown, NY 10591-
(718) 817-5636-**B**, (914) 591-7697-**H**, (914) 524-0586-**F**
zayas@murray.fordham.edu
Ethnicity: Hispanic/Latino
Languages: Spanish
Degree and Year: PhD 1986
Major Field: Developmental Psychology
Specialty: Adolescent Therapy;Child & Pediatric Psychology;Ethnic Minorities;Child Development;Parent-Child Interaction

ZAYAS, Maria A.
225 South Front Street
Wilmington, NC 28401
Ethnicity: Hispanic/Latino
Languages: French, Spanish
Degree and Year: EdD 1989
Major Field: Counseling Psychology
Specialty: Individual Psychotherapy;Child Therapy;Family Therapy

ZEPEDA, Marlene
12574 Woodgreen St
Los Angeles, CA 90066-2724
(323) 343-4643-**B**, (310) 398-2314-**H**, (323) 343-4770-**F**
mzepeda@calstatela.edu
Ethnicity: Hispanic/Latino
Languages: Spanish
Degree and Year: PhD 1984
Major Field: Developmental Psychology
Specialty: Child Development;Cultural & Social Processes;Developmental Psychology;Ethnic Minorities;Family Processes

ZHU, Jiajun
The Psychological Corporation
555 Academic Court
San Antonio, TX 78204-2498
(210) 949-4437-**B**, (210) 949-4475-**F**
jj_zhu@hbtpc.com
Ethnicity: Asian-American/Asian/Pacific Islander
Languages: Chinese
Degree and Year: PhD 1993
Major Field: Developmental Psychology
Specialty: Intelligence;Research Design & Methodology;Quantitative/ Mathematical, Psychometrics;Child Development;Cognitive Development;Measurement

ZIGHELBOIM, Vivien A.
9100 Wilshire Boulevard #605
Beverly Hills, CA 90212-3415

(213) 277-4389-**B**
Ethnicity: Hispanic/Latino
Degree and Year: PhD 1986
Major Field: Clinical Psychology
Specialty: Psychotherapy

ZUERCHER-WHITE, Elke
Kaiser Permanente Medical Center
Psychiatry Department
San Francisco, CA 94080
(415) 742-2553-**B**
Ethnicity: Hispanic/Latino
Degree and Year: PhD 1977
Major Field: Clinical Psychology
Specialty: Psychotherapy;Cognitive Behavioral Therapy

ZURIFF, Gerald E.
Wheaton College
Norton, MA 02766
(508) 286-3692-**B**, (617) 868-7806-**H**
gzurigg@wheatonma.edu
Ethnicity: Hispanic/Latino
Degree and Year: PhD 1968
Major Field: Experimental Psychology
Specialty: Psychoanalysis;Philosophy of Science;Behavior
Therapy;Systems, Methods & Issues

Ethnic Group Listing

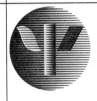

Psychologists of color are listed alphabetically
under one of six self-reported categories
of ethnic group membership:

African American/Black

American Indian/Alaska Native

Asian American/Asian/Pacific Islander

Hispanic/Latino

Multiethnic
(i.e., persons of self-reported multiple ethnicity)

No Information

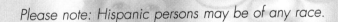

Please note: Hispanic persons may be of any race.

ETHNIC GROUP LISTING

AFRICAN AMERICAN/BLACK

Abercombie, Delrita
Abernethy, Alexis D.
Abston, Jr., Nathaniel
Adams, Jr., Clarence L.
Adams, Afesa M.
Adams, C. Jama
Aldrich, John W.
Alexander, Allen T.
Alexander, Charlene M.
Allen-Claiborne, Joyce G.
Allen, Christeen
Allen, Jane E.
Allen, Winnie M.
Allen, Wise E.
Allgood-Hill, Barbara A.
Allsopp, Ralph N
Alston, Denise A.
Anderson, Linda
Anderson, Louis P.
Anderson, Norman B.
Anderson, Shirley G.
Anderson, William H.
Anthony, Bobbie M.
Apenahier, Leonard
Aradom, Tesfay A
Archibald, Eloise M.
Artis, Daphne J.
Asbury, Charles A.
Asbury, Jo-Ellen
Ashmore-Hudson, Anne
Atwell, Robert L.
Bailey, Joan W.
Baker, III, Carl E.
Baker, Christine
Baker, Octave V.
Baly, Iris E.
Bamgbose, Olujiimi O.
Banks, Hobart M.
Banks, Karel L.
Banks, Martha E.
Barbarin, Oscar A.
Barber, Kevin V.
Barker-Hackett, Lori
Barner, II, Pearl
Barnes, Denise R.
Barnes, Michael J.

Bartee, Robert L.
Bartholomew, Charles
Bastien, Rochelle T.
Battiest, William V.
Baxley, Gladys B.
Baxter, Anthony G.
Baxter, Bernice K.
Beam, Micheline
Beatty, Lula A.
Beckles, Nicola
Belgrave, Faye Z
Belgrave, Jeffrey
Bell, Anita G.
Bell, K. Pat
Belton, Monique
Bennett, Maisha H.
Berry, Joyce Hamilton
Biggs, Bradley
Bingham, Rosie P.
Binion, Victoria J.
Binns, Derrick
Blackett-Sullivan, Gwendolyn A.
Blanding, Benjamin
Block, Carolyn B.
Bolden, Wiley S.
Bostick, Rosie M.
Bowen, Tanya U.
Bowman, Sharon L.
Boxley, Russell L.
Boyd, Naughne L.
Boyd, Vivian S.
Boyer, Michele C.
Brannon, Lorraine
Brice, Janet R.
Briggs, Felicia H.
Brinson, Les
Broadfield, Charles S.
Brodie, Debra A.
Brookins, Geraldine K
Brooks, Lewis A.
Brown, Anita B.
Brown, Barbara J.
Browne, Ronald H.
Brown, John R.
Brown, Marilyn F.
Brown, Michael T.
Brown, Pamela
Bryant-Tuckett, Rose M.

Bryant, Gerard W.
Buffin, Janice E.
Burchell, Charles R.
Burks, Eura O.
Burnett Young, Myra N.
Burnett, John H.
Burnett, Judith A.
Burnham, Lem
Burr, Sharon S.
Butler, B. LaConyea
Bynum, Edward B.
Cade, Bonita G.
Caesar, Robert
Caldwell-Colbert, A. Toy
Caldwell, Barrett S.
Callahan, Michelle R.
Cameron, Linda S.
Campbell-Flint, Maxine E
Campbell, Barbara L.
Campbell, Stephen N.
Capp, Larry D.
Carey, Patricia M.
Carrington, Christine H.
Carter, Allen C.
Carter, Charles A.
Carter, Lamore J.
Carter, Lonnie T.
Carter, Robert T.
Cason, Valerie K.
Cathcart, Conrad W.
Chatman, Vera A
Chesnutt, James H.
Chisum, Gloria T.
Clansy, Pauline A.
Clark, Jr., Eddie M.
Clark, Brenda A.
Clark, Kenneth B.
Clark, Marie
Coates, Deborah L.
Coelho, Richard J.
Coffey, Maryann B.
Cohen, Isadora
Coleburn, Lila A.
Coleman, Hardin L.
Coleman, Philip P.
Coleman, Willie J.
Collins, Edsmond J.
Collins, William

Cone-Dekle, Cynthia A.
Congo, Carroll A.
Connor, Michael E.
Constantine, Madonna G.
Cook, Donelda
Cook, Rudolf E.
Cooper, Alan
Cooper, Colin
Cooper, Donna M.
Copeland, Jr., E. Thomas
Copemann, Chester D.
Copher-Haynes, Harriett
Cornwell, Henry G.
Corr, Donald
Cotterell, Norman
Cottingham, Alice L.
Craig, U-Shaka
Crawford, Monica L.
Critton, Barbara L.
Crockett, Deborah P.
Crowder, Virginia B.
Cunningham, Michael
Cunningham, Wayman B.
Curry, Alpha O.
Curry, Bonita Pope
Dalhouse, A. Derick
Daly, Frederica Y.
Davis-Russell, Elizabeth
Davis, Annette E.
Davis, Bernice M.
Davis, Charles E.
Davis, Cheryl L.
Davis, Jerry H.
Dawkins, Arthur C.
Dawkins, Marva P.
Dawson, Harriett E.
De Leaire, Robert
DeBardelaben, Garfield
DeFour, Darlene C.
Deleaire, Robert N.
Dennis, Dothlyn J.G.
Denson, Eric L.
Derrick, Sara M.
Derrickson, Kimberly B.
Devezin, Armond A.
DeWindt-Robson, L. Kimberly
Dingus, C. Mary
Dixon, Carrie B.

Dixon, J. Faye	Friday, Jennifer C.	Gump, Janice P.	Hunt, Wilson L.
Dobbins, James E.	Frisby, Craig L.	Gunn, Robert L.	Hurst, Jurlene
Dockett, Kathleen H.	Fullilove, Constance	Haggins, Kristee L.	Hutchinson, Kim M.
Donahue, Pamela J.	Fulton, Aubyn	Hall, Howard	Ike, Chris A.
Donald, Liz	Fulton, Wayne M.	Hall, Juanita L.	Ingram, Jesse C.
Donnella, John	Gadson, Eugene J.	Hall, Ruth L.	Ingram, Winifred
Doris, Terri M.	Gaines, Stanley O.	Hall, William A.	Ireland Hurd, Evelyn C.
Dorr, Bernadette	Gardner, Lamaurice H.	Hambrick-Dixon, Priscilla J.	Isaacs, Owen K.
Doss, Juanita K.	Garner, Edward L.	Hambright, Jerold E.	Jackson-Davis, Brandi
Douglas, Byron C.	Garnes, Delbert F.	Hamer, Forrest M.	Jackson, Anna M.
Dozier, Arthur L.	Garrett-Akinsanya, BraVada	Hammond, Gladys	Jackson, Helen L.
Dudley-Grant, G. Rita	Garrett, Aline M.	Hammond, W. Rodney	Jackson, Jacquelyne F.
Dudley, Charma D.	Gary, Juneau M.	Hampton, Juanita R.	Jackson, James S.
Duncan, Bessie A.	Gayle, Michael C.	Hanley, Jerome H.	Jackson, John H.
Dunston, Patricia	Gayles, Joyce M.	Hardin, Jr., Oscar A.	Jackson, Joyce Taborn
Dyson, Vida	Gay, Patricia L.	Hare, Nathan	Jackson, Leslie C.
Eberhardt, Carolyn A.	Geter-douglas, Beth	Harleston, Bernard W.	Jackson, Ronald A.
Edelin, Patricia	Gibbons-Carr, Michele V.	Harper, Frederick	Jacobs-Jr., Walter R.
Edwards, Karen L.	Gibbs, Charles C.	Harper, Mary S.	James, Jr., Earnest
El-Amin, Debra El-Amin	Gibbs, Jewelle Taylor	Harrell, Shelly P.	James-Parker, Magna M.
Elder, Patricia	Gibson, Ralph M.	Harris, Jasper W.	James, Lainee M.
Elion, Victor H.	Gibson, Rose C.	Harris, Michelle F.	James, Larry C.
Elligan, Don G.	Giles, Cheryl A.	Harris, Shanette M.	James, Michelle D.
Elligen, Don G.	Gillem, Angela R	Harris, William G.	James, Norman L.
Elliott, Vanessa E.	Gloster, Janice L.	Hart, Allen J.	Jemmott, III, John B.
Ellis, Rosita P.	Glover, O.S.	Harte, Lisa M.	Jenkins-Monroe, Valata
Emory, Eugene K.	Gordon, Kimberly A.	Hawkins, Ioma L.	Jenkins, Adelbert H
Epps, Pamela J.	Gordon, LaFaune Y.	Hawkins, James Leon	Jenkins, Sheila A.
Ervin, Betty J.	Gordon, Rhea J.	Hayles, V. Robert	Jenkins, Susan M.
Escoffery, Aubrey S.	Gordon, Ruth H.	Henderson Daniel, Jessica	Jenkins, Yvonne M
Essandoh, Pius K.	Graddick, Miriam M.	Henderson, Brenda A.	Jennings, Jr., Wilmar A.
Evans, Helen L.	Graham, Quentin	Henry, Rolando R.	Jennings, Lesajean M.
Everett, Moses L.	Graham, Sandra	Henry, Vincent dePaul	Jennings, Valdea D.
Ezeilo, Bernice N.	Granberry, Dorothy	Hernandez, Michael	Johnson, David L.
Fairchild, Halford H.	Grant, Kim D.	Hestick, Henrietta	Johnson, Denise MW
Farley, Florence S.	Grant, Wanda F.	Hicks, Laurabeth	Johnson, Edward E.
Fields, Anika C.	Graves-Cooper, Phyllis J.	Hicks, Leslie H.	Johnson, Eugene H.
Fields, Richard L.	Graves, Kenneth J.	Hill, Anthony L	Johnson, Fern M.
Finley, Laurene Y.	Graves, Sherryl B.	Hilton, William F.	Johnson, Fred A.
Fisher, Patricia A.	Gray-Little, Bernadette	Hines, Laura M.	Johnson, Joan J.
Fleming, Andrea L.	Gray, Arthur A.	Hines, Paulette M.	Johnson, Johnny
Fletcher, Betty A.	Green, Charles A.	Holliday, Bertha G.	Johnson, Lawrence B.
Flowers, Jana D.	Greene, Anthony F.	Holmes, Dorothy E.	Johnson, Marjorie
Floyd, Bridget J.	Greene, Beverly	Holsey, Chandra V.	Johnson, Matthew B.
Floyd, James A.	Greene, Clifford	Hooker, Olivia J.	Johnson, Sylvia T
Ford, Deshay D.	Greene, Lorraine	Hopkins, Kenneth	Johnson, W. Roy
Ford, Fatima Y	Green, Theophilus E.	Hopson, Ronald E.	Johnson, William L.
Ford, Leon I.	Grier, Priscilla E.	Horsford, Bernard I.	Johnson, Zonya
Forrester, Bettye J.	Griffin, Patricia L.	Horton, Carrell	Jones, Annie Lee
Foster, Jr., Hilliard G.	Griffith, Albert R.	Houston, Holly O.	Jones, Arthur C.
Foster, Evelyn L.	Griffith, Marlin S.	Houston, Lawrence N.	Jones, Cynthia A.
Foster, Robert	Griffith, Stanford	Howard, Mary T.	Jones, Elaine F.
Francisco, Richard P.	Grimes, Tresmaine R	Hudley, Cynthia	Jones, Ferdinand
Francois, Theodore V.	Grinstead, Olga A.	Hughes-Wheatland, Roxanne	Jones, George L.
Fraser, Kathryn P.	Grych, Diane S.	Hughes, Anita L.	Jones, Hugh E.
Freeman, Charlotte M.	Guevarra, Josephine S.	Hunter, Knoxice C	Jones, James M.
Freeman, James E.	Guillory, Paul T.	Hunt, Portia	Jones, Paulette
Fresh, Edith M.	Gulley, Silas	Hunt, William K.	Jones, Reginald

Jones, Reginald L.
Jones, Ruby M.
Jones, Russell T.
Jordan, Albert K.
Joseph, Jr., Herbert M.
June, Lee N.
Keglar, Shelvy H.
Keita, Gwendolyn P.
Kelly-Radford, Lily M.
Kelly, Jennifer F.
Kemp, Arthur D.
Kennedy, Clive D.
King, Valerie
Kirklen, Leonard E.
Klopner, Michele C.
Lambert, Michael C.
Lampkin, Emmett C.
Langley, Merlin R
Lawrence, Stephen N.
Lawrence, Valerie W.
Lawson, Jasper J.
Leary, Kimberlyn
Lee, Yolanda W.
Lessing, Elise E.
LeSure-Lester, G. Evelyn
Levermore, Monique A.
Lewis, Brenda J.
Lewis, George R.
Lewis, Marva L
Lineberger, Marilyn H.
Lipson, Diane R.
Liston, Hattye H.
London, Dyanne P.
London, Lorna H.
Louden, Delroy M.
Lovelace, Valeria O.
Luke, Equilla
Lyles, William B.
Mack, Delores E.
Mack, Faite R. P.
Mahy, Yvonne C.
Mallisham, Ivy J.
Mann, Coramae R.
Mars, Raymond G.
Mate-Kole, C. Charles
Matthews, Belvia W.
Maynard, Edward S.
Mayo, Benjamin F.
Mays, Vickie M.
Mccain, Lillie W.
McCandies, Terry T
McCarley, Victor J.
McClure, Faith H.
McCombs, Harriet G.
McDonald, II, Ozzie H.
McGowan, Eugene
McIntyre, Lorna A.
McKenzie, Jr., Loratuis L.

McLean, Jr, Alvin
Mcloyd, Vonnie C.
McMillan, Robert
McNeal, Meryl
McNeill, Earle
McRae, Mary B.
Meadows-Yancey, Dorothy
Merritt, Marcellus M.
Milburn, Norweeta G.
Miles, Gary T.
Millard, Wilbur A.
Miller, Fayneese
Miller, Robin L.
Miller, S. Walden
Mills, Marcia C.
Mindingall, Marilyn P.
Mitchell, Horace
Mitchell, Howard E.
Mobley, Brenda D.
Molden, Sabrina
Monteiro, Kenneth P.
Monteiro, Rita C.
Moody, Helaine L.
Moore, C. L.
Moore, Carolyn D.
Moore, Cleo H.
Moore, Helen B.
Moore, Sandra
Moorman-Lewis, Deborah A.
Morgan, Cynthia L.
Morris, Dolores O.
Morris, Edward F.
Morris, Joseph R.
Morse, Roberta N.
Mosley-Howard, Gerri S.
Motes, Patricia S.
Mouzon, Richard R.
Muir-Malcolm, Joan A.
Muiu, Charles
Munford, Paul R.
Murfree, Jr., Joshua W.
Murray, James L.
Musgrove, Barbara J.
Myers, Ernest R.
Myers, Hector F.
Myers, Linda J.
Nabors, Nina A.
Neal-Barnett, Angela M.
Nelson-Goedert, Carolyn Y
Nelson-le, Sharon A.
Nesbitt, Eric B.
Nettles, Arie L.
Nicholson, Liston O.
Nickerson, Kim J.
Nicks, T. Leon
Nix-Early, Vivian
Noel, Winifred
Nolan, Jr., Benjamin C.

Nolan, Beverly D.
Norman-Jackson, Jacquelyn
Norman, William H.
Norton, A. Evangeline
Nzewi, Esther N.
Okonji, Jacques A.
Okorodudu, Corahann
Oshodi, John
Outlaw, Patricia A.
Owens-Lane, Jan
Ozuzu, Sam
Parham, Patricia A.
Parham, Thomas A.
Parham, William D.
Parks, Carlton
Parks, Fayth M.
Parks, Gregory S.
Paster, Vera S.
Patrice, David
Patterson, Drayton R.
Patton, Kenneth
Payton, Carolyn R.
Peavyhouse, Betty M.
Peniston, Eugene G.
Penn, Nolan E.
Peoples, Kathleen
Peoples, Napoleon L.
Pernell, Eugene
Perry, Cereta E.
Perry, Jeanell
Peters, James S.
Pettigrew, Dorothy C.
Phelps, C. K.
Phelps, Rosemary E.
Phillips, Campbell C.
Philp, Frederick W.
Pierce, William D.
Piercy, Patricia A.
Pinder-Amaker, Stephanie L.
Pinderhughes, Ellen B.
Pinderhughes, Victoria A.
Polite, Craig K.
Polite, Kenneth
Pope-Davis, Donald B.
Pope-Tarrence, Jacqueline R.
Porche-Burke, Lisa M.
Porter, Julia
Poston, II, Walker S.
Powell, Lois
Prelow, Hazel M.
Price, Gregory E.
Price, Linda A.
Pruitt, Jr., Joseph H.
Pugh, Roderick W.
Pulliam, Barbara A.
Rambo, Lewis M.
Ramseur, Howard P.
Ray, Jacqueline W.

Ray, Vivian D.
Reams, Bennie P
Reaves, Andrew L
Reaves, Juanita Y.
Redd-Barnes, Renee A.
Reed, III, Jesse A.
Reed, James D.
Reeves, Alan
Reid, Pamela T
Reilly, Patrick M.
Rice, Donadrian
Richard, Harriette W.
Richards, Henry J.
Richardson, Frederick
Riddle, P. Elayne
Ridley, Charles R.
Rivers, Miriam W.
Roberts, Albert
Roberts, Harrell B.
Robertson, John F.
Roberts, Terrence J.
Robinson, Gregory F.
Robinson, Jane A.
Robinson, John D
Robinson, W. LaVome
Rogers, Melvin L.
Rollock, David
Romero, Regina E.
Romney, Patricia
Ross, Sandra I.
Rouce, Sandra
Rountree, Yvonne B.
Ruffins, Stephen A.
Russell, David M.
Salter, Beatrice R.
Salter, Dianne S.
Samaan, Makram K.
Sampson, Myrtle B.
Samuels, Robert M.
Samuel, Valerie J.
Sanchez-Hucles, Janis V.
Sanders-Thompson, Vetta L.
Sanders, Betty M.
Sanders, Daniel W.
Sapp, Marty
Savage, Jr., James E.
Scott-Jones, Diane
Scott, Linda D.
Scott, Merilla M.
Searcy, Mary L.
Seymour, Guy O.
Sharp, Jude C.
Shaw, Paula
Shell, Juanita
Shipp, Pamela L.
Sikes, Melvin P.
Simms Puig, Jan
Simpson, Adelaide W.

Sims-Patterson, Sandra
Singleton, Edward G.
Slaughter-Defoe, Diana T.
Smedley, Joseph W.
Smith, Jr., Theodore R.
Smith, Althea
Smith, Alvin E.
Smith, Benjamin
Smith, Carol Y.
Smith, Charles E.
Smith, Cherryl R.
Smith, Iola R.
Smith, Walanda W.
Smith, William
Smith, William F.
Snowden, Lonnie R.
Solomon, Sondra E.
Southerland, Deborah L.
Speight, Suzette L.
Spencer, Margaret B.
Spidell Helms, Dorothy J.
Spivey, Philop B.
Spraings, Violet E.
Sprouse, Agnes A.
St. Leger, Sidney C.
Stallworth, Lisa M.
Starks-Williams, Mary L.
Steele, Marilyn
Steele, Robert E.
Stevenson, Jr., Edward E.
Stewart, Vlenaetha
Stokes, Devon R.
Stone, Lynn J.
Strickland, Tony L
Stringer, Anthony Y.
Stroud, Barbara
Sutton, Sharon E.
Swanston, Melvon C.
Tapo, Linda J.
Tate, Donald
Tatum, Beverly D.
Taylor, Palmeda D.
Thomas, Jr., Charles B.
Thomas, Anita J.
Thomas, Hilton T.
Thompson, Chalmer E.
Thompson, Veronique L.
Thornton, Dozier W.
Tiggle, Ronald B.
Toldson, Ivory L.
Tomes, Henry
Tomlinson-Clarke, Saundra M.
Toms, Esther C.
Toomer, Jethro W.
Treadwell, Marsha J.
Triplett, Sheila J.
Trotman, Frances K.
Troutt, Bobbye V.

Trufant, Carol A.
Tucker, Dorothy M.
Tucker, James L.
Tucker, Samuel J.
Turner, Alvin L.
Turner, Castellano
Turner, Samuel M.
Twe, Boikai S.
Ugwuegbu, Denis C.
Underwood, Robert J.
Vance, Marilyn M.
Vanderhost, Leonette
Vanderpool, Andrea T.
Vaughan, Elaine
Vaughans, Kirkland C.
Vontress, Clemmont E.
Walcott, Delores D.
Walker, Lila K.
Walker, Lola '.
Walker, O'Neal A.
Walton, Duncan E.
Ward, Alan J.
Ward, Connie M.
Ward, Lucretia M.
Washington, Anita C.
Washington, Dianna E.
Washington, Robert A.
Watts, Charlotte B.
Watts, Roderick J.
Webb, Wanda
Webster, E. Carol
Wellons, Retha V.
Wells, Annie M.
West, Gerald I.
West, James E.
Weston, Raymond E.
Whisenton, Joffre T.
Whitaker, Arthur L.
Whitehead, Barry X.
Whitehead, Jesse
Whitehurst, Jr., William H.
White, Joseph L.
White, Voncile
Whitten, Lisa A.
Williams-Markum, Deirdre
Williams-Petersen, Janice
Williams, Carrolyn N.
Williams, Daniel E.
Williams, David R.
Williams, Eddie E.
Williams, Estelle M.
Williams, Everett B.
Williams, Indy J.
Williams, Karen P. W.
Williams, Medria L.
Williams, Michael A.
Williams, Phyllis J.
Williams, Steve

Williams, Victoria F.
Williams, Willie S.
Wilson, Margaret
Wilson, Melvin N.
Wilson, Shirley B.
Wilson, Susan B.
Wilson, Woodrow
Winfrey, Angela D.
Winfrey, LaPearl L.
Wisner, Roscoe W.
Witter, Jeanette M.
Wood, Jr., Nollie P.
Wood, Keith A.
Woodland, Calvin E.
Woods, Delma M.
Wooten, William
Word, James C.
Worrell, Frank C.
Wright, Doris J.
Wright, Michael F.
Wyatt, Gail E.
Wyche, Sr., LaMonte G.
Wyche, Karen F.
Wynne, Michael
Yancey, Angela L.
York, Joan E. S.

AMERICAN INDIAN/ALASKA NATIVE

Arnold, John F.
Atkinson, Michael B.
Babb, Harold
Ballering, Lawrence R.
Blair, Deborah G.
Blubaugh, Victoria G.
Blue, Arthur W.
Bostwick, Allen D.
Bouffard, R. Gerard
Bowen, Peggy C.
Brooks, Jr., Glenwood C.
Byrd, Robert D.
Campos, Peter E.
Carter, William J.
Chapman, Nancy G.
Choney, John M.
Church, June S.
Coats, Gary L.
Cummings, Joseph D.
Daisy, Fransing
DeGraff, Christopher D.
Derocher, Terry L.
Durant, Jr., Adrian J.
Eaton, Sheila J.
Ertz, Dewey J.
Everson, Howard T.

Fain, Thomas C.
Fields, Amanda H.
Fleming, Candace M.
Foster, Daniel V.
Foster, Rachel A.
Gant, Bob L.
Gladue, Brian A.
Goffin, Richard D.
Gregory, Robert A.
Haddock, Dean M.
Hartzell, Richard E.
Hayes, Forrest L.
Hillabrant, Walter J.
Horvat, Jr., Joseph J.
Hui, Len Dang
James, Steven E
Joesting-Goodwoman, Joan A.
Jones-Saumty, Deborah J.
Joure, Sylvia A.
Jun, Heesoon
Karson, Samuel
Knapp, W. Mace
LaDue, Robin A.
LaFromboise, Teresa
Lashley, Karen H.
Love, Craig T.
Lucas, Jay H.
Matheson, Charlene
McCoy, George F.
McDonald, Arthur L.
Mellor, Catherine A.
Miller, Sarah S.
Milner, Joel S.
Mink, Oscar G.
Mizwa, Martine M.
Montgomery, Robert L.
Moynihan, Kelly L.
Muller, Terry P.
Nolley, David A.
Paige, Roger
Pine, Charles J.
Pope, Mark
Prutsman, Thomas D.
Quinn, Lisa
Rainwater, III, Avie J.
Reandeau, Sharon L
Reisinger, Curtis W.
Richardson, E. Strong-Legs
Robey, Dale L.
Ryan, Loye M.
Ryan, Robert A.
Sadler, Mark S.
Samford, Judith A.
Sanders, Gilbert O.
Sellards, Robert
Shaw, Terry G.
Shohet, Jacqueline M.
Silling, S. Marc

Stewart, G. Keith
Stone, G. Vaughn
Sutton, David
Swaney, Gyda
Taylor, Gary
Taylor, Peggy S.
Thomas, Thomas J.
Thorson, Billie J.
Thurman, Pamela J.
Trimble, Joseph E.
Turnbough, P. Diane
Uzzell, Barbara P.
Valley, John A.
Vraniak, Damian A.
Williams, Mary Beth
Williamson, Diane H.
Willis, Cynthia E.
Willis, Diane J.
Wilson, Jennifer
Wilson, Lloyd K.
York, Mary J.
Young, Kimberly S.

ASIAN AMERICAN/ASIAN/ PACIFIC ISLANDER

Abudabbeh, Nuha
Acka-Pope, Zeynep K
Advani, Nisha
Ahana, Ellen
Ahmed, Mohiuddin
Ahsen, Akhter
Ahuja, Harmeen
Ai, Amy L.
Akamatsu, T. John
Akimoto, Sharon A
Akiyama, M. Michael
Akutagawa, Donald
Akutsu, Phillip D.
Al-tai, Nazar M.
Aldaba-Lim, Estefania
Amawattana, Tipawadee
Ambady, Nalina
Amin, Kiran
Anand, Shashi
Anselmo, Fe
Anzai, Yuichiro
Aoki, Bart K.
Aoki, Melanie F.
Aoki, Wayne T.
Arana, Olga R.
Armilla, Jose
Asamen, Joy K.
Ascano, Ricardo
Asghar, Anila
Ashida, Sachio

Attore, Lois
Atwal, Baljit K,
Austria, Asuncion M.
Baba, Masao
Baba, Vishwanath V.
Bainum, Charlene K.
Banaji, Mahzarin R.
Banik, Sambhu N.
Beattie, Muriel Y.
Belzunce, Philip R.
Bhanthumnavin, Duangduen
Bhatia, Kiran
Birky, Ian
Blackburn, Winona K.
Boggs, Minnie
Boodoo, Gwyneth M.
Bradshaw, Carla K.
Caberto, Steven C.
Campbell, Kamal E.
Campos, Joseph J.
Catarina, Mathilda B.
Chan, Adrian
Chan, Connie S.
Chan, Daniel S.
Chan, Darrow A.
Chan, David C.
Chang, Alice F.
Chang, Barbara
Chang, Bradford W.
Chang, Theodore C. H.
Chang, Thomas M.C.
Chang, Weining C.
Chan, Kenyon S.
Chan, Paul K.
Chan, Paul K. F.
Chan, Samuel Q.
Chao, Christine M.
Chao, Georgia T.
Chao, Janet
Chen, Eric C
Cheng, W. David
Chen, Hongjen
Chen, S. Andrew
Chew, Marion W.
Chiang, Grace CT
Chia, Rosina
Ching-Yang Hsu, Chris
Ching, June W. J.
Chin, James
Chin, Jean L
Chin, Lemin
Chinn, Roberta N.
Chino, Allan F.
Chin, Raymond J.
Chin, Sandra B
Chiu, Lian-Hwam
Chiu, Loanne
Choi, George C.

Chou, Thomas T.
Choy, Catherine L.
Choy, Stephen S.F.
Chu, Lily
Chung, Edith C.
Chung, Moon Ja
Chung, Rita L.
Chung, Y. Barry
Chun, Marvin M.
Clarke-Pine, Dora D.
Coelho, George V.
Coggins, Margaret H.
Collins, James F.
D'Heurle, Adma J.
Das, Ajit K.
Das, Jagannath P.
Das, Manju P.
Dave, Jagdish P.
Dawis, Rene V.
DeMeis, Debra K.
Deshmukh, Mukund
Dias, Milagres C.
Dong, Tim T.
Drieberg, Keith L
Duan, Changming
Ebreo, Angela
Eng, Albert M.
Eskandari, Esfandiar
Fanibanda, Darius K.
Fergus, Esther O.
Field, Lucy F.
Fong, Donald L.
Fong, Geoffrey T.
Fong, Jane Y.
Fong, Larry
Foo, Koong H.
Foo, Rebecca E.
Fo, Walter S O
Fry, Prem S.
Fugita, Stephen S.
Fujii, Daryl E M
Fujimura, Laura E.
Fujinaka, Larry H.
Fujioka, Terry Ann T.
Fujita, George T.
Fujitsubo, Lani C.
Fukuyama, Mary A.
Funabiki, Dean
Fung, Hellen C.
Fung, Samuel
Furukawa, James M.
Furuno, Setsu
Gam, John
Garg, Mithlesh
Gasquoine, Philip G.
Gee, Carol S.
Ghalib, Nadeem
Ghassemzadeh, Habib

Gironella, Oliva C.
Goburdhun, Sara S.
Gock, Terry S.
Goh, David S.
Gong-Guy, Elizabeth
Gong, Susan M.
Grant, Swadesh S.
Gui, Chui-Liu Serena
Guo, Trudy Narikiyo
Gutterman, Carmen Y.
Hall, Christine I.
Hamada, Roger S.
Hamdani-Raab, Asma J.
Hamid, Mohammad
Ham, MaryAnna D.
Han, Yu Ling
Hao, Judy Y.
Harper, Renuka R.
Harris, William W.
Hartanto, Frans
Hartka, Elizabeth
Hashimoto, Jerry S.
Hass, Giselle A.
Hatsukami, Dorothy K.
Henson, Ramon M.
Heras, Patricia
Higashi, Wilfred H.
Higa, William R.
Hiroto, Donald S.
Ho, Chin-Chin
Ho, Christine K.
Hojat, Mohammadr
Ho, John E.
Ho, Kay
Hom, Harry L.
Hom, Jim
Hong, Barry A.
Hong, Eunsook
Hong, George K.
Hoshiko, Michael
Hoshino, Frank
Hoshmand, Lisa T.
Hossain, Ziarat
Hser, Yih-Ing
Hsia, Heidi
Hsu, Louis M.
Hsu, Shang H.
Huang, Karen H C
Huang, Larke N.
Huang, Wei-Jen William
Hufano, Linda D.
Hu, Li-Tze
Huset, Martha K.
Hu, Trudy HC
Hwee, Elsa
Hyde, Elsie HA
Ibrahim, Farah A.
Ichiyama, Michael A.

Iguchi, Martin Y.	Kim, Seock-Ho	Liem, Ramsay	Miyahira, Sarah D.
Inoue, Sachi	Kim, Sook K.	Lie, Rudolph T.B	Miyake, Steven M.
Ip, Sau Mei V.	Kim, Sung C.	Lim, Hoili C.	Mizokawa, Donald T.
Iqbal, S. Mohammed	Kim, Yang Ja	Lim, Patricia J.	Mock, Matthew R.
Ishida, Taeko H.	Kim, Yung Che	Lin, Hsin-Tai	Mody, Zarin R.
Ishikawa-Fullmer, Janet	Kitano, Margie K.	Lin, J.C. Gisela G.	Moideen, Yasmine
Ishiyama, Toaru	Kitayama, Shinobu	Lin, Jeanne L.	Mondol, Merlyn D.
Itatani, Robert M.	Kobayashi, Steve K.	Lin, Marie K.	Moon, Tae-Hyun
Ito, Elaine S.	Koh, Tong-He	Linn, Nancy SC	Mori, DeAnna L.
Iwai, Charles T.	Ko, Hwawei	Lin, Thung-Rung	Mori, Lisa T.
Iwamasa, Gayle Y.	Kondo, Charles Y.	Liu, An-Yen	Morishige, Howard H.
Iyengar, Shanto	Kop, Tim M.	Liu, Joseph C.	Morishima, James K.
Izawa, Chizuko	Koshino, Hideya	Li, Xiaoming	Morita, Denise N.
Izutsu, Satoru	Kothandapani, Virupaksha	Loo, Chalsa M.	Moritsugu, John
Ja, Davis Y.	Kuan, Yie-Wen Y.	Loong, James	Mo, Suchoon
Jain, Sharat K.	Kumar, Santosh	Loo, Russell	Moy, Samuel
Jaitly, Kailash N.	Kumar, V. K.	Low, Benson P.	Mukherjee, Subhash C.
Jani, Aurobindo J.	Kunitake, Yutaka	Lowe, Susana M.	Muradian, Mark G.
Japzon Gillum, Debra	Kupur, Veena	Lu, Elsie G.	Murakami, Janice
Jay, Milton T.	Kurato, Yoshiya	Lui, Barbara J.	Murakami, Sharon
Jew, Wing	Kurosawa, Kaoru	Lukman, Roy L.	Murakawa, Fay
Jin, Young-Sun	Kwei-Levy, Carol	Lum, Rodger G.	Nagamoto, Alan
Joshi, Sheila	Kwon, Paul H.	Luthar, Suniya S.	Nagata, Donna K.
Jue, Ronald W.	Lam, Chow S.	Macaranas, Eduarda A.	Nagayama Hall, Gordon C.
Junn, Ellen	Lau, Godwin	Machida, Sandra K.	Nagy, Vivian T.
Jurilla-Pastrana, Lina L.	Lau, Lavay	Majumder, Ranjit K.	Naidoo, Josephine C.
Kagehiro, Dorthy K.	Laviena, Luis	Malancharuvil, Joseph M.	Nakagawa, Janice Y.
Kakaiya, Divya	Le-Xuan-Hy, G. M.	Mane, Kamille L.	Nakamura, Charles Y.
Kamano, Dennis K.	Ledesma, Lourdes K.	Manese, Jeanne E.	Nakamura, Linda K
Kame'enui, Edward J.	Lee-Richter, Julie	Manese, Wilfredo R.	Navarro Foley, Gloria L.
Kameshima, Shinya	Lee, Anna C.	Manuel, Gerdenio M.	Nayak, Madhabika B.
Kamii, Constance	Lee, C. Jarnie W J	Mar, Harvey H.	Nemoto, Tooru
Kam, Sherilyn M.	Lee, D. John	Mariano, Tomas V.	Nezu, Arthur M.
Kaneshige, Edward	Lee, Daniel D.	Ma, Rita J.	Ng, James T.
Kang, Tai Lydia	Lee, David Y. K.	Mar, Norman J.	Ng, Pak C.
Kannarkat, Joy P.	Lee, Hing-Chu B.	Maruyama, Geoffrey	Nguyen, Dao Q.
Kanungo, Rabindra	Lee, Howard B.	Maruyama, Magoroh	Nhan, Nguyen
Kao, Barbara T.	Lee, Jerome	Matsui, Wesley T.	Nihira, Kazuo
Kashikar-Zuck, Susmita M.	Lee, Jo Ann	Matsumiya, Yoichi	Ninonuevo, Fred
Kato, Takashi	Lee, Julie C.	Matsumoto, David	Nishi-Strattner, Linda
Kau, Alice S. M.	Lee, Jung K.	Matsumoto, Gregory Y.	Nishio, Kazumi
Kawahara, Yoshito	Lee, Margaret	Matsumoto, Roy T.	Niwa, John S.
Kee, Daniel W.	Lee, Ronald W.	Matsuura, Larry N.	Noronha, Greta A.
Keefe, Keunho	Lee, See-Woo S.	Maung, Iqbal T.	Nowatari, Masahiro
Kee, PooKong	Lee, Seong S.	Ma, Yat-Ming C.	Oana, Leilani K.
Khalili, Hassan	Lee, Thomas W.	McCann, Robin S.	Oda, Ethel Aiko
Khan, Badrul A.	Lee, Wanda M. L.	McWilliams, Junko O.	Oh, Jungyeol L.
Khan, Kanwar H.	Lee, William W.	Mehrotra, Chandra M.N.	Ohwaki, Sonoko
Khanna, Jaswant L.	Lee, Yueh-Ting	Mehta, Kripal K.	Ohye, Bonnie Y.
Khanna, Mukti	Leong, Che K.	Mellot, Ramona N.	Oka, Evelyn R.
Khorakiwala, Durriyah	Leong, Deborah J.	Mikamo, Akiko	Okagaki, Lynn
Kich, George K.	Leong, Frederick T. T.	Minagawa, Rahn Y.	Okazaki, Sumie
Kich, George Kitahara	Le, Trinh To	Mink, Iris T.	Okiyama, Stephen L.
Kimbauer, Elli M.	Leung, Alex C. N.	Mino, Itsuko	Omizo, Michael M.
Kim, Chang-Dai	Leung, Paul	Minturn, Robin H.	Omoto, Allen M.
Kim, Elizabeth J.	Leung, S. Alvin	Mio, Jeffery S.	Ong, Eddie N.
Kim, Mary Ann Y.	Lew, Wei M.	Misra, Rajendra K.	Onizuka, Richard K.
Kim, Randi I.	Licuanan, Patricia	Miura, Irene T.	Onoda, Lawrence

Oommen Thomas, Susy
Osato, Sheryl
Otani, Akira
Ou, Young-Shi
Owyang, Walter
Ozaki, Mona M.
Pang, Dawn
Parasnis, Ila
Parasuraman, Raja
Park, Eyoungsoo
Patel, Sanjiv A.
Patterson, Mayin Lau
Perez, Ruperto M.
Poon, Leonard W.
Powers, Keiko I.
Pullium, Rita M.
Purochit, Arjun P.
Quijano, Walter Y.
Rajaram, Suparna
Ramaswami, Sundar
Randhawa, Bikkar S.
Rangoonwala, Rafique
Rattenbury, Francie R.
Raval, Bina D.
Ray, Arun B.
Rhee, Susan B.
Rigrish, Diana
Rohila, Pritam K.
Root, Maria P. P.
Roque, Sylvia A.
Rosenquist, Henry S.
Roy, Swati
Saito, Gloria C.
Sakamoto, Katsuyuki
Sakata, Robert T.
Sakurai, Mariko
Saleem, Rakhshanda
Salway, Milton R.
San Luis, Roberto R.
Saner-Yiu, Li-Chia
Saraf, Komal C.
Sasao, Toshiaki
Sato, Susan D.
Saul, Tuck T.
Sax, Kenji W.
Sayama, Mike K.
Schlesinger, Laura Ann
Schroff, Kamal
Seitz, Kathleen
Sen, Tapas K.
Serafica, Felicisima C.
Shahani-denning, Comila
Shah, Vasantkumar B.
Sharma, Greesh C.
Sharma, Satanand

Sharma, Vijai P.
Shen, John
Shima, Fred M.
Shimizu, Annette A.
Shimoda, Kim C.
Shing, Marn-Ling
Shirakawa, Patti
Shires, Michael R.
Shon, Elizbabeth
Shopshire, Michael S.
Shroff, Kamal
Shum, Hilda B.
Shum, Hilda B.
Sikka, Anjoo
Singg, Sangeeta
Singh, Darshan
Singh, Nirbhay N.
Singh, R. K. Janmeha
Singh, Ramadhar
Singh, Silvija S.
Sinha, Birendra
Sinha, Sachchida
Sison, Cecile E.
Sitharthan, Thiagarajan
Smith, Michael C.
Smith, Teresa D.
Sodowsky, Gargi R.
Somjee, Lubna
Somwaru, Jwalla P.
Srinivasan, Sampurna
Srivastva, Suresh
Stephens, Dorothy W.
Sterling, Sharon E.
Stewart, Sunita M.
Sudevan, Padmanbhan
Sue, David
Sue, Derald W.
Sue, Stanley
Sugai, Don P.
Sugawara, Hazuki M.
Suinn, Richard M.
Sundararajan, Louise-
  Kuen-Wei L.
Sung, Yong H.
Sun, Irene L.
Suzuki, Lisa A.
Swan, June A.
Sy, Michael J.
Tai, Chun-Nan
Takahashi, Lorey K.
Takamine, Sandra
Takanishi, Ruby
Takemoto-Chock, Naomi
Tamayo, Federico M. V.
Tamura, Leonard J.

Tana, Joseph
Tanaka-Matsumi, Junko
Tanaka, Koji
Tanaka, Yasumasa
Tan, Gabriel
Tang, Terry
Tang, Thomas L P
Tan, Josephine
Tan, Rowena N.
Tan, Siang-Yang Y.
Tatara, Mikihachiro
Tatsuguchi, Rosalie K.
Teng, Evelyn L.
Teng, L. Neal
Teo, Thomas
Thimotheose, K. G.
Thomas, Joseph E.
Tien, Liang
Ting-Chau, Theodora
Tobias, Manuel D.
Tom, Agnes
Torigoe, Rodney Y.
Toshima, Tamotsu
True, Reiko Homma
Tsai, Mavis
Tsang, Michael Hing- Pui
Tsui, Alice M.
Tsui, Ellen C.
Tsujimoto, Richard N.
Tsukamoto, Donna E.
Tsushima, William T.
Tung, May
Uno, Elizabeth
Upadhyaya, Shripati
Uyeda, Arthur A.
Vaid, Jyotsna
Vakhariya, Sobha
Valdez, Jr., Romulo
Valentiner, David P.
Vance, Ellen B.
Varki, C. Paily
Velayo, Richard S.
Verghese, Cherian
Villejo, Ron E.
Viswesvaran, Chockalingam
Wagner, Aureen Pinto
Wakeman, Richard J.
Walia, Kusum
Wang, Alvin
Wang, Edward S.
Wang, James D.
Wang, Margaret C.
Wang, Paul H.
Wang, Richard S.
Wang, Wen-Hsiu

Wang, Youde
Watanabe-Muraoka, Agnes M.
Whang, Patricia A.
Wibberly, Kathy H.
Wickramasekera, Ian E.
Wilkinson, H. Sook
Winter, Amal
Win, U. Kyaw
Wong-Ngan, Julia A.
Wong-Rieger, Durhane
Wong, Deborah A.
Wong, Dorothy L.
Wong, Florence C
Wong, Frankie Y.
Wong, Hermund
Wong, Jane L.
Wong, Jessie
Wong, Kit L.
Wong, Lily Y.S
Wong, Lily H.
Wong, Martin R.
Wong, Philip S
Wong, Roderick
Wong, Tony M.
Wong, Wilson
Woo, Rose
Woo, Tae O.
Wu, Jing-Jyi
Wu, Li-Chuan
Wu, Sheila T.
Wu, Shi-Jiuan
Xu, Gang
Yabusaki, Ann S.
Yamada, Elaine M.
Yamaguchi, Harry G.
Yamaguchi, Mitsue Y.
Yamamura, Lorraine M.
Yanagida, Evelyn H.
Yan, Bernice
Yang, Raymond K.
Yap, Kim O.
Yasutake, Joseph Y.
Yee, Albert H.
Yee, Barbara W. K.
Yee, Brian W.
Yee, Jane K.
Yee, Jennie Hy
Yee, Randall W.
Yee, Tina T.
Yi, Kris Y.
Ying, Yu-Wen
Yoshimura, G. Joji
Yoshimura, Kari K.
Young, David A.
Yu, Angelita M.
Yuen, Lenora L.
Yu, Howard K.
Yun, S.B.

Yu, Pamela
Zane, Nolan W.S
Zhu, Jiajun

HISPANIC/LATINO

Abello, Ana L.
Abercrombie, Maria M.
Abordo, Enrique J.
Abraido-Lanza, Ana F
Acosta, Frank X.
Adams-Esquivel, Henry
Adler, Peter J.
Aguilar, Martha C.
Aguilera, David M.
Aguirre-Deandreis, Ana I.
Ainslie, Ricardo C.
Albert, Rosita D.
Alfaro-Garcia, Rafael A.
Alonso, Mario
Alonso, Martha R.
Altarriba, Jeanette
Alvarez, Blanca M. De
Alvarez, Carlos M.
Alvarez, Gary L.
Alvarez, Manuel E.
Alvarez, Maria D.
Alvarez, Mauricia
Alvarez, Mildred M.
Alvarez, Paul A.
Alvarez, Roland
Alvarez, Rosaligia
Alvarez, Vivian
Amaro, Hortensia
Amezaga, Jr., Alfredo M.
Amezcua, Charlie A.
Anderson, Claudia J.
Andujar, Carlos A.
Antokoletz, Juana C.
Antonuccio, David
Anton, William D.
Aponte, Evelyn I.
Aponte, Joseph F.
Araoz, Daniel L.
Arboleda, Catalina
Arbona, Consuelo
Arcaya, Jose M.
Ardila, Ruben
Arellano-Lopez, Juan
Arellano, Charleanea
Arenas, Jr., Silverio
Arevalo, Luis E.
Ariza-Menedez, Maria
Arizmeudi, Thomas
Armengol, Carmen G.
Arnau-Gras, Jamie

Arredondo, Patricia
Arreola-Rockwell, Fran-
Pepitone-
Arriso, Roberta H
Arroyo, Judith A.
Arroyo, Patricia M.
Arsuaga, Enrique N.
Artiles, Alfredo J.
Artiles, Laura M.
Artiola, Lydia
Arvelo, Luis E.
Ascencao, Erlete M.
Atilano, Raymond B.
Auuilas-Gaxiola, Sergio A.
Aviera, Arlene T.
Aviles, Alice A.
Ayllon, Teodoro
Ayoub, Catherine C.
Azaret, Marisa
Azcarate, Eduardo M.
Azevedo, Don Fernando
Azmitia, Margarita
Bacal, Sergio
Baca, Sandra G.
Bacigalupe, Gonzalo M.
Badillo, Diana
Baez, Luis
Balbona, Manuel
Balcazar, Fabricio E.
Balderrama, Sylvia R.
Baratta, Frank S.
Bardenstein, Karen K.
Barnes, Charles A.
Barona, Andres
Baron, Augustine
Barrera, Jr., Manuel
Barrera, Francisco J.
Barrios, Francisco X.
Barry, Martha J.
Basco, Monica A.
Bascuas, Joseph W.
Bastien, IV, Samuel A.
Bauermeisten, Jose J.
Bavon, Moises
Baxter-Boehm, Alva
Bayon, E. Paul
Beato-Smith, Vera
Belen, Ines I.
Beliz, Jr., Efrain A.
Beltran, Joe
Benamu, Icem
Benavides, Jr., Robert
Bencomo, Armando A.
Benet-Martinez, Veronica
Benitez, John C.
Bennasar, Mari C.
Benzaquen, Isaac
Bernal, Alberto J.

Bernal, Guillermo A.
Bernal, Guillermo
Bernal, Martha E
Bernat, Gloria S.
Berrill, Naftali G.
Berrios, Zaida R.
Bersing, Doris S.
Betancourt, Hector
Bild-Libbin, Raguel
Blanco-Beledo, Ricardo
Blandino, Ramon A.
Boone, Martin
Borgatta, Edgar F.
Borrego, Richard L.
Borrero-Hernandez, Alejo
Bosch, Isora
Boulette, Tersea R.
Boulon-Diaz, Frances E.
Bracero, William
Bradman, Leo H.
Brandenburg, Carlos E.
Brattesami, Karen A.
Bruguera, Mark R.
Bueno, Luis F.
Buki, Lydia P.
Burciaga, Lawrence E.
Bursztyn, Alberto M.
Bustamante, Eduardo M.
Caetano, Elizabeth
Caldera, Yvonne M.
Calderon, Vivian
Camargo, Robert J.
Camarillo, Max
Campos, Leonard P.
Canedo, Angelo R.
Canovas Welles, Nydia L.
Cappon, Jorge
Caraveo, Libardo E.
Carballo-Dieguez, Alex
Carcas, Marilyn B.
Cardalda, Elsa B.
Cardena, Etzel A.
Cardona, Gilbert
Cardoza, Desdemona
Caro, Yvette
Carpenter, Gerald A.
Carr-Casanova, Rosario
Carra, Sylvia F.
Carr, Paquita R.
Casas, Eduardo F.
Cascallar, Eduardo C.
Castillo, Diane T.
Castro-Blanco, David R.
Cebollero, Ana Margarita
Cepeda-Benito, Antonio
Cereijido, Margarita
Cervantes, Joseph M.
Chapa, Joel R.

Chatigny, Anita L.
Chaves, John F.
Chavez, Ernest L.
Cherbosque, Jorge
Chiriboga, David A.
Choca, James
Chriss, Gloria M.
Cimino, Cynthia R.
Cirino, Gabriel
Cleveland, Adriana F.
Coes, Maria R.
Collado, Armando
Colon, Ana I.
Colon, Luis H.
Colon, R. Phillip
Colotla, Victor A.
Comas-Diaz, Lillian
Constanzo, Magda S.
Contreras, Raquel J.
Cordero, Fernando
Cornide, Carmen R.
Correa, Martha L.
Corte, Henry E.
Cortese, Margaret
Costa, Armenio S.
Crane, Rosario S.
Credidio, Vivian F.
Crespo, Alfredo E.
Crespo, Gloria M.
Cruz-Lopez, Miguel
Cruz, Albert R.
Cruz, Arnold de la
Cruz, Maria C.
Cruz, Vivian A.
Cuesta, George M.
Cunha, Maria I.
Dallas, Mercedes
Daruna, Jorge H.
Davila, Joanne
De Apodaca, Roberto F.
De Armas, Armando
de Fuentes, Nanette
de Jesus, Nelson H.
De La Cancela, Victor
de la Pena, Augustin M.
De la Serna, Marcelo
de la Sota, Elizanda M.
De Las Fuentes, Cynthia
de Llano, Carmen
De Louredes Mattei, Maria
De Queiroz, Aidyl M.
De Varona, M .
DeBlassie, III, Paul A.
DeFerreire, Mary Elizabeth
Dehmer-Abalo, Elena M.
Del Rio, Augusto B.
Delgado-Hachey, Maria
Dendaluce, Inaki

Marrero, Bernie	Munoz, Marisol	Pincheira, Juan A.	Rodriguez, Maria A.
Marroquin, Arthur R.	Munoz, Nina R.	Pinto, Alcides	Rodriguez, Ramon O.
Martinez, Jr., Joe L.	Munoz, Ricardo F.	Pita, Marcia E.	Rodriguez, Richard A.
Martinez-Lugo, Miguel E.	Murillo, Nathan	Pizano-Thomen, Margarita	Rodriguez, Rogelio E.
Martinez-Urrutia, Angel C.	Mussenden, Gerald	Plazas, Carlos A.	Rodriguez, Wilfredo
Martinez, Alejandro M.	Nadal-Vazquez, Vilma Y.	Poal, Pilar	Roehlke, Helen J.
Martinez, Cynthia	Narvaez, Darcia F.	Pompa, Janiece L.	Rogler, Lloyd H.
Martinez, Eduardo M.	Natalicio, Luiz	Pons, Michael B.	Roig, Miguel
Martinez, Floyd H.	Navas-Robleto, Jose J.	Ponton, Marcel O.	Roll, Samuel
Martinez, Gabriel P.	Navedo, Christella N.	Porges, Carlos R.	Roman, Hugo
Martinez, Maria J.	Nazario, Jr., Andres	Posner, Carmen A.	Romero, Arturo
Martinez, Raul	Netter, Beatriz E. C.	Praderas, Kim	Romero, Augusto
Martinez, Sergio I.	Netter, Roberto	Prado, Haydee	Romero, Jose
Martin, Laura P.	Niemann, Yolanda F	Prado, William M.	Romey, Carol M.
Martorell, Mario F.	Nieto-Cardoso, Ezequiel	Prendes-Lintel, Maria L.	Rosado, John W.
Masini, Angela	Nieves-Grafals, Sara	Price, Alicia A.	Rosales, Israel B.
Mastrapa, Selma A.	Nieves, Luis R.	Prieto, Addys	Rosario, Margaret
McNeill, Elizabeth M.	Nogales, Ana	Prieto, Susan L.	Rosin, Susana A.
Mejia, Juan A.	Nunez, Narina N	Puente, Antonio E.	Rossello, Jeannette
Melgoza, Bertha	Nuttall, Ena V.	Puertas, Lorenzo	Rubio, Charles T.
Mellor-Crummey, Cynthia A.	O'Brien, B. Marco	Puig, Ange	Ruiz, Fernando
Menchaca, Victoria A.	O'Neill-dePumarada, Celeste	Puig, Hector	Ruiz, Nicholas J.
Mendelberg, Hava E.	Ocasio-Garcia, Ketty	Quintana, Stephen M.	Ruiz, Sonia I.
Mendez, Gloria I.	Olguin, Arthur	Ramirez-Cancel, Carlos M.	Ruth, Richard
Mendoza, Jorge L.	Olivas, Romeo A.	Ramirez, David E.	Sacasa, Rafael E.
Miccio-Fonseca, L. C.	Olivero, Gerald	Ramirez, John/Juan	Saenz, Javier
Millan, Fred	Olmedo, Esteban L.	Ramirez, Sylvia Z.	Saenz, Karol K.
Miranda, David J.	Olmo, Manuel C.	Ramos-Grenier, Julia	Salais, A. Joseph
Miranda, Jose P.	Orabona, Elaine	Ramos, Arnaldo J.	Salas, Eduardo
Miranda, M.	Ortega, Richard J.	Reisinger, Mercedes C.	Salas, Jesus A.
Miranda, Manuel R.	Ortega, Robert M.	Rey-Casserly, Celiane M.	Saldana, Delia H.
Modiano, Rachel	Ortiz, Berta S.	Reyes-Mayer, Erwin	Salgado de Snyder, V. Nelly S.
Mogro, Ana Klatt	Ortiz, Vilma	Reyes, Carla J.	Salganicoff, Matilde
Mondragon, Nathan J.	Otero, Rafael F.	Reyna, Valerie F.	Samaniego, Sandra
Monguio, Ines	Ovide, Christopher R.	Reza, Ernesto M.	Samano, Italo A.
Monserrat, Laura	Pacheco, Angel E.	Rezentes, III, William C.	San Miguel, Christopher L.
Montalvo, Roberto E.	Palomares, Ronald S.	Ribera-Gonzalez, Julio C.	Sanchez-Caso, Luis M.
Montemayor, Raymond	Panciera, Lawrence A.	Rigual-Lynch, Lourdes	Sanchez-Torrento, Eugenio
Montes, Francisco	Paniagua, Freddy A.	Rivas-Vazquez, Ana A.	Sanchez, David M.
Montesi, Alexandra Saba	Pardo, Ruben C.	Rivera-Lopez, Hector	Sanchez, Debra A.
Montijo, Jorge A.	Paredes, Jr., Frank C.	Rivera-Medina, Eduardo J.	Sanchez, H.G.
Montoya, E. Carolina	Parlade, Rafael J.	Rivera-Molina, Elba	Sanchez, Juan
Morales-Barreto, Gisela	Pasamonte, Ana M.	Rivera-Sinclair, Elsa A.	Sanchez, Victor C.
Morales, Cynthia T.	Patrick, Carol L.	Rivera, Beatriz D.	Sanchez, William
Morales, Eduardo S.	Pedemonte, Monica	Rivera, Carmen J.	Sancho, Ana M.
Morales, Elias	Pelaez, Carmen	Rivera, Enrique	Sandoval, Jonathan
Morales, Pamilla V.	Peralta, Carmelina	Rivera, Jo Ann M.	Santiago-Negron, Salvador
Mora, Ralph	Pereira, Glona M.	Rivera, Miquela	Santiago, Lydia V.
Mordka, Irwin	Perez Ebrahimi, Concepcion	Rivera, Nelson E.	Santini-Hernandez, Ernesto
Morones, Pete A.	Perez-Arce, Patricia	Rivero, Estela M.	Santos de Barona, Maryann
Morote, Gloria	Perez-Ramos, Juan	Robertin, Hector	Sanua, Victor D.
Mortimer, Joan R.	Perez, Carlos A.	Rodriguez, Carlos J.	Sarmiento, Robert F.
Muga, Joe	Perez, Cecilia M.	Rodriguez, Carmen G.	Sasscer-Burgos, Julie
Mujica, Ernesto	Perez, Fred M.	Rodriguez, David A.	Saucedo, Carlos
Munoz, Daniel G	Perez, Juan C.	Rodriguez, Ester R.	Saucedo, Carlos
Munoz, John A.	Perilla, Julia L.	Rodriguez, Lavinia	Saunders, Walter C.
Munoz, Leticia S.	Pflaum, John H.	Rodriguez, Luis J.	Schacht, Thomas E.
Munoz, Luis A.	Pico, Daima	Rodriguez, Manuel D.	Schenquerman, Berta N.

Schlesinger, Susana J.
Schmajuk, Nestor
Schreier, Raquel L.
Seda, Gilbert
Sedo, Manuel A.
Serrano-Garcia, Irma
Shapiro, Ester R.
Shea-Martinez, Herminia E.
Shuffer, Jr., Jacob M.
Silva, Santiago
Sloan, R. Lloyd
Sobrino, James F.
Softas, Basilia C.
Soler, Robin E
Somodevilla, S. A.
Sonneborn, Dean R.
Soriano, Fernando I.
Soriano, Marcel
Sosa, Juan N.
Soto, Elaine
Soto, George M.
Soto, Tomas A.
Soza, Anthony M.
Stasson, Mark F.
Stern, Marilyn
Stewart, Arleen R.
Suarez-Balcazar, Yolanda
Suarez-Crowe, Yolanda
Suarez, Alejandra
Suarez, Carlota
Suarez, Enrique M.
Suarez, Miguel G.
Suarez, Susan D.
Szapocznik, Jose
Tabachnik, Samuel
Takushi, Ruby Y.
Tamayo, Jose M.
Taylor, Stephen Q.
Tazeau, Yvette N.
Teitel, Raquel S.
Teixeira, Michael A.
Tejeda, Manuel J.
Thorn, Isabel M.
Tirado, John
Tirado, Linda Ann
Tischer, Hans
Todd-Mancillas, William R.
Topolski, James M.
Toro-Alfonso, Jose
Toro, Carlos A.
Toro, Haydee
Torres-Saenz, Jorge
Torres, Mario A.
Tostado, John F.
Towns-Miranda, Luz
Turner, Darrell D.
Urbina, Susana P.
Urquiza, Anthony J.

Vada, Alejo
Valdes, Luis F.
Valdes, Maria
Valdes, Thusnelda M.
Valdez-Menchaca, Marta C.
Valdez, Jesse N.
Valdivia, Lino
Valencia-Laver, Debra
Valtierra, Mary
Vargas, Luis A.
Vargas, M. Angelica
Vargas, Manuel J.
Vasquez, Melba
Vasquez, Michael B.
Vazquez-Ruiz, Francisco
Vazquez, Carlos D.
Vazquez, Cesar D.
Vazquez, Rosa
Vega, Jose G.
Vega, Star
Vegega, Maria E.
Velasco, Frank E.
Velasquez, John M.
Velasquez, Roberto J.
Velez-Diaz, Angel
Velez, Maria T.
Vera, Elizabeth M.
Viale-val, Graciela
Vicente, Peter J.
Vigil, Patricia L.
Villegas, Orlando L.
Villela, Leopoldo F.
Whitaker, Sandra V.
Yniguez, Linda E.
Zaldivar, Luis R.
Zamudio, Anthony
Zaragoza, Maria S.
Zavala-Martinez, Iris
Zavala, Albert
Zayas-Bazan, Carmen
Zayas, Luis H.
Zayas, Maria A.
Zepeda, Marlene
Zighelboim, Vivien A.
Zuercher-White, Elke
Zuriff, Gerald E.

AFRICAN AMERICAN/ BLACK, AND AMERICAN INDIAN/ALASKA NATIVE
Newburgh, Tracey LS
Andrieu, Brenda J.
Branche, Leota Susan
Brooks, Juanita O.
Dent, Harold E.
Gist, Marilyn E.

Grubb, Henry J.
Hargrove, Jr., Jerry E.
Hart, Anton H.
Hightower, Eugene
McCombs, Daniel
Rivers, Marie D.
Somerville, Addison W.
Taylor, Flor N.
Windham, Thomas L.

AFRICAN AMERICAN/ BLACK, AND ASIAN AMERICAN/ASIAN/PACIFIC ISLANDER
Hargrow, Mary E.
Lewis, Page
Salone, Lavorial

AFRICAN AMERICAN/ BLACK, AND HISPANIC/ LATINO
Mahabee-Harris, Marilyn M.
Martin, William F.
Moss, Ramona J.
Parson, Erwin R.
Peart-Newkirk, Natalia J.
Williams, Rebecca E.

AFRICAN AMERICAN/ BLACK, AND WHITE/ EUROPEAN
Greene, Karen J.
Walker, L. Gorman

AMERICAN INDIAN/ALASKA NATIVE, AND HISPANIC/ LATINO
Rojas, Rebecca S
Vargas, Alice M.

AMERICAN INDIAN/ALASKA NATIVE, AND WHITE/ EUROPEAN
Hough, Sigmund
Natani, Kirmach

ASIAN AMERICAN/ASIAN/ PACIFIC ISLANDER, AND HISPANIC/LATINO
Akca, Zeynep K.
Bonal, Kathleen A.
Fernandez, Ephrem
Garcia, Melinda A.
Jew, Cynthia L.
Mehta, Sheila
Osorno, Wendell A.
Ozoa, Claudette
Pang, Mark G.
Pirhekayaty-Soriano, Tahereh
Unson, Delia C. O.

HISPANIC/LATINO, AND WHITE/EUROPEAN
Burton, Roger V.
Edwards, Henry P.
Llorca, Arthur L.
McNeill, Brian
Mendez-Calderon, Luis M.
Selgas, James W.

Geographical Listing

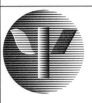

Geographical listings are divided into two major subsections:

Foreign Countries of domicile and

U.S. States or Possessions of residence.

Within each of these subsections,

psychologists of color are listed alphabetically by:

Specific Foreign Country or

U.S. State/Possession

(and within each of these by)

Ethnic Group

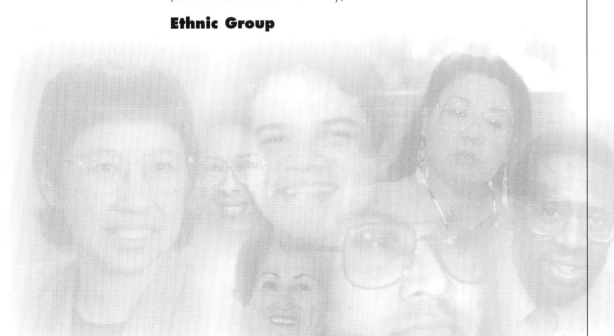

GEOGRAPHICAL LISTING

FOREIGN COUNTRIES

ARGENTINA

-Hispanic/Latino

Insua, Ana Maria

AUSTRALIA

-Asian American/AsianPacific Islander

Kee, PooKong
Leung, Paul
Sitharthan, Thiagarajan

BERMUDA

-African American/Black

Binns, Derrick

BRAZIL

-Hispanic/Latino

De Queiroz, Aidyl M.
Lemos-Mettel, Thereza P. De
Perez-Ramos, Juan

CANADA

-American Indian/Alaska Native

Blue, Arthur W.
Bouffard, R. Gerard

-Asian American/Asian/Pacific Islander

Al-tai, Nazar M.
Baba, Vishwanath V.
Chan, David C.
Das, Jagannath P.
Fong, Geoffrey T.
Fong, Larry
Fry, Prem S.
Gironella, Oliva C.
Ip, Sau Mei V.
Kanungo, Rabindra
Khalili, Hassan
Khan, Badrul A.
Lau, Godwin
Lee, Seong S.
Leong, Che K.
Naidoo, Josephine C.
Purochit, Arjun P.
Randhawa, Bikkar S.
Sinha, Birendra
Sy, Michael J.
Tan, Josephine
Teo, Thomas
Wong-Rieger, Durhane
Wong, Jessie
Wong, Roderick
Yan, Bernice

-Hispanic/Latino

Bacal, Sergio
Barrera, Francisco J.
Camargo, Robert J.
Casas, Eduardo F.
Colotla, Victor A.

-Hispanic/Latino, White/ European

Edwards, Henry P.

EL SALVADOR

-Hispanic/Latino

Gaborit, Mauricio

FRANCE

-African American/Black

Donnella, John

HONG KONG

-Asian American/Asian/Pacific Islander

Lee, Hing-Chu B.
Tsang, Michael Hing- Pui

INDIA

-Asian American/Asian/Pacific Islander

Sinha, Sachchida

INDONESIA

-Asian American/Asian/Pacific Islander

Hartanto, Frans

IRAN

-Asian American/Asian/Pacific Islander

Ghassemzadeh, Habib

JAPAN

-Asian American/Asian/Pacific Islander

Anzai, Yuichiro
Baba, Masao
Kameshima, Shinya
Kato, Takashi
Kitayama, Shinobu
Kurato, Yoshiya
Kurosawa, Kaoru
Maruyama, Magoroh
Nowatari, Masahiro
Sasao, Toshiaki
Sugawara, Hazuki M.
Tanaka, Koji
Tanaka, Yasumasa
Tatara, Mikihachiro
Toshima, Tamotsu
Watanabe-Muraoka, Agnes M.

KOREA

-Asian American/Asian/Pacific Islander

Jin, Young-Sun

KUWAIT

-Asian American/Asian/Pacific Islander

Nayak, Madhabika B.

MALAYSIA

-Asian American/Asian/Pacific Islander

Chin, Sandra B

MEXICO

-Hispanic/Latino

Alvarez, Blanca M. De
Blanco-Beledo, Ricardo
Cappon, Jorge
Diaz-Guerrero, Rogelio
Garza, Alicia de la
Lafarga-Corona, Juan B.
Nieto-Cardoso, Ezequiel
Salgado de Snyder, V. Nelly S.

NIGERIA

-African American/Black

Ezeilo, Bernice N.
Ugwuegbu, Denis C.

AKISTAN

**-Asian American/Asian/
Pacific Islander**

Ghalib, Nadeem

PHILIPPINES

**-Asian American/Asian/
Pacific Islander**

Aldaba-Lim, Estefania
Ledesma, Lourdes K.
Licuanan, Patricia

PORTUGAL

**-Asian American/Asian/
Pacific Islander**

Lee, Anna C.

SINGAPORE

**-Asian American/Asian/
Pacific Islander**

Chang, Weining C.
Foo, Koong H.
Singh, Ramadhar
Wong, Lily H.

SOUTH KOREA

**-Asian American/Asian/
Pacific Islander**

Chung, Moon Ja
Kim, Chang-Dai
Kim, Yung Che

SPAIN

-Hispanic/Latino

Arnau-Gras, Jamie
Dendaluce, Inaki
Garriga-Trillo, Ana J.

SWITZERLAND

**-Asian American/Asian/
Pacific Islander**

Saner-Yiu, Li-Chia

TAIWAN

**-Asian American/Asian/
Pacific Islander**

Chiang, Grace CT
Hsu, Shang H.
Ko, Hwawei
Lin, Hsin-Tai
Shing, Marn-Ling
Tai, Chun-Nan
Wang, Wen-Hsiu
Wu, Li-Chuan

THAILAND

**-Asian American/Asian/
Pacific Islander**

Amawattana, Tipawadee
Bhanthumnavin, Duangduen

TRINIDAD

-African American/Black

Phillips, Campbell C.

UNITED KINGDOM

-African American/Black

Horsford, Bernard I.

**-Asian American/Asian/
Pacific Islander**

Upadhyaya, Shripati

VENEZUELA

-Hispanic/Latino

Garcia-Gonzalez, Jose A.

-African American/Black

Levermore, Monique A.

U.S. STATES AND POSSESSIONS

ALABAMA

-African American/Black

Abston, Jr., Nathaniel
Floyd, Bridget J.
Gordon, Ruth H.
Graves, Kenneth J.

Matthews, Belvia W.
Reaves, Andrew L
Wells, Annie M.

**-Asian American/Asian/
Pacific Islander**

Gam, John
Kamii, Constance
Kothandapani, Virupaksha
Whang, Patricia A.

-Hispanic/Latino

Beltran, Joe
Borrero-Hernandez, Alejo
Labbe, Elise E.
Rubio, Charles T.
Suarez-Crowe, Yolanda

**-Asian American/Asian/
Pacific Islander and White/
European**

Mehta, Sheila

ALASKA

-African American/Black

Jennings, Jr., Wilmar A.

**-American Indian/Alaska
Native**

Hayes, Forrest L.
Sanders, Gilbert O.

-Hispanic/Latino

McNeill, Elizabeth M.

ARIZONA

-African American/Black

Battiest, William V.
Hardin, Jr., Oscar A.
Prelow, Hazel M.
Smith, Walanda W.

**-Asian American/Asian/
Pacific
Islander**

Amin, Kiran
Chang, Alice F.
Chao, Janet
Hall, Christine I.
Khan, Kanwar H.
Mellot, Ramona N.
Tsui, Alice M.
Yee, Brian W.

-Hispanic/Latino

Artiola, Lydia
Barona, Andres
Barrera, Jr., Manuel
Bencomo, Armando A.
Bernal, Martha E
Bernat, Gloria S.
Caraveo, Libardo E.
de Jesus, Nelson H.
Martinez, Floyd H.
Martinez, Sergio I.
Mordka, Irwin
Reyna, Valerie F.
Rodriguez, Ester R.
Santos de Barona, Maryann
Velez, Maria T.

ARKANSAS

-African American/Black

Griffin, Patricia L.

-Hispanic/Latino

Prado, William M.

CALIFORNIA

-African American/Black

Abernethy, Alexis D.
Allen, Winnie M.
Allen, Wise E.
Artis, Daphne J.
Baker, Octave V.
Baly, Iris E.
Bamgbose, Olujiimi O.
Banks, Hobart M.
Barker-Hackett, Lori
Bartee, Robert L.
Bastien, Rochelle T.
Beam, Micheline
Block, Carolyn B.
Boxley, Russell L.
Browne, Ronald H.
Brown, Marilyn F.
Brown, Michael T.
Campbell, Barbara L.
Cohen, Isadora
Coleman, Philip P.
Collins, Edsmond J.
Connor, Michael E.
Cook, Rudolf E.
Craig, U-Shaka
Curry, Alpha O.
Davis-Russell, Elizabeth

Ervin, Betty J.
Fairchild, Halford H.
Ford, Deshay D.
Ford, Fatima Y
Francisco, Richard P.
Fulton, Aubyn
Fulton, Wayne M.
Gaines, Stanley O.
Garner, Edward L.
Gay, Patricia L.
Gibbs, Jewelle Taylor
Glover, O.S.
Gordon, LaFaune Y.
Graham, Sandra
Griffith, Marlin S.
Grinstead, Olga A.
Guillory, Paul T.
Gulley, Silas
Gunn, Robert L.
Haggins, Kristee L.
Hamer, Forrest M.
Harrell, Shelly P.
Hawkins, Ioma L.
Hawkins, James Leon
Hudley, Cynthia
Hunt, William K.
Jackson, Jacquelyne F.
Jackson, Leslie C.
Jenkins-Monroe, Valata
Johnson, Zonya
Kennedy, Clive D.
LeSure-Lester, G. Evelyn
Lipson, Diane R.
Luke, Equilla
Lyles, William B.
Mack, Delores E.
Mayo, Benjamin F.
Mays, Vickie M.
McClure, Faith H.
McLean, Jr, Alvin
Milburn, Norweeta G.
Miles, Gary T.
Miller, S. Walden
Mills, Marcia C.
Mitchell, Horace
Monteiro, Kenneth P.
Monteiro, Rita C.
Moore, Sandra
Morgan, Cynthia L.
Munford, Paul R.
Myers, Hector F.
Noel, Winifred
Nzewi, Esther N.
Parham, Thomas A.
Parham, William D.
Parks, Carlton
Patton, Kenneth
Penn, Nolan E.

Pierce, William D.
Polite, Kenneth
Porche-Burke, Lisa M.
Pruitt, Jr., Joseph H.
Reams, Bennie P
Reilly, Patrick M.
Richardson, Frederick
Roberts, Terrence J.
Samaan, Makram K.
Scott, Merilla M.
Sharp, Jude C.
Smith, Charles E.
Smith, William
Snowden, Lonnie R.
Spraings, Violet E.
Steele, Marilyn
Strickland, Tony L
Stroud, Barbara
Thompson, Veronique L.
Treadwell, Marsha J.
Trufant, Carol A.
Tucker, Dorothy M.
Underwood, Robert J.
Vaughan, Elaine
Walker, Lola '.
Washington, Anita C.
Wellons, Retha V.
West, Gerald I.
White, Joseph L.
Williams, Estelle M.
Williams, Karen P. W.
Williams, Medria L.
Wright, Michael F.
Wyatt, Gail E.
Wynne, Michael

-American Indian/Alaska Native

Byrd, Robert D.
Cummings, Joseph D.
Gregory, Robert A.
Haddock, Dean M.
LaFromboise, Teresa
Miller, Sarah S.
Nolley, David A.
Pine, Charles J.
Quinn, Lisa
Shohet, Jacqueline M.
Taylor, Peggy S.
York, Mary J.

-Asian American/Asian/Pacific Islander

Advani, Nisha
Akutsu, Phillip D.
Aoki, Bart K.
Aoki, Wayne T.

Asamen, Joy K.
Attore, Lois
Atwal, Baljit K,
Bainum, Charlene K.
Campos, Joseph J.
Chan, Daniel S.
Chan, Kenyon S.
Chan, Samuel Q.
Chinn, Roberta N.
Chung, Edith C.
Clarke-Pine, Dora D.
Deshmukh, Mukund
Dias, Milagres C.
Dong, Tim T.
Drieberg, Keith L
Eng, Albert M.
Eskandari, Esfandiar
Fanibanda, Darius K.
Fong, Donald L.
Fong, Jane Y.
Foo, Rebecca E.
Fugita, Stephen S.
Gock, Terry S.
Gong-Guy, Elizabeth
Gong, Susan M.
Hao, Judy Y.
Hartka, Elizabeth
Heras, Patricia
Hiroto, Donald S.
Hong, George K.
Hoshino, Frank
Hser, Yih-Ing
Hu, Li-Tze
Ichiyama, Michael A.
Iguchi, Martin Y.
Inoue, Sachi
Ishida, Taeko H.
Itatani, Robert M.
Iyengar, Shanto
Ja, Davis Y.
Jew, Wing
Joshi, Sheila
Jue, Ronald W.
Junn, Ellen
Jurilla-Pastrana, Lina L.
Kakaiya, Divya
Kam, Sherilyn M.
Kang, Tai Lydia
Kawahara, Yoshito
Kee, Daniel W.
Keefe, Keunho
Khorakiwala, Durriyah
Kich, George K.
Kich, George Kitahara
Kimbauer, Elli M.
Kim, Elizabeth J.
Kim, Mary Ann Y.
Kim, Randi I.

Kim, Sung C.
Kitano, Margie K.
Kobayashi, Steve K.
Koshino, Hideya
Kumar, Santosh
Kunitake, Yutaka
Lee, Daniel D.
Lee, Howard B.
Lee, Julie C.
Lee, See-Woo S.
Lee, Wanda M. L.
Lew, Wei M.
Lin, Jeanne L.
Lin, Marie K.
Linn, Nancy SC
Lin, Thung-Rung
Liu, Joseph C.
Lu, Elsie G.
Lum, Rodger G.
Machida, Sandra K.
Malancharuvil, Joseph M.
Mane, Kamille L.
Manese, Jeanne E.
Manuel, Gerdenio M.
Ma, Rita J.
Matsumoto, David
Matsumoto, Gregory Y.
Matsumoto, Roy T.
Maung, Iqbal T.
Mikamo, Akiko
Minagawa, Rahn Y.
Mink, Iris T.
Mio, Jeffery S.
Miura, Irene T.
Mock, Matthew R.
Moon, Tae-Hyun
Mori, Lisa T.
Murakawa, Fay
Nagamoto, Alan
Nagy, Vivian T.
Nakagawa, Janice Y.
Nakamura, Charles Y.
Nakamura, Linda K
Nemoto, Tooru
Ng, James T.
Nguyen, Dao Q.
Nihira, Kazuo
Nishio, Kazumi
Oh, Jungyeol L.
Ohwaki, Sonoko
Okiyama, Stephen L.
Ong, Eddie N.
Onoda, Lawrence
Osato, Sheryl
Owyang, Walter
Park, Eyoungsoo
Powers, Keiko I.
Rangoonwala, Rafique

Roy, Swati
Saito, Gloria C.
Sakamoto, Katsuyuki
Salway, Milton R.
Sharma, Satanand
Shima, Fred M.
Shon, Elizbabeth
Shopshire, Michael S.
Shum, Hilda B.
Shum, Hilda B.
Singh, R. K. Janmeha
Sue, Derald W.
Sue, Stanley
Sun, Irene L.
Swan, June A.
Tang, Terry
Tan, Siang-Yang Y.
Teng, Evelyn L.
Ting-Chau, Theodora
Tobias, Manuel D.
True, Reiko Homma
Tsujimoto, Richard N.
Tung, May
Uno, Elizabeth
Uyeda, Arthur A.
Wickramasekera, Ian E.
Win, U. Kyaw
Wong, Hermund
Wong, Lily Y.S
Woo, Rose
Wu, Sheila T.
Yabusaki, Ann S.
Yamaguchi, Mitsue Y.
Yamamura, Lorraine M.
Yasutake, Joseph Y.
Yee, Jane K.
Yee, Jennie Hy
Yee, Randall W.
Yee, Tina T.
Yi, Kris Y.
Ying, Yu-Wen
Yoshimura, G. Joji
Yoshimura, Kari K.
Young, David A.
Yuen, Lenora L.
Yu, Howard K.
Zane, Nolan W.S

-Hispanic/Latino

Abordo, Enrique J.
Acosta, Frank X.
Adams-Esquivel, Henry
Adler, Peter J.
Aguilera, David M.
Alvarez, Mildred M.
Alvarez, Paul A.
Alvarez, Vivian

Amezcua, Charlie A.
Arevalo, Luis E.
Arizmeudi, Thomas
Arreola-Rockwell, Fran
Pepitone-
Artiles, Alfredo J.
Arvelo, Luis E.
Auuilas-Gaxiola, Sergio A.
Aviera, Arlene T.
Azmitia, Margarita
Baca, Sandra G.
Baratta, Frank S.
Barnes, Charles A.
Bavon, Moises
Bayon, E. Paul
Beliz, Jr., Efrain A.
Benavides, Jr., Robert
Bersing, Doris S.
Betancourt, Hector
Boulette, Tersea R.
Bruguera, Mark R.
Caetano, Elizabeth
Calderon, Vivian
Camarillo, Max
Campos, Leonard P.
Cardona, Gilbert
Cardoza, Desdemona
Carr-Casanova, Rosario
Cervantes, Joseph M.
Chatigny, Anita L.
Cherbosque, Jorge
Cordero, Fernando
Cortese, Margaret
Credidio, Vivian F.
Crespo, Alfredo E.
Cruz, Arnold de la
Davila, Joanne
De Apodaca, Roberto F.
De Armas, Armando
de Fuentes, Nanette
de la Pena, Augustin M.
de Llano, Carmen
Dehmer-Abalo, Elena M.
Del Rio, Augusto B.
Dosamantes-Beaudry, Irma
Dunbar, Waldo
Duran, Richard P.
Espin, Oliva M.
Falicov, Celia J.
Fayard, Carlos
Ferdman, Bernardo M.
Fils, David H.
Flaherty, Maria Y.
Flores de Apodaca, Roberto
Flores, Elena
Fuhrmann, Max E.
Gamez, George L.
Garcia, Betty

Genhart, Michael J.
Gomez, Jr., Francisco C.
Gonsalves, Carlos J.
Gonzales, Michael
Gonzalez-Huss, Mary
Gonzalez, Alexander
Gonzalez, Gerardo M
Grosso, Federico C.
Grunhaus-Belzer, Rosa
Guanipa, Carmen L.
Guerra, Anna Maria
Guerra, Julio J.
Hall, M. Elizabeth L.
Hearn, Kathleen E.
Heller, Beatriz
Hernandez, Maria G.
Hofer, Ricardo
Hyman, Edward J.
Jaimez, T. Lanac
Jimenez-Safir, Paula B.
Juarez, Reina M.
Kelly, Tara L.
Kirst, Stephen P.
Kolt, Laurie
Lawson, Gary W.
Lein, H. Beatriz
Leon, Ruben
Lifur-Bennett, Linda
Lopez, Anthony A.
Lopez, Steven R.
Lowman, Rodney
Lozano, Irma
Luna, Donna J.
Majesty, Melvin S.
Mancillas, Paul
Marin, Gerardo
Martinez, Alejandro M.
Martinez, Cynthia
Martin, Laura P.
Melgoza, Bertha
Menchaca, Victoria A.
Miccio-Fonseca, L. C.
Miranda, Manuel R.
Mogro, Ana Klatt
Monguio, Ines
Montalvo, Roberto E.
Montesi, Alexandra Saba
Morales, Cynthia T.
Morales, Eduardo S.
Muga, Joe
Munoz, Daniel G
Munoz, Luis A.
Munoz, Marisol
Munoz, Nina R.
Munoz, Ricardo F.
Murillo, Nathan
Netter, Beatriz E. C.
Netter, Roberto

Nogales, Ana
Olguin, Arthur
Olmedo, Esteban L.
Ortiz, Berta S.
Ortiz, Vilma
Pardo, Ruben C.
Perez-Arce, Patricia
Perez, Juan C.
Pons, Michael B.
Ponton, Marcel O.
Reza, Ernesto M.
Rodriguez, Richard A.
Romero, Arturo
Romero, Augusto
Rosales, Israel B.
Ruiz, Fernando
Salais, A. Joseph
Sanchez, H.G.
Sanchez, Victor C.
Sandoval, Jonathan
Santiago, Lydia V.
Saucedo, Carlos
Saucedo, Carlos
Saunders, Walter C.
Schenquerman, Berta N.
Shea-Martinez, Herminia E.
Shuffer, Jr., Jacob M.
Sonneborn, Dean R.
Soriano, Fernando I.
Soriano, Marcel
Soza, Anthony M.
Stewart, Arleen R.
Tabachnik, Samuel
Tazeau, Yvette N.
Tirado, Linda Ann
Todd-Mancillas, William R.
Tostado, John F.
Urquiza, Anthony J.
Valdez-Menchaca, Marta C.
Valdivia, Lino
Valencia-Laver, Debra
Valtierra, Mary
Vasquez, Michael B.
Vega, Star
Velasco, Frank E.
Velasquez, Roberto J.
Villela, Leopoldo F.
Yniguez, Linda E.
Zamudio, Anthony
Zavala, Albert
Zepeda, Marlene
Zighelboim, Vivien A.
Zuercher-White, Elke

-Asian American/Asian/Pacific Islander

Leung, Alex C. N.

-Hispanic/Latino
Gonzalez, Rocio R
Rivera-Lopez, Hector

-African American/Black, and
American Indian/Alaska Native
Hightower, Eugene
Rivers, Marie D.
Somerville, Addison W.

-African American/Black, and
Asian American/Asian/Pacific
Islander
Hargrow, Mary E.
Lewis, Page

-African American/Black, and
Hispanic/Latino
Williams, Rebecca E.

-African American/Black, and
White/European
Walker, L. Gorman

-American Indian/Alaska
Native, and Hispanic/Latino
Rojas, Rebecca S

-Asian American/Asian/Pacific
Islander, and Hispanic/Latino
Jew, Cynthia L.

-Asian American/Asian/Pacific
Islander, and White/European
Pirhekayaty-Soriano, Tahereh

COLORADO

-African American/Black
Atwell, Robert L.
Brown, John R.
Jones, Arthur C.
Okonji, Jacques A.
Shipp, Pamela L.
Stone, Lynn J.
Tucker, James L.

-American Indian/Alaska
Native
Coats, Gary L.
Fleming, Candace M.
Thurman, Pamela J.

-Asian American/Asian/Pacific
Islander
Chao, Christine M.
Hashimoto, Jerry S.
Hossain, Ziarat
Iwai, Charles T.
Jaitly, Kailash N.
Lee-Richter, Julie
Lee, Ronald W.
Leong, Deborah J.
Manese, Wilfredo R.
McCann, Robin S.
Mo, Suchoon
Onizuka, Richard K.
Saleem, Rakhshanda
Suinn, Richard M.
Tamura, Leonard J.
Yang, Raymond K.

-Hispanic/Latino
Aguilar, Martha C.
Arellano, Charleanea
Borrego, Richard L.
Carpenter, Gerald A.
Chapa, Joel R.
Chavez, Ernest L.
Esparza, Ricardo
Figueroa, Jorge L.
Garza, Joe G.
Gomez, Ana L
Harris, Josette G
Irueste-Montes, Ana M.
Lujan, Cleo C.
Manzanares, Dan L.
Montes, Francisco
Rodriguez, Carlos J.
Rodriguez, Manuel D.
Softas, Basilia C.
Valdes, Maria
Valdez, Jesse N.
Vega, Jose G.
Vigil, Patricia L.

-African American/Black, and
American Indian/Alaska Native
Windham, Thomas L.

-Asian American/Asian/Pacific
Islander, and Hispanic/Latino
Osorno, Wendell A.

CONNECTICUT

-African American/Black
Aldrich, John W.
Banks, Karel L.

Callahan, Michelle R.
Coleman, Willie J.
Foster, Jr., Hilliard G.
Mate-Kole, C. Charles
Nolan, Jr., Benjamin C.
Owens-Lane, Jan
Peters, James S.
Russell, David M.

-Asian American/Asian/Pacific
Islander
Banaji, Mahzarin R.
Chun, Marvin M.
Ibrahim, Farah A.
Moy, Samuel
Muradian, Mark G.
Ramaswami, Sundar
Somjee, Lubna

-Hispanic/Latino
Badillo, Diana
Guzman, L. Philip
Losada-Paisey, Gloria
Ramos-Grenier, Julia
Rivera, Nelson E.
Suarez, Miguel G.

-Asian American/Asian/Pacific
Islander, and White/European
Bonal, Kathleen A.

DELAWARE

-African American/Black
Denson, Eric L.
McGowan, Eugene
Turner, Alvin L.
Williams, Phyllis J.

-Asian American/Asian/Pacific
Islander
Iqbal, S. Mohammed

-Hispanic/Latino
Ferreira, Pedro M.

DISTRICT OF COLUMBIA
-African American/Black
Alston, Denise A.
Asbury, Charles A.
Ashmore-Hudson, Anne
Baxley, Gladys B.
Belgrave, Faye Z
Brannon, Lorraine

Brown, Barbara J.
Carter, Charles A.
Cooper, Donna M.
Davis, Annette E.
Dockett, Kathleen H.
Dunston, Patricia
Ellis, Rosita P.
Fisher, Patricia A.
Graham, Quentin
Gump, Janice P.
Harper, Mary S.
Hicks, Leslie H.
Hill, Anthony L
Holliday, Bertha G.
Holmes, Dorothy E.
Hughes, Anita L.
Ireland Hurd, Evelyn C.
Johnson, Sylvia T
Keita, Gwendolyn P.
Millard, Wilbur A.
Musgrove, Barbara J.
Myers, Ernest R.
Nickerson, Kim J.
Payton, Carolyn R.
Peoples, Kathleen
Perry, Cereta E.
Porter, Julia
Reaves, Juanita Y.
Robinson, John D
Romero, Regina E.
Savage, Jr., James E.
Shaw, Paula
Smith, Cherryl R.
Tomes, Henry
Toms, Esther C.
Vontress, Clemmont E.
Washington, Robert A.
Whitehurst, Jr., William H.
Williams, Steve

-American Indian/Alaska
Native
Hillabrant, Walter J.

-Asian American/Asian/Pacific
Islander
Abudabbeh, Nuha
Blackburn, Winona K.
Coggins, Margaret H.
Huang, Larke N.
Parasuraman, Raja
Shimoda, Kim C.
Wu, Jing-Jyi

-Hispanic/Latino
Buki, Lydia P.
Carr, Paquita R.

Cereijido, Margarita
Comas-Diaz, Lillian
Marotta, Sylvia A.
Miranda, M.
Nieves-Grafals, Sara
Sloan, R. Lloyd

-African American/Black, and American Indian/Alaska Native

Hargrove, Jr., Jerry E.

FLORIDA

-African American/Black

Adams, Afesa M.
Allen, Jane E.
Bell, K. Pat
Campbell, Stephen N.
Capp, Larry D.
Eberhardt, Carolyn A.
Fields, Anika C.
Fraser, Kathryn P.
Gibbs, Charles C.
Greene, Anthony F.
Kirklen, Leonard E.
Mahy, Yvonne C.
Muir-Malcolm, Joan A.
Nelson-Goedert, Carolyn Y
Oshodi, John
Ozuzu, Sam
Smith, Jr., Theodore R.
Smith, William F.
Toomer, Jethro W.
Webster, E. Carol
Williams-Petersen, Janice
Wilson, Woodrow
Wooten, William

-American Indian/Alaska Native

Hui, Len Dang
Joesting-Goodwoman, Joan A.

-Asian American/Asian/Pacific Islander

Fukuyama, Mary A.
Gui, Chui-Liu Serena
Jani, Aurobindo J.
Kashikar-Zuck, Susmita M.
Lukman, Roy L.
San Luis, Roberto R.
Viswesvaran, Chockalingam
Wang, Alvin
Yee, Albert H.

-Hispanic/Latino

Abello, Ana L.
Alonso, Martha R.
Alvarez, Carlos M.
Alvarez, Manuel E.
Alvarez, Maria D.
Alvarez, Roland
Anton, William D.
Ariza-Menedez, Maria
Artiles, Laura M.
Azaret, Marisa
Bernal, Alberto J.
Bild-Libbin, Raguel
Bradman, Leo H.
Carcas, Marilyn B.
Carra, Sylvia F.
Cimino, Cynthia R.
Collado, Armando
Constanzo, Magda S.
Cornide, Carmen R.
Crane, Rosario S.
Cruz, Vivian A.
Desdin, Roberto
Diaz-Machado, Carmen B.
Diaz, Eduardo I.
Diaz, Raul
Dos Santos, John F.
Echavarria, David
Escovar, Luis A.
Faraci, Ana M.
Fazzano, Catalina U.
Feldman, Esther
Fernandez, Maria C.
Figueredo, Migdalia I.
Fuentes, Dainery M.
Gallardo-Cooper, Maria M.
Garcia-Abid, Calixto
Garcia, Hector D.
Garcia, Jose L.
Garcia, Lazaro
Gonzalez, Hector P.
Grabau, David
Healy, James M.
Hernandez, Cibeles
Herrera-Pino, Jorge A.
Hevia, Modesto J.
Incera, Armando
Joffe, Vera
Kelton-Brand, Ana
Labarta, Margarita M.
Lasaga, Agueda M.
Lasaga, Jose I.
Leon, Yolanda C.
Lequerica, Martha
Lorenzo, Gladys
Maldonado, Loretto
Manruque-Reichard, Marta E.

Marina, Dorita
Marrero, Bernie
Montoya, E. Carolina
Morales, Elias
Mora, Ralph
Mussenden, Gerald
Nazario, Jr., Andres
Pacheco, Angel E.
Parlade, Rafael J.
Pedemonte, Monica
Perez, Fred M.
Pico, Daima
Pita, Marcia E.
Porges, Carlos R.
Prado, Haydee
Price, Alicia A.
Prieto, Addys
Reyes-Mayer, Erwin
Rivas-Vazquez, Ana A.
Rivera, Enrique
Rodriguez, Lavinia
Rodriguez, Luis J.
Ruiz, Sonia I.
Salas, Eduardo
Sanchez-Torrento, Eugenio
Sanchez, Juan
Suarez, Enrique M.
Szapocznik, Jose
Toro, Haydee
Urbina, Susana P.
Vada, Alejo
Velez-Diaz, Angel
Zaldivar, Luis R.
Zayas-Bazan, Carmen

-African American/Black and American Indian/Alaska Native

Brooks, Juanita O.

GEORGIA

-African American/Black

Allen-Claiborne, Joyce G.
Allsopp, Ralph N
Anderson, Louis P.
Bartholomew, Charles
Bolden, Wiley S.
Burnett Young, Myra N.
Butler, B. LaConyea
Carter, Allen C.
Cone-Dekle, Cynthia A.
Crockett, Deborah P.
Davis, Jerry H.
Emory, Eugene K.
Epps, Pamela J.
Fleming, Andrea L.
Fresh, Edith M.

Friday, Jennifer C.
Gordon, Rhea J.
Grant, Kim D.
Hammond, W. Rodney
Hunter, Knoxice C
Jacobs-Jr., Walter R.
James-Parker, Magna M.
Johnson, Marjorie
Kelly, Jennifer F.
Lawrence, Valerie W.
Lineberger, Marilyn H.
Mallisham, Ivy J.
McNeal, Meryl
Mindingall, Marilyn P.
Mouzon, Richard R.
Murfree, Jr., Joshua W.
Phelps, Rosemary E.
Rice, Donadrian
Richard, Harriette W.
Seymour, Guy O.
Sims-Patterson, Sandra
Stringer, Anthony Y.
Tucker, Samuel J.
Walker, Lila K.
Ward, Connie M.
Whisenton, Joffre T.
Wood, Keith A.

-American Indian/Alaska Native

Campos, Peter E.
Thorson, Billie J.

-Asian American/Asian/Pacific Islander

Asghar, Anila
Campbell, Kamal E.
Chung, Y. Barry
Kagehiro, Dorthy K.
Kim, Seock-Ho
Perez, Ruperto M.
Poon, Leonard W.

-Hispanic/Latino

Ayllon, Teodoro
Bascuas, Joseph W.
De la Serna, Marcelo
Figueroa, Rolando G.
Flores, Philip J.
Gonzalez, Fernando
Lopez, Sarah C.
Perilla, Julia L.
Soler, Robin E
Valdes, Luis F.

-African American/Black and Hispanic/Latino

Mahabee-Harris, Marilyn M.

HAWAII

-African American/Black

James, Larry C.

-American Indian/Alaska Native

Samford, Judith A.

-Asian American/Asian/Pacific Islander

Boggs, Minnie
Chang, Thomas M.C.
Ching, June W. J.
Choi, George C.
Choy, Stephen S.F.
Fo, Walter S O
Fujii, Daryl E M
Fujinaka, Larry H.
Fujioka, Terry Ann T.
Fujita, George T.
Furuno, Setsu
Guo, Trudy Narikiyo
Hamada, Roger S.
Higa, William R.
Hufano, Linda D.
Hyde, Elsie HA
Ishikawa-Fullmer, Janet
Izutsu, Satoru
Kaneshige, Edward
Kop, Tim M.
Lau, Lavay
Lee, C. Jarnie W J
Lim, Hoili C.
Loo, Chalsa M.
Loo, Russell
Matsuura, Larry N.
Miyahira, Sarah D.
Miyake, Steven M.
Murakami, Sharon
Oda, Ethel Aiko
Omizo, Michael M.
Pang, Dawn
Sayama, Mike K.
Schlesinger, Laura Ann
Shimizu, Annette A.
Shirakawa, Patti
Takamine, Sandra
Takemoto-Chock, Naomi
Tatsuguchi, Rosalie K.
Torigoe, Rodney Y.

Tsukamoto, Donna E.
Tsushima, William T.
Yanagida, Evelyn H.

-Hispanic/Latino

Lopez-Reyes, Ramon
Rezentes, III, William C.
Robertin, Hector

ILLINOIS

-African American/Black

Anthony, Bobbie M.
Bennett, Maisha H.
Burnett, John H.
Caldwell-Colbert, A. Toy
Davis, Charles E.
Dawkins, Marva P.
Dyson, Vida
Evans, Helen L.
Fullilove, Constance
Gordon, Kimberly A.
Green, Theophilus E.
Hall, Juanita L.
Hampton, Juanita R.
Henderson, Brenda A.
Houston, Holly O.
James, Michelle D.
Lessing, Elise E.
Lewis, George R.
London, Lorna H.
Miller, Robin L.
Moody, Helaine L.
Parham, Patricia A.
Patterson, Drayton R.
Peavyhouse, Betty M.
Pugh, Roderick W.
Reeves, Alan
Robinson, W. LaVome
Speight, Suzette L.
St. Leger, Sidney C.
Thomas, Anita J.
Ward, Alan J.
Watts, Roderick J.
Whitehead, Barry X.
Williams, Eddie E.

-American Indian/Alaska Native

Durant, Jr., Adrian J.
Goffin, Richard D.
Milner, Joel S.

-Asian American/Asian/Pacific Islander

Ahuja, Harmeen

Anand, Shashi
Aoki, Melanie F.
Choy, Catherine L.
Dave, Jagdish P.
Hamid, Mohammad
Hoshiko, Michael
Huang, Wei-Jen William
Kamano, Dennis K.
Koh, Tong-He
Lam, Chow S.
Lee, William W.
Lim, Patricia J.
Ma, Yat-Ming C.
Rattenbury, Francie R.
Rhee, Susan B.
Roque, Sylvia A.
Smith, Michael C.
Sung, Yong H.
Thomas, Joseph E.
Tom, Agnes
Valentiner, David P.
Villejo, Ron E.
Wang, James D.

-Hispanic/Latino

Baez, Luis
Balcazar, Fabricio E.
Benitez, John C.
Canovas Welles, Nydia L.
Choca, James
Elena Lee, Karen
Gallagher, Rosina M.
Gomez, Madeleine Y.
Lopez, Martita A.
Machabanski, Hector
Manghi, Elina R.
Plazas, Carlos A.
Posner, Carmen A.
Rodriguez, Rogelio E.
Schlesinger, Susana J.
Schmajuk, Nestor
Soto, Tomas A.
Suarez-Balcazar, Yolanda
Tamayo, Jose M.
Tirado, John
Turner, Darrell D.
Vera, Elizabeth M.
Viale-val, Graciela
Whitaker, Sandra V.

-Asian American/Asian/Pacific Islander and White/European

Akca, Zeynep K.

INDIANA

-African American/Black

Alexander, Charlene M.
Bowman, Sharon L.
Boyer, Michele C.
Critton, Barbara L.
Dixon, Carrie B.
Jordan, Albert K.
Keglar, Shelvy H.
Mann, Coramae R.
Ridley, Charles R.
Rollock, David
Smedley, Joseph W.
Thompson, Chalmer E.
West, James E.

-Asian American/Asian/Pacific Islander

Chiu, Lian-Hwam
Field, Lucy F.
Iwamasa, Gayle Y.
Minturn, Robin H.
Okagaki, Lynn
Stephens, Dorothy W.
Yamaguchi, Harry G.

-Hispanic/Latino

Alvarez, Gary L.
Goltz, Sonia
Hernandez, Vivian O.
Prieto, Susan L.
Vargas, Manuel J.

-African American/Black

Triplett, Sheila J.

IOWA

-African American/Black

Jackson, Ronald A.
Johnson, W. Roy
Lampkin, Emmett C.
Pope-Davis, Donald B.

-American Indian/Alaska Native

Moynihan, Kelly L.

-Asian American/Asian/Pacific Islander

Chang, Theodore C. H.
Singh, Darshan
Tan, Rowena N.
Wong, Jane L.

-Hispanic/Latino

Barrios, Francisco X.
Gonzalez-Forestier, Tomas
Grajales, Elisa M.

KANSAS

-African American/Black

Lawrence, Stephen N.

**-Asian American/Asian/Pacific
Islander**

Jain, Sharat K.
Omoto, Allen M.

KENTUCKY

-African American/Black

Pope-Tarrence, Jacqueline R.
Wright, Doris J.

**-American Indian/Alaska
Native**

Blair, Deborah G.

**-Asian American/Asian/Pacific
Islander**

Ebreo, Angela
Srinivasan, Sampurna
Wong, Wilson

-Hispanic/Latino

Aponte, Joseph F.
Balbona, Manuel

LOUISIANA

-African American/Black

Burchell, Charles R.
Campbell-Flint, Maxine E
Cunningham, Michael
Devezin, Armond A.
Garrett, Aline M.
Hicks, Laurabeth
Lewis, Marva L
Tapo, Linda J.
Toldson, Ivory L.

**-American Indian/Alaska
Native**

Atkinson, Michael B.
Fain, Thomas C.
Sellards, Robert

**-Asian American/Asian/Pacific
Islander**

Ho, Chin-Chin
Ho, Kay
Izawa, Chizuko
Wakeman, Richard J.
Winter, Amal

-Hispanic/Latino

Daruna, Jorge H.

MAINE

-African American/Black

Hambright, Jerold E.

-Hispanic/Latino

Barry, Martha J.

MARYLAND

-African American/Black

Allen, Christeen
Allgood-Hill, Barbara A.
Anderson, Norman B.
Apenahier, Leonard
Beatty, Lula A.
Berry, Joyce Hamilton
Boyd, Vivian S.
Briggs, Felicia H.
Carrington, Christine H.
Cason, Valerie K.
Chesnutt, James H.
Cook, Donelda
Cooper, Colin
Cunningham, Wayman B.
Derrickson, Kimberly B.
Edelin, Patricia
Fletcher, Betty A.
Foster, Robert
Geter-douglas, Beth
Hall, William A.
Hammond, Gladys
Hestick, Henrietta
Hughes-Wheatland, Roxanne
Johnson, Eugene H.
Johnson, Fern M.
Johnson, Lawrence B.
Jones, James M.
Jones, Ruby M.
Joseph, Jr., Herbert M.
McCombs, Harriet G.
Moorman-Lewis, Deborah A.
Outlaw, Patricia A.
Powell, Lois
Richards, Henry J.

Roberts, Albert
Searcy, Mary L.
Singleton, Edward G.
Smith, Benjamin
Smith, Iola R.
Steele, Robert E.
Tiggle, Ronald B.
Turner, Samuel M.
Vanderpool, Andrea T.
Washington, Dianna E.
Wilson, Shirley B.
Witter, Jeanette M.
Wood, Jr., Nollie P.
Wyche, Sr., LaMonte G.
Yancey, Angela L.

**-American Indian/Alaska
Native**

Brooks, Jr., Glenwood C.
Chapman, Nancy G.
Hartzell, Richard E.
Karson, Samuel
McCoy, George F.

**-Asian American/Asian/Pacific
Islander**

Banik, Sambhu N.
Coelho, George V.
Furukawa, James M.
Han, Yu Ling
Hsia, Heidi
Kau, Alice S. M.
Kupur, Veena
Li, Xiaoming
McWilliams, Junko O.
Nhan, Nguyen
Oommen Thomas, Susy
Otani, Akira
Ou, Young-Shi
Raval, Bina D.
Tamayo, Federico M. V.
Verghese, Cherian
Yamada, Elaine M.
Yu, Angelita M.

-Hispanic/Latino

Aguirre-Deandreis, Ana I.
Cardena, Etzel A.
Cruz, Albert R.
Dallas, Mercedes
Fernandez, M. Isabel
Gardano, Anna C.
Gurri Glass, Margarita E.
Lancaster, JoAnn
Mastrapa, Selma A.
Miranda, David J.
Nadal-Vazquez, Vilma Y.

Ortega, Richard J.
Pinto, Alcides
Rivera-Sinclair, Elsa A.
Ruth, Richard
Sasscer-Burgos, Julie
Teitel, Raquel S.
Thorn, Isabel M.

**-African American/Black,
Hispanic/Latino**

Martin, William F.
Parson, Erwin R.

MASSACHUSETTS

-African American/Black

Aradom, Tesfay A
Baxter, Anthony G.
Bynum, Edward B.
Cade, Bonita G.
Doris, Terri M.
Elligan, Don G.
Elligen, Don G.
Gibbons-Carr, Michele V.
Giles, Cheryl A.
Harleston, Bernard W.
Hart, Allen J.
Henderson Daniel, Jessica
Hunt, Wilson L.
Jenkins, Yvonne M
Langley, Merlin R
Lawson, Jasper J.
London, Dyanne P.
Moore, Helen B.
Nicks, T. Leon
Patrice, David
Rambo, Lewis M.
Ramseur, Howard P.
Romney, Patricia
Samuel, Valerie J.
Scott-Jones, Diane
Smith, Althea
Stallworth, Lisa M.
Tatum, Beverly D.
Turner, Castellano
Whitaker, Arthur L.
White, Voncile

**-American Indian/Alaska
Native**

James, Steven E

-Asian American/Asian/Pacific Islander

Ahmed, Mohiuddin
Ambady, Nalina
Chan, Connie S.
Chin, Jean L
Garg, Mithlesh
Ham, MaryAnna D.
Hoshmand, Lisa T.
Ito, Elaine S.
Jay, Milton T.
Lee, Yueh-Ting
Liem, Ramsay
Lowe, Susana M.
Mino, Itsuko
Mori, DeAnna L.
Mukherjee, Subhash C.
Ohye, Bonnie Y.
Sakurai, Mariko
Sugai, Don P.
Wang, Edward S.
Wong, Frankie Y.
Wu, Shi-Jiuan

-Hispanic/Latino

Albert, Rosita D.
Alvarez, Mauricia
Amaro, Hortensia
Arboleda, Catalina
Armengol, Carmen G.
Arredondo, Patricia
Ayoub, Catherine C.
Bacigalupe, Gonzalo M.
Bennasar, Mari C.
Bustamante, Eduardo M.
Cebollero, Ana Margarita
De Louredes Mattei, Maria
Dhimitri, Patricio
Figler, Clare S.
Garrido-Castillo, Pedro
Genero, Nancy P.
Hermenet, Argelia B.
Jette, Carmen CB
Lagomasino, Andrew J.
Linares, Lourdes O.
Morales-Barreto, Gisela
Munoz, Leticia S.
Nuttall, Ena V.
Rey-Casserly, Celiane M.
Sanchez, William
Sedo, Manuel A.
Shapiro, Ester R.
Taylor, Stephen Q.
Torres, Mario A.
Zuriff, Gerald E.

-Hispanic/Latino

Kochevar-Sukkarie, Renee J.

-African American/Black and American Indian/Alaska Native

Newburgh, Tracey LS

-American Indian/Alaska Native, White/European

Hough and Sigmund

MICHIGAN

-African American/Black

Barbarin, Oscar A.
Barber, Kevin V.
Binion, Victoria J.
Brodie, Debra A.
Brookins, Geraldine K
Coelho, Richard J.
Collins, William
Curry, Bonita Pope
Doss, Juanita K.
Douglas, Byron C.
Everett, Moses L.
Gardner, Lamaurice H.
Gibson, Ralph M.
Gibson, Rose C.
Green, Charles A.
Hurst, Jurlene
Jackson, James S.
Johnson, Joan J.
Jones, Hugh E.
June, Lee N.
Lambert, Michael C.
Leary, Kimberlyn
Lewis, Brenda J.
Mack, Faite R. P.
Mccain, Lillie W.
McKenzie, Jr., Loratuis L.
Mcloyd, Vonnie C.
Morris, Joseph R.
Nabors, Nina A.
Nettles, Arie L.
Pernell, Eugene
Reed, James D.
Reid, Pamela T
Robinson, Jane A.
Spidell Helms, Dorothy J.
Starks-Williams, Mary L.
Stewart, Vlenaetha
Sutton, Sharon E.
Tate, Donald
Thomas, Jr., Charles B.
Thomas, Hilton T.
Thornton, Dozier W.

Walcott, Delores D.
Ward, Lucretia M.
Williams, David R.

-American Indian/Alaska Native

Derocher, Terry L.
Eaton, Sheila J.
Foster, Rachel A.

-Asian American/Asian/Pacific Islander

Ai, Amy L.
Akiyama, M. Michael
Anselmo, Fe
Chao, Georgia T.
Fergus, Esther O.
Goburdhun, Sara S.
Lee, D. John
Mondol, Merlyn D.
Nagata, Donna K.
Oka, Evelyn R.
Seitz, Kathleen
Thimotheose, K. G.
Vakhariya, Sobha
Wilkinson, H. Sook
Wong, Martin R.

-Hispanic/Latino

Arellano-Lopez, Juan
Benet-Martinez, Veronica
Dooley, John A.
Flachier, Roberto
Garcia-Shelton, Linda M.
Gomez, John P
Gonzalez, Matthew B.
Madrid, Raul P.
Marroquin, Arthur R.
Martinez, Gabriel P.
Ortega, Robert M.
Schreier, Raquel L.
Teixeira, Michael A.
Villegas, Orlando L.

MINNESOTA

-African American/Black

Barner, II, Pearl
Copher-Haynes, Harriett
Dalhouse, A. Derick
Hayles, V. Robert
Howard, Mary T.
Jackson, Joyce Taborn
James, Norman L.
Moore, C. L.

-American Indian/Alaska Native

Lucas, Jay H.
Wilson, Jennifer

-Asian American/Asian/Pacific Islander

Akimoto, Sharon A
Ascano, Ricardo
Das, Ajit K.
Dawis, Rene V.
Gutterman, Carmen Y.
Hatsukami, Dorothy K.
Lee, Margaret
Maruyama, Geoffrey
Mehrotra, Chandra M.N.
Moideen, Yasmine
Ninonuevo, Fred
Somwaru, Jwalla P.

-Hispanic/Latino

Garcia-Peltoniemi, Rosa E.
Narvaez, Darcia F.
Ruiz, Nicholas J.

-African American/Black and Asian American/Asian/Pacific Islander

Salone, Lavorial

MISSISSIPPI

-Asian American/Asian/Pacific Islander

Liu, An-Yen

-Hispanic/Latino

Orabona, Elaine

-Asian American/Asian/Pacific Islander and Hispanic/Latino

Pang, Mark G.

MISSOURI

-African American/Black

Clark, Jr., Eddie M.
Clark, Marie
Copeland, Jr., E. Thomas
Frisby, Craig L.
Grier, Priscilla E.
Harris, Jasper W.

Jones, Elaine F.
Kemp, Arthur D.
Phelps, C. K.
Sanders-Thompson, Vetta L.
Wilson, Susan B.

-American Indian/Alaska Native

Montgomery, Robert L.
Paige, Roger
Pope, Mark

-Asian American/Asian/Pacific Islander

Acka-Pope, Zeynep K
Duan, Changming
Hom, Harry L.
Hong, Barry A.
Wang, Paul H.

-Hispanic/Latino

Chaves, John F.
Roehlke, Helen J.
Sancho, Ana M.
Topolski, James M.

-American Indian/Alaska Native and White/European

Natani, Kirmach

MONTANA

-American Indian/Alaska Native

Foster, Daniel V.
McDonald, Arthur L.
Swaney, Gyda

-Asian American/Asian/Pacific Islander

Lie, Rudolph T.B

-Hispanic/Latino

Sanchez, Debra A.

NEBRASKA

-African American/Black

Muiu, Charles

-American Indian/Alaska Native

Willis, Cynthia E.

-Asian American/Asian/Pacific Islander

Sodowsky, Gargi R.

-Hispanic/Latino

Madison, James K.
Prendes-Lintel, Maria L.

NEVADA

-American Indian/Alaska Native

DeGraff, Christopher D.
Knapp, W. Mace
Mellor, Catherine A.
Turnbough, P. Diane

-Asian American/Asian/Pacific Islander

Chino, Allan F.
Hong, Eunsook

-Hispanic/Latino

Amezaga, Jr., Alfredo M.
Antonuccio, David
Brandenburg, Carlos E.
Sanchez, David M.

NEW HAMPSHIRE

-American Indian/Alaska Native

Blubaugh, Victoria G.

-Asian American/Asian/Pacific Islander

Chin, Raymond J.
Valdez, Jr., Romulo

-Hispanic/Latino

Arroyo, Patricia M.

NEW JERSEY

-African American/Black

Bailey, Joan W.
Baker, Christine
Belgrave, Jeffrey
Blanding, Benjamin
Brice, Janet R.
Burnham, Lem
Cameron, Linda S.
Coffey, Maryann B.
Corr, Donald

Davis, Bernice M.
Essandoh, Pius K.
Floyd, James A.
Gary, Juneau M.
Graddick, Miriam M.
Grant, Wanda F.
Greene, Clifford
Griffith, Albert R.
Hall, Ruth L.
Henry, Vincent dePaul
Hines, Paulette M.
Isaacs, Owen K.
Jemmott, III, John B.
Johnson, Denise MW
Johnson, Edward E.
Johnson, Matthew B.
McMillan, Robert
Nolan, Beverly D.
Okorodudu, Corahann
Pinder-Amaker, Stephanie L.
Simms Puig, Jan
Sprouse, Agnes A.
Tomlinson-Clarke, Saundra M.
Trotman, Frances K.
Walton, Duncan E.
Whitehead, Jesse
Williams, Carrolyn N.
Williams, Daniel E.
Williams, Everett B.
Woodland, Calvin E.
York, Joan E. S.

-American Indian/Alaska Native

Reisinger, Curtis W.

-Asian American/Asian/Pacific Islander

Boodoo, Gwyneth M.
Catarina, Mathilda B.
Chin, Lemin
Henson, Ramon M.
Ho, John E.
Hsu, Louis M.
Kim, Yang Ja
Matsui, Wesley T.
Patel, Sanjiv A.
Saraf, Komal C.
Schroff, Kamal
Sen, Tapas K.
Shah, Vasantkumar B.
Shroff, Kamal
Wong, Kit L.

-Hispanic/Latino

Bosch, Isora
Escudero, Micaela

Esquivel, Giselle B.
Fernandez, Rosemary
Finkel, Eva
Garcia, Luis T.
Garcia, Margarita
Gonzalez, Haydee M.
Gonzalez, Maria L.
Kramer, Diana R.
Laosa, Luis M.
Latorre, Miriam D.
Lewis, Carmelita M.
Lijtmaer, Ruth M
Ludmer, Alba
Martorell, Mario F.
Modiano, Rachel
Nieves, Luis R.
Pelaez, Carmen
Perez, Cecilia M.
Puertas, Lorenzo
Puig, Ange
Rodriguez, David A.
Roig, Miguel
Rosado, John W.
Samaniego, Sandra

-African American/Black, American Indian/Alaska Native

Taylor, Flor N.

NEW MEXICO

-African American/Black

Daly, Frederica Y.
Jackson, Helen L.

-Asian American/Asian/Pacific Islander

Chan, Paul K.
Chan, Paul K. F.
Chu, Lily

-Hispanic/Latino

Arroyo, Judith A.
Castillo, Diane T.
Coes, Maria R.
DeBlassie, III, Paul A.
Dennedy-Frank, David P.
Gonzales, Ricardo R.
Marquez, E. Mario
Rivera, Miquela
Roll, Samuel
Sosa, Juan N.
Vargas, Luis A.

-American Indian/Alaska Native, Hispanic/Latino

Vargas, Alice M.

-Asian American/Asian/Pacific Islander and Hispanic/Latino

Garcia, Melinda A.

NEW YORK

-African American/Black

Abercombie, Delrita
Adams, Jr., Clarence L.
Adams, C. Jama
Alexander, Allen T.
Anderson, Linda
Archibald, Eloise M.
Barnes, Michael J.
Baxter, Bernice K.
Beckles, Nicola
Belton, Monique
Biggs, Bradley
Blackett-Sullivan, Gwendolyn A.
Bowen, Tanya U.
Brooks, Lewis A.
Bryant-Tuckett, Rose M.
Buffin, Janice E.
Carey, Patricia M.
Carter, Robert T.
Cathcart, Conrad W.
Clark, Brenda A.
Clark, Kenneth B.
Coates, Deborah L.
Coleburn, Lila A.
Congo, Carroll A.
Constantine, Madonna G.
Cottingham, Alice L.
Crowder, Virginia B.
Dawson, Harriett E.
De Leaire, Robert
DeFour, Darlene C.
Deleaire, Robert N.
Dennis, Dothlyn J.G.
Dozier, Arthur L.
Duncan, Bessie A.
Francois, Theodore V.
Gayle, Michael C.
Graves-Cooper, Phyllis J.
Graves, Sherryl B.
Gray, Arthur A.
Greene, Beverly
Griffith, Stanford
Guevarra, Josephine S.
Hambrick-Dixon, Priscilla J.
Hare, Nathan
Harte, Lisa M.

Hilton, William F.
Hines, Laura M.
Hooker, Olivia J.
Jenkins, Adelbert H
Johnson, William L.
Jones, Annie Lee
Jones, Paulette
King, Valerie
Louden, Delroy M.
Lovelace, Valeria O.
Maynard, Edward S.
McIntyre, Lorna A.
McRae, Mary B.
Morris, Dolores O.
Nesbitt, Eric B.
Nicholson, Liston O.
Norman-Jackson, Jacquelyn
Parks, Gregory S.
Paster, Vera S.
Perry, Jeanell
Pinderhughes, Victoria A.
Polite, Craig K.
Pulliam, Barbara A.
Ray, Jacqueline W.
Robertson, John F.
Ross, Sandra I.
Rountree, Yvonne B.
Ruffins, Stephen A.
Shell, Juanita
Smith, Alvin E.
Spivey, Philop B.
Stevenson, Jr., Edward E.
Swanston, Melvon C.
Troutt, Bobbye V.
Vanderhost, Leonette
Vaughans, Kirkland C.
Weston, Raymond E.
Whitten, Lisa A.
Wisner, Roscoe W.
Wyche, Karen F.

-American Indian/Alaska Native

Babb, Harold
Everson, Howard T.

-Asian American/Asian/Pacific Islander

Ahsen, Akhter
Ashida, Sachio
Beattie, Muriel Y.
Chang, Barbara
Chen, Eric C
Cheng, W. David
Chin, James
Chou, Thomas T.
D'Heurle, Adma J.

Das, Manju P.
DeMeis, Debra K.
Goh, David S.
Grant, Swadesh S.
Harris, William W.
Laviena, Luis
Luthar, Suniya S.
Mar, Harvey H.
Mehta, Kripal K.
Mody, Zarin R.
Morita, Denise N.
Parasnis, Ila
Rajaram, Suparna
Shahani-denning, Comila
Sison, Cecile E.
Sterling, Sharon E.
Sundararajan, Louise Kuen-Wei
Suzuki, Lisa A.
Takanishi, Ruby
Tana, Joseph
Tanaka-Matsumi, Junko
Tsui, Ellen C.
Velayo, Richard S.
Wagner, Aureen Pinto
Walia, Kusum
Wang, Richard S.
Wong, Florence C
Wong, Philip S
Wong, Tony M.

-Hispanic/Latino

Abraido-Lanza, Ana F
Altarriba, Jeanette
Aponte, Evelyn I.
Araoz, Daniel L.
Arcaya, Jose M.
Arriso, Roberta H
Aviles, Alice A.
Balderrama, Sylvia R.
Bastien, IV, Samuel A.
Baxter-Boehm, Alva
Beato-Smith, Vera
Benamu, Icem
Benzaquen, Isaac
Berrill, Naftali G.
Blandino, Ramon A.
Bracero, William
Bursztyn, Alberto M.
Canedo, Angelo R.
Carballo-Dieguez, Alex
Caro, Yvette
Cleveland, Adriana F.
Colon, R. Phillip
Correa, Martha L.
Cuesta, George M.
De La Cancela, Victor
Detres, Michael P.

Fleisher, Nancy F.
Foster, RoseMarie P.
Garcia, Michael A.
Gubler, Lyle W.
Gular, Enrique
Haley, Adriana R.
Inclan, Jaime
Javier, Rafael A.
Jove-Altman, Jacqueline
Kahan, Harry
Langrod, John
Lopez, Emilia
Lopez, Thomas W.
Madrazo-Peterson, Rita
Martinez-Urrutia, Angel C.
Martinez, Maria J.
Millan, Fred
Monserrat, Laura
Mujica, Ernesto
Munoz, John A.
Olivero, Gerald
Pasamonte, Ana M.
Peralta, Carmelina
Perez Ebrahimi, Concepcion
Pizano-Thomen, Margarita
Ramos, Arnaldo J.
Rigual-Lynch, Lourdes
Rivera, Carmen J.
Rivera, Jo Ann M.
Rivero, Estela M.
Rodriguez, Carmen G.
Rodriguez, Maria A.
Rogler, Lloyd H.
Romero, Jose
Rosario, Margaret
Sanua, Victor D.
Sobrino, James F.
Soto, Elaine
Stern, Marilyn
Suarez, Carlota
Suarez, Susan D.
Towns-Miranda, Luz
Vazquez, Rosa
Zayas, Luis H.

-African American/Black, American Indian/Alaska Native

Branche, Leota Susan
Hart, Anton H.

-African American/Black, White/European

Greene, Karen J.

-Asian American/Asian/Pacific
Islander, Hispanic/Latino

Ozoa, Claudette

-Hispanic/Latino, White/
European

Burton, Roger V.

NORTH CAROLINA

-African American/Black

Anderson, Shirley G.
Barnes, Denise R.
Brinson, Les
DeWindt-Robson, L. Kimberly
Fields, Richard L.
Gray-Little, Bernadette
Harris, William G.
Hutchinson, Kim M.
Ike, Chris A.
Kelly-Radford, Lily M.
Liston, Hattye H.
McCandies, Terry T
Merritt, Marcellus M.
Molden, Sabrina
Roberts, Harrell B.
Sampson, Myrtle B.
Webb, Wanda
Williams, Victoria F.

-American Indian/Alaska
Native

Taylor, Gary

-Asian American/Asian/Pacific
Islander

Chia, Rosina
Lee, Jo Ann
Pullium, Rita M.
Sakata, Robert T.

-Hispanic/Latino

Azevedo, Don Fernando
De Varona, M .
Johnson, Melissa R.
Puente, Antonio E.
San Miguel, Christopher L.
Zayas, Maria A.

-Hispanic/Latino, White/
European

Llorca, Arthur L.

NORTH DAKOTA

-Asian American/Asian/Pacific
Islander

Huset, Martha K.

OHIO

-African American/Black

Banks, Martha E.
Derrick, Sara M.
Dobbins, James E.
Dorr, Bernadette
Edwards, Karen L.
El-Amin, Debra El-Amin
Freeman, James E.
Hall, Howard
Harris, Michelle F.
Hernandez, Michael
James, Jr., Earnest
Johnson, David L.
Jones, Reginald
Lee, Yolanda W.
McCarley, Victor J.
Mobley, Brenda P.
Mosley-Howard, Gerri S.
Myers, Linda J.
Neal-Barnett, Angela M.
Norton, A. Evangeline
Robinson, Gregory F.
Sanders, Daniel W.
Southerland, Deborah L.
Twe, Boikai S.
Vance, Marilyn M.
Williams, Michael A.
Williams, Willie S.

-American Indian/Alaska
Native

Gladue, Brian A.
Silling, S. Marc
Valley, John A.

-Asian American/Asian/Pacific
Islander

Akamatsu, T. John
Belzunce, Philip R.
Chung, Rita L.
Fujimura, Laura E.
Gee, Carol S.
Ishiyama, Toaru
Lee, Jung K.
Leong, Frederick T. T.
Misra, Rajendra K.
Nagayama Hall, Gordon C.
Ray, Arun B.

Rigrish, Diana
Saul, Tuck T.
Sax, Kenji W.
Serafica, Felicisima C.
Shen, John
Srivastva, Suresh
Wong, Deborah A.
Yun, S.B.

-Hispanic/Latino

Bardenstein, Karen K.
Bernal, Guillermo A.
Fliman, Vivian P.
Lopez-Baez, Sandra I.
Montemayor, Raymond
Mortimer, Joan R.
Patrick, Carol L.
Vicente, Peter J.
Zaragoza, Maria S.

OKLAHOMA

-American Indian/Alaska
Native

Bowen, Peggy C.
Choney, John M.
Jones-Saumty, Deborah J.
Lashley, Karen H.
Robey, Dale L.
Sadler, Mark S.
Shaw, Terry G.
Williamson, Diane H.
Willis, Diane J.

-Hispanic/Latino

Kranau, Edgar J.
Mendoza, Jorge L.

OREGON

-African American/Black

DeBardelaben, Garfield
Morris, Edward F.

-American Indian/Alaska
Native

Reandeau, Sharon L

-Asian American/Asian/Pacific
Islander

Fujitsubo, Lani C.
Kame'enui, Edward J.
Nishi-Strattner, Linda
Ozaki, Mona M.

Rohila, Pritam K.
Wong-Ngan, Julia A.
Yap, Kim O.

-Hispanic/Latino

Gonzales, Linda R.
Marmol, Leonardo M.
Morones, Pete A.
Torres-Saenz, Jorge

PENNSYLVANIA

-African American/Black

Baker, III, Carl E.
Bell, Anita G.
Brown, Pamela
Bryant, Gerard W.
Chisum, Gloria T.
Cornwell, Henry G.
Cotterell, Norman
Dixon, J. Faye
Donahue, Pamela J.
Dudley, Charma D.
Elder, Patricia
Finley, Laurene Y.
Ford, Leon I.
Gadson, Eugene J.
Gillem, Angela R
Hopkins, Kenneth
Houston, Lawrence N.
Hunt, Portia
Jennings, Valdea D.
McNeill, Earle
Mitchell, Howard E.
Moore, Cleo H.
Nelson-le, Sharon A.
Nix-Early, Vivian
Piercy, Patricia A.
Ray, Vivian D.
Rogers, Melvin L.
Salter, Beatrice R.
Salter, Dianne S.
Slaughter-Defoe, Diana T.
Spencer, Margaret B.
Winfrey, Angela D.
Worrell, Frank C.

-American Indian/Alaska
Native

Prutsman, Thomas D.
Young, Kimberly S.

-Asian American/Asian/Pacific Islander

Birky, Ian
Chen, Hongjen
Chen, S. Andrew
Hojat, Mohammadr
Huang, Karen H C
Kumar, V. K.
Kwei-Levy, Carol
Lee, David Y. K.
Lee, Jerome
Nezu, Arthur M.
Sharma, Greesh C.
Shires, Michael R.
Singh, Silvija S.
Varki, C. Paily
Wang, Margaret C.
Woo, Tae O.
Xu, Gang

-Hispanic/Latino

Alonso, Mario
Castro-Blanco, David R.
Crespo, Gloria M.
Droz, Elizabeth
Echemendia, Ruben J.
Ellis, Edwin E.
Ficher, Ilda V.
Fried-Cassorla, Martha J.
Gutierrez, Manuel J.
Jemail, Jay A.
Laguna, John N.
Louredes Mattei, Maria De
Loyola, Jaime L.
Lugo, Daisy R.
Magran, Betty A.
Perez, Carlos A.
Pincheira, Juan A.
Poal, Pilar
Ramirez, David E.
Rodriguez, Wilfredo
Salas, Jesus A.
Salganicoff, Matilde
Soto, George M.
Tejeda, Manuel J.

-Hispanic/Latino, White/ European

Selgas, James W.

PUERTO RICO

-Hispanic/Latino

Alfaro-Garcia, Rafael A.
Alvarez, Rosaligia
Andujar, Carlos A.
Ardila, Ruben
Arsuaga, Enrique N.
Bauermeisten, Jose J.
Belen, Ines I.
Bernal, Guillermo
Berrios, Zaida R.
Boulon-Diaz, Frances E.
Cardalda, Elsa B.
Cirino, Gabriel
Colon, Ana I.
Colon, Luis H.
Cruz-Lopez, Miguel
Fankhanel, Edward H.
Garcia, Agustin
Garcia, Pedro I.
Gonzalez-Pabon, Jose F.
Gonzalez, Laura A.
Gonzalez, Max A.
Guzman, Milagros
Herrans, Laura L.
Huergo, Mayra
Llado, Sarah L.
Llanos, Aracely B.
Margarida, Maria T.
Martinez-Lugo, Miguel E.
Martinez, Eduardo M.
Montijo, Jorge A.
Navas-Robleto, Jose J.
Navedo, Christella N.
O'NeilldePumaradaCelest
OcasioGarcia,Ketty
Olmo, Manuel C.
Puig, Hector
Ramirez-Cancel, Carlos M.
Ribera-Gonzalez, Julio C.
Rivera-Medina, Eduardo J.
Rivera-Molina, Elba
Rivera, Beatriz D.
Rodriguez, Ramon O.
Roman, Hugo
Romey, Carol M.
Rossello, Jeannette
Sanchez-Caso, Luis M.
Santiago-Negron, Salvador
Santini-Hernandez, Ernesto
Serrano-Garcia, Irma
Toro-Alfonso, Jose
Toro, Carlos A.
Vazquez-Ruiz, Francisco
Vazquez, Carlos D.
Vazquez, Cesar D.
Zavala-Martinez, Iris

-Hispanic/Latino and White/ European

Mendez-Calderon, Luis M.

RHODE ISLAND

-African American/Black

Harris, Shanette M.
Jones, Ferdinand
Miller, Fayneese
Norman, William H.
Samuels, Robert M.

-American Indian/Alaska Native

Love, Craig T.

-Asian American/Asian/Pacific Islander

Kao, Barbara T.
Matsumiya, Yoichi

-Hispanic/Latino

Costa, Armenio S.
Garcia-Coll; Cynthia
Garrido, Maria

-African American/Black, American Indian/Alaska Native

McCombs, Daniel

SOUTH CAROLINA

-African American/Black

Caesar, Robert
Foster, Evelyn L.
Grimes, Tresmaine R
Hanley, Jerome H.
Jones, George L.
Motes, Patricia S.
Parks, Fayth M.
Walker, O'Neal A.
Woods, Delma M.

-American Indian/Alaska Native

Rainwater, III, Avie J.

-Asian American/Asian/Pacific Islander

Harper, Renuka R.
Sato, Susan D.

SOUTH DAKOTA

-American Indian/Alaska Native

Ertz, Dewey J.

TENNESSEE

-African American/Black

Bingham, Rosie P.
Burnett, Judith A.
Chatman, Vera A
Donald, Liz
Elliott, Vanessa E.
Forrester, Bettye J.
Freeman, Charlotte M.
Granberry, Dorothy
Greene, Lorraine
Henry, Rolando R.
Hopson, Ronald E.
Horton, Carrell
Jackson, Anna M.
Johnson, Johnny
Mars, Raymond G.
Pinderhughes, Ellen B.
Taylor, Palmeda D.

-American Indian/Alaska Native

Joure, Sylvia A.

-Asian American/Asian/Pacific Islander

Fung, Samuel
Khanna, Jaswant L.
Khanna, Mukti
Sharma, Vijai P.
Tang, Thomas L P

-Hispanic/Latino

Abercrombie, Maria M.
Ascencao, Erlete M.
Bueno, Luis F.
Corte, Henry E.
Masini, Angela
Schacht, Thomas E.

-African American/Black and American Indian/Alaska Native

Grubb, Henry J.

TEXAS

-African American/Black

Bostick, Rosie M.
Burks, Eura O.
Burr, Sharon S.
Carter, Lamore J.
Clansy, Pauline A.
Cooper, Alan
Flowers, Jana D.
Garnes, Delbert F.

Garrett-Akinsanya, BraVada
Gayles, Joyce M.
Gloster, Janice L.
Ingram, Jesse C.
Jackson-Davis, Brandi
Jenkins, Sheila A.
Jennings, Lesajean M.
Klopner, Michele C.
Murray, James L.
Peniston, Eugene G.
Pettigrew, Dorothy C.
Philp, Frederick W.
Poston, II, Walker S.
Reed, III, Jesse A.
Rouce, Sandra
Sanders, Betty M.
Sikes, Melvin P.
Williams-Markum, Deirdre

-American Indian/Alaska Native

Ballering, Lawrence R.
Carter, William J.
Gant, Bob L.
Mink, Oscar G.
Stewart, G. Keith
Sutton, David
Thomas, Thomas J.
Uzzell, Barbara P.
Wilson, Lloyd K.

-Asian American/Asian/Pacific Islander

Arana, Olga R.
Bhatia, Kiran
Caberto, Steven C.
Chiu, Loanne
Gasquoine, Philip G.
Hom, Jim
Hu, Trudy HC
Kim, Sook K.
Le, Trinh To
Leung, S. Alvin
Lin, J.C. Gisela G.
Navarro Foley, Gloria L.
Oana, Leilani K.
Patterson, Mayin Lau
Quijano, Walter Y.
Rosenquist, Henry S.
Sikka, Anjoo
Singg, Sangeeta
Stewart, Sunita M.
Tan, Gabriel
Vaid, Jyotsna
Wong, Dorothy L.
Yee, Barbara W. K.
Yu, Pamela

Zhu, Jiajun

-Hispanic/Latino

Ainslie, Ricardo C.
Anderson, Claudia J.
Antokoletz, Juana C.
Arbona, Consuelo
Atilano, Raymond B.
Baron, Augustine
Basco, Monica A.
Burciaga, Lawrence E.
Caldera, Yvonne M.
Cepeda-Benito, Antonio
Chiriboga, David A.
Chriss, Gloria M.
Contreras, Raquel J.
Cruz, Maria C.
de la Sota, Elizanda M.
De Las Fuentes, Cynthia
DeFerreire, Mary Elizabeth
Delgado-Hachey, Maria
Escandell, Vincent A.
Fernandez, Peter
Galaz, Alfred
Galue, Alberto I.
Garcia, Teresa
Gonzalez-Sorensen, Anna G.
Gonzalez, John
Hammond, Evelyn S.
Hill, Jr., Sam S.
Lerma, Joe L.
Llorente, Antolin M.
Loredo, Carlos M.
Marrach, Alexa
Martinez, Jr., Joe L.
Martinez, Raul
Mellor-Crummey, Cynthia A.
Miranda, Jose P.
Morales, Pamilla V.
Natalicio, Luiz
Niemann, Yolanda F
Otero, Rafael F.
Palomares, Ronald S.
Paniagua, Freddy A.
Paredes, Jr., Frank C.
Pereira, Glona M.
Praderas, Kim
Ramirez, Sylvia Z.
Rosin, Susana A.
Sacasa, Rafael E.
Saldana, Delia H.
Samano, Italo A.
Sarmiento, Robert F.
Silva, Santiago
Somodevilla, S. A.
Valdes, Thusnelda M.
Vargas, M. Angelica
Vasquez, Melba

Velasquez, John M.

-Asian American/Asian/Pacific Islander and Hispanic/Latino

Fernandez, Ephrem

UTAH
-American Indian/Alaska Native

Horvat, Jr., Joseph J.

-Asian American/Asian/Pacific Islander

Higashi, Wilfred H.
Kondo, Charles Y.
Loong, James

-Hispanic/Latino

Mejia, Juan A.
Pompa, Janiece L.
Reisinger, Mercedes C.
Reyes, Carla J.
Saenz, Javier
Saenz, Karol K.

VERMONT
-African American/Black

Solomon, Sondra E.

-Asian American/Asian/Pacific Islander

Murakami, Janice

-African American/Black and American Indian/Alaska Native

Andrieu, Brenda J.

VIRGIN ISLANDS
-African American/Black

Copemann, Chester D.
Dudley-Grant, G. Rita

-Hispanic/Latino

Mendez, Gloria I.

-African American/Black, Hispanic/Latino

Moss, Ramona J.

VIRGINIA
-Hispanic/Latino

Hass, Giselle A

-African American/Black

Anderson, William H.
Broadfield, Charles S.
Brown, Anita B.
Crawford, Monica L.
Dawkins, Arthur C.
Elion, Victor H.
Escoffery, Aubrey S.
Farley, Florence S.
Harper, Frederick
Holsey, Chandra V.
James, Lainee M.
Jenkins, Susan M.
Johnson, Fred A.
Jones, Cynthia A.
Jones, Reginald L.
Jones, Russell T.
Meadows-Yancey, Dorothy
Moore, Carolyn D.
Morse, Roberta N.
Peoples, Napoleon L.
Price, Gregory E.
Price, Linda A.
Riddle, P. Elayne
Rivers, Miriam W.
Sanchez-Hucles, Janis V.
Simpson, Adelaide W.
Watts, Charlotte B.
Williams, Indy J.
Wilson, Margaret
Wilson, Melvin N.
Winfrey, LaPearl L.
Word, James C.

-American Indian/Alaska Native

Fields, Amanda H.
Muller, Terry P.
Richardson, E. Strong-Legs
Williams, Mary Beth

-Asian American/Asian/Pacific Islander

Armilla, Jose
Chew, Marion W.
Ching-Yang Hsu, Chris
Hamdani-Raab, Asma J.
Hass, Giselle A.
Kannarkat, Joy P.
Le-Xuan-Hy, G. M.
Macaranas, Eduarda A.
Mariano, Tomas V.

Ng, Pak C.
Noronha, Greta A.
Singh, Nirbhay N.
Wang, Youde
Wibberly, Kathy H.

-Hispanic/Latino

Azcarate, Eduardo M.
Cascallar, Eduardo C.
Giraldo, Macario
Goebes, Diane D.
Jarama, S. Lisbeth
Morote, Gloria
Olivas, Romeo A.
Seda, Gilbert
Stasson, Mark F.
Tischer, Hans
Vegega, Maria E.

-African American/Black, American Indian/Alaska Native

Dent, Harold E.

-African American/Black, Hispanic/Latino

Peart-Newkirk, Natalia J.

WASHINGTON

-African American/Black

Boyd, Naughne L.
Dingus, C. Mary
Ingram, Winifred
Stokes, Devon R.

-American Indian/Alaska Native

Arnold, John F.
Bostwick, Allen D.
Daisy, Fransing
Jun, Heesoon
LaDue, Robin A.
Matheson, Charlene
Ryan, Loye M.
Ryan, Robert A.
Trimble, Joseph E.

-Asian American/Asian/Pacific Islander

Ahana, Ellen
Akutagawa, Donald
Bradshaw, Carla K.
Chan, Darrow A.
Chang, Bradford W.
Collins, James F.

Funabiki, Dean
Fung, Hellen C.
Ho, Christine K.
Hwee, Elsa
Kuan, Yie-Wen Y.
Kwon, Paul H.
Lee, Thomas W.
Low, Benson P.
Lui, Barbara J.
Mar, Norman J.
Mizokawa, Donald T.
Morishige, Howard H.
Morishima, James K.
Moritsugu, John
Niwa, John S.
Root, Maria P. P.
Sue, David
Teng, L. Neal
Tien, Liang
Tsai, Mavis
Vance, Ellen B.

-Hispanic/Latino

Arenas, Jr., Silverio
Borgatta, Edgar F.
Brattesami, Karen A.
Ginorio, Angela B.
Johnson, Paul W.
Kramer, Harry M. O.
Marquez, Steven
Ramirez, John/Juan
Suarez, Alejandra
Takushi, Ruby Y.

-African American/Black, American Indian/Alaska Native

Gist, Marilyn E.

-Hispanic/Latino, White/ European

McNeill, Brian

WEST VIRGINIA

-African American/Black

Asbury, Jo-Ellen
Grych, Diane S.

-American Indian/Alaska Native

Church, June S.

-Asian American/Asian/Pacific Islander

Majumder, Ranjit K.

Smith, Teresa D.

-Hispanic/Latino

Boone, Martin

WISCONSIN

-African American/Black

Caldwell, Barrett S.
Carter, Lonnie T.
Coleman, Hardin L.
Jackson, John H.
Redd-Barnes, Renee A.
Sapp, Marty
Smith, Carol Y.

-American Indian/Alaska Native

Mizwa, Martine M.
Stone, G. Vaughn
Vraniak, Damian A.

-Asian American/Asian/Pacific Islander

Austria, Asuncion M.
Chan, Adrian
Okazaki, Sumie
Sudevan, Padmanbhan
Takahashi, Lorey K.

- Hispanic/Latino

Cunha, Maria I.
Donate-Bartfield, Evelyn
Fouad, Nadya A.
Gloria, Alberta M.
Mendelberg, Hava E.
O'Brien, B. Marco
Ovide, Christopher R.
Panciera, Lawrence A.
Pflaum, John H.
Quintana, Stephen M.

-Asian American/Asian/Pacific Islander, Hispanic/Latino

Unson and Delia C. O.

WYOMING

-Hispanic/Latino

Mondragon, Nathan J.
Nunez, Narina N

Division Listing

APA has 53 divisions. Divisions represent subdisciplines, specialty areas, and special interests groups. Psychologists of color are represented among the membership of nearly every division. In the following section, each APA division is numerically ordered and identified. For each division, the names of members of color are alphabetically arranged within the major ethnic group categories. Persons are listed under each division with which they are actively affiliated.

THE APA DIVISIONS

1   General Psychology
2   Teaching of Psychology
3   Experimental Psychology
5   Evaluation, Measurement, and Statistics
6   Physiological and Comparative Psychology
7   Developmental Psychology
8   The Society of Personality and Social Psychology
9   The Society for the Psychological Study of Social Issues
10 Psychology and the Arts
12 Clinical Psychology
13 Consulting Psychology
14 The Society for Industrial and Organizational Psychology, Inc.
15 Educational Psychology
16 School Psychology
17 Counseling Psychology
18 Psychologists in Public Service
19 Military Psychology
20 Adult Development and Aging
21 Applied Experimental and Engineering Psychologists
22 Rehabilitation Psychology
23 Consumer Psychology
24 Theoretical and Philosophical Psychology
25 Division of Behavior Analysis
26 History of Psychology
27 Society for Community Research and Action: The Division of Community Psychology
28 Psychopharmacology
29 Psychotherapy
30 Psychological Hypnosis
31 State Psychological Association Affairs
32 Humanistic Psychology
33 Mental Retardation and Developmental Disabilities
34 Population and Environmental Psychology
35 Psychology of Women
36 Psychologists Interested in Religious Issues
37 Child, Youth, and Family Services
38 Health Psychology
39 Psychoanalysis
40 Clinical Neuropsychology
41 American Psychology—Law Society
42 Psychologists in Independent Practice
43 Family Psychology
44 The Society for the Psychological Study of Lesbian, Gay, and Bisexual Issues
45 Society for the Psychological Study of Ethnic Minority Issues
46 Media Psychology
47 Exercise and Sport Psychology
48 Peace Psychology
49 Group Psychology and Group Psychotherapy
50 Addictions
51 Society for the Psychological Study of Men and Masculinity
52 International Psychology
53 Clinical Child Psychology
54 Society of Pediatric Psychology
55 American Society for the Advancement of Pharmacotherapy

APA DIVISION LISTING

01 GENERAL PSYCHOLOGY

-African American/Black

Barnes, Michael J.
Chesnutt, James H.
Chisum, Gloria T.
Dalhouse, A. Derick
Francisco, Richard P.
Hall, William A.
McMillan, Robert
Mindingall, Marilyn P.
Penn, Nolan E.
Sampson, Myrtle B.
Samuel, Valerie J.
Sanders-Thompson, Vetta L.
Slaughter-Defoe, Diana T.
Vontress, Clemmont E.
Whitehead, Jesse

-American Indian/Alaska Native

Atkinson, Michael B.
Babb, Harold
Everson, Howard T.
LaDue, Robin A.

-Asian American/Asian/Pacific Islander

Ahmed, Mohiuddin
Amawattana, Tipawadee
Ashida, Sachio
Blackburn, Winona K.
Chen, Hongjen
Hojat, Mohammadr
Hyde, Elsie HA
Izawa, Chizuko
Lukman, Roy L.
Maung, Iqbal T.
Mio, Jeffery S.
Misra, Rajendra K.
Mondol, Merlyn D.
Moritsugu, John
Omizo, Michael M.
Parasuraman, Raja
Randhawa, Bikkar S.
Sax, Kenji W.
Sharma, Satanand
Sue, Derald W.
Suinn, Richard M.
Sundararajan, Louise Kuen-Wei L.
Swan, June A.
Velayo, Richard S.

-Hispanic/Latino

Adler, Peter J.
Alfaro-Garcia, Rafael A.
Aponte, Joseph F.
Benavides, Jr., Robert
Betancourt, Hector
Blanco-Beledo, Ricardo
Camarillo, Max
Chriss, Gloria M.
Dhimitri, Patricio
Gonsalves, Carlos J.
Latorre, Miriam D.
Martinez, Jr., Joe L.
Puertas, Lorenzo
Reyna, Valerie F.
Rivera-Molina, Elba
Rodriguez, Luis J.
Roig, Miguel
Sanua, Victor D.
Schreier, Raquel L.
Torres, Mario A.
Vada, Alejo
Vasquez, Melba

02 SOCIETY FOR THE TEACHING OF PSYCHOLOGY

-African American/Black

Anderson, Linda
Anderson, Shirley G.
Butler, B. LaConyea
Caldwell-Colbert, A. Toy
Fulton, Aubyn
Gillem, Angela R
Granberry, Dorothy
Grimes, Tresmaine R
Horton, Carrell
Lampkin, Emmett C.
Penn, Nolan E.
Porche-Burke, Lisa M.
Prelow, Hazel M.
Reid, Pamela T
Richard, Harriette W.
Smith, William F.
Stallworth, Lisa M.
Swanston, Melvon C.
Tatum, Beverly D.
Twe, Boikai S.
Whitten, Lisa A.
Wynne, Michael

-American Indian/Alaska Native

Horvat, Jr., Joseph J.
Karson, Samuel

-Asian American/Asian/Pacific Islander

Akimoto, Sharon A
Amawattana, Tipawadee
Austria, Asuncion M.
Collins, James F.
Fujinaka, Larry H.
Fujitsubo, Lani C.
Junn, Ellen
Khanna, Mukti
Kim, Randi I.
Leong, Frederick T. T.
Manuel, Gerdenio M.
Mehrotra, Chandra M.N.
Mio, Jeffery S.
Sasao, Toshiaki
Serafica, Felicisima C.
Velayo, Richard S.
Wang, Alvin

-Hispanic/Latino

Ascencao, Erlete M.
Cuesta, George M.
Diaz-Guerrero, Rogelio
Lafarga-Corona, Juan B.
Puente, Antonio E.
Roig, Miguel
Roll, Samuel
Serrano-Garcia, Irma
Stasson, Mark F.
Tazeau, Yvette N.

-African American/Black and American Indian/Alaska Native

Somerville, Addison W.

-Hispanic/Latino, White/ European

Edwards, Henry P.

03 EXPERIMENTAL PSYCHOLOGY

-African American/Black

Penn, Nolan E.

-American Indian/Alaska Native

Babb, Harold

-Asian American/Asian/Pacific Islander

Banaji, Mahzarin R.
Blackburn, Winona K.
Izawa, Chizuko
Mio, Jeffery S.
Parasuraman, Raja
Sax, Kenji W.
Velayo, Richard S.
Yu, Howard K.

-Hispanic/Latino

Arnau-Gras, Jamie
Cascallar, Eduardo C.
Garriga-Trillo, Ana J.
Narvaez, Darcia F.
Roig, Miguel

05 EVALUATION, MEASUREMENT AND STATISTICS

-African American/Black

Apenahier, Leonard
Baxter, Anthony G.
Burnham, Lem
Harris, William G.
Hilton, William F.
Louden, Delroy M.
Morris, Dolores O.
Prelow, Hazel M.
Sapp, Marty

-American Indian/Alaska Native

Everson, Howard T.
Goffin, Richard D.
Karson, Samuel
Love, Craig T.
Pope, Mark

-Asian American/Asian/Pacific Islander

Boodoo, Gwyneth M.
Chiang, Grace CT
Goh, David S.
Hartka, Elizabeth
Hojat, Mohammadr
Hu, Li-Tze
Hyde, Elsie HA
Ja, Davis Y.
Kameshima, Shinya
Kim, Seock-Ho
Lin, Hsin-Tai
Liu, An-Yen
Li, Xiaoming
Mehrotra, Chandra M.N.
Murakawa, Fay
Powers, Keiko I.
Sikka, Anjoo
Tai, Chun-Nan
Watanabe-Muraoka, Agnes M.
Yap, Kim O.
Yu, Howard K.
Zhu, Jiajun

-Hispanic/Latino

Andujar, Carlos A.
Barnes, Charles A.
Borgatta, Edgar F.
Dendaluce, Inaki
Garcia, Jose L.
Garriga-Trillo, Ana J.
Mendoza, Jorge L.
Olmedo, Esteban L.

Tejeda, Manuel J.
Topolski, James M.
Urbina, Susana P.

06 BEHAVIORAL NEUROSCIENCE AND COMPARATIVE PSYCHOLOGY

-American Indian/Alaska Native

Nolley, David A.

-Asian American/Asian/Pacific Islander

Lim, Patricia J.
Takahashi, Lorey K.

-Hispanic/Latino

Bracero, William
Kirst, Stephen P.
Martinez, Jr., Joe L.
Puente, Antonio E.
Sanua, Victor D.

07 DEVELOPMENTAL PSYCHOLOGY

-African American/Black

Brookins, Geraldine K
Cunningham, Michael
Flowers, Jana D.
Floyd, Bridget J.
Jackson, Jacquelyne F.
Jones, Elaine F.
Jones, Reginald L.
Nelson-le, Sharon A.
Okorodudu, Corahann
Parks, Carlton
Scott-Jones, Diane
Slaughter-Defoe, Diana T.
Spencer, Margaret B.
Wyche, Karen F.

-Asian American/Asian/Pacific Islander

Blackburn, Winona K.
Collins, James F.
Kameshima, Shinya
Luthar, Suniya S.
Machida, Sandra K.
Oka, Evelyn R.
Sax, Kenji W.
Serafica, Felicisima C.
Takanishi, Ruby

Yang, Raymond K.

-Hispanic/Latino

Alvarez, Mildred M.
Azmitia, Margarita
Bracero, William
Linares, Lourdes O.
Reyna, Valerie F.
Zepeda, Marlene

-Hispanic/Latino and White/European

Burton, Roger V.

08 SOCIETY FOR PERSONALITY AND SOCIAL PSYCHOLOGY

-African American/Black

Bailey, Joan W.
Belgrave, Faye Z
Clark, Jr., Eddie M.
Collins, William
Dunston, Patricia
Garrett-Akinsanya, BraVada
Graham, Sandra
Green, Charles A.
Harris, William G.
Jackson, James S.
Jemmott, III, John B.
Jones, James M.
Parks, Carlton
Pope-Tarrence, Jacqueline R.
Reaves, Andrew L
Stallworth, Lisa M.
Ugwuegbu, Denis C.
Vaughan, Elaine
Ward, Alan J.

-American Indian/Alaska Native

Bowen, Peggy C.
Foster, Rachel A.
Pope, Mark

-Asian American/Asian/Pacific Islander

Akimoto, Sharon A
Banaji, Mahzarin R.
Beattie, Muriel Y.
Bhanthumnavin, Duangduen
Chen, Hongjen
Chia, Rosina
Fong, Geoffrey T.
Fugita, Stephen S.
Fung, Samuel

Hom, Harry L.
Hu, Li-Tze
Hyde, Elsie HA
Kothandapani, Virupaksha
Kurosawa, Kaoru
Lin, Hsin-Tai
Maruyama, Geoffrey
Matsumoto, David
Nagy, Vivian T.
Ng, Pak C.
Omoto, Allen M.
Serafica, Felicisima C.
Singh, Ramadhar
Tanaka-Matsumi, Junko
Viswesvaran, Chockalingam

-Hispanic/Latino

Alfaro-Garcia, Rafael A.
Benet-Martinez, Veronica
Betancourt, Hector
Borgatta, Edgar F.
Camargo, Robert J.
Diaz-Guerrero, Rogelio
Diaz-Machado, Carmen B.
Gaborit, Mauricio
Garcia, Teresa
Jarama, S. Lisbeth
Munoz, Luis A.
Narvaez, Darcia F.
Niemann, Yolanda F
Olmedo, Esteban L.
Pons, Michael B.
Santini-Hernandez, Ernesto
Sanua, Victor D.
Soriano, Fernando I.
Soriano, Marcel
Stasson, Mark F.
Whitaker, Sandra V.

-African American/Black, American Indian/Alaska Native

Hightower, Eugene

09 SOCIETY FOR THE PSYCHOLOGICAL STUDY OF SOCIAL ISSUES - SPSSI

-African American/Black

Alston, Denise A.
Ashmore-Hudson, Anne
Beatty, Lula A.
Brookins, Geraldine K
Clark, Jr., Eddie M.
Collins, William
Cook, Rudolf E.
Copher-Haynes, Harriett

Davis, Bernice M.
Dawkins, Marva P.
DeFour, Darlene C.
Deleaire, Robert N.
Dudley-Grant, G. Rita
Dunston, Patricia
Fairchild, Halford H.
Gaines, Stanley O.
Graham, Sandra
Granberry, Dorothy
Greene, Beverly
Hanley, Jerome H.
Harrell, Shelly P.
Hayles, V. Robert
Hill, Anthony L
Holliday, Bertha G.
Hooker, Olivia J.
Jackson, Anna M.
Jackson, James S.
Jemmott, III, John B.
Jones, Ferdinand
Jones, James M.
Jones, Reginald L.
Keita, Gwendolyn P.
Moore, Sandra
Morris, Dolores O.
Nolan, Jr., Benjamin C.
Okorodudu, Corahann
Parks, Carlton
Paster, Vera S.
Peters, Sheila
Price, Linda A.
Pugh, Roderick W.
Ramseur, Howard P.
Reid, Pamela T
Robinson, Jane A.
Salter, Beatrice R.
Scott-Jones, Diane
Sims-Patterson, Sandra
Smith, Althea
Smith, William F.
Solomon, Sondra E.
Spencer, Margaret B.
Stallworth, Lisa M.
Tatum, Beverly D.
Thompson, Chalmer E.
Wilson, Melvin N.
Wyche, Karen F.

-American Indian/Alaska Native

Foster, Rachel A.
Knapp, W. Mace
LaFromboise, Teresa
Love, Craig T.
Richardson, E. Strong-Legs
Ryan, Loye M.

Ryan, Robert A.
Trimble, Joseph E.

-Asian American/Asian/Pacific Islander

Advani, Nisha
Ambady, Nalina
Banaji, Mahzarin R.
Beattie, Muriel Y.
Chan, Connie S.
Chen, Hongjen
Chia, Rosina
D'Heurle, Adma J.
Ebreo, Angela
Fong, Geoffrey T.
Fugita, Stephen S.
Fung, Samuel
Iguchi, Martin Y.
Ja, Davis Y.
Kee, PooKong
Khanna, Jaswant L.
Khanna, Mukti
Le-Xuan-Hy, G. M.
Low, Benson P.
Maruyama, Geoffrey
Moritsugu, John
Nagata, Donna K.
Oda, Ethel Aiko
Omoto, Allen M.
Sasao, Toshiaki
Suinn, Richard M.
Takanishi, Ruby
Teo, Thomas
Tsui, Alice M.

-Hispanic/Latino

Aguilera, David M.
Alfaro-Garcia, Rafael A.
Amaro, Hortensia
Bacigalupe, Gonzalo M.
Balcazar, Fabricio E.
Betancourt, Hector
Boulon-Diaz, Frances E.
Castro-Blanco, David R.
Chiriboga, David A.
De La Cancela, Victor
Diaz-Guerrero, Rogelio
Ferdman, Bernardo M.
Garcia, Betty
Ginorio, Angela B.
Inclan, Jaime
Morales, Eduardo S.
Mortimer, Joan R.
O'Neill-dePumarada, Celeste
Olguin, Arthur
Olmedo, Esteban L.
Olmo, Manuel C.

Rigual-Lynch, Lourdes
Rivera, Nelson E.
Sanua, Victor D.
Serrano-Garcia, Irma
Soriano, Fernando I.
Soriano, Marcel
Stasson, Mark F.
Topolski, James M.
Vasquez, Melba

-African American/Black, American Indian/Alaska Native

Dent, Harold E.
Rivers, Marie D.
Windham, Thomas L.

10 PSYCHOLOGY AND THE ARTS

-African American/Black

Alexander, Charlene M.
Lawson, Jasper J.

-Asian American/Asian/Pacific Islander

Khanna, Jaswant L.
Sundararajan, Louise Kuen-Wei L.

-Hispanic/Latino

Barnes, Charles A.
Berrill, Naftali G.
Bracero, William
Cruz, Albert R.
Lowman, Rodney
Mujica, Ernesto

-African American/Black, American Indian/Alaska Native

Hart, Anton H.

12 CLINICAL PSYCHOLOGY

-African American/Black

Archibald, Eloise M.
Atwell, Robert L.
Bamgbose, Olujiimi O.
Banks, Martha E.
Barker-Hackett, Lori
Brown, Anita B.
Browne, Ronald H.
Caesar, Robert
Caldwell-Colbert, A. Toy
Cathcart, Conrad W.
Cook, Rudolf E.

Cooper, Donna M.
Crawford, Monica L.
Davis-Russell, Elizabeth
Davis, Charles E.
Dingus, C. Mary
Dixon, J. Faye
Epps, Pamela J.
Floyd, Bridget J.
Fulton, Aubyn
Graves-Cooper, Phyllis J.
Gray-Little, Bernadette
Greene, Beverly
Greene, Clifford
Gulley, Silas
Hall, Ruth L.
Harper, Mary S.
Harris, Michelle F.
Harris, Shanette M.
Henderson Daniel, Jessica
Holmes, Dorothy E.
Hooker, Olivia J.
Houston, Lawrence N.
Hunt, William K.
Hunt, Wilson L.
Jackson, Anna M.
Jackson, Leslie C.
James, Larry C.
Jenkins, Adelbert H.
Jones, Ruby M.
Jones, Russell T.
Kennedy, Clive D.
Klopner, Michele C.
Langley, Merlin R
Lawson, Jasper J.
London, Dyanne P.
Mallisham, Ivy J.
Maynard, Edward S.
McClure, Faith H.
Miles, Gary T.
Mindingall, Marilyn P.
Mobley, Brenda D.
Morris, Dolores O.
Muir-Malcolm, Joan A.
Myers, Linda J.
Nettles, Arie L.
Nolan, Jr., Benjamin C.
Penn, Nolan E.
Prelow, Hazel M.
Pruitt, Jr., Joseph H.
Pugh, Roderick W.
Richards, Henry J.
Rivers, Miriam W.
Robinson, John D.
Robinson, W. LaVome
Rollock, David
Sanchez-Hucles, Janis V.
Singleton, Edward G.
Smith, Alvin E.

Stokes, Devon R.
Stringer, Anthony Y.
Taylor, Palmeda D.
Thomas, Hilton T.
Tomes, Henry
Trufant, Carol A.
Tucker, James L.
Turner, Samuel M.
Walker, Lila K.
Ward, Alan J.
Watts, Charlotte B.
White, Joseph L.
Williams-Markum, Deirdre
Williams, Medria L.
Wilson, Melvin N.
Wilson, Woodrow
Wyatt, Gail E.
Wyche, Karen F.

-American Indian/Alaska Native

Bostwick, Allen D.
Campos, Peter E.
DeGraff, Christopher D.
Fain, Thomas C.
Gant, Bob L.
Haddock, Dean M.
Karson, Samuel
Pine, Charles J.
Rainwater, III, Avie J.
Richardson, E. Strong-Legs
Willis, Diane J.

-Asian American/Asian/Pacific Islander

Ahmed, Mohiuddin
Akamatsu, T. John
Austria, Asuncion M.
Chan, Darrow A.
Chin, Jean L
Chin, Raymond J.
Chin, Sandra B
Choi, George C.
Fujioka, Terry Ann T.
Gam, John
Gee, Carol S.
Gock, Terry S.
Gong-Guy, Elizabeth
Gong, Susan M.
Guo, Trudy Narikiyo
Hamada, Roger S.
Han, Yu Ling
Huang, Wei-Jen William
Itatani, Robert M.
Iwamasa, Gayle Y.
Jain, Sharat K.
Koh, Tong-He

Kothandapani, Virupaksha
Kuan, Yie-Wen Y.
Lee, Anna C.
Lu, Elsie G.
Manuel, Gerdenio M.
Morishige, Howard H.
Moritsugu, John
Nezu, Arthur M.
Nishi-Strattner, Linda
Oana, Leilani K.
Quijano, Walter Y.
Root, Maria P. P.
Serafica, Felicisima C.
Sue, Stanley
Suinn, Richard M.
Tanaka-Matsumi, Junko
Tan, Josephine
Tsang, Michael Hing- Pui
Tsujimoto, Richard N.
Wagner, Aureen Pinto
Wickramasekera, Ian E.
Yanagida, Evelyn H.
Ying, Yu-Wen

-Hispanic/Latino

Abercrombie, Maria M.
Aguilera, David M.
Alvarez, Manuel E.
Amezaga, Jr., Alfredo M.
Anderson, Claudia J.
Antonuccio, David
Arellano, Charleanea
Bascuas, Joseph W.
Bastien, IV, Samuel A.
Bayon, E. Paul
Bernal, Guillermo
Berrill, Naftali G.
Berrios, Zaida R.
Camargo, Robert J.
Camarillo, Max
Caro, Yvette
Carpenter, Gerald A.
Carra, Sylvia F.
Castro-Blanco, David R.
Chavez, Ernest L.
Cimino, Cynthia R.
Comas-Diaz, Lillian
Dooley, John A.
Echemendia, Ruben J.
Fuentes, Dainery M.
Garcia-Abid, Calixto
Garrido, Maria
Gomez, Ana L
Gomez, John P
Gular, Enrique

Hill, Jr., Sam S.
Hyman, Edward J.
Incera, Armando
Javier, Rafael A.
Kelton-Brand, Ana
Kirst, Stephen P.
Lopez, Steven R.
Lowman, Rodney
Madison, James K.
Miranda, David J.
Miranda, M.
Montes, Francisco
Montijo, Jorge A.
Morones, Pete A.
Nieves, Luis R.
Paredes, Jr., Frank C.
Ramos-Grenier, Julia
Roll, Samuel
Romero, Jose
Ruth, Richard
Salais, A. Joseph
Santini-Hernandez, Ernesto
Sanua, Victor D.
Tazeau, Yvette N.
Tostado, John F.
Towns-Miranda, Luz
Turner, Darrell D.
Vargas, Luis A.
Vazquez, Rosa
Velasquez, John M.
Velasquez, Roberto J.

-African American/Black

Triplett, Sheila J.

-African American/Black American Indian/Alaska Native

Grubb, Henry J.
Hart, Anton H.
Hightower, Eugene
Somerville, Addison W.

-American Indian/Alaska Native and White/European

Hough, Sigmund

-Asian American/Asian/Pacific Islander, Hispanic/Latino

Garcia, Melinda A.

13 CONSULTING PSYCHOLOGY

-African American/Black

Baxter, Anthony G.

Cook, Rudolf E.
Copher-Haynes, Harriett
Dunston, Patricia
Hunt, Wilson L.
Jackson, John H.
Morris, Joseph R.
Tucker, Dorothy M.
Ugwuegbu, Denis C.
Ward, Alan J.
West, Gerald I.
Williams, Everett B.
Wilson, Susan B.*
Wright, Doris J.

-American Indian/Alaska Native

Karson, Samuel

-Asian American/Asian/Pacific Islander

Chan, Adrian
Hamdani-Raab, Asma J.
Heras, Patricia
Khanna, Jaswant L.
Lukman, Roy L.
Matsumoto, Gregory Y.
Ng, James T.
Salway, Milton R.
Tai, Chun-Nan
Wong-Rieger, Durhane
Yu, Howard K.

-Hispanic/Latino

Aguilera, David M.
Amezaga, Jr., Alfredo M.
Cherbosque, Jorge
Crane, Rosario S.
Incera, Armando
Lawson, Gary W.
Lowman, Rodney
Valdes, Luis F.

-Asian American/Asian/Pacific Islandet

Leung, Alex C. N.

14 SOCIETY FOR INDUSTRIAL AND ORGANIZATIONAL PSYCHOLOGY

-African American/Black

Abernethy, Alexis D.
Allen, Jane E.
Caldwell-Colbert, A. Toy
Cooper, Colin

Hayles, V. Robert
Horsford, Bernard I.
James, Jr., Earnest
Smedley, Joseph W.
Wellons, Retha V.

-American Indian/Alaska Native

Everson, Howard T.
Goffin, Richard D.
Hui, Len Dang
Mink, Oscar G.

-Asian American/Asian/Pacific Islander

Al-tai, Nazar M.
Aldaba-Lim, Estefania
Baba, Vishwanath V.
Chan, Paul K.
Chan, Paul K. F.
Chao, Georgia T.
Ching-Yang Hsu, Chris
Henson, Ramon M.
Kam, Sherilyn M.
Lee, Thomas W.
Lin, Thung-Rung
Saner-Yiu, Li-Chia
Sen, Tapas K.
Shahani-denning, Comila
Singh, Ramadhar
Tang, Thomas L P
Viswesvaran, Chockalingam
Wong-Rieger, Durhane

-Hispanic/Latino

Alfaro-Garcia, Rafael A.
Betancourt, Hector
Boulon-Diaz, Frances E.
Cherbosque, Jorge
Del Rio, Augusto B.
Diaz, Raul
Ferdman, Bernardo M.
Galue, Alberto I.
Goltz, Sonia
Gonsalves, Carlos J.
Hyman, Edward J.
Kramer, Diana R.
Lowman, Rodney
Mendoza, Jorge L.
Mondragon, Nathan J.
Navedo, Christella N.
Nieves, Luis R.
Reyes-Mayer, Erwin
Rodriguez, David A.
Salas, Eduardo
Tazeau, Yvette N.
Tejeda, Manuel J.

Thorn, Isabel M.
Topolski, James M.

-African American/Black, American Indian/Alaska Native

Gist, Marilyn E.

-Asian American/Asian/Pacific Islander and Hispanic/Latino

Pang, Mark G.

15 EDUCATIONAL PSYCHOLOGY

-African American/Black

Anderson, Shirley G.
Apenahier, Leonard
Baxter, Anthony G.
Davis, Annette E.
Graham, Sandra
Hill, Anthony L
Hilton, William F.
Johnson, Sylvia T.
Mosley-Howard, Gerri S.
Nelson-le, Sharon A.
Price, Linda A.
Scott-Jones, Diane
Spencer, Margaret B.
Stone, Lynn J.
Sutton, Sharon E.
Swanston, Melvon C.
Twe, Boikai S.
Williams, Michael A.

-American Indian/Alaska Native

Carter, William J.
Durant, Jr., Adrian J.
Everson, Howard T.

-Asian American/Asian/Pacific Islander

Boodoo, Gwyneth M.
Chiang, Grace CT
Collins, James F.
Goh, David S.
Kame'enui, Edward J.
Leong, Che K.
Leong, Deborah J.
Maruyama, Geoffrey
Mondol, Merlyn D.
Oka, Evelyn R.
Okagaki, Lynn
Randhawa, Bikkar S.
Serafica, Felicisima C.
Sikka, Anjoo

Velayo, Richard S.
Wong, Lily H.
Yu, Howard K.

-Hispanic/Latino

Boulon-Diaz, Frances E.
Coes, Maria R.
Garcia, Teresa
Genero, Nancy P.
Narvaez, Darcia F.
Pita, Marcia E.
Reyna, Valerie F.
Sandoval, Jonathan
Tamayo, Jose M.

-African American/Black and Asian American/Asian/Pacific Islander

Salone, Lavorial

-African American/Black, Hispanic/Latino

Mahabee-Harris, Marilyn M.

-Hispanic/Latino and White/ European

Mendez-Calderon, Luis M.

16 SCHOOL PSYCHOLOGY

-African American/Black

Barnes, Michael J.
Bartholomew, Charles
Crockett, Deborah P.
Dawson, Harriett E.
Hampton, Juanita R.
Hines, Laura M.
Jackson, John H.
Mack, Faite R. P.
Millard, Wilbur A.
Morris, Dolores O.
Nettles, Arie L.
Parks, Carlton
Rivers, Miriam W.
Slaughter-Defoe, Diana T.
Whitehead, Jesse
Williams, Michael A.
Wyche, Sr., LaMonte G.

-American Indian/Alaska Native

Durant, Jr., Adrian J.
Ertz, Dewey J.
Haddock, Dean M.
Mellor, Catherine A.

-Asian American/Asian/Pacific Islander

Chao, Janet
Khan, Kanwar H.
Oka, Evelyn R.

-Hispanic/Latino

Alvarez, Maria D.
Barona, Andres
Boulon-Diaz, Frances E.
Bursztyn, Alberto M.
Esquivel, Giselle B.
Lopez, Emilia
Loyola, Jaime L.
Marquez, E. Mario
Nuttall, Ena V.
Pompa, Janiece L.
Ramirez, Sylvia Z.
Rosado, John W.
Sandoval, Jonathan
Santos de Barona, Maryann

-Asian American/Asian/Pacific Islander and Hispanic/Latino

Jew, Cynthia L.

-Hispanic/Latino, White/ European

Selgas, James W.

17 COUNSELING PSYCHOLOGY

-African American/Black

Alexander, Charlene M.
Allsopp, Ralph N
Bingham, Rosie P.
Bowman, Sharon L.
Boyd, Vivian S.
Brown, Michael T.
Carey, Patricia M.
Carter, Robert T.
Coleman, Hardin L.
Constantine, Madonna G.
Cook, Donelda
Cook, Rudolf E.
Copher-Haynes, Harriett
Essandoh, Pius K.
Griffith, Albert R.
Haggins, Kristee L.
Howard, Mary T.
Jackson, Anna M.
James, Larry C.

James, Norman L.
Johnson, David L.
Kemp, Arthur D.
Langley, Merlin R
Luke, Equilla
McRae, Mary B.
Morris, Joseph R.
Parham, Thomas A.
Parks, Fayth M.
Phelps, Rosemary E.
Pope-Davis, Donald B.
Poston, II, Walker S.
Robinson, Gregory F.
Robinson, John D
Sapp, Marty
Shipp, Pamela L.
Speight, Suzette L.
Tatum, Beverly D.
Thomas, Anita J.
Thompson, Chalmer E.
Tomlinson-Clarke, Saundra M.
Tucker, Dorothy M.
Ward, Connie M.
Watts, Charlotte B.
Webb, Wanda
West, Gerald I.
Whitehead, Barry X.
Whitehead, Jesse
Wright, Doris J.

-American Indian/Alaska Native

Carter, William J.
LaFromboise, Teresa
Mink, Oscar G.
Pope, Mark
Sanders, Gilbert O.

-Asian American/Asian/Pacific Islander

Acka-Pope, Zeynep K
Amawattana, Tipawadee
Chen, Eric C
Chung, Y. Barry
Dawis, Rene V.
Fukuyama, Mary A.
Ham, MaryAnna D.
Hoshmand, Lisa T.
Ibrahim, Farah A.
Khanna, Jaswant L.
Koh, Tong-He
Leong, Frederick T. T.
Leung, Paul
Lin, J.C. Gisela G.
Manese, Jeanne E.
Mellot, Ramona N.
Morishige, Howard H.

Moritsugu, John
Ng, James T.
Omizo, Michael M.
Perez, Ruperto M.
Saito, Gloria C.
Sodowsky, Gargi R.
Sue, Derald W.
Suinn, Richard M.
Suzuki, Lisa A.
Tanaka, Koji
Tan, Rowena N.
Watanabe-Muraoka, Agnes M.

-Hispanic/Latino

Arbona, Consuelo
Ardila, Ruben
Balderrama, Sylvia R.
Baron, Augustine
Barry, Martha J.
Bursztyn, Alberto M.
Canedo, Angelo R.
Contreras, Raquel J.
Fankhanel, Edward H.
Flores, Elena
Fouad, Nadya A.
Gloria, Alberta M.
Gonzales, Michael
Lopez-Baez, Sandra I.
Ludmer, Alba
Marotta, Sylvia A.
Millan, Fred
Nadal-Vazquez, Vilma Y.
Nazario, Jr., Andres
Nuttall, Ena V.
Ovide, Christopher R.
Prendes-Lintel, Maria L.
Prieto, Susan L.
Quintana, Stephen M.
Ramirez, John/Juan
Rodriguez, Richard A.
Roehlke, Helen J.
Ruiz, Nicholas J.
Silva, Santiago
Softas, Basilia C.
Stern, Marilyn
Valdez, Jesse N.
Vasquez, Melba
Vazquez, Cesar D.
Vera, Elizabeth M.

-African American/Black and American Indian/Alaska Native

Rivers, Marie D.
Somerville, Addison W.

-African American/Black and Asian American/Asian/Pacific Islander

Salone, Lavorial

-Asian American/Asian/Pacific Islander and White/European

Akca, Zeynep K.

-Hispanic/Latino, White/European

McNeill, Brian
Selgas, James W.

18 PSYCHOLOGISTS IN PUBLIC SERVICE

-African American/Black

Abernethy, Alexis D.
Archibald, Eloise M.
Barber, Kevin V.
Binns, Derrick
Burchell, Charles R.
Tucker, Dorothy M.

-American Indian/Alaska Native

Hui, Len Dang
Pine, Charles J.
Sanders, Gilbert O.
Williams, Mary Beth

-Asian American/Asian/Pacific Islander

Lu, Elsie G.
Mar, Norman J.
Smith, Teresa D.
Torigoe, Rodney Y.
True, Reiko Homma

-Hispanic/Latino

Antonuccio, David
Bracero, William
Diaz, Raul
Lowman, Rodney
Parlade, Rafael J.
Pons, Michael B.
Rodriguez, Manuel D.
Somodevilla, S. A.

19 MILITARY PSYCHOLOGY

-African American/Black

James, Larry C.

Johnson, Lawrence B.
Reed, James D.

-Asian American/Asian/Pacific Islander

Caberto, Steven C.

-Hispanic/Latino

Salas, Eduardo
Seda, Gilbert

20 ADULT DEVELOPMENT AND AGING

-African American/Black

Forrester, Bettye J.
Garrett, Aline M.
Harper, Mary S.
Jackson, James S.
Parks, Carlton

-American Indian/Alaska Native

McDonald, Arthur L.
Montgomery, Robert L.

-Asian American/Asian/Pacific Islander

Chew, Marion W.
Fry, Prem S.
Gam, John
Izutsu, Satoru
Mehrotra, Chandra M.N.
Nagy, Vivian T.
Poon, Leonard W.
Sato, Susan D.
Teng, Eveiyn L.
Yee, Barbara W. K.

-Hispanic/Latino

Camarillo, Max
Chiriboga, David A.
Fils, David H.
Fuhrmann, Max E.
Garza, Alicia de la
Gonzales, Linda R.
Johnson, Paul W.
Laguna, John N.
Lopez, Martita A.
Miranda, Manuel R.
Mussenden, Gerald
Olivas, Romeo A.
Prieto, Addys
Romero, Arturo
Romero, Jose

Saunders, Walter C.
Soriano, Fernando I.
Tazeau, Yvette N.
Topolski, James M.
Towns-Miranda, Luz
Vada, Alejo
Valencia-Laver, Debra

21 APPLIED EXPERIMENTAL AND ENGINEERING PSYCHOLOGY

-African American/Black

Caldwell, Barrett S.
Johnson, Lawrence B.

-American Indian/Alaska Native

Pine, Charles J.

-Asian American/Asian/Pacific Islander

Hsu, Shang H.
Parasuraman, Raja
Sen, Tapas K.

-Hispanic/Latino

Gonzalez, Fernando
Salas, Eduardo

22 REHABILITATION PSYCHOLOGY

-African American/Black

Abercombie, Delrita
Allen, Christeen
Banks, Martha E.
Critton, Barbara L.
Dingus, C. Mary
Howard, Mary T.
Poston, II, Walker S.

-American Indian/Alaska Native

Uzzell, Barbara P.

-Asian American/Asian/Pacific Islander

Fergus, Esther O.
Izutsu, Satoru
Khanna, Jaswant L.
Kothandapani, Virupaksha
Lam, Chow S.
Leung, Paul
Oda, Ethel Aiko

Sax, Kenji W.
Tobias, Manuel D.
Yu, Howard K.

-Hispanic/Latino

Armengol, Carmen G.
Balcazar, Fabricio E.
Berrill, Naftali G.
Canedo, Angelo R.
Castro-Blanco, David R.
Comas-Diaz, Lillian
Elena Lee, Karen
Ferreira, Pedro M.
Incera, Armando
Kranau, Edgar J.
Pedemonte, Monica
Perez, Juan C.
Porges, Carlos R.

23 SOCIETY FOR CONSUMER PSYCHOLOGY

-African American/Black

Johnson, Lawrence B.

-Asian American/Asian/Pacific Islander

Austria, Asuncion M.
Kee, PooKong
Nagy, Vivian T.
Powers, Keiko I.

-Hispanic/Latino

Alfaro-Garcia, Rafael A.
Barrera, Francisco J.
Brattesami, Karen A.
Sanchez, Juan
Towns-Miranda, Luz
Zuriff, Gerald E.

24 THEORETICAL AND PHILOSOPHICAL PSYCHOLOGY

-African American/Black

Cook, Rudolf E.
Jenkins, Adelbert H.
Williams, Everett B.

-American Indian/Alaska Native

Pine, Charles J.

-Asian American/Asian/Pacific Islander

D'Heurle, Adma J.
Fanibanda, Darius K.
Hoshmand, Lisa T.
Sundararajan, Louise Kuen-Wei L.
Teo, Thomas

-Hispanic/Latino

Alfaro-Garcia, Rafael A.
Arcaya, Jose M.
Bayon, E. Paul
Blanco-Beledo, Ricardo
Canedo, Angelo R.
Comas-Diaz, Lillian
Ferreira, Pedro M.
Hill, Jr., Sam S.
Natalicio, Luiz
Perez, Juan C.
Villela, Leopoldo F.
Zuriff, Gerald E.

25 DIVISION OF BEHAVIOR ANALYSIS

-African American/Black

Hammond, W. Rodney
Turner, Samuel M.

-American Indian/Alaska Native

Nolley, David A.
Pope, Mark

-Asian American/Asian/Pacific Islander

Kameshima, Shinya
Nezu, Arthur M.
Tanaka-Matsumi, Junko

-Hispanic/Latino

Abordo, Enrique J.
Corte, Henry E.
Garcia, Hector D.
Goltz, Sonia
Irueste-Montes, Ana M.
Montes, Francisco
Natalicio, Luiz
Paniagua, Freddy A.
Pinto, Alcides
Zuriff, Gerald E.

26 HISTORY OF PSYCHOLOGY

-African American/Black

Asbury, Jo-Ellen
Howard, Mary T.
Hunt, Wilson L.
Jackson, James S.
Pugh, Roderick W.

-American Indian/Alaska Native

Durant, Jr., Adrian J.
Foster, Rachel A.
Karson, Samuel

-Hispanic/Latino

Colon, Ana I.
Martinez, Jr., Joe L.
Natalicio, Luiz
Puente, Antonio E.
Sanua, Victor D.

27 SOCIETY FOR COMMUNITY RESEARCH AND ACTION: DIVISION OF COMMUNITY PSYCHOLOGY

-African American/Black

Barbarin, Oscar A.
Cameron, Linda S.
Cook, Rudolf E.
DeFour, Darlene C.
Dockett, Kathleen H.
Floyd, James A.
Harrell, Shelly P.
Hines, Paulette M.
Holliday, Bertha G.
Jones, Ferdinand
Klopner, Michele C.
Milburn, Norweeta G.
Miller, Robin L.
Motes, Patricia S.
Myers, Hector F.
Nickerson, Kim J.
Parks, Carlton
Penn, Nolan E.*
Peters, Sheila
Prelow, Hazel M.
Reid, Pamela T
Robinson, W. LaVome
Smith, William F.
Steele, Robert E.
Tomes, Henry
Watts, Roderick J.
Wilson, Melvin N.

Wyatt, Gail E.
Wynne, Michael

-American Indian/Alaska Native

Trimble, Joseph E.

-Asian American/Asian/Pacific Islander

Fergus, Esther O.
Ja, Davis Y.
Mar, Norman J.
Moritsugu, John
Nemoto, Tooru
Root, Maria P. P.
Sasao, Toshiaki
Singh, R. K. Janmeha
Sue, Stanley
Wong-Rieger, Durhane
Wong, Frankie Y.
Ying, Yu-Wen
Zane, Nolan W.S

-Hispanic/Latino

Ainslie, Ricardo C.
Aponte, Joseph F.
Balcazar, Fabricio E.
Bernal, Guillermo
Genero, Nancy P.
Inclan, Jaime
Munoz, Ricardo F.
Rosario, Margaret
Sanua, Victor D.
Serrano-Garcia, Irma
Suarez-Balcazar, Yolanda

**28
PSYCHOPHARMACOLOGY
AND SUBSTANCE ABUSE**

-African American/Black

Blanding, Benjamin
Johnson, David L.
Singleton, Edward G.
Ward, Alan J.

American Indian/Alaska Native

Haddock, Dean M.
Knapp, W. Mace

-Asian American/Asian/Pacific Islander

Chan, Daniel S.
Iguchi, Martin Y.

-Hispanic/Latino

Alvarez, Manuel E.
Badillo, Diana
Benzaquen, Isaac
Marin, Gerardo
Martinez, Jr., Joe L.
Munoz, Luis A.
Perez-Arce, Patricia
Pinto, Alcides
Puertas, Lorenzo
Rosario, Margaret

29 PSYCHOTHERAPY

-African American/Black

Allsopp, Ralph N
Bastien, Rochelle T.
Belton, Monique
Binns, Derrick
Brice, Janet R.
Bryant-Tuckett, Rose M.
Buffin, Janice E.
Cook, Rudolf E.
Crowder, Virginia B.
Dudley-Grant, G. Rita
Green, Charles A.
Greene, Beverly
Harris, Michelle F.
Henry, Vincent dePaul
Holmes, Dorothy E.
Hunt, Wilson L.
Jackson, Anna M.
Jackson, John H.
Jackson, Leslie C.
Jenkins, Adelbert H.
Johnson, Zonya
Jones, Ferdinand
Jones, Ruby M.
Maynard, Edward S.
McMillan, Robert
Molden, Sabrina
Nolan, Jr., Benjamin C.
Paster, Vera S.
Pernell, Eugene
Perry, Cereta E.
Phelps, C. K.
Porche-Burke, Lisa M.
Pugh, Roderick W.
Richardson, Frederick
Roberts, Harrell B.
Robinson, Jane A.
Rountree, Yvonne B.
Thomas, Hilton T.
Vanderhost, Leonette
Vaughans, Kirkland C.
Ward, Alan J.
White, Voncile

Williams, Michael A.
Witter, Jeanette M.
Wyatt, Gail E.

-American Indian/Alaska Native

Blue, Arthur W.
LaFromboise, Teresa
Williamson, Diane H.
Willis, Diane J.

-Asian American/Asian/Pacific Islander

Ahana, Ellen
Anand, Shashi
Birky, Ian
Campbell, Kamal E.
Chin, Jean L
Choi, George C.
Gui, Chui-Liu Serena
Hong, George K.
Ibrahim, Farah A.
Itatani, Robert M.
Iwamasa, Gayle Y.
Jain, Sharat K.
Khanna, Jaswant L.
Malancharuvil, Joseph M.
Miyahira, Sarah D.
Morishige, Howard H.
Onizuka, Richard K.
Saito, Gloria C.
Saul, Tuck T.
Sue, Stanley
Suinn, Richard M.
Tamura, Leonard J.
Valdez, Jr., Romulo
Young, David A.

-Hispanic/Latino

Aguilera, David M.
Aguirre-Deandreis, Ana I.
Antonuccio, David
Arreola-Rockwell, Fran
   Pepitone-
Azcarate, Eduardo M.
Bayon, E. Paul
Bernal, Guillermo A.
Bracero, William
Camarillo, Max
Castro-Blanco, David R.
Cherbosque, Jorge
Comas-Diaz, Lillian
Diaz, Raul
Fankhanel, Edward H.
Flores, Philip J.
Garrido-Castillo, Pedro
Hill, Jr., Sam S.

Javier, Rafael A.
Machabanski, Hector
Martinez, Cynthia
Mortimer, Joan R.
Nieves, Luis R.
Ovide, Christopher R.
Rivera-Molina, Elba
Roehlke, Helen J.
Rosado, John W.
Santiago, Lydia V.
Santini-Hernandez, Ernesto
Soriano, Marcel
Teixeira, Michael A.
Tostado, John F.
Viale-val, Graciela
Yniguez, Linda E.

-African American/Black, American Indian/Alaska Native

Hart, Anton H.
Somerville, Addison W.

-Asian American/Asian/Pacific Islander, White/European

Bonal, Kathleen A.

30 PSYCHOLOGICAL HYPNOSIS

-African American/Black

Artis, Daphne J.
Bamgbose, Olujiimi O.
Blanding, Benjamin
Bryant-Tuckett, Rose M.
Dawson, Harriett E.
Green, Charles A.
Hammond, Gladys
Johnson, David L.
Sapp, Marty
Ward, Alan J.

-Asian American/Asian/Pacific Islander

Hojat, Mohammadr
Hong, George K.
Jain, Sharat K.
Kothandapani, Virupaksha
Lau, Lavay
Otani, Akira
Sax, Kenji W.
Wickramasekera, Ian E.

-Hispanic/Latino

Araoz, Daniel L.
Arellano-Lopez, Juan
Bernal, Guillermo A.
Cardena, Etzel A.
Figueredo, Migdalia I.
Hall, M. Elizabeth L.
Kranau, Edgar J.
Monguio, Ines
Ortiz, Berta S.

31 STATE PSYCHOLOGICAL ASSOCIATION AFFAIRS

-African American/Black

Howard, Mary T.
Phelps, C. K.
Sanders, Daniel W.

-Asian American/Asian/Pacific Islander

Lu, Elsie G.
Suinn, Richard M.

-Hispanic/Latino

De La Cancela, Victor
Vega, Star

32 HUMANISTIC PSYCHOLOGY

-African American/Black

Cook, Rudolf E.
Crowder, Virginia B.
Jenkins, Adelbert H.
Paster, Vera S.
Perry, Cereta E.
Price, Linda A.
Robertson, John F.

-Asian American/Asian/Pacific Islander

Khanna, Jaswant L.
Manuel, Gerdenio M.
Singh, Nirbhay N.
Srivastva, Suresh
Sundararajan, Louise Kuen-Wei L.
Wang, Wen-Hsiu

-Hispanic/Latino

Dendaluce, Inaki
Fankhanel, Edward H.
Fried-Cassorla, Martha J.

Sanua, Victor D.
Soriano, Marcel

33 MENTAL RETARDATION AND DEVELOPMENTAL DISABILITIES

-African American/Black

Brooks, Lewis A.
Derrick, Sara M.
Dunston, Patricia
Hammond, W. Rodney
Hooker, Olivia J.
Jones, Reginald L.

-American Indian/Alaska Native

Blubaugh, Victoria G.
Durant, Jr., Adrian J.
Nolley, David A.

-Asian American/Asian/Pacific Islander

Mar, Harvey H.
Nezu, Arthur M.
Singh, Nirbhay N.

-Hispanic/Latino

Abordo, Enrique J.
Armengol, Carmen G.
Barrera, Francisco J.
De La Cancela, Victor
Figueroa, Rolando G.
Garcia, Hector D.
Ramirez, Sylvia Z.

-American Indian/Alaska Native, White/European

Hough, Sigmund

34 POPULATION AND ENVIRONMENTAL PSYCHOLOGY

-African American/Black

Hilton, William F.
Vaughan, Elaine

-Asian American/Asian/Pacific Islander

Beattie, Muriel Y.
Ebreo, Angela
Kee, PooKong

-Hispanic/Latino

Borgatta, Edgar F.

35 PSYCHOLOGY OF WOMEN

-African American/Black

Alston, Denise A.
Anderson, Linda
Anthony, Bobbie M.
Banks, Martha E.
Bingham, Rosie P.
Binion, Victoria J.
Brookins, Geraldine K
Brown, Anita B.
Butler, B. LaConyea
Caldwell-Colbert, A. Toy
Carey, Patricia M.
Constantine, Madonna G.
Crawford, Monica L.
Daly, Frederica Y.
Davis-Russell, Elizabeth
Dawson, Harriett E.
DeFour, Darlene C.
Dudley-Grant, G. Rita
Dunston, Patricia
Friday, Jennifer C.
Garrett-Akinsanya, BraVada
Gillem, Angela R
Gordon, Rhea J.
Granberry, Dorothy
Greene, Beverly
Gump, Janice P.
Harris, Shanette M.
Henderson Daniel, Jessica
Hines, Laura M.
Howard, Mary T.
Jackson, Jacquelyne F.
Keita, Gwendolyn P.
Moore, Sandra
Okorodudu, Corahann
Outlaw, Patricia A.
Parham, Patricia
Parks, Carlton
Peters, Sheila
Phelps, Rosemary E.
Porche-Burke, Lisa M.
Porter, Julia
Reaves, Juanita Y.
Reid, Pamela T.
Salter, Beatrice R.
Sampson, Myrtle B.
Sanchez-Hucles, Janis V.
Scott-Jones, Diane
Smith, Althea
Solomon, Sondra E.
Tatum, Beverly D.

Trotman, Frances K.
Tucker, Dorothy M.
White, Voncile
Whitten, Lisa A.
Wilson, Margaret
Wilson, Shirley B.
Witter, Jeanette M.
Wyatt, Gail E.
Wyche, Karen F.

-American Indian/Alaska Native

Blubaugh, Victoria G.
Eaton, Sheila J.
Foster, Rachel A.
LaFromboise, Teresa
Mizwa, Martine M.
Thurman, Pamela J.

-Asian American/Asian/Pacific Islander

Austria, Asuncion M.
Bainum, Charlene K.
Beattie, Muriel Y.
Chin, Jean L.
Chin, Sandra B.
Gong-Guy, Elizabeth
Gui, Chui-Liu Serena
Guo, Trudy Narikiyo
Hall, Christine I.
Hass, Giselle A.
Ho, Christine K.
Izawa, Chizuko
Kakaiya, Divya
Lee, Wanda M. L.
Lu, Elsie G.
Lui, Barbara J.
Miyahira, Sarah D.
Oda, Ethel Aiko
Root, Maria P. P.
Takanishi, Ruby
Tien, Liang
True, Reiko Homma
Tsui, Alice M.
Wong, Frankie Y.
Yee, Barbara W. K.

-Hispanic/Latino

Amaro, Hortensia
Anderson, Claudia J.
Arellano, Charleanea
Arredondo, Patricia
Arreola-Rockwell, Fran
Pepitone-
Arroyo, Patricia M.
Barry, Martha J.
Comas-Diaz, Lillian

De Las Fuentes, Cynthia
Flaherty, Maria Y.
Fouad, Nadya A.
Garcia, Betty
Ginorio, Angela B.
Gloria, Alberta M.
Kelton-Brand, Ana
Marotta, Sylvia A.
Miranda, David J.
Nuttall, Ena V.
Roehlke, Helen J.
Saldana, Delia H.
Santos de Barona, Maryann
Serrano-Garcia, Irma
Softas, Basilia C.
Towns-Miranda, Luz
Urbina, Susana P.
Urquiza, Anthony J.
Vasquez, Melba
Vazquez, Rosa
Zepeda, Marlene

-African American/Black and White/European

Greene, Karen J.

36 PSYCHOLOGY OF RELIGION

-African American/Black

Dockett, Kathleen H.
Henry, Vincent dePaul
Steele, Robert E.
Williams, Michael A.

-American Indian/Alaska Native

Foster, Rachel A.
Gant, Bob L.
Haddock, Dean M.
Sanders, Gilbert O.

-Asian American/Asian/Pacific Islander

Al-tai, Nazar M.
Austria, Asuncion M.
Manuel, Gerdenio M.
Moritsugu, John
Okagaki, Lynn
Tai, Chun-Nan
Tamura, Leonard J.
Tan, Siang-Yang Y.
Valdez, Jr., Romulo

-Hispanic/Latino

Azcarate, Eduardo M.

de Fuentes, Nanette
DeBlassie, III, Paul A.
Fayard, Carlos
Olmo, Manuel C.

37 CHILD, YOUTH, AND FAMILY SERVICES

-African American/Black

Beam, Micheline
Coleman, Hardin L.
Davis, Charles E.
Floyd, Bridget J.
Gulley, Silas
Hammond, W. Rodney
Jackson, John H.
King, Valerie
Louden, Delroy M.
Nesbitt, Eric B.
Parks, Carlton
Paster, Vera S.
Peters, Sheila
Samuel, Valerie J.
Scott-Jones, Diane
Slaughter-Defoe, Diana T.
Smith, Alvin E.
Ward, Alan J.

-American Indian/Alaska Native

Willis, Diane J.

-Asian American/Asian/Pacific Islander

Chan, Samuel Q.
Chew, Marion W.
Low, Benson P.
Luthar, Suniya S.
Serafica, Felicisima C.
Singh, Nirbhay N.
Takanishi, Ruby
Villejo, Ron E.
Yang, Raymond K.
Yoshimura, G. Joji

-Hispanic/Latino

Anderson, Claudia J.
Ayoub, Catherine C.
Azcarate, Eduardo M.
Carra, Sylvia F.
Castro-Blanco, David R.
Modiano, Rachel
Munoz, Luis A.
Santini-Hernandez, Ernesto
Towns-Miranda, Luz
Vargas, Luis A.

Zayas, Luis H.
Zepeda, Marlene

-American Indian/Alaska Native, Hispanic/Latino

Vargas, Alice M.

38 HEALTH PSYCHOLOGY

-African American/Black

Anderson, Norman B.
Belgrave, Faye Z
Collins, Edsmond J.
Collins, William
DeBardelaben, Garfield
Dingus, C. Mary
Greene, Anthony F.
Hall, Howard
Hammond, W. Rodney
Harris, Shanette M.
Hilton, William F.
Hunt, William K.
James, Larry C.
Jemmott, III, John B.
Keita, Gwendolyn P.
Louden, Delroy M.
Merritt, Marcellus M.
Miller, Robin L.
Myers, Hector F.
Poston, II, Walker S.
Robinson, John D
Solomon, Sondra E.
Steele, Robert E.
Vaughan, Elaine

-American Indian/Alaska Native

Campos, Peter E.
Sanders, Gilbert O.

-Asian American/Asian/Pacific Islander

Ahana, Ellen
Aoki, Melanie F.
Beattie, Muriel Y.
Chan, Daniel S.
Chin, Lemin
Chino, Allan F.
Chin, Sandra B
Fong, Geoffrey T.
Itatani, Robert M.
Kothandapani, Virupaksha
Lee, William W.
Leung, Paul
Lukman, Roy L.
Manese, Jeanne E.

Miyake, Steven M.
Mori, DeAnna L.
Nagy, Vivian T.
Nezu, Arthur M.
Oda, Ethel Aiko
Sasao, Toshiaki
Sato, Susan D.
Sitharthan, Thiagarajan
Wickramasekera, Ian E.
Yamaguchi, Mitsue Y.
Yee, Barbara W. K.
Young, David A.

-Hispanic/Latino

Abraido-Lanza, Ana F.
Amaro, Hortensia
Bernal, Guillermo A.
Boulon-Diaz, Frances E.
Carpenter, Gerald A.
Castro-Blanco, David R.
Chiriboga, David A.
Dooley, John A.
Hill, Jr., Sam S.
Incera, Armando
Maldonado, Loretto
Miranda, M.
Munoz, Luis A.
Munoz, Nina R.
Ortiz, Berta S.
Ovide, Christopher R.
Puente, Antonio E.
Romero, Augusto
Santini-Hernandez, Ernesto
Stern, Marilyn
Towns-Miranda, Luz
Velasquez, John M.
Vicente, Peter J.

39 PSYCHOANALYSIS

-African American/Black

Adams, C. Jama
Coleburn, Lila A.
Dunston, Patricia
Gump, Janice P.
Hamer, Forrest M.
Holmes, Dorothy E.
Howard, Mary T.
Hunt, Wilson L.
Johnson, David L.
Johnson, Zonya
Jones, Annie Lee
Leary, Kimberlyn
McIntyre, Lorna A.
Morris, Dolores O.
Ruffins, Stephen A.
Troutt, Bobbye V.

Vaughans, Kirkland C.

-American Indian/Alaska Native
Blue, Arthur W.
Eaton, Sheila J.

-Asian American/Asian/Pacific Islander
Campbell, Kamal E.
Ishida, Taeko H.
Khanna, Jaswant L.
Lee, Anna C.
Manuel, Gerdenio M.
Mody, Zarin R.
Tobias, Manuel D.
Wong, Philip S

-Hispanic/Latino
Ainslie, Ricardo C.
Arboleda, Catalina
Aviera, Arlene T.
Beato-Smith, Vera
Bernat, Gloria S.
Blanco-Beledo, Ricardo
De Louredes Mattei, Maria
DeBlassie, III, Paul A.
Dosamantes-Beaudry, Irma
Garrido-Castillo, Pedro
Genhart, Michael J.
Hill, Jr., Sam S.
Javier, Rafael A.
Lagomasino, Andrew J.
Lijtmaer, Ruth M.
Louredes Mattei, Maria De
Marina, Dorita
Mujica, Ernesto
Paredes, Jr., Frank C.
Peralta, Carmelina
Perez, Juan C.
Ramirez, David E.
Rigual-Lynch, Lourdes
Roll, Samuel
Ruth, Richard
Teixeira, Michael A.
Towns-Miranda, Luz
Vazquez, Rosa

-African American/Black and American Indian/Alaska Native
Hart, Anton H.

-Asian American/Asian/Pacific Islander and White/European
Pirhekayaty-Soriano, Tahereh

40 CLINICAL NEUROPSYCHOLOGY

-African American/Black
Allen, Christeen
Blanding, Benjamin
Caesar, Robert
Collins, Edsmond J.
Cook, Rudolf E.
Grant, Wanda F.
Hughes-Wheatland, Roxanne
Hunt, William K.
Johnson, David L.
Kemp, Arthur D.
Louden, Delroy M.
Miles, Gary T.
Nolan, Jr., Benjamin C.
Sapp, Marty
Solomon, Sondra E.
Strickland, Tony L.
Stringer, Anthony Y.
Trufant, Carol A.
Walker, Lila K.

-American Indian/Alaska Native
Bostwick, Allen D.
Durant, Jr., Adrian J.
Ertz, Dewey J.
Fain, Thomas C.
Haddock, Dean M.
Nolley, David A.
Richardson, E. Strong-Legs
Uzzell, Barbara P.
Williamson, Diane H.

-Asian American/Asian/Pacific Islander
Attore, Lois
Chang, Bradford W.
Chin, Raymond J.
Drieberg, Keith L
Fujii, Daryl E. M.
Gam, John
Gasquoine, Philip G.
Gutterman, Carmen Y.
Hom, Jim
Hoshino, Frank
Itatani, Robert M.
Jay, Milton T.
Jin, Young-Sun
Kothandapani, Virupaksha
Lau, Godwin
Leung, Paul
Lim, Patricia J.
Loong, James

Minturn, Robin H.
Rohila, Pritam K.
Sax, Kenji W.
Sitharthan, Thiagarajan
Sy, Michael J.
Tobias, Manuel D.
Tsang, Michael Hing-Pui
Wong-Ngan, Julia A.
Wong, Jane L.

-Hispanic/Latino
Alvarez, Manuel E.
Armengol, Carmen G.
Artiola, Lydia
Badillo, Diana
Barnes, Charles A.
Bastien, IV, Samuel A.
Benzaquen, Isaac
Berrill, Naftali G.
Boone, Martin
Borrego, Richard L.
Camargo, Robert J.
Canedo, Angelo R.
Carpenter, Gerald A.
Carra, Sylvia F.
Castro-Blanco, David R.
Chavez, Ernest L.
Cimino, Cynthia R.
Colon, Luis H.
Cuesta, George M.
De la Serna, Marcelo
Del Rio, Augusto B.
Diaz-Machado, Carmen B.
Diaz, Raul
Echemendia, Ruben J.
Feldman, Esther
Ferreira, Pedro M.
Garrido-Castillo, Pedro
Harris, Josette G
Herrera-Pino, Jorge A.
Javier, Rafael A.
Kirst, Stephen P.
Llorente, Antolin M.
Marmol, Leonardo M.
Monguio, Ines
Monserrat, Laura
Montijo, Jorge A.
Morales, Pamilla V.
Morote, Gloria
Natalicio, Luiz
Otero, Rafael F.
Perez-Arce, Patricia
Pompa, Janiece L.
Porges, Carlos R.
Puente, Antonio E.
Ramos-Grenier, Julia
Rey-Casserly, Celiane M.

Rodriguez, Carlos J.
Salais, A. Joseph
Sanchez-Caso, Luis M.
Saucedo, Carlos
Sedo, Manuel A.
Suarez, Enrique M.
Tamayo, Jose M.
Urbina, Susana P.
Valdivia, Lino
Vega, Jose G.
Vega, Star
Villela, Leopoldo F.

-Asian American/Asian/Pacific Islander
Garg, Mithlesh

-American Indian/Alaska Native, White/European
Hough, Sigmund

41 AMERICAN PSYCHOLOGY-LAW SOCIETY

-African American/Black
Atwell, Robert L.
Coleburn, Lila A.
Elion, Victor H.
Everett, Moses L.
Hart, Allen J.
Johnson, Matthew B.
Lewis, George R.
Pope-Tarrence, Jacqueline R.
Seymour, Guy O.
Tucker, James L.
Williams, Eddie E.
Wright, Michael F.

-American Indian/Alaska Native
Bowen, Peggy C.
Fain, Thomas C.
Foster, Daniel V.
James, Steven E
Willis, Cynthia E.

-Asian American/Asian/Pacific Islander
Ascano, Ricardo
Coggins, Margaret H.
Fong, Larry
Gock, Terry S.
Itatani, Robert M.
Kagehiro, Dorthy K.
Khorakiwala, Durriyah

Kop, Tim M.
Kothandapani, Virupaksha
Minagawa, Rahn Y.
Nagayama Hall, Gordon C.
Quijano, Walter Y.
Smith, Teresa D.
Tsushima, William T.

-Hispanic/Latino

Alfaro-Garcia, Rafael A.
Alvarez, Manuel E.
Aviera, Arlene T.
Ayoub, Catherine C.
Beliz, Jr., Efrain A.
Bencomo, Armando A.
Benzaquen, Isaac
Boulon-Diaz, Frances E.
Campos, Leonard P.
Caraveo, Libardo E.
Chatigny, Anita L.
Collado, Armando
De Apodaca, Roberto F.
De Armas, Armando
de Jesus, Nelson H.
Diaz, Raul
Echavarria, David
Fankhanel, Edward H.
Garcia, Lazaro
Grosso, Federico C.
Hill, Jr., Sam S.
Huergo, Mayra
Llanos, Aracely B.
Marmol, Leonardo M.
Morales, Elias
Mussenden, Gerald
Natalicio, Luiz
Nunez, Narina N.
Ovide, Christopher R.
Panciera, Lawrence A.
Paredes, Jr., Frank C.
Ramos-Grenier, Julia
Reisinger, Mercedes C.
Roll, Samuel
Romey, Carol M.
Rosado, John W.
Sanchez-Caso, Luis M.
Sanchez, H.G.
Santini-Hernandez, Ernesto
Schacht, Thomas E.
Suarez, Enrique M.
Towns-Miranda, Luz
Viale-val, Graciela
Zaragoza, Maria S.

42 PSYCHOLOGISTS IN INDEPENDENT PRACTICE

-African American/Black

Adams, Jr., Clarence L.
Allsopp, Ralph N.
Artis, Daphne J.
Bamgbose, Olujiimi O.
Banks, Karel L.
Belton, Monique
Bennett, Maisha H.
Block, Carolyn B.
Boxley, Russell L.
Brice, Janet R.
Briggs, Felicia H.
Brodie, Debra A.
Browne, Ronald H.
Bryant-Tuckett, Rose M.
Buffin, Janice E.
Burchell, Charles R.
Cameron, Linda S.
Carter, Allen C.
Coleman, Willie J.
Davis-Russell, Elizabeth
Dawson, Harriett E.
Dudley-Grant, G. Rita
Elion, Victor H.
Evans, Helen L.
Farley, Florence S.
Fleming, Andrea L.
Freeman, Charlotte M.
Greene, Clifford
Griffin, Patricia L.
Guillory, Paul T.
Hall, Juanita L.
Hammond, Gladys
Hammond, W. Rodney
Hare, Nathan
Henry, Vincent dePaul
Houston, Holly O.
Jackson, Helen L.
James, Lainee M.
Jennings, Valdea D.
Jones, Ferdinand
King, Valerie
LeSure-Lester, G. Evelyn
Lewis, Brenda J.
Mobley, Brenda D.
Musgrove, Barbara J.
Nicholson, Liston O.
Payton, Carolyn R.
Peters, James S.
Pettigrew, Dorothy C.
Pinderhughes, Ellen B.
Powell, Lois
Savage, Jr., James E.
Searcy, Mary L.
Stringer, Anthony Y.

Swanston, Melvon C.
Tate, Donald
Trufant, Carol A.
Tucker, Dorothy M.
Tucker, Samuel J.
Turner, Alvin L.
Vanderhost, Leonette
Ward, Alan J.
Whitehead, Jesse
Whitten, Lisa A.
Williams, Karen P. W.
Williams, Michael A.
Wilson, Shirley B.

-American Indian/Alaska Native

Brooks, Jr., Glenwood C.
Cummings, Joseph D.
Durant, Jr., Adrian J.
Fields, Amanda H.
Pine, Charles J.
Prutsman, Thomas D.
Rainwater, III, Avie J.
Sadler, Mark S.
Sanders, Gilbert O.
Willis, Diane J.

-Asian American/Asian/Pacific Islander

Ahana, Ellen
Chan, Darrow A.
Chang, Bradford W.
Chang, Theodore C. H.
Chin, Sandra B.
Chiu, Loanne
Fong, Jane Y.
Fujioka, Terry Ann T.
Fujita, George T.
Fung, Hellen C.
Gee, Carol S.
Gong, Susan M.
Higashi, Wilfred H.
Higa, William R.
Hiroto, Donald S.
Ho, Chin-Chin
Kupur, Veena
Lau, Lavay
Loo, Russell
Lu, Elsie G.
Matsumoto, Gregory Y.
Matsuura, Larry N.
Minagawa, Rahn Y.
Moon, Tae-Hyun
Moy, Samuel
Nishi-Strattner, Linda
Rangoonwala, Rafique
Saraf, Komal C.

Sharma, Satanand
Sharma, Vijai P.
Sun, Irene L.
Takemoto-Chock, Naomi
Torigoe, Rodney Y.
Valdez, Jr., Romulo
Vance, Ellen B.
Villejo, Ron E.
Wagner, Aureen Pinto
Wong, Dorothy L.
Young, David A.
Yuen, Lenora L.
Yu, Pamela

-Hispanic/Latino

Abordo, Enrique J.
Arcaya, Jose M.
Arsuaga, Enrique N.
Azcarate, Eduardo M.
Azevedo, Don Fernando
Barry, Martha J.
Basco, Monica A.
Bascuas, Joseph W.
Beliz, Jr., Efrain A.
Bernat, Gloria S.
Berrill, Naftali G.
Bracero, William
Burciaga, Lawrence E.
Canovas Welles, Nydia L.
Chapa, Joel R.
Cherbosque, Jorge
Chriss, Gloria M.
Colon, R. Phillip
Comas-Diaz, Lillian
Cruz, Vivian A.
de Jesus, Nelson H.
Diaz, Raul
Elena Lee, Karen
Ellis, Edwin E.
Escandell, Vincent A.
Escovar, Luis A.
Esparza, Ricardo
Ficher, Ilda V.
Garcia, Michael A.
Giraldo, Macario
Goebes, Diane D.
Gonzalez, Laura A.
Gubler, Lyle W.
Hammond, Evelyn S.
Healy, James M.
Incera, Armando
Johnson, Paul W.
Kelton-Brand, Ana
Kolt, Laurie
Laguna, John N.
Lerma, Joe L.
Manghi, Elina R.

Martinez, Alejandro M.
Masini, Angela
Mellor-Crummey, Cynthia A.
Munoz, John A.
Nieves, Luis R.
Ortiz, Berta S.
Pincheira, Juan A.
Pompa, Janiece L.
Ramirez-Cancel, Carlos M.
Rivera, Miquela
Rubio, Charles T.
Sarmiento, Robert F.
Saunders, Walter C.
Schlesinger, Susana J.
Teitel, Raquel S.
Towns-Miranda, Luz
Turner, Darrell D.
Vargas, Manuel J.
Vasquez, Melba
Vazquez, Carlos D.
Villela, Leopoldo F.
Whitaker, Sandra V.

-Asian American/Asian/Pacific Islander
Leung, Alex C. N.

-Hispanic/Latin
Rivera-Lopez, Hector

-African American/Black and American Indian/Alaska Native
Brooks, Juanita O.

-African American/Black and Hispanic/Latino
Martin, William F.

43 FAMILY PSYCHOLOGY

-African American/Black
Baly, Iris E.
Brice, Janet R.
Dobbins, James E.
Griffith, Stanford
McMillan, Robert
Moore, C. L.
Roberts, Harrell B.
Rountree, Yvonne B.
Stokes, Devon R.
Williams, Michael A.

-American Indian/Alaska Native
Blair, Deborah G.
Carter, William J.

James, Steven E.
Williams, Mary Beth

-Asian American/Asian/Pacific Islander
Anand, Shashi
Ham, MaryAnna D.
Hong, George K.
Lukman, Roy L.
Ma, Yat-Ming C.
Mock, Matthew R.
Nishi-Strattner, Linda
Seitz, Kathleen
Tien, Liang
Vance, Ellen B.

-Hispanic/Latino
Anderson, Claudia J.
Araoz, Daniel L.
Atilano, Raymond B.
Bacigalupe, Gonzalo M.
Cardona, Gilbert
Carra, Sylvia F.
Cervantes, Joseph M.
Falicov, Celia J.
Gardano, Anna C.
Inclan, Jaime
Mellor-Crummey, Cynthia A.
Montes, Francisco
Nazario, Jr., Andres
Ruiz, Nicholas J.
Tostado, John F.
Towns-Miranda, Luz
Vazquez, Cesar D.
Vazquez, Rosa

-American Indian/Alaska Native, White/European
Hough, Sigmund

44 SOCIETY FOR THE PSYCHOLOGICAL STUDY OF LESBIAN, GAY AND BISEXUAL ISSUES

-African American/Black
Campbell-Flint, Maxine E.
Gillem, Angela R.
Greene, Beverly
Hall, Ruth L.
Johnson, Johnny
Lawson, Jasper J.
Parks, Carlton
Robinson, John D
Scott, Linda D.
Smith, Alvin E.

White, Voncile

-American Indian/Alaska Native
Blubaugh, Victoria G.
Campos, Peter E.
James, Steven E
Pope, Mark

-Asian American/Asian/Pacific Islander
Chan, Connie S.
Chung, Y. Barry
Fukuyama, Mary A.
Gock, Terry S.
Kich, George K.
Kich, George Kitahara
Omoto, Allen M.
Root, Maria P. P.
Sue, Derald W.
Wong, Frankie Y.

-Hispanic/Latino
Amaro, Hortensia
Arellano, Charleanea
Baron, Augustine
Benitez, John C.
Carballo-Dieguez, Alex
Diaz-Machado, Carmen B.
Gonzales, Michael
Lawson, Gary W.
Morales, Eduardo S.
Nazario, Jr., Andres
Rodriguez, Richard A.
Roehlke, Helen J.
Rosario, Margaret
Vasquez, Melba

45 SOCIETY FOR THE PSYCHOLOGICAL STUDY OF ETHNIC MINORITY ISSUES

-African American/Black
Abernethy, Alexis D.
Abston, Jr., Nathaniel
Alston, Denise A.
Anderson, Linda
Anderson, Louis P.
Anderson, Norman B.
Artis, Daphne J.
Asbury, Jo-Ellen
Atwell, Robert L.
Bamgbose, Olujiimi O.
Banks, Martha E.
Barbarin, Oscar A.
Barker-Hackett, Lori

Barnes, Michael J.
Bastien, Rochelle T.
Baxter, Anthony G.
Beckles, Nicola
Belgrave, Faye Z.
Belton, Monique
Bingham, Rosie P.
Binion, Victoria J.
Block, Carolyn B.
Brice, Janet R.
Brookins, Geraldine K
Brown, John R.
Burnett Young, Myra N.
Caldwell-Colbert, A. Toy
Carter, Robert T.
Coleburn, Lila A.
Coleman, Hardin L.
Coleman, Willie J.
Constantine, Madonna G.
Cook, Donelda
Cunningham, Michael
Curry, Alpha O.
Davis-Russell, Elizabeth
Dawson, Harriett E.
DeFour, Darlene C.
Dobbins, James E.
Dockett, Kathleen H.
Dudley-Grant, G. Rita
Epps, Pamela J.
Essandoh, Pius K.
Everett, Moses L.
Fairchild, Halford H.
Floyd, Bridget J.
Francisco, Richard P.
Friday, Jennifer C.
Gaines, Stanley O.
Garner, Edward L.
Gillem, Angela R.
Gloster, Janice L.
Gordon, Kimberly A.
Graham, Sandra
Greene, Anthony F.
Greene, Beverly
Greene, Clifford
Greene, Lorraine
Gulley, Silas
Gump, Janice P.
Hall, Ruth L.
Hammond, Gladys
Hammond, W. Rodney
Hanley, Jerome H.
Harrell, Shelly P.
Hayles, V. Robert
Henderson Daniel, Jessica
Hines, Laura M.
Holliday, Bertha G.
Hooker, Olivia J.
Howard, Mary T.

Hughes-Wheatland, Roxanne
Hunt, Wilson L.
Jackson, Anna M.
Jackson, Jacquelyne F.
Jackson, James S.
Jackson, Leslie C.
Jemmott, III, John B.
Jenkins-Monroe, Valata
Jenkins, Adelbert H
Jenkins, Yvonne M
Johnson, Zonya
Jones, Elaine F.
Jones, Hugh E.
Jones, James M.
Joseph, Jr., Herbert M.
Keita, Gwendolyn P.
Kennedy, Clive D.
King, Valerie
Langley, Merlin R.
Lawrence, Stephen N.
Lawson, Jasper J.
LeSure-Lester, G. Evelyn
Levermore, Monique A.
London, Dyanne P.
Luke, Equilla
Mack, Delores E.
Maynard, Edward S.
McClure, Faith H.
McRae, Mary B.
Milburn, Norweeta G.
Miller, Fayneese
Monteiro, Rita C.
Moore, Sandra
Morris, Joseph R.
Mosley-Howard, Gerri S.
Munford, Paul R.
Myers, Hector F.
Nettles, Arie L.
Nickerson, Kim J.
Nzewi, Esther N.
Okorodudu, Corahann
Parham, Thomas A.
Parks, Carlton
Parks, Fayth M.
Paster, Vera S.
Penn, Nolan E.
Phelps, Rosemary E.
Pinderhughes, Ellen B.
Pope-Davis, Donald B.
Porche-Burke, Lisa M.
Porter, Julia
Pugh, Roderick W.
Reid, Pamela T.
Richard, Harriette W.
Roberts, Harrell B.
Robertson, John F.
Robinson, Gregory F.
Robinson, John D.

Robinson, W. LaVome
Rollock, David
Ross, Sandra I.
Samuels, Robert M.
Samuel, Valerie J.
Sanders-Thompson, Vetta L.
Sanders, Daniel W.
Scott-Jones, Diane
Scott, Linda D.
Seymour, Guy O.
Shaw, Paula
Simpson, Adelaide W.
Singleton, Edward G.
Slaughter-Defoe, Diana T.
Smith, William F.
Speight, Suzette L.
Spencer, Margaret B.
Spivey, Philop B.
Steele, Robert E.
Stewart, Vlenaetha
Stokes, Devon R.
Swanston, Melvon C.
Tatum, Beverly D.
Thomas, Anita J.
Thomas, Hilton T.
Thompson, Chalmer E.
Tomes, Henry
Trufant, Carol A.
Tucker, Dorothy M.
Turner, Castellano
Turner, Samuel M.
Vontress, Clemmont E.
Watts, Roderick J.
Webb, Wanda
Weston, Raymond E.
Whitten, Lisa A.
Williams, Medria L.
Williams, Michael A.
Wilson, Melvin N.
Wilson, Susan B.
Wilson, Woodrow
Winfrey, LaPearl L.
Wright, Doris J.
Wyatt, Gail E.
Wyche, Karen F.
Wynne, Michael

-American Indian/Alaska Native

Blue, Arthur W.
Derocher, Terry L.
Durant, Jr., Adrian J.
Fain, Thomas C.
Fleming, Candace M.
Foster, Daniel V.
Foster, Rachel A.
Haddock, Dean M.

Horvat, Jr., Joseph J.
James, Steven E.
LaDue, Robin A.
LaFromboise, Teresa
Lashley, Karen H.
Love, Craig T.
McDonald, Arthur L.
Pine, Charles J.
Pope, Mark
Quinn, Lisa
Ryan, Loye M.
Ryan, Robert A.
Trimble, Joseph E.
Vraniak, Damian A.
Willis, Diane J.

-Asian American/Asian/Pacific Islander

Abudabbeh, Nuha
Akimoto, Sharon A.
Asamen, Joy K.
Austria, Asuncion M.
Bradshaw, Carla K.
Chan, Connie S.
Chan, Darrow A.
Chan, Samuel Q.
Chao, Christine M.
Chew, Marion W.
Chin, Jean L.
Collins, James F.
Dong, Tim T.
Fergus, Esther O.
Fugita, Stephen S.
Fukuyama, Mary A.
Gock, Terry S.
Goh, David S.
Hall, Christine I.
Hamada, Roger S.
Ham, MaryAnna D.
Hass, Giselle A.
Ho, Christine K.
Hong, George K.
Hsia, Heidi
Huang, Larke N.
Ichiyama, Michael A.
Itatani, Robert M.
Iwamasa, Gayle Y.
Izawa, Chizuko
Ja, Davis Y.
Junn, Ellen
Kao, Barbara T.
Kee, PooKong
Khanna, Jaswant L.
Khanna, Mukti
Kich, George K.
Kich, George Kitahara
Kim, Elizabeth J.
Koh, Tong-He

Kwon, Paul H.
Lau, Lavay
Lee, Wanda M. L.
Leong, Frederick T. T.
Leung, Paul
Leung, S. Alvin
Lin, J.C. Gisela G.
Lin, Jeanne L.
Lu, Elsie G.
Lui, Barbara J.
Manese, Jeanne E.
Mar, Norman J.
Maruyama, Geoffrey
Mio, Jeffery S.
Miyahira, Sarah D.
Mock, Matthew R.
Morishige, Howard H.
Moritsugu, John
Murakawa, Fay
Nagata, Donna K.
Nakagawa, Janice Y.
Nemoto, Tooru
Nezu, Arthur M.
Ng, James T.
Nguyen, Dao Q.
Oda, Ethel Aiko
Okiyama, Stephen L.
Omoto, Allen M.
Onizuka, Richard K.
Ozaki, Mona M.
Root, Maria P. P.
Sakamoto, Katsuyuki
Sasao, Toshiaki
Shirakawa, Patti
Sodowsky, Gargi R.
Stewart, Sunita M.
Sue, Derald W.
Sue, Stanley
Tamayo, Federico M. V.
Tamura, Leonard J.
Teo, Thomas
Torigoe, Rodney Y.
True, Reiko Homma
Tsukamoto, Donna E.
Wong, Frankie Y.
Yabusaki, Ann S.
Yee, Barbara W. K.
Yee, Jennie Hy
Ying, Yu-Wen
Young, David A.
Zane, Nolan W.S

-Hispanic/Latino

Abraido-Lanza, Ana F.
Adler, Peter J.
Alfaro-Garcia, Rafael A.
Alvarez, Gary L.
Alvarez, Maria D.

Amaro, Hortensia
Anderson, Claudia J.
Aponte, Joseph F.
Arbona, Consuelo
Ardila, Ruben
Arellano, Charleanea
Arenas, Jr., Silverio
Arredondo, Patricia
Arreola-Rockwell, Fran
     Pepitone-
Arroyo, Judith A.
Ascencao, Erlete M.
Auuilas-Gaxiola, Sergio A.
Balderrama, Sylvia R.
Barona, Andres
Baron, Augustine
Basco, Monica A.
Beato-Smith, Vera
Benitez, John C.
Bernal, Guillermo
Bernal, Martha E.
Betancourt, Hector
Blandino, Ramon A.
Boulon-Diaz, Frances E.
Bracero, William
Bruguera, Mark R.
Bursztyn, Alberto M.
Camarillo, Max
Canovas Welles, Nydia L.
Cardalda, Elsa B.
Caro, Yvette
Castro-Blanco, David R.
Chavez, Ernest L.
Colon, Luis H.
Comas-Diaz, Lillian
Contreras, Raquel J.
Cordero, Fernando
Crespo, Gloria M.
Cruz, Vivian A.
De La Cancela, Victor
de Llano, Carmen
De Lourdes Mattei, Maria
Dhimitri, Patricio
Diaz, Eduardo I.
Falicov, Celia J.
Flores, Elena
Garcia-Coll, Cynthia
Garcia-Gonzalez, Jose A.
Garcia, Betty
Garcia, Luis T.
Garrido-Castillo, Pedro
Ginorio, Angela B.
Gloria, Alberta M.
Gomez, Ana L.
Gomez, John P.
Gomez, Madeleine Y.
Gonsalves, Carlos J.
Gonzales, Michael

Gonzales, Ricardo R.
Gonzalez, Gerardo M
Gonzalez, Haydee M.
Grajales, Elisa M.
Grunhaus-Belzer, Rosa
Guzman, L. Philip
Harris, Josette G
Herrera-Pino, Jorge A.
Hill, Jr., Sam S.
Inclan, Jaime
Jarama, S. Lisbeth
Javier, Rafael A.
Juarez, Reina M.
Lijtmaer, Ruth M
Linares, Lourdes O.
Lopez-Baez, Sandra I.
Lopez, Emilia
Lopez, Steven R.
Lorenzo, Gladys
Louredes Mattei, Maria De
Loyola, Jaime L.
Machabanski, Hector
Marin, Gerardo
Marmol, Leonardo M.
Martinez, Jr., Joe L.
Martinez, Raul
Millan, Fred
Miranda, Manuel R.
Morales-Barreto, Gisela
Morales, Eduardo S.
Morales, Pamilla V.
Mujica, Ernesto
Munoz, Ricardo F.
Nazario, Jr., Andres
Niemann, Yolanda F
Nieves, Luis R.
Olivero, Gerald
Olmedo, Esteban L.
Paniagua, Freddy A.
Paredes, Jr., Frank C.
Peralta, Carmelina
Prendes-Lintel, Maria L.
Puente, Antonio E.
Quintana, Stephen M.
Ramirez, John/Juan
Ramos, Arnaldo J.
Rezentes, III, William C.
Rivera, Nelson E.
Rivera-Lopez, Hector
Rodriguez, Luis J.
Rodriguez, Richard A.
Roehlke, Helen J.
Rogler, Lloyd H.
Roll, Samuel
Rosado, John W.
Rosario, Margaret
Ruth, Richard
Saenz, Javier

Saldana, Delia H.
Santiago-Negron, Salvador
Santos de Barona, Maryann
Serrano-Garcia, Irma
Soriano, Fernando I.
Tabachnik, Samuel
Takushi, Ruby Y.
Tazeau, Yvette N.
Towns-Miranda, Luz
Urquiza, Anthony J.
Valdivia, Lino
Vargas, Luis A.
Vasquez, Melba
Vega, Star
Velasquez, Roberto J.
Vera, Elizabeth M.
Yniguez, Linda E.
Zavala-Martinez, Iris
Zayas, Luis H.
Zepeda, Marlene

-African American/Black and American Indian/Alaska Native
Dent, Harold E.
Hargrove, Jr., Jerry E.
Somerville, Addison W.

-African American/Black and Hispanic/Latino
Parson, Erwin R.

-American Indian/Alaska Native, Hispanic/Latino
Vargas, Alice M.

-Asian American/Asian/Pacific Islander, Hispanic/Latino
Garcia, Melinda A.
Unson, Delia C. O.

-Hispanic/Latino, White/ European
McNeill, Brian

46 MEDIA PSYCHOLOGY

-African American/Black
Brodie, Debra A.
Johnson, Zonya
Walcott, Delores D.

-Asian American/Asian/Pacific Islander
Villejo, Ron E.

-Hispanic/Latino
Berrill, Naftali G.
Comas-Diaz, Lillian
Garcia, Pedro I.
Gardano, Anna C.
Santiago-Negron, Salvador
Towns-Miranda, Luz

47 EXERCISE AND SPORT PSYCHOLOGY

-African American/Black
Allen, Jane E.
Bamgbose, Olujiimi O.
Barber, Kevin V.
Hall, Ruth L.
Stewart, Vlenaetha
Thomas, Hilton T.
Wilson, Woodrow

-American Indian/Alaska Native
Everson, Howard T.
Hartzell, Richard E.

-Asian American/Asian/Pacific Islander
Birky, Ian
Caberto, Steven C.
Chan, Connie S.
Hom, Harry L.
Sax, Kenji W.
Tamura, Leonard J.
Wang, Youde
Young, David A.

-Hispanic/Latino
Arellano-Lopez, Juan
Kelly, Tara L.
Labbe, Elise E.
Madison, James K.
Valdivia, Lino

48 PEACE PSYCHOLOGY

-African American/Black
Fairchild, Halford H.
Okorodudu, Corahann
Price, Linda A.
Trufant, Carol A.

-Asian American/Asian/Pacific Islander
D'Heurle, Adma J.
Khanna, Mukti

-Hispanic/Latino

Alvarez, Carlos M.
Betancourt, Hector
Diaz-Machado, Carmen B.
Kelton-Brand, Ana
Lopez, Sarah C.
Schlesinger, Susana J.

**-African American/Black and
American Indian/Alaska Native**

Hart, Anton H.

49 GROUP PSYCHOLOGY AND GROUP PSYCHOTHERAPY

-African American/Black

Hambright, Jerold E.
Howard, Mary T.
Isaacs, Owen K.
Jones, Ruby M.
Muiu, Charles
Penn, Nolan E.
Peters, Sheila
Robinson, John D.
Rountree, Yvonne B.
Sampson, Myrtle B.
Stallworth, Lisa M.
Wilson, Shirley B.

-American Indian/Alaska Native

Atkinson, Michael B.
Blair, Deborah G.
Fain, Thomas C.

-Asian American/Asian/Pacific Islander

Ahmed, Mohiuddin
Chen, Eric C.
Khanna, Jaswant L.
Kothandapani, Virupaksha
Morishige, Howard H.
Verghese, Cherian

-Hispanic/Latino

Bernat, Gloria S.
Bracero, William
Flachier, Roberto
Flores, Philip J.
Lerma, Joe L.
Marotta, Sylvia A.
Nadal-Vazquez, Vilma Y.
Rivera, Jo Ann M.
Saenz, Karol K.

Stasson, Mark F.
Vasquez, Melba

**-African American/Black and
American Indian/Alaska Native**

Hart, Anton H.

**-American Indian/Alaska
Native, White/European**

Hough, Sigmund

50 ADDICTIONS

-African American/Black

Collins, Edsmond J.
Greene, Lorraine
Johnson, David L.
Jones, Ruby M.
Kennedy, Clive D.
Robertson, John F.
Singleton, Edward G.
Spivey, Philop B.
Strickland, Tony L.

-American Indian/Alaska Native

Love, Craig T.
Pope, Mark
Reandeau, Sharon L
Sanders, Gilbert O.
Young, Kimberly S.

-Asian American/Asian/Pacific Islander

Ichiyama, Michael A.
Iguchi, Martin Y.
Ja, Davis Y.
Jay, Milton T.
Kothandapani, Virupaksha
Powers, Keiko I.
Tamura, Leonard J.

-Hispanic/Latino

Alvarez, Paul A.
Antonuccio, David
Flores, Philip J.
Gonzales, Ricardo R.
Laguna, John N.
Morales, Eduardo S.
Santiago-Negron, Salvador

**-African American/Black,
American Indian/Alaska Native**

Somerville, Addison W.

51 SOCIETY FOR THE PSYCHOLOGICAL STUDY OF MEN AND MASCULINITY

-African American/Black

Allsopp, Ralph N.
Bingham, Rosie P.
Cunningham, Michael
Lawson, Jasper J.
Robinson, John D.
Smith, Alvin E.
Wilson, Melvin N.

-American Indian/Alaska Native

Silling, S. Marc

-Asian American/Asian/Pacific Islander

Perez, Ruperto M.

-Hispanic/Latino

Boulon-Diaz, Frances E.
De La Cancela, Victor
Inclan, Jaime
Morales, Eduardo S.
Munoz, Luis A.
Olguin, Arthur
Tostado, John F.

52 INTERNATIONAL PSYCHOLOGY

-African American/Black

Dudley-Grant, G. Rita
Jackson, James S.
Johnson, Sylvia T
Keita, Gwendolyn P.
Okorodudu, Corahann
Oshodi, John
Penn, Nolan E.
Price, Linda A.
Robinson, John D.
Ruffins, Stephen A.

-American Indian/Alaska Native

Pope, Mark

-Asian American/Asian/Pacific Islander

Abudabbeh, Nuha
Chia, Rosina
Gock, Terry S.
Hass, Giselle A.
Joshi, Sheila

Kannarkat, Joy P.
Khanna, Jaswant L.
Lee, Anna C.
Leong, Frederick T. T.
Leung, Paul
Lu, Elsie G.
Miyahira, Sarah D.
Sasao, Toshiaki
Schroff, Kamal
Stewart, Sunita M.
Suinn, Richard M.
Tanaka-Matsumi, Junko
Tan, Josephine
Torigoe, Rodney Y.
Tung, May
Velayo, Richard S.

-Hispanic/Latino

Amezaga, Jr., Alfredo M.
Bascuas, Joseph W.
Betancourt, Hector
Cardena, Etzel A.
Comas-Diaz, Lillian
de Fuentes, Nanette
De La Cancela, Victor
Diaz-Guerrero, Rogelio
Javier, Rafael A.
Marmol, Leonardo M.
Mejia, Juan A.
Puente, Antonio E.
Quintana, Stephen M.
Santiago-Negron, Salvador
Sanua, Victor D.
Soriano, Marcel
Tazeau, Yvette N.

53 CLINICAL CHILD PSYCHOLOGY

-African American/Black

Floyd, Bridget J.
Scott-Jones, Diane

-Asian American/Asian/Pacific Islander

Aoki, Wayne T.
Chin, Raymond J.
Shum, Hilda B.
Shum, Hilda B.
Singh, Nirbhay N.

-Hispanic/Latino

Aguilera, David M.
Kelton-Brand, Ana
Tazeau, Yvette N.
Urquiza, Anthony J.

**-African American/Black,
American Indian/Alaska Native**

    Somerville, Addison W.

54 THE SOCIETY OF PEDIATRIC PSYCHOLOGY

-African American/Black

    Nettles, Arie L.
    Strickland, Tony L
    Treadwell, Marsha J.
    Wilson, Melvin N.

-Asian American/Asian/Pacific Islander

    Chan, Daniel S.
    Chin, Raymond J.
    Lee, William W.
    Mar, Harvey H.
    Mori, DeAnna L.
    Shum, Hilda B.
    Shum, Hilda B.

-Hispanic/Latino

    Alvarez, Maria D.
    Cervantes, Joseph M.
    Comas-Diaz, Lillian
    Fernandez, Maria C.
    Hall, M. Elizabeth L.
    Modiano, Rachel
    Munoz, Luis A.
    Pompa, Janiece L.
    Rey-Casserly, Celiane M.
    Stern, Marilyn

**-African American/Black,
American Indian/Alaska Native**

    Somerville, Addison W.

55 AMERICAN SOCIETY FOR THE ADVANCEMENT OF PHARMACOTHERAPY

-American Indian/Alaska Native

    Love, Craig T.

APA Division
Fellow Listing

Qualified APA members may, on nomination by an APA division and election by the APA Council of Representatives, become Fellows of the APA. Fellows must "...present evidence of unusual or outstanding contribution or performance in the field of psychology."

Information in this section is listed in the following order:

Divisions (numerically ordered; and under each:)

Ethnic Group (and under each:)

Names (alphabetized)

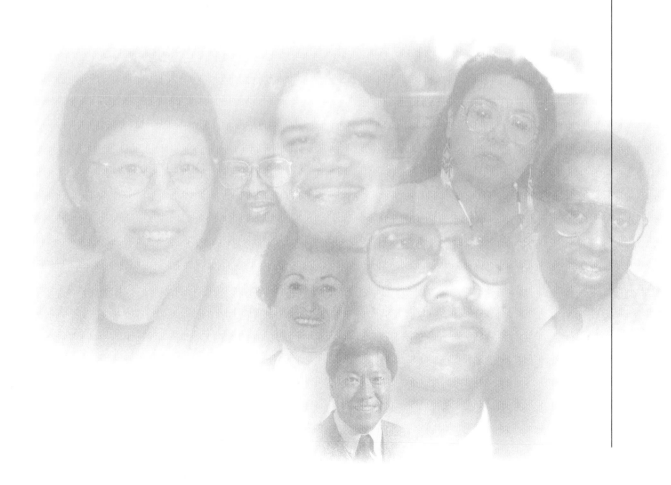

APA DIVISION FELLOW LISTING

01 GENERAL PSYCHOLOGY

-American Indian/Alaska Native
Babb, Harold

-Asian American/Asian/Pacific Islander
Izawa, Chizuko
Randhawa, Bikkar S.
Sax, Kenji W.
Sue, Derald W.

-Hispanic/Latino
Sanua, Victor D.
Vasquez, Melba

02 SOCIETY FOR THE TEACHING OF PSYCHOLOGY

-African American/Black
Porche-Burke, Lisa M.

-Asian American/Asian/Pacific Islander
Mehrotra, Chandra M.N.

-Hispanic/Latino
Puente, Antonio E.
Serrano-Garcia, Irma

03 EXPERIMENTAL PSYCHOLOGY

-African American/Black
Penn, Nolan E.

-Asian American/Asian/Pacific Islander
Izawa, Chizuko

05 EVALUATION, MEASUREMENT AND STATISTICS

-Asian American/Asian/Pacific Islander
Goh, David S.

06 BEHAVIORAL NEUROSCIENCE AND COMPARATIVE PSYCHOLOGY

-Hispanic/Latino
Bracero, William
Sanua, Victor D.

07 DEVELOPMENTAL PSYCHOLOGY

-Asian American/Asian/Pacific Islander
Sax, Kenji W.

-Hispanic/Latino
Bracero, William

-Hispanic/Latino and White/European
Burton, Roger V.

08 SOCIETY FOR PERSONALITY AND SOCIAL PSYCHOLOGY

-Hispanic/Latino
Sanua, Victor D.

09 SOCIETY FOR THE PSYCHOLOGICAL STUDY OF SOCIAL ISSUES - SPSSI

-African American/Black
Jackson, Anna M.
Pugh, Roderick W.

-American Indian/Alaska Native
Trimble, Joseph E.

-Asian American/Asian/Pacific Islander
Maruyama, Geoffrey

-Hispanic/Latino
Chiriboga, David A.
Morales, Eduardo S.
Sanua, Victor D.

10 PSYCHOLOGY AND THE ARTS

-African American/Black
Lawson, Jasper J.

-Hispanic/Latino
Bracero, William

12 CLINICAL PSYCHOLOGY

-African American/Black
Caldwell-Colbert, A. Toy
Gray-Little, Bernadette
Greene, Beverly
Jenkins, Adelbert H
Lawson, Jasper J.
Penn, Nolan E.
Pugh, Roderick W.
Rivers, Miriam W.
Robinson, John D.
Turner, Samuel M.

-American Indian/Alaska Native
Willis, Diane J.

-Asian American/Asian/Pacific Islander
Austria, Asuncion M.
Nezu, Arthur M.
Sue, Stanley
Tanaka-Matsumi, Junko

-Hispanic/Latino
Lopez, Steven R.
Sanua, Victor D.

13 CONSULTING PSYCHOLOGY

-African American/Black
Jackson, John H.
Wilson, Susan B.

15 EDUCATIONAL PSYCHOLOGY

-African American/Black
Johnson, Sylvia T

-Asian American/Asian/Pacific Islander
Goh, David S.
Randhawa, Bikkar S.

-Hispanic/Latino
Reyna, Valerie F.

16 SCHOOL PSYCHOLOGY

-African American/Black
Hines, Laura M.
Jackson, John H.
Rivers, Miriam W.

-Asian American/Asian/Pacific Islander

Goh, David S.

-Hispanic/Latino

Barona, Andres

17 COUNSELING PSYCHOLOGY

-African American/Black

Bingham, Rosie P.
Carter, Robert T.
Howard, Mary T.
Jackson, Anna M.
Parham, Thomas A.

-American Indian/Alaska Native

LaFromboise, Teresa

-Asian American/Asian/Pacific Islander

Dawis, Rene V.
Sue, Derald W.

-Hispanic/Latino

Fouad, Nadya A.
Roehlke, Helen J.
Stern, Marilyn
Vasquez, Melba

18 PSYCHOLOGISTS IN PUBLIC SERVICE

-Hispanic/Latino

Bracero, William

19 MILITARY PSYCHOLOGY

20 ADULT DEVELOPMENT AND AGING

-Asian American/Asian/Pacific Islander

Mehrotra, Chandra M.N.

-Hispanic/Latino

Chiriboga, David A.

21 APPLIED EXPERIMENTAL AND ENGINEERING PSYCHOLOGY

22 REHABILITATION PSYCHOLOGY

-American Indian/Alaska Native

Uzzell, Barbara P.

-Asian American/Asian/Pacific Islander

Lam, Chow S.
Sax, Kenji W.

23 CONSUMER PSYCHOLOGY

24 THEORETICAL AND PHILOSOPHICAL PSYCHOLOGY

-African American/Black

Jenkins, Adelbert H

-Hispanic/Latino

Zuriff, Gerald E.

25 DIVISION OF BEHAVIOR ANALYSIS

-African American/Black

Turner, Samuel M.

26 HISTORY OF PSYCHOLOGY

27 SOCIETY FOR COMMUNITY RESEARCH AND ACTION: DIVISION OF COMMUNITY PSYCHOLOGY

-African American/Black

Barbarin, Oscar A.
Myers, Hector F.
Penn, Nolan E.

-American Indian/Alaska Native

Trimble, Joseph E.

-Asian American/Asian/Pacific Islander

Sue, Stanley
Ying, Yu-Wen

-Hispanic/Latino

Bernal, Guillermo
Munoz, Ricardo F.
Serrano-Garcia, Irma

28 PSYCHOPHARMACOLOGY AND SUBSTANCE ABUSE

-Hispanic/Latino

Marin, Gerardo

29 PSYCHOTHERAPY

-African American/Black

Greene, Beverly
Holmes, Dorothy E.
Jackson, Anna M.
Jenkins, Adelbert H
Porche-Burke, Lisa M.
Pugh, Roderick W.

-American Indian/Alaska Native

Willis, Diane J.

-Asian American/Asian/Pacific Islander

Sue, Stanley

-Hispanic/Latino

Roehlke, Helen J.

30 PSYCHOLOGICAL HYPNOSIS

-Asian American/Asian/Pacific Islander

Sax, Kenji W.

31 STATE PSYCHOLOGICAL ASSOCIATION AFFAIRS

32 HUMANISTIC PSYCHOLOGY

-African American/Black

Jenkins, Adelbert H

33 MENTAL RETARDATION AND DEVELOPMENTAL DISABILITIES

-African American/Black

Hooker, Olivia J.
Jones, Reginald L.

34 POPULATION & ENVIRONMENTAL PSYCHOLOGY

35 PSYCHOLOGY OF WOMEN

-African American/Black

Greene, Beverly
Hines, Laura M.
Wyche, Karen F.

-Asian American/Asian/Pacific Islander

Hall, Christine I.
Takanishi, Ruby
True, Reiko Homma

-Hispanic/Latino

Ginorio, Angela B.
Roehlke, Helen J.
Vasquez, Melba

36 PSYCHOLOGISTS INTERESTED IN RELIGIOUS ISSUES

37 CHILD, YOUTH, AND FAMILY SERVICES

-African American/Black

Jackson, John H.
Paster, Vera S.
Slaughter-Defoe, Diana T.

-American Indian/Alaska Native

Willis, Diane J.

38 HEALTH PSYCHOLOGY

-African American/Black

Jemmott, III, John B.

-Asian American/Asian/Pacific Islander

Nezu, Arthur M.

-Hispanic/Latino

Chiriboga, David A.

39 PSYCHOANALYSIS

40 CLINICAL NEUROPSYCHOLOGY

-American Indian/Alaska Native

Uzzell, Barbara P.

-Hispanic/Latino

Puente, Antonio E.

41 AMERICAN PSYCHOLOGY LAW SOCIETY

42 PSYCHOLOGISTS IN INDEPENDENT PRACTICE

43 FAMILY PSYCHOLOGY

-Hispanic/Latino

Inclan, Jaime

44 SOCIETY FOR THE PSYCHOLOGICAL STUDY OF LESBIAN, GAY AND BISEXUAL ISSUES

-African American/Black

Greene, Beverly
Lawson, Jasper J.

-Asian American/Asian/Pacific Islander

Sue, Derald W.

-Hispanic/Latino

Morales, Eduardo S.
Roehlke, Helen J.

45 SOCIETY FOR THE PSYCHOLOGICAL STUDY OF ETHNIC MINORITY ISSUES

-African American/Black

Block, Carolyn B.
Caldwell-Colbert, A. Toy
Carter, Robert T.
Greene, Beverly
Henderson Daniel, Jessica
Hines, Laura M.
Jackson, Anna M.
Jenkins, Adelbert H
Lawson, Jasper J.
Myers, Hector F.
Parham, Thomas A.
Porche-Burke, Lisa M.
Robinson, John D
Slaughter-Defoe, Diana T.
Turner, Samuel M.
Wilson, Susan B.

-American Indian/Alaska Native

LaFromboise, Teresa
Trimble, Joseph E.
Willis, Diane J.

-Asian American/Asian/Pacific Islander

Austria, Asuncion M.
Goh, David S.
Hall, Christine I.
Nagata, Donna K.
Sue, Derald W.
Sue, Stanley
True, Reiko Homma
Zane, Nolan W.S

-Hispanic/Latino

Arredondo, Patricia
Bernal, Guillermo
Ginorio, Angela B.
Lopez, Steven R.
Marin, Gerardo
Morales, Eduardo S.
Munoz, Ricardo F.
Roehlke, Helen J.
Vasquez, Melba

46 MEDIA PSYCHOLOGY

47 EXERCISE AND SPORT PSYCHOLOGY

-Asian American/Asian/Pacific Islander

Sax, Kenji W.

-African American/Black

Penn, Nolan E.

48 SOCIETY FOR THE STUDY OF PEACE, CONFLICT & VIOLENCE: PEACE PSYCHOLOGY

49 GROUP PSYCHOLOGY & GROUP PSYCHOTHERAPY

50 ADDICTIONS

51 SOCIETY FOR THE PSYCHOLOGICAL STUDY OF MEN AND MASCULINITY

-African American/Black

Lawson, Jasper J.

52 INTERNATIONAL PSYCHOLOGY

-African American/Black

Oshodi, John

53 CLINICAL CHILD PSYCHOLOGY

54 THE SOCIETY OF PEDIATRIC PSYCHOLOGY

55 AMERICAN SOCIETY FOR THE ADVANCEMENT OF PHARMACOTHERAPY

Major Field/ Professional Role

The OEMA Survey requests respondents to identify
their Major Field (from among a list of 21) and to rank order (relative to "time
and effort") their involvement in six major professional roles (i.e., Academician,
Administrator, Consultant, Practitioner, Researcher, and Other**).

Information in this section is listed in the following order:

Major Field (Alphabetically ordered and under each:)

Professional Roles (Six role types and under each:)

Primary Role and Associated Names (Alphabetized)

Secondary Role and Associated Names (Alphabetized)

** Examples of "Other" roles identified by OEMA Survey Respondents are: Test Developer,
Publisher/Author, Clinical Supervisor/Manager, Human Resources Staff, Psychological
Examiner, Program Developer, Talk Show Host, Trainer, and Parent Educator.

THE MAJOR FIELDS

Clinical Child Psychology
Clinical Psychology
Cognitive Psychology
Community Psychology
Comparative Psychology
Counseling Psychology
Developmental Psychology
Educational Psychology
Environmental Psychology
Experimental Psychology
General Psychology/Methods & Systems
Geropsychology
Health Psychology
Industrial Organizational Psychology
Neurosciences
Personality Psychology
Physiological Psychology/Psychobiology
Psychopharmacology
Quantitative/Mathematical & Psychometrics/Statistics
School Psychology
Social Psychology

MAJOR FIELDS AND PROFESSIONAL ROLE LISTING

CLINICAL CHILD PSYCHOLOGY

-Academician-

Primary Role

Bauermeisten, Jose J.
Floyd, Bridget J.
Hill, Jr., Sam S.
Jones, Russell T.
Paniagua, Freddy A.
Ramos, Arnaldo J.
Reyes, Carla J.
Williams, Michael A.
Willis, Diane J.

Secondary Role

Arellano, Charleanea
Beam, Micheline
Grant, Wanda F.
Moideen, Yasmine
Villejo, Ron E.

-Administrator-

Primary Role

Corte, Henry E.
Foo, Rebecca E.
Hanley, Jerome H.
Hashimoto, Jerry S.
Henderson, Brenda A.
Lessing, Elise E.
Stroud, Barbara
Villejo, Ron E.

Secondary Role

Arroyo, Patricia M.
Davis, Cheryl L.
Freeman, Charlotte M.

-Consultant-

Primary Role

Gonzalez, Max A.

Secondary Role

Azaret, Marisa
Baker, Christine
Chan, Darrow A.
Gordon, LaFaune Y.
Gutterman, Carmen Y.
Hanley, Jerome H.
Hashimoto, Jerry S.
Henderson, Brenda A.
Ito, Elaine S.
Japzon Gillum, Debra
Lein, H. Beatriz
Leon, Yolanda C.
Low, Benson P.

Marquez, Steven
Perry, Jeanell
Rosin, Susana A.
Santiago, Lydia V.
Steele, Marilyn
Tucker, James L.
Wagner, Aureen Pinto
Wilkinson, H. Sook
Williams, Karen P. W.

-Practitioner-

Primary Role

Arroyo, Patricia M.
Azaret, Marisa
Baker, Christine
Beam, Micheline
Byrd, Robert D.
Chan, Darrow A.
Davis, Cheryl L.
Freeman, Charlotte M.
Gordon, LaFaune Y.
Grant, Wanda F.
Gutterman, Carmen Y.
Hamada, Roger S.
Ito, Elaine S.
Japzon Gillum, Debra
Lee-Richter, Julie
Lein, H. Beatriz
Leon, Yolanda C.
Lui, Barbara J.
Mar, Harvey H.
Marquez, Steven
Moideen, Yasmine
Morote, Gloria
Patton, Kenneth
Perry, Jeanell
Rosin, Susana A.
Santiago, Lydia V.
Shimoda, Kim C.
Sugai, Don P.
Treadwell, Marsha J.
Tucker, James L.
Wagner, Aureen Pinto
Wilkinson, H. Sook
Williams, Karen P. W.

Secondary Role

Bauermeisten, Jose J.
Byrd, Robert D.
Corte, Henry E.
Foo, Rebecca E.
Hill, Jr., Sam S.
Luthar, Suniya S.
Paniagua, Freddy A.
Ramos, Arnaldo J.
Samuel, Valerie J.

Stroud, Barbara
Urquiza, Anthony J.
Williams, Michael A.
Willis, Diane J.

-Researcher-

Primary Role

Arellano, Charleanea
Luthar, Suniya S.
Samuel, Valerie J.
Urquiza, Anthony J.

Secondary Role

Hamada, Roger S.
Jones, Russell T.
Lessing, Elise E.
Lui, Barbara J.
Mar, Harvey H.
Patton, Kenneth
Reyes, Carla J.
Sugai, Don P.
Treadwell, Marsha J.

-Other-

Primary Role

Steele, Marilyn

CLINICAL PSYCHOLOGY

-Academician-

Primary Role

Abernethy, Alexis D.
Ainslie, Ricardo C.
Akamatsu, T. John
Akutsu, Phillip D.
Allsopp, Ralph N
Alvarez, Carlos M.
Anderson, Louis P.
Aoki, Wayne T.
Arcaya, Jose M.
Armengol, Carmen G.
Arreola-Rockwell, Fran Pepitone-
Arroyo, Judith A.
Ascencao, Erlete M.
Austria, Asuncion M.
Auuilas-Gaxiola, Sergio A.
Barrera, Jr., Manuel
Belen, Ines I.
Bernal, Guillermo A.
Bernal, Guillermo
Bernal, Martha E
Binion, Victoria J.

Blackett-Sullivan, Gwendolyn
Boone, Martin
Caldwell-Colbert, A. Toy
Cardena, Etzel A.
Cervantes, Joseph M.
Chan, Connie S.
Chavez, Ernest L.
Choney, John M.
Cimino, Cynthia R.
Collins, James F.
Connor, Michael E.
Dave, Jagdish P.
Davila, Joanne
Davis-Russell, Elizabeth
Dixon, J. Faye
Dobbins, James E.
Donate-Bartfield, Evelyn
Dosamantes-Beaudry, Irma
Evans, Helen L.
Ezeilo, Bernice N.
Falicov, Celia J.
Fernandez, Ephrem
Flores, Elena
Ford, Deshay D.
Fujitsubo, Lani C.
Fulton, Aubyn
Garnes, Delbert F.
Gary, Juneau M.
Gillem, Angela R
Glover, O.S.
Gonzalez, Gerardo M
Graves-Cooper, Phyllis J.
Gray-Little, Bernadette
Greene, Beverly
Grosso, Federico C.
Guanipa, Carmen L.
Hall, Ruth L.
Harrell, Shelly P.
Harris, Shanette M.
Hass, Giselle A
Hass, Giselle A.
Higa, William R.
Hightower, Eugene
Hong, George K.
Ichiyama, Michael A.
Ike, Chris A.
Ingram, Winifred
Iwamasa, Gayle Y.
Jackson, Leslie C.
Jaimez, T. Lanac
James, Michelle D.
James, Steven E
Javier, Rafael A.
Jenkins, Adelbert H
Johnson, Fred A.

Johnson, Zonya
Jones, Arthur C.
Jones, George L.
Joseph, Jr., Herbert M.
Kashikar-Zuck, Susmita M.
Khanna, Jaswant L.
Khanna, Mukti
Kwon, Paul H.
Labbe, Elise E.
Lambert, Michael C.
Langley, Merlin R
Lee, Hing-Chu B.
Lee, Wanda M. L.
LeSure-Lester, G. Evelyn
Levermore, Monique A.
Liem, Ramsay
Lijtmaer, Ruth M
Liston, Hattye H.
Llanos, Aracely B.
Llorente, Antolin M.
London, Lorna H.
Lopez, Martita A.
Machabanski, Hector
Mate-Kole, C. Charles
Matthews, Belvia W.
Maynard, Edward S.
McClure, Faith H.
McKenzie, Jr., Loratuis L.
Mehta, Sheila
Mio, Jeffery S.
Miranda, M.
Mitchell, Howard E.
Mobley, Brenda D.
Montesi, Alexandra Saba
Mori, Lisa T.
Moritsugu, John
Morris, Edward F.
Munoz, Ricardo F.
Myers, Hector F.
Myers, Linda J.
Nabors, Nina A.
Nagayama Hall, Gordon C.
Nakamura, Charles Y.
Nayak, Madhabika B.
Nettles, Arie L.
Nix-Early, Vivian
Nzewi, Esther N.
Okazaki, Sumie
Paige, Roger
Penn, Nolan E.
Perez Ebrahimi, Concepcion
Pinder-Amaker, Stephanie L.
Polite, Kenneth
Pugh, Roderick W.
Rainwater, III, Avie J.
Rivera, Jo Ann M.
Robinson, W. LaVome
Rollock, David
Roll, Samuel
Romney, Patricia
San Luis, Roberto R.
Sanders-Thompson, Vetta L.
Sanua, Victor D.

Schacht, Thomas E.
Serafica, Felicisima C.
Shopshire, Michael S.
Smith, Michael C.
Snowden, Lonnie R.
Solomon, Sondra E.
Stewart, Sunita M.
Suarez-Crowe, Yolanda
Suarez, Carlota
Sue, David
Sue, Stanley
Suinn, Richard M.
Tanaka-Matsumi, Junko
Tan, Josephine
Tan, Siang-Yang Y.
Tatum, Beverly D.
Thompson, Veronique L.
Thornton, Dozier W.
Tsang, Michael Hing- Pui
Tsujimoto, Richard N.
Turnbough, P. Diane
Valentiner, David P.
Vargas, Luis A.
Varki, C. Paily
Velasquez, John M.
Velasquez, Roberto J.
Vraniak, Damian A.
Walcott, Delores D.
Walton, Duncan E.
Whitaker, Sandra V.
White, Joseph L.
Whitten, Lisa A.
Wilson, Melvin N.
Wong, Jane L.
Wong, Philip S
Wright, Michael F.
Wyatt, Gail E.
Wyche, Karen F.
Wynne, Michael
Ying, Yu-Wen
Zamudio, Anthony
Zane, Nolan W.S

Secondary Role
Abercombie, Delrita
Abston, Jr., Nathaniel
Adams, C. Jama
Anderson, Linda
Antonuccio, David
Artis, Daphne J.
Barbarin, Oscar A.
Basco, Monica A.
Bascuas, Joseph W.
Bavon, Moises
Blanding, Benjamin
Bowen, Tanya U.
Bracero, William
Carr-Casanova, Rosario
Carter, Allen C.
Cepeda-Benito, Antonio
Chin, Sandra B
Coats, Gary L.
Collins, Edsmond J.
Colon, Ana I.

Colotla, Victor A.
Comas-Diaz, Lillian
Cordero, Fernando
Costa, Armenio S.
Credidio, Vivian F.
Crowder, Virginia B.
Cruz-Lopez, Miguel
Cuesta, George M.
Davis, Charles E.
De Louredes Mattei, Maria
Devezin, Armond A.
Dixon, J. Faye
Echemendia, Ruben J.
Flaherty, Maria Y.
Foster, Evelyn L.
Foster, RoseMarie P.
Fresh, Edith M.
Garcia-Abid, Calixto
Giles, Cheryl A.
Gonzales, Michael
Graves, Sherryl B.
Grier, Priscilla E.
Hamer, Forrest M.
Hart, Anton H.
Herrera-Pino, Jorge A.
Holmes, Dorothy E.
Hooker, Olivia J.
Hoshmand, Lisa T.
Huang, Karen H C
Huang, Larke N.
Hyman, Edward J.
Ishida, Taeko H.
Jackson, Anna M.
Ja, Davis Y.
June, Lee N.
Kich, George K.
King, Valerie
Leary, Kimberlyn
Lew, Wei M.
Loo, Chalsa M.
Louredes Mattei, Maria De
Lum, Rodger G.
Maldonado, Loretto
Manuel, Gerdenio M.
Manzanares, Dan L.
Margarida, Maria T.
Marmol, Leonardo M.
Matsui, Wesley T.
Milner, Joel S.
Mujica, Ernesto
Nagata, Donna K.
Netter, Beatriz E. C.
Ninonuevo, Fred
Oshodi, John
Paster, Vera S.
Perilla, Julia L.
Ponton, Marcel O.
Powell, Lois
Price, Alicia A.
Richardson, E. Strong-Legs
Rivera-Lopez, Hector
Romey, Carol M.
Rouce, Sandra

Ruiz, Sonia I.
Saldana, Delia H.
Santini-Hernandez, Ernesto
Seda, Gilbert
Shea-Martinez, Herminia E.
Stevenson, Jr., Edward E.
Suarez, Alejandra
Swaney, Gyda
Szapocznik, Jose
Tien, Liang
Torres, Mario A.
Towns-Miranda, Luz
Tucker, Dorothy M.
Turner, Samuel M.
Vance, Ellen B.
Vargas, Manuel J.
Winfrey, LaPearl L.
Woo, Rose
Yoshimura, G. Joji

-Administrator-

Primary Role
Aguilar, Martha C.
Alvarez, Gary L.
Anderson, Norman B.
Anton, William D.
Aoki, Bart K.
Archibald, Eloise M.
Baron, Augustine
Bascuas, Joseph W.
Bastien, IV, Samuel A.
Binns, Derrick
Boulette, Tersea R.
Brandenburg, Carlos E.
Buffin, Janice E.
Burnett, Judith A.
Campbell, Kamal E.
Campbell, Stephen N.
Campos, Peter E.
Church, June S.
Crowder, Virginia B.
Cruz, Albert R.
Davis, Charles E.
Echemendia, Ruben J.
Eng, Albert M.
Epps, Pamela J.
Everett, Moses L.
Faraci, Ana M.
Fields, Anika C.
Floyd, James A.
Francois, Theodore V.
Fresh, Edith M.
Fuentes, Dainery M.
Gallagher, Rosina M.
Gant, Bob L.
Garg, Mithlesh
Garrett-Akinsanya, BraVada
Garza, Joe G.
Gonzalez, Rocio R
Graves, Sherryl B.
Green, Theophilus E.
Gulley, Silas
Guzman, L. Philip

Hawkins, Ioma L.
Hines, Paulette M.
Hoshmand, Lisa T.
Hsia, Heidi
Hunter, Knoxice C
Ishiyama, Toaru
Jackson, Anna M.
June, Lee N.
Klopner, Michele C.
Lie, Rudolph T.B
London, Dyanne P.
Lum, Rodger G.
Mack, Delores E.
Marmol, Leonardo M.
Martinez, Alejandro M.
Montoya, E. Carolina
Morishige, Howard H.
Muga, Joe
Nezu, Arthur M.
Onizuka, Richard K.
Ozaki, Mona M.
Pang, Dawn
Peniston, Eugene G.
Peoples, Kathleen
Perez-Arce, Patricia
Pinto, Alcides
Reisinger, Curtis W.
Rivera, Carmen J.
Rivera, Nelson E.
Rivero, Estela M.
Shah, Vasantkumar B.
Soto, Tomas A.
Tate, Donald
Tomes, Henry
Torigoe, Rodney Y.
Toro-Alfonso, Jose
True, Reiko Homma
Velasco, Frank E.
Velez, Maria T.
Viale-val, Graciela
Washington, Robert A.
Williams, Everett B.
Williams, Indy J.
Williams, Rebecca E.
Williams, Steve
Winfrey, LaPearl L.
Wood, Jr., Nollie P.
Woodland, Calvin E.
Word, James C.
Yabusaki, Ann S.
Yanagida, Evelyn H.
Yee, Tina T.
Young, David A.

Secondary Role

Akamatsu, T. John
Allen-Claiborne, Joyce G.
Amezaga, Jr., Alfredo M.
Anderson, William H.
Aoki, Wayne T.
Arreola-Rockwell, Fran
    Pepitone-
Atkinson, Michael B.
Aviles, Alice A.

Azevedo, Don Fernando
Belgrave, Jeffrey
Bennett, Maisha H.
Bernat, Gloria S.
Birky, Ian
Bonal, Kathleen A.
Bradman, Leo H.
Brooks, Juanita O.
Browne, Ronald H.
Bryant-Tuckett, Rose M.
Bueno, Luis F.
Caldwell-Colbert, A. Toy
Caro, Yvette
Chapman, Nancy G.
Chavez, Ernest L.
Chino, Allan F.
Clark, Brenda A.
Cohen, Isadora
Coleman, Willie J.
Colon, R. Phillip
Copemann, Chester D.
Craig, U-Shaka
Cummings, Joseph D.
Das, Manju P.
Davis-Russell, Elizabeth
Davis, Bernice M.
Dobbins, James E.
Dooley, John A.
Dudley-Grant, G. Rita
Eaton, Sheila J.
Elena Lee, Karen
Eskandari, Esfandiar
Ezeilo, Bernice N.
Figueroa, Jorge L.
Ford, Deshay D.
Fo, Walter S O
Fujii, Daryl E M
Gock, Terry S.
Gonzalez-Huss, Mary
Gray-Little, Bernadette
Green, Charles A.
Greene, Clifford
Griffith, Marlin S.
Griffith, Stanford
Haddock, Dean M.
Hough, Sigmund
Incera, Armando
Javier, Rafael A.
Johnson, Matthew B.
Jurilla-Pastrana, Lina L.
Keglar, Shelvy H.
Kochevar-Sukkarie, Renee J.
Lagomasino, Andrew J.
Laguna, John N.
Lau, Godwin
Magran, Betty A.
Mallisham, Ivy J.
Martinez, Raul
Martin, Laura P.
Martin, William F.
Matthews, Belvia W.
McCarley, Victor J.
Mellor-Crummey, Cynthia A.

Mills, Marcia C.
Mobley, Brenda D.
Molden, Sabrina
Munoz, Marisol
Nakamura, Linda K
Nix-Early, Vivian
Ohye, Bonnie Y.
Pacheco, Angel E.
Peart-Newkirk, Natalia J.
Piercy, Patricia A.
Pinderhughes, Victoria A.
Polite, Kenneth
Prieto, Addys
Richards, Henry J.
Rivera, Enrique
Rivera, Jo Ann M.
Rodriguez, Manuel D.
Sasscer-Burgos, Julie
Savage, Jr., James E.
St. Leger, Sidney C.
Stephens, Dorothy W.
Stokes, Devon R.
Tan, Siang-Yang Y.
Taylor, Palmeda D.
Thompson, Veronique L.
Thornton, Dozier W.
Vaughans, Kirkland C.
Vega, Star
Walker, Lola '.
Wu, Sheila T.
Yancey, Angela L.
Zayas-Bazan, Carmen

-Consultant-

Primary Role

Alonso, Mario
Balbona, Manuel
Beliz, Jr., Efrain A.
Berrios, Zaida R.
Bolden, Wiley S.
Bowen, Tanya U.
Carr, Paquita R.
Chapman, Nancy G.
Doss, Juanita K.
Elligen, Don G.
Esparza, Ricardo
Fo, Walter S O
Fullilove, Constance
Gibbons-Carr, Michele V.
Harper, Mary S.
Hooker, Olivia J.
Incera, Armando
Ireland Hurd, Evelyn C.
Ja, Davis Y.
Khan, Badrul A.
Kich, George Kitahara
King, Valerie
Kirst, Stephen P.
Kolt, Laurie
Lawson, Gary W.
Llado, Sarah L.
Matsumoto, Gregory Y.
Mellor-Crummey, Cynthia A.

Menchaca, Victoria A.
Mills, Marcia C.
Mora, Ralph
Nesbitt, Eric B.
Nicks, T. Leon
Phillips, Campbell C.
Richards, Henry J.
Richardson, E. Strong-Legs
Sharp, Jude C.
Smith, Jr., Theodore R.
Takamine, Sandra
Tucker, Dorothy M.
Upadhyaya, Shripati
Williams, Victoria F.
Young, Kimberly S.

Secondary Role

Abello, Ana L.
Aguilar, Martha C.
Aguilera, David M.
Ahana, Ellen
Ahmed, Mohiuddin
Alonso, Martha R.
Alvarez, Carlos M.
Alvarez, Manuel E.
Alvarez, Mauricia
Alvarez, Vivian
Anderson, Claudia J.
Arenas, Jr., Silverio
Arevalo, Luis E.
Arnold, John F.
Ascano, Ricardo
Ashmore-Hudson, Anne
Azcarate, Eduardo M.
Bacal, Sergio
Bamgbose, Olujiimi O.
Banks, Karel L.
Barber, Kevin V.
Baron, Augustine
Bartee, Robert L.
Bastien, IV, Samuel A.
Bastien, Rochelle T.
Beato-Smith, Vera
Belen, Ines I.
Bell, K. Pat
Belton, Monique
Beltran, Joe
Benavides, Jr., Robert
Bencomo, Armando A.
Benitez, John C.
Benzaquen, Isaac
Berrill, Naftali G.
Berry, Joyce Hamilton
Bhatia, Kiran
Blackett-Sullivan, Gwendolyn A.
Blair, Deborah G.
Block, Carolyn B.
Borrego, Richard L.
Bostwick, Allen D.
Boulette, Tersea R.
Boxley, Russell L.
Boyd, Naughne L.
Branche, Leota Susan
Brannon, Lorraine

Brown, Barbara J.	Gardano, Anna C.	Khorakiwala, Durriyah	Nishi-Strattner, Linda
Brown, Pamela	Gardner, Lamaurice H.	Kim, Mary Ann Y.	Nogales, Ana
Bustamante, Eduardo M.	Garnes, Delbert F.	Kobayashi, Steve K.	Nolan, Jr., Benjamin C.
Caberto, Steven C.	Garrido, Maria C.	Koh, Tong-He	Oana, Leilani K.
Cade, Bonita G.	Garrido, Maria	Lancaster, JoAnn	Oh, Jungyeol L.
Camarillo, Max	Gee, Carol S.	Lawson, Jasper J.	Okiyama, Stephen L.
Campos, Leonard P.	Ghalib, Nadeem	Lee, Anna C.	Olmo, Manuel C.
Cappon, Jorge	Goebes, Diane D.	Lee, Daniel D.	Ortega, Richard J.
Carpenter, Gerald A.	Gong, Susan M.	Lee, Julie C.	Otero, Rafael F.
Cason, Valerie K.	Gonzales, Ricardo R.	Lee, Jung K.	Outlaw, Patricia A.
Chan, Daniel S.	Gonzalez, Haydee M.	Lee, Ronald W.	Owens-Lane, Jan
Chang, Barbara	Gonzalez, Matthew B.	Le, Trinh To	Paredes, Jr., Frank C.
Chang, Bradford W.	Grabau, David	Leung, Alex C. N.	Patel, Sanjiv A.
Chao, Christine M.	Graham, Quentin	Lewis, Page	Patterson, Mayin Lau
Chapa, Joel R.	Griffin, Patricia L.	Lie, Rudolph T.B	Pelaez, Carmen
Chesnutt, James H.	Grosso, Federico C.	Lijtmaer, Ruth M	Peralta, Carmelina
Chiu, Loanne	Grubb, Henry J.	Lin, Jeanne L.	Perez, Juan C.
Choi, George C.	Guerra, Julio J.	Llorca, Arthur L.	Pettigrew, Dorothy C.
Choy, Stephen S.F.	Gulley, Silas	Loo, Russell	Pierce, William D.
Clark, Marie	Guo, Trudy Narikiyo	Loredo, Carlos M.	Pirhekayaty-Soriano, Tahereh
Coleburn, Lila A.	Gurri Glass, Margarita E.	Losada-Paisey, Gloria	Plazas, Carlos A.
Coleman, Philip P.	Gutierrez, Manuel J.	Lozano, Irma	Poal, Pilar
Constanzo, Magda S.	Guzman, L. Philip	Lucas, Jay H.	Pompa, Janiece L.
Cooper, Donna M.	Harper, Renuka R.	Lujan, Cleo C.	Porges, Carlos R.
Cornide, Carmen R.	Harris, William W.	Madrid, Raul P.	Porter, Julia
Cottingham, Alice L.	Hass, Giselle A	Malancharuvil, Joseph M.	Prado, Haydee
Crespo, Alfredo E.	Hass, Giselle A.	Mancillas, Paul	Prado, William M.
Crespo, Gloria M.	Heller, Beatriz	Manghi, Elina R.	Prutsman, Thomas D.
Cruz, Maria C.	Henry, Vincent dePaul	Mar, Norman J.	Pulliam, Barbara A.
Cunha, Maria I.	Higashi, Wilfred H.	Marroquin, Arthur R.	Quijano, Walter Y.
Daruna, Jorge H.	Ho, Christine K.	Martinez-Urrutia, Angel C.	Ramos-Grenier, Julia
Dawkins, Marva P.	Ho, John E.	Martinez, Eduardo M.	Rattenbury, Francie R.
De Apodaca, Roberto F.	Holsey, Chandra V.	Martinez, Gabriel P.	Ray, Arun B.
de Fuentes, Nanette	Hong, George K.	Matheson, Charlene	Rigual-Lynch, Lourdes
de Llano, Carmen	Houston, Holly O.	McCombs, Daniel	Rivas-Vazquez, Ana A.
DeGraff, Christopher D.	Huang, Wei-Jen William	McWilliams, Junko O.	Rivera-Molina, Elba
Donald, Liz	Hunter, Knoxice C	Mehta, Kripal K.	Rivera, Carmen J.
Dosamantes-Beaudry, Irma	Hunt, Wilson L.	Mejia, Juan A.	Rivera, Miquela
Duncan, Bessie A.	Hwee, Elsa	Mendelberg, Hava E.	Rodriguez, Lavinia
Echavarria, David	Inclan, Jaime	Miccio-Fonseca, L. C.	Rodriguez, Ramon O.
El-Amin, Debra El-Amin	Iqbal, S. Mohammed	Mikamo, Akiko	Rogers, Melvin L.
Elion, Victor H.	Ishikawa-Fullmer, Janet	Miranda, David J.	Romero, Augusto
Ellis, Edwin E.	Ishiyama, Toaru	Mitchell, Howard E.	Romero, Jose
Eng, Albert M.	Itatani, Robert M.	Monguio, Ines	Romero, Regina E.
Fain, Thomas C.	Jackson-Davis, Brandi	Montijo, Jorge A.	Roque, Sylvia A.
Fanibanda, Darius K.	Jackson, Helen L.	Moon, Tae-Hyun	Ross, Sandra I.
Fernandez, Ephrem	James, Steven E	Morita, Denise N.	Roy, Swati
Fernandez, Peter	Jenkins, Adelbert H	Morones, Pete A.	Ruth, Richard
Figueroa, Rolando G.	Jennings, Lesajean M.	Morris, Dolores O.	Sacasa, Rafael E.
Fils, David H.	Jimenez-Safir, Paula B.	Morris, Edward F.	Salais, A. Joseph
Flachier, Roberto	Johnson, Denise MW	Motes, Patricia S.	Salganicoff, Matilde
Fleisher, Nancy F.	Johnson, Joan J.	Muller, Terry P.	Salter, Dianne S.
Fliman, Vivian P.	Jones, Annie Lee	Munoz, John A.	Salway, Milton R.
Flores de Apodaca, Roberto	Jones, Reginald	Munoz, Leticia S.	Samford, Judith A.
Fong, Jane Y.	Jones, Ruby M.	Munoz, Nina R.	Sanchez-Torrento, Eugenio
Fong, Larry	Joshi, Sheila	Murakami, Janice	Sanchez, H.G.
Ford, Leon I.	Jue, Ronald W.	Murillo, Nathan	Saraf, Komal C.
Francois, Theodore V.	Kahan, Harry	Myers, Linda J.	Saunders, Walter C.
Fuentes, Dainery M.	Kakaiya, Divya	Neal-Barnett, Angela M.	Schenquerman, Berta N.
Fujioka, Terry Ann T.	Kelly, Jennifer F.	Nesbitt, Eric B.	Schreier, Raquel L.
Gamez, George L.	Kelly, Tara L.	Netter, Roberto	Schroff, Kamal
Garcia, Melinda A.	Kennedy, Clive D.	Nguyen, Dao Q.	Scott, Linda D.
Garcia, Pedro I.	Khalili, Hassan	Nieves-Grafals, Sara	Searcy, Mary L.

Shah, Vasantkumar B.
Sharma, Vijai P.
Shaw, Paula
Shen, John
Shon, Elizbabeth
Shum, Hilda B.
Shum, Hilda B.
Simpson, Adelaide W.
Singh, R. K. Janmeha
Sitharthan, Thiagarajan
Smith, Carol Y.
Smith, Walanda W.
Smith, William
Sobrino, James F.
Somodevilla, S. A.
Sosa, Juan N.
Southerland, Deborah L.
Spivey, Philop B.
Stewart, Arleen R.
Suinn, Richard M.
Swan, June A.
Sy, Michael J.
Tabachnik, Samuel
Tamura, Leonard J.
Tapo, Linda J.
Tazeau, Yvette N.
Teng, L. Neal
Thorson, Billie J.
Tomes, Henry
Toro-Alfonso, Jose
Triplett, Sheila J.
True, Reiko Homma
Tsushima, William T.
Tung, May
Uzzell, Barbara P.
Valdivia, Lino
Vazquez, Carlos D.
Vazquez, Rosa
Velasco, Frank E.
Villela, Leopoldo F.
Wakeman, Richard J.
Washington, Anita C.
Washington, Dianna E.
Weston, Raymond E.
White, Joseph L.
Whitten, Lisa A.
Williams, Everett B.
Williams, Mary Beth
Wilson, Susan B.
Wilson, Woodrow
Winter, Amal
Witter, Jeanette M.
Wong-Ngan, Julia A.
Wong, Kit L.
Wood, Jr., Nollie P.
Woodland, Calvin E.
Wynne, Michael
Yniguez, Linda E.
Yoshimura, Kari K.
Yu, Pamela

-Practitioner-

<u>Primary Role</u>

Abello, Ana L.
Abercombie, Delrita
Abercrombie, Maria M.
Abston, Jr., Nathaniel
Adams, Jr., Clarence L.
Adams, C. Jama
Aguilera, David M.
Aguirre-Deandreis, Ana I.
Ahana, Ellen
Ahmed, Mohiuddin
Ahuja, Harmeen
Akutagawa, Donald
Allen-Claiborne, Joyce G.
Allen, Christeen
Alonso, Martha R.
Alvarez, Manuel E.
Alvarez, Mauricia
Alvarez, Vivian
Amezaga, Jr., Alfredo M.
Anderson, Claudia J.
Anderson, Linda
Anderson, William H.
Antonuccio, David
Arana, Olga R.
Arellano-Lopez, Juan
Arenas, Jr., Silverio
Arevalo, Luis E.
Arizmeudi, Thomas
Arnold, John F.
Arsuaga, Enrique N.
Artiles, Laura M.
Artis, Daphne J.
Ascano, Ricardo
Ashmore-Hudson, Anne
Atkinson, Michael B.
Atwal, Baljit K,
Aviles, Alice A.
Azcarate, Eduardo M.
Azevedo, Don Fernando
Bacal, Sergio
Bamgbose, Olujiimi O.
Banks, Karel L.
Barber, Kevin V.
Barnes, Charles A.
Bartee, Robert L.
Bastien, Rochelle T.
Bavon, Moises
Bayon, E. Paul
Beato-Smith, Vera
Belgrave, Jeffrey
Bell, Anita G.
Bell, K. Pat
Belton, Monique
Beltran, Joe
Benavides, Jr., Robert
Bencomo, Armando A.
Benitez, John C.
Bennasar, Mari C.
Bennett, Maisha H.
Benzaquen, Isaac
Bernat, Gloria S.
Berrill, Naftali G.
Berry, Joyce Hamilton

Bhatia, Kiran
Birky, Ian
Blair, Deborah G.
Blanding, Benjamin
Block, Carolyn B.
Bonal, Kathleen A.
Borrego, Richard L.
Bostick, Rosie M.
Bostwick, Allen D.
Boxley, Russell L.
Boyd, Naughne L.
Bracero, William
Bradman, Leo H.
Branche, Leota Susan
Brannon, Lorraine
Briggs, Felicia H.
Brooks, Juanita O.
Brown, Barbara J.
Browne, Ronald H.
Brown, Pamela
Bryant-Tuckett, Rose M.
Bueno, Luis F.
Burr, Sharon S.
Bustamante, Eduardo M.
Bynum, Edward B.
Caberto, Steven C.
Cade, Bonita G.
Camargo, Robert J.
Camarillo, Max
Cameron, Linda S.
Campos, Leonard P.
Canedo, Angelo R.
Cappon, Jorge
Cardona, Gilbert
Caro, Yvette
Carpenter, Gerald A.
Carr-Casanova, Rosario
Carra, Sylvia F.
Carter, Allen C.
Cason, Valerie K.
Cathcart, Conrad W.
Cebollero, Ana Margarita
Chan, Daniel S.
Chang, Alice F.
Chang, Barbara
Chang, Bradford W.
Chang, Theodore C. H.
Chao, Christine M.
Chapa, Joel R.
Chatigny, Anita L.
Chesnutt, James H.
Chew, Marion W.
Ching, June W. J.
Chin, Lemin
Chino, Allan F.
Chin, Sandra B
Chiu, Loanne
Choca, James
Choi, George C.
Choy, Stephen S.F.
Clark, Brenda A.
Clark, Marie
Coats, Gary L.

Cohen, Isadora
Coleburn, Lila A.
Coleman, Philip P.
Coleman, Willie J.
Collado, Armando
Collins, Edsmond J.
Colon, Ana I.
Colon, R. Phillip
Colotla, Victor A.
Comas-Diaz, Lillian
Constanzo, Magda S.
Cooper, Alan
Cooper, Donna M.
Copemann, Chester D.
Cordero, Fernando
Cornide, Carmen R.
Correa, Martha L.
Costa, Armenio S.
Cotterell, Norman
Cottingham, Alice L.
Craig, U-Shaka
Crane, Rosario S.
Crawford, Monica L.
Credidio, Vivian F.
Crespo, Alfredo E.
Crespo, Gloria M.
Critton, Barbara L.
Cruz-Lopez, Miguel
Cruz, Maria C.
Cuesta, George M.
Cummings, Joseph D.
Cunha, Maria I.
Daruna, Jorge H.
Das, Manju P.
Davis, Bernice M.
Dawkins, Marva P.
De Apodaca, Roberto F.
de Fuentes, Nanette
de Llano, Carmen
DeFerreire, Mary Elizabeth
DeGraff, Christopher D.
Dehmer-Abalo, Elena M.
Denson, Eric L.
Detres, Michael P.
Devezin, Armond A.
Donald, Liz
Dooley, John A.
Dudley-Grant, G. Rita
Duncan, Bessie A.
Eaton, Sheila J.
Echavarria, David
El-Amin, Debra El-Amin
Elena Lee, Karen
Elion, Victor H.
Ellis, Edwin E.
Eskandari, Esfandiar
Fain, Thomas C.
Fanibanda, Darius K.
Fayard, Carlos
Fernandez, Maria C.
Fernandez, Peter
Figueroa, Jorge L.
Figueroa, Rolando G.

Fils, David H.	Hao, Judy Y.	Lau, Godwin	Molden, Sabrina
Flachier, Roberto	Harper, Renuka R.	Lau, Lavay	Monguio, Ines
Flaherty, Maria Y.	Harris, William W.	Lawson, Jasper J.	Monserrat, Laura
Fleisher, Nancy F.	Hart, Anton H.	Leary, Kimberlyn	Montalvo, Roberto E.
Fletcher, Betty A.	Heller, Beatriz	Lee, Anna C.	Montijo, Jorge A.
Fliman, Vivian P.	Henry, Vincent dePaul	Lee, Daniel D.	Moody, Helaine L.
Flores de Apodaca, Roberto	Heras, Patricia	Lee, Julie C.	Moon, Tae-Hyun
Fong, Jane Y.	Hernandez, Cibeles	Lee, Jung K.	Morita, Denise N.
Fong, Larry	Herrera-Pino, Jorge A.	Lee, Ronald W.	Morones, Pete A.
Ford, Leon I.	Higashi, Wilfred H.	Le, Trinh To	Morris, Dolores O.
Foster, Evelyn L.	Ho, Christine K.	Leung, Alex C. N.	Moss, Ramona J.
Foster, RoseMarie P.	Hofer, Ricardo	Lewis, Carmelita M.	Motes, Patricia S.
Fried-Cassorla, Martha J.	Ho, John E.	Lewis, Page	Mujica, Ernesto
Fujii, Daryl E M	Holmes, Dorothy E.	Lew, Wei M.	Muller, Terry P.
Fujioka, Terry Ann T.	Holsey, Chandra V.	Lin, Jeanne L.	Munoz, John A.
Fung, Hellen C.	Hough, Sigmund	Liu, Joseph C.	Munoz, Leticia S.
Gamez, George L.	Houston, Holly O.	Llorca, Arthur L.	Munoz, Marisol
Garcia-Abid, Calixto	Huang, Karen H C	Loong, James	Munoz, Nina R.
Garcia, Melinda A.	Huang, Wei-Jen William	Loo, Russell	Murakami, Janice
Garcia, Pedro I.	Hunt, Wilson L.	Lopez, Sarah C.	Murillo, Nathan
Gardano, Anna C.	Hwee, Elsa	Loredo, Carlos M.	Mussenden, Gerald
Gardner, Lamaurice H.	Hyman, Edward J.	Losada-Paisey, Gloria	Nakagawa, Janice Y.
Garrido, Maria C.	Inclan, Jaime	Lozano, Irma	Nakamura, Linda K
Garrido, Maria	Ip, Sau Mei V.	Lucas, Jay H.	Netter, Beatriz E. C.
Gayles, Joyce M.	Iqbal, S. Mohammed	Lujan, Cleo C.	Netter, Roberto
Gee, Carol S.	Ishida, Taeko H.	Macaranas, Eduarda A.	Nguyen, Dao Q.
Ghalib, Nadeem	Ishikawa-Fullmer, Janet	Madrid, Raul P.	Nieves-Grafals, Sara
Gibbs, Charles C.	Itatani, Robert M.	Magran, Betty A.	Ninonuevo, Fred
Giles, Cheryl A.	Jackson, Helen L.	Malancharuvil, Joseph M.	Nishi-Strattner, Linda
Gock, Terry S.	Jain, Sharat K.	Maldonado, Loretto	Nogales, Ana
Goebes, Diane D.	Jennings, Lesajean M.	Mallisham, Ivy J.	Nolan, Jr., Benjamin C.
Gomez, Jr., Francisco C.	Jette, Carmen CB	Mancillas, Paul	Norman, William H.
Gong, Susan M.	Jimenez-Safir, Paula B.	Manghi, Elina R.	Norton, A. Evangeline
Gonsalves, Carlos J.	Johnson, Denise MW	Manruque-Reichard, Marta E.	Oana, Leilani K.
Gonzales, Michael	Johnson, Joan J.	Manzanares, Dan L.	Oh, Jungyeol L.
Gonzales, Ricardo R.	Johnson, Matthew B.	Margarida, Maria T.	Okiyama, Stephen L.
Gonzalez-Pabon, Jose F.	Jones, Annie Lee	Ma, Rita J.	Olmo, Manuel C.
Gonzalez, Haydee M.	Jones, Reginald	Mar, Norman J.	Oommen Thomas, Susy
Gonzalez, Maria L.	Jones, Ruby M.	Marrach, Alexa	Ortega, Richard J.
Gonzalez, Matthew B.	Joshi, Sheila	Marroquin, Arthur R.	Oshodi, John
Gordon, Rhea J.	Jue, Ronald W.	Martinez-Urrutia, Angel C.	Otero, Rafael F.
Grabau, David	Jurilla-Pastrana, Lina L.	Martinez, Eduardo M.	Outlaw, Patricia A.
Graham, Quentin	Kahan, Harry	Martinez, Gabriel P.	Owens-Lane, Jan
Grant, Kim D.	Kakaiya, Divya	Martinez, Raul	Pacheco, Angel E.
Greene, Clifford	Kao, Barbara T.	Martin, Laura P.	Paredes, Jr., Frank C.
Greene, Karen J.	Keglar, Shelvy H.	Martin, William F.	Paster, Vera S.
Grier, Priscilla E.	Kelly, Jennifer F.	Masini, Angela	Patel, Sanjiv A.
Griffin, Patricia L.	Kelly, Tara L.	Matheson, Charlene	Patterson, Mayin Lau
Griffith, Marlin S.	Kennedy, Clive D.	Matsui, Wesley T.	Peart-Newkirk, Natalia J.
Griffith, Stanford	Khalili, Hassan	McCann, Robin S.	Peavyhouse, Betty M.
Grubb, Henry J.	Khorakiwala, Durriyah	McCarley, Victor J.	Pelaez, Carmen
Grunhaus-Belzer, Rosa	Kich, George K.	McCombs, Daniel	Peralta, Carmelina
Guerra, Anna Maria	Kim, Mary Ann Y.	McNeill, Elizabeth M.	Perez, Juan C.
Guerra, Julio J.	Kim, Sung C.	McWilliams, Junko O.	Pettigrew, Dorothy C.
Gular, Enrique	Kobayashi, Steve K.	Mehta, Kripal K.	Pico, Daima
Gump, Janice P.	Koh, Tong-He	Mejia, Juan A.	Pierce, William D.
Guo, Trudy Narikiyo	Kuan, Yie-Wen Y.	Melgoza, Bertha	Piercy, Patricia A.
Gurri Glass, Margarita E.	Kupur, Veena	Mendelberg, Hava E.	Pinderhughes, Victoria A.
Haddock, Dean M.	Kwei-Levy, Carol	Miccio-Fonseca, L. C.	Pita, Marcia E.
Hall, Howard	Lagomasino, Andrew J.	Mikamo, Akiko	Plazas, Carlos A.
Hamer, Forrest M.	Laguna, John N.	Miles, Gary T.	Poal, Pilar
Hamid, Mohammad	Lancaster, JoAnn	Miranda, David J.	Pompa, Janiece L.
Han, Yu Ling	Latorre, Miriam D.	Mock, Matthew R.	Ponton, Marcel O.

Porges, Carlos R.
Porter, Julia
Posner, Carmen A.
Powell, Lois
Praderas, Kim
Prado, Haydee
Prado, William M.
Price, Alicia A.
Prieto, Addys
Prutsman, Thomas D.
Pulliam, Barbara A.
Quijano, Walter Y.
Ramos-Grenier, Julia
Rattenbury, Francie R.
Ray, Arun B.
Reed, III, Jesse A.
Rey-Casserly, Celiane M.
Rigrish, Diana
Rigual-Lynch, Lourdes
Rivas-Vazquez, Ana A.
Rivera-Lopez, Hector
Rivera-Molina, Elba
Rivera, Enrique
Rivera, Miquela
Robinson, Jane A.
Rodriguez, Lavinia
Rodriguez, Ramon O.
Rodriguez, Rogelio E.
Rogers, Melvin L.
Roman, Hugo
Romero, Augusto
Romero, Jose
Romero, Regina E.
Romey, Carol M.
Root, Maria P. P.
Roque, Sylvia A.
Rosales, Israel B.
Ross, Sandra I.
Rouce, Sandra
Roy, Swati
Ruiz, Sonia I.
Russell, David M.
Ruth, Richard
Sacasa, Rafael E.
Saito, Gloria C.
Salais, A. Joseph
Salas, Jesus A.
Salganicoff, Matilde
Salter, Dianne S.
Salway, Milton R.
Samaniego, Sandra
Samford, Judith A.
Sanchez-Torrento, Eugenio
Sanchez, Debra A.
Sanchez, H.G.
Sanchez, William
Santini-Hernandez, Ernesto
Saraf, Komal C.
Sasscer-Burgos, Julie
Saucedo, Carlos
Saunders, Walter C.
Savage, Jr., James E.
Schenquerman, Berta N.

Schreier, Raquel L.
Schroff, Kamal
Scott, Linda D.
Searcy, Mary L.
Seda, Gilbert
Sharma, Greesh C.
Sharma, Vijai P.
Shaw, Paula
Shea-Martinez, Herminia E.
Shell, Juanita
Shen, John
Shon, Elizbabeth
Shroff, Kamal
Shum, Hilda B.
Shum, Hilda B.
Simpson, Adelaide W.
Singh, R. K. Janmeha
Singh, Silvija S.
Sison, Cecile E.
Smith, Carol Y.
Smith, Cherryl R.
Smith, Walanda W.
Smith, William
Sobrino, James F.
Somjee, Lubna
Somodevilla, S. A.
Sosa, Juan N.
Soto, Elaine
Southerland, Deborah L.
Soza, Anthony M.
Spidell Helms, Dorothy J.
Spivey, Philop B.
Srinivasan, Sampurna
St. Leger, Sidney C.
Stephens, Dorothy W.
Stevenson, Jr., Edward E.
Stewart, Arleen R.
Stewart, Vlenaetha
Suarez, Alejandra
Swaney, Gyda
Swan, June A.
Sy, Michael J.
Tabachnik, Samuel
Takemoto-Chock, Naomi
Tamura, Leonard J.
Tan, Gabriel
Tapo, Linda J.
Taylor, Palmeda D.
Taylor, Peggy S.
Tazeau, Yvette N.
Teng, L. Neal
Thorson, Billie J.
Tien, Liang
Torres-Saenz, Jorge
Torres, Mario A.
Tostado, John F.
Towns-Miranda, Luz
Triplett, Sheila J.
Tsai, Mavis
Tsushima, William T.
Tung, May
Uzzell, Barbara P.
Vakhariya, Sobha

Valdivia, Lino
Valtierra, Mary
Vance, Ellen B.
Vance, Marilyn M.
Vanderhost, Leonette
Vargas, M. Angelica
Vargas, Manuel J.
Vaughans, Kirkland C.
Vazquez, Rosa
Vega, Star
Velez-Diaz, Angel
Villela, Leopoldo F.
Wakeman, Richard J.
Walker, L. Gorman
Walker, Lola '.
Ward, Alan J.
Washington, Anita C.
Washington, Dianna E.
Webster, E. Carol
Wickramasekera, Ian E.
Williams-Markum, Deirdre
Williams, Mary Beth
Williams, Medria L.
Wilson, Susan B.
Wilson, Woodrow
Winter, Amal
Witter, Jeanette M.
Wong-Ngan, Julia A.
Wong, Kit L.
Woo, Rose
Wu, Sheila T.
Yamaguchi, Mitsue Y.
Yancey, Angela L.
Yee, Jane K.
Yi, Kris Y.
Yniguez, Linda E.
Yoshimura, G. Joji
Yoshimura, Kari K.
Yuen, Lenora L.
Yu, Pamela
Zaldivar, Luis R.
Zayas-Bazan, Carmen

Secondary Role

Abernethy, Alexis D.
Ainslie, Ricardo C.
Allsopp, Ralph N
Alonso, Mario
Alvarez, Gary L.
Anton, William D.
Aoki, Bart K.
Arcaya, Jose M.
Archibald, Eloise M.
Austria, Asuncion M.
Balbona, Manuel
Beliz, Jr., Efrain A.
Bernal, Guillermo A.
Berrios, Zaida R.
Binns, Derrick
Brandenburg, Carlos E.
Buffin, Janice E.
Burnett, Judith A.
Campbell, Kamal E.
Campbell, Stephen N.

Campos, Peter E.
Carr, Paquita R.
Cervantes, Joseph M.
Choney, John M.
Church, June S.
Connor, Michael E.
Dave, Jagdish P.
Doss, Juanita K.
Emory, Eugene K.
Epps, Pamela J.
Evans, Helen L.
Everett, Moses L.
Falicov, Celia J.
Faraci, Ana M.
Fields, Anika C.
Floyd, James A.
Fujitsubo, Lani C.
Fullilove, Constance
Fulton, Aubyn
Gallagher, Rosina M.
Gant, Bob L.
Garg, Mithlesh
Garrett-Akinsanya, BraVada
Gary, Juneau M.
Garza, Joe G.
Gillem, Angela R
Glover, O.S.
Gonzalez, Rocio R
Graves-Cooper, Phyllis J.
Greene, Beverly
Green, Theophilus E.
Grinstead, Olga A.
Hawkins, Ioma L.
Hernandez, Cibeles
Higa, William R.
Hsia, Heidi
Ingram, Winifred
Inoue, Sachi
Jackson, Leslie C.
James, Michelle D.
Johnson, Fred A.
Johnson, Zonya
Jones, George L.
Joseph, Jr., Herbert M.
Kashikar-Zuck, Susmita M.
Khan, Badrul A.
Khanna, Jaswant L.
Klopner, Michele C.
Kolt, Laurie
Langley, Merlin R
Lawson, Gary W.
LeSure-Lester, G. Evelyn
Llado, Sarah L.
Llanos, Aracely B.
Llorente, Antolin M.
London, Dyanne P.
Lopez, Martita A.
Machabanski, Hector
Mack, Delores E.
Martinez, Alejandro M.
Matsumoto, Gregory Y.
Maynard, Edward S.
McKenzie, Jr., Loratuis L.

Menchaca, Victoria A.
Montesi, Alexandra Saba
Montoya, E. Carolina
Mora, Ralph
Morishige, Howard H.
Moritsugu, John
Muga, Joe
Muir-Malcolm, Joan A.
Murakawa, Fay
Nabors, Nina A.
Onizuka, Richard K.
Osato, Sheryl
Paige, Roger
Pang, Dawn
Peniston, Eugene G.
Penn, Nolan E.
Peoples, Kathleen
Perez-Arce, Patricia
Phillips, Campbell C.
Pinder-Amaker, Stephanie L.
Pinto, Alcides
Pugh, Roderick W.
Rainwater, III, Avie J.
Rivera, Nelson E.
Rivero, Estela M.
Romney, Patricia
Ruiz, Fernando
Schacht, Thomas E.
Sharp, Jude C.
Smith, Jr., Theodore R.
Smith, Michael C.
Soto, Tomas A.
Strickland, Tony L
Stringer, Anthony Y.
Suarez-Crowe, Yolanda
Suarez, Carlota
Takamine, Sandra
Takushi, Ruby Y.
Tate, Donald
Thurman, Pamela J.
Torigoe, Rodney Y.
Turnbough, P. Diane
Upadhyaya, Shripati
Vargas, Luis A.
Velez, Maria T.
Walcott, Delores D.
Walker, O'Neal A.
Walton, Duncan E.
Whitaker, Sandra V.
Williams, Indy J.
Williams, Rebecca E.
Williams, Victoria F.
Wong, Philip S
Word, James C.
Yabusaki, Ann S.
Yanagida, Evelyn H.
Yee, Tina T.
Young, David A.
Zamudio, Anthony

-Researcher-

Primary Role
Barbarin, Oscar A.

Basco, Monica A.
Carballo-Dieguez, Alex
Cepeda-Benito, Antonio
Emory, Eugene K.
Gomez, John P
Green, Charles A.
Grinstead, Olga A.
Gutierrez, Manuel J.
Inoue, Sachi
Kochevar-Sukkarie, Renee J.
LaDue, Robin A.
Lopez, Steven R.
Milner, Joel S.
Muir-Malcolm, Joan A.
Nagata, Donna K.
Neal-Barnett, Angela M.
Osato, Sheryl
Perilla, Julia L.
Pinderhughes, Ellen B.
Prelow, Hazel M.
Saldana, Delia H.
Sitharthan, Thiagarajan
Strickland, Tony L
Stringer, Anthony Y.
Szapocznik, Jose
Takushi, Ruby Y.
Thurman, Pamela J.
Turner, Samuel M.
Weston, Raymond E.

Secondary Role
Adams, Jr., Clarence L.
Akutsu, Phillip D.
Anderson, Louis P.
Anderson, Norman B.
Arellano-Lopez, Juan
Armengol, Carmen G.
Arroyo, Judith A.
Ascencao, Erlete M.
Auuilas-Gaxiola, Sergio A.
Barnes, Charles A.
Barrera, Jr., Manuel
Bernal, Guillermo
Bernal, Martha E
Binion, Victoria J.
Boone, Martin
Bynum, Edward B.
Camargo, Robert J.
Cardena, Etzel A.
Cebollero, Ana Margarita
Chang, Alice F.
Chang, Theodore C. H.
Chin, Lemin
Choca, James
Cimino, Cynthia R.
Cruz, Albert R.
DeFerreire, Mary Elizabeth
Flores, Elena
Fried-Cassorla, Martha J.
Gomez, Jr., Francisco C.
Gonsalves, Carlos J.
Gonzalez, Gerardo M
Guanipa, Carmen L.
Gular, Enrique

Hall, Howard
Hall, Ruth L.
Han, Yu Ling
Harper, Mary S.
Harrell, Shelly P.
Harris, Shanette M.
Hightower, Eugene
Ichiyama, Michael A.
Ike, Chris A.
Iwamasa, Gayle Y.
Jain, Sharat K.
Jones, Arthur C.
Kao, Barbara T.
Kich, George Kitahara
Kuan, Yie-Wen Y.
Kwon, Paul H.
Labbe, Elise E.
Lambert, Michael C.
Lee, Hing-Chu B.
Lee, Wanda M. L.
Liem, Ramsay
Liston, Hattye H.
London, Lorna H.
Manruque-Reichard, Marta E.
Mate-Kole, C. Charles
McCann, Robin S.
McClure, Faith H.
Miles, Gary T.
Mio, Jeffery S.
Miranda, M.
Mori, Lisa T.
Munoz, Ricardo F.
Myers, Hector F.
Nagayama Hall, Gordon C.
Nakamura, Charles Y.
Nayak, Madhabika B.
Nettles, Arie L.
Nezu, Arthur M.
Norman, William H.
Okazaki, Sumie
Reisinger, Curtis W.
Robinson, W. LaVome
Rodriguez, Rogelio E.
Rollock, David
Roll, Samuel
Root, Maria P. P.
Russell, David M.
Sanders-Thompson, Vetta L.
Sanua, Victor D.
Serafica, Felicisima C.
Shell, Juanita
Shopshire, Michael S.
Sison, Cecile E.
Snowden, Lonnie R.
Solomon, Sondra E.
Somjee, Lubna
Spidell Helms, Dorothy J.
Stewart, Sunita M.
Sue, David
Sue, Stanley
Takemoto-Chock, Naomi
Tanaka-Matsumi, Junko
Tan, Gabriel

Tan, Josephine
Tatum, Beverly D.
Tsang, Michael Hing- Pui
Tsujimoto, Richard N.
Valentiner, David P.
Valtierra, Mary
Velasquez, John M.
Velasquez, Roberto J.
Viale-val, Graciela
Vraniak, Damian A.
Ward, Alan J.
Wickramasekera, Ian E.
Williams, Steve
Wilson, Melvin N.
Wong, Jane L.
Wyche, Karen F.
Ying, Yu-Wen
Young, Kimberly S.
Zane, Nolan W.S

-Other-

Primary Role
De Louredes Mattei, Maria
Huang, Larke N.
Jackson-Davis, Brandi
Kimbauer, Elli M.
Louredes Mattei, Maria De
Murakawa, Fay
Ohye, Bonnie Y.
Pirhekayaty-Soriano, Tahereh
Rodriguez, Manuel D.
Ruiz, Fernando
Stokes, Devon R.
Vazquez, Carlos D.

COGNITIVE PSYCHOLOGY

-Academician-

Primary Role
Chun, Marvin M.
Jin, Young-Sun
Monteiro, Kenneth P.
Roig, Miguel
Sudevan, Padmanbhan
Valencia-Laver, Debra

Secondary Role
Altarriba, Jeanette
Gonzalez, Fernando
Kim, Yung Che
Monteiro, Kenneth P.
Rajaram, Suparna

-Administrator-

Primary Role
Cleveland, Adriana F.
Dong, Tim T.
Jones, Paulette
Koshino, Hideya

Secondary Role

Reyna, Valerie F.

-Consultant-

Primary Role
Laviena, Luis

Secondary Role
Cleveland, Adriana F.

-Practitioner-

Primary Role
Benamu, Icem
Ho, Kay

Secondary Role
Laviena, Luis

-Researcher-

Primary Role
Altarriba, Jeanette
Chiang, Grace CT
Gonzalez, Fernando
Kim, Yung Che
Rajaram, Suparna
Reyna, Valerie F.

COMMUNITY PSYCHOLOGY

-Academician-

Primary Role
Chung, Rita L.
Dockett, Kathleen H.
Fergus, Esther O.
Milburn, Norweeta G.
Miller, Robin L.
Moore, Sandra
Myers, Ernest R.
Sasao, Toshiaki
Serrano-Garcia, Irma
Suarez-Balcazar, Yolanda
Watts, Roderick J.

Secondary Role
Nemoto, Tooru
Ray, Jacqueline W.
Rogler, Lloyd H.
Rosario, Margaret

-Administrator-

Primary Role
Blandino, Ramon A.
Hernandez, Maria G.
Holliday, Bertha G.
McNeal, Meryl
Nickerson, Kim J.
Ray, Jacqueline W.

Secondary Role
Valdes, Maria

-Consultant-

Primary Role
Valdes, Maria

Secondary Role
Coelho, Richard J.
Elligan, Don G.
Friday, Jennifer C.
Garcia, Hector D.
Holliday, Bertha G.
Hernandez, Maria G.
Myers, Ernest R.
Watts, Roderick J.

-Practitioner-

Primary Role
Elligan, Don G.
Garcia, Hector D.

Secondary Role
Blandino, Ramon A.
Fergus, Esther O.

-Researcher-

Primary Role
Coelho, Richard J.
Friday, Jennifer C.
Nemoto, Tooru
Rogler, Lloyd H.
Rosario, Margaret

COMPARATIVE PSYCHOLOGY

-Academician-

Primary Role
Suarez, Susan D.

-Researcher-

Primary Role
Uyeda, Arthur A.

COUNSELING PSYCHOLOGY

-Academician-

Primary Role
Alexander, Charlene M.
Amawattana, Tipawadee
Araoz, Daniel L.
Arbona, Consuelo
Ayoub, Catherine C.
Bacigalupe, Gonzalo M.
Bowman, Sharon L.
Boyer, Michele C.
Brown, Michael T.
Buki, Lydia P.
Bursztyn, Alberto M.
Butler, B. LaConyea
Chang, Thomas M.C.
Chen, Eric C
Chung, Y. Barry
Clarke-Pine, Dora D.
Coleman, Hardin L.

Constantine, Madonna G.
Dawis, Rene V.
De Las Fuentes, Cynthia
Duan, Changming
Espin, Oliva M.
Essandoh, Pius K.
Finley, Laurene Y.
Fouad, Nadya A.
Fraser, Kathryn P.
Garcia-Shelton, Linda M.
Gloria, Alberta M.
Gui, Chui-Liu Serena
Ham, MaryAnna D.
Hunt, Portia
Ibrahim, Farah A.
Jun, Heesoon
Kim, Randi I.
LaFromboise, Teresa
Lam, Chow S.
Leong, Frederick T. T.
Leung, Paul
Lopez-Baez, Sandra I.
Lowe, Susana M.
Marotta, Sylvia A.
McMillan, Robert
McNeill, Brian
McRae, Mary B.
Mellot, Ramona N.
Millan, Fred
Morales, Pamilla V.
Nadal-Vazquez, Vilma Y.
Oda, Ethel Aiko
Owyang, Walter
Perez, Carlos A.
Phelps, Rosemary E.
Philp, Frederick W.
Pope-Davis, Donald B.
Pope, Mark
Quintana, Stephen M.
Rhee, Susan B.
Ridley, Charles R.
Rivera, Beatriz D.
Robinson, John D
Rodriguez, Ester R.
Ruiz, Nicholas J.
Sapp, Marty
Selgas, James W.
Sodowsky, Gargi R.
Soriano, Marcel
Speight, Suzette L.
Sue, Derald W.
Suzuki, Lisa A.
Tai, Chun-Nan
Tan, Rowena N.
Thomas, Anita J.
Thompson, Chalmer E.
Tomlinson-Clarke, Saundra M.
Valdez, Jesse N.
Vargas, Alice M.
Vazquez, Cesar D.
Vera, Elizabeth M.
Wang, Wen-Hsiu

Watanabe-Muraoka, Agnes M.
Whitaker, Arthur L.
Wright, Doris J.
Wu, Li-Chuan
Wu, Shi-Jiuan

Secondary Role
Amezcua, Charlie A.
Barry, Martha J.
Blanco-Beledo, Ricardo
Chan, Adrian
Cook, Donelda
Dias, Milagres C.
Doris, Terri M.
Ervin, Betty J.
Fukuyama, Mary A.
Hammond, Gladys
Howard, Mary T.
Kemp, Arthur D.
Ledesma, Lourdes K.
Lee, C. Jarnie W J
Mitchell, Horace
Morales, Eduardo S.
Morris, Joseph R.
Omizo, Michael M.
Ovide, Christopher R.
Perez, Ruperto M.
Peters, James S.
Porche-Burke, Lisa M.
Poston, II, Walker S.
Ramirez-Cancel, Carlos M.
Reyes-Mayer, Erwin
Rodriguez, Richard A.
Sakata, Robert T.
Sancho, Ana M.
Sedo, Manuel A.
Silva, Santiago
Toldson, Ivory L.
Tucker, Samuel J.
Valdes, Thusnelda M.
Vega, Jose G.
Vigil, Patricia L.
York, Mary J.

-Administrator-

Primary Role
Alvarez, Paul A.
Bingham, Rosie P.
Borrero-Hernandez, Alejo
Carter, William J.
Chan, Adrian
Clansy, Pauline A.
Copher-Haynes, Harriett
De Leaire, Robert
Deleaire, Robert N.
Dias, Milagres C.
Kim, Elizabeth J.
Martinez, Floyd H.
Mitchell, Horace
Miyahira, Sarah D.
Morales-Barreto, Gisela
Morris, Joseph R.
Omizo, Michael M.
Parham, Thomas A.

Parks, Fayth M.
Payton, Carolyn R.
Peoples, Napoleon L.
Peters, James S.
Porche-Burke, Lisa M.
Reed, James D.
Reilly, Patrick M.
Riddle, P. Elayne
Rodriguez, Carmen G.
Sakata, Robert T.
Salone, Lavorial
Sanders, Gilbert O.
Silva, Santiago
West, Gerald I.
Whitehead, Barry X.
White, Voncile
Wibberly, Kathy H.
York, Joan E. S.

Secondary Role
Abudabbeh, Nuha
Asghar, Anila
Balderrama, Sylvia R.
Bursztyn, Alberto M.
Contreras, Raquel J.
Droz, Elizabeth
Fisher, Patricia A.
Haggins, Kristee L.
James, Larry C.
Jones-Saumty, Deborah J.
Lin, J.C. Gisela G.
Mastrapa, Selma A.
Mellot, Ramona N.
Noel, Winifred
Oda, Ethel Aiko
Owyang, Walter
Parham, William D.
Perez, Carlos A.
Philp, Frederick W.
Prendes-Lintel, Maria L.
Prieto, Susan L.
Ramirez, John/Juan
Robinson, Gregory F.
Roehlke, Helen J.
Sanders, Daniel W.
Silling, S. Marc
Williams, Eddie E.
Wu, Shi-Jiuan
Yu, Angelita M.

-Consultant-

Primary Role
Arredondo, Patricia
Carter, Lonnie T.
Cook, Donelda
Fankhanel, Edward H.
Jones-Saumty, Deborah J.
Morales, Eduardo S.
Rojas, Rebecca S
Valdes, Luis F.
Wang, Richard S.
Webb, Wanda

Secondary Role
Alvarez, Paul A.
Amawattana, Tipawadee
Anand, Shashi
Araoz, Daniel L.
Barner, II, Pearl
Biggs, Bradley
Boyer, Michele C.
Bruguera, Mark R.
Cherbosque, Jorge
Chung, Edith C.
Cook, Rudolf E.
Copher-Haynes, Harriett
de la Sota, Elizanda M.
Derrickson, Kimberly B.
Espin, Oliva M.
Field, Lucy F.
Garcia-Shelton, Linda M.
Garrido-Castillo, Pedro
Gonzalez-Sorensen, Anna G.
Griffith, Albert R.
Hargrow, Mary E.
Hartzell, Richard E.
Houston, Lawrence N.
Jackson, Joyce Taborn
Jenkins, Yvonne M
Johnson, Johnny
Kramer, Harry M. O.
Lashley, Karen H.
Lee, D. John
Lerma, Joe L.
Ludmer, Alba
Luke, Equilla
Marquez, E. Mario
Mars, Raymond G.
McNeill, Earle
Miyahira, Sarah D.
Morales-Barreto, Gisela
Newburgh, Tracey LS
Onoda, Lawrence
Ortiz, Berta S.
Puig, Ange
Ramirez, David E.
Riddle, P. Elayne
Rivera-Sinclair, Elsa A.
Robertson, John F.
Rodriguez, Carmen G.
Rohila, Pritam K.
Sadler, Mark S.
Saul, Tuck T.
Schlesinger, Susana J.
Shipp, Pamela L.
Shires, Michael R.
Tan, Rowena N.
Taylor, Flor N.
Trotman, Frances K.
Turner, Alvin L.
Valdez, Jr., Romulo
Valley, John A.
Vasquez, Melba
Vazquez, Cesar D.
Vicente, Peter J.
Ward, Connie M.

Watts, Charlotte B.
West, Gerald I.
Zayas, Maria A.

-Practitioner-

Primary Role
Abudabbeh, Nuha
Acka-Pope, Zeynep K
Akca, Zeynep K.
Amezcua, Charlie A.
Anand, Shashi
Andrieu, Brenda J.
Asghar, Anila
Balderrama, Sylvia R.
Baly, Iris E.
Barner, II, Pearl
Barry, Martha J.
Biggs, Bradley
Bild-Libbin, Raguel
Blanco-Beledo, Ricardo
Bruguera, Mark R.
Canovas Welles, Nydia L.
Castillo, Diane T.
Cherbosque, Jorge
Chung, Edith C.
Contreras, Raquel J.
Cook, Rudolf E.
de la Sota, Elizanda M.
Derrickson, Kimberly B.
Doris, Terri M.
Droz, Elizabeth
Ervin, Betty J.
Fernandez, Rosemary
Field, Lucy F.
Fisher, Patricia A.
Francisco, Richard P.
Fukuyama, Mary A.
Garrido-Castillo, Pedro
Gironella, Oliva C.
Gonzalez-Sorensen, Anna G.
Grajales, Elisa M.
Griffith, Albert R.
Haggins, Kristee L.
Haley, Adriana R.
Hambright, Jerold E.
Hammond, Gladys
Hargrow, Mary E.
Hartzell, Richard E.
Hernandez, Vivian O.
Houston, Lawrence N.
Howard, Mary T.
Hu, Trudy HC
Jackson, Joyce Taborn
James-Parker, Magna M.
James, Larry C.
Jenkins, Sheila A.
Jenkins, Yvonne M
Kemp, Arthur D.
Kramer, Harry M. O.
Lashley, Karen H.
Ledesma, Lourdes K.
Lee, C. Jarnie W J
Lee, D. John

Lee, Margaret
Lerma, Joe L.
Lin, J.C. Gisela G.
Ludmer, Alba
Luke, Equilla
Manese, Jeanne E.
Marquez, E. Mario
Mars, Raymond G.
Martinez, Cynthia
Mastrapa, Selma A.
McNeill, Earle
Minturn, Robin H.
Nazario, Jr., Andres
Newburgh, Tracey LS
Nieto-Cardoso, Ezequiel
Noel, Winifred
Onoda, Lawrence
Ortiz, Berta S.
Ovide, Christopher R.
Parham, William D.
Perez, Ruperto M.
Prendes-Lintel, Maria L.
Prieto, Susan L.
Puig, Ange
Ramirez-Cancel, Carlos M.
Ramirez, David E.
Ramirez, John/Juan
Reams, Bennie P
Ribera-Gonzalez, Julio C.
Rivera-Sinclair, Elsa A.
Robertson, John F.
Robinson, Gregory F.
Rodriguez, Richard A.
Roehlke, Helen J.
Rohila, Pritam K.
Ryan, Robert A.
Sadler, Mark S.
Saenz, Karol K.
Sampson, Myrtle B.
Sancho, Ana M.
Sanders, Daniel W.
Saul, Tuck T.
Schlesinger, Susana J.
Sedo, Manuel A.
Shipp, Pamela L.
Shires, Michael R.
Silling, S. Marc
Stone, G. Vaughn
Sundararajan, Louise Kuen-Wei
Sutton, David
Taylor, Flor N.
Toldson, Ivory L.
Trotman, Frances K.
Tucker, Samuel J.
Turner, Alvin L.
Valdes, Thusnelda M.
Valdez, Jr., Romulo
Valley, John A.
Vasquez, Melba
Vega, Jose G.
Vicente, Peter J.
Vigil, Patricia L.
Ward, Connie M.

Watts, Charlotte B.
  West, James E.
  Williams, Eddie E.
  Wong, Martin R.
  York, Mary J.
  Yu, Angelita M.
  Yun, S.B.
  Zayas, Maria A.
Secondary Role
  Arredondo, Patricia
  Ayoub, Catherine C.
  Bingham, Rosie P.
  Borrero-Hernandez, Alejo
  Bowman, Sharon L.
  Buki, Lydia P.
  Carter, Lonnie T.
  Carter, William J.
  Chang, Thomas M.C.
  Clansy, Pauline A.
  Clarke-Pine, Dora D.
  Fankhanel, Edward H.
  Finley, Laurene Y.
  Fraser, Kathryn P.
  Gui, Chui-Liu Serena
  Hargrove, Jr., Jerry E.
  Hunt, Portia
  Ibrahim, Farah A.
  Kim, Elizabeth J.
  Lopez-Baez, Sandra I.
  McMillan, Robert
  Millan, Fred
  Parham, Thomas A.
  Payton, Carolyn R.
  Peoples, Napoleon L.
  Reed, James D.
  Reilly, Patrick M.
  Rhee, Susan B.
  Rivera, Beatriz D.
  Robinson, John D.
  Ruiz, Nicholas J.
  Salone, Lavorial
  Sanders, Gilbert O.
  Selgas, James W.
  Sue, Derald W.
  Tai, Chun-Nan
  Thomas, Anita J.
  Vargas, Alice M.
  Webb, Wanda
  Whitaker, Arthur L.
  Whitehead, Barry X.
  White, Voncile
  Wu, Li-Chuan
  York, Joan E. S.

-Researcher-

Primary Role
  Battiest, William V.
  Johnson, Johnny
  Poston, II, Walker S.
  Reyes-Mayer, Erwin

Secondary Role
  Arbona, Consuelo
  Bacigalupe, Gonzalo M.
  Castillo, Diane T.
  Chung, Y. Barry
  Coleman, Hardin L.
  Constantine, Madonna G.
  Dawis, Rene V.
  De Las Fuentes, Cynthia
  De Leaire, Robert
  Deleaire, Robert N.
  Duan, Changming
  Essandoh, Pius K.
  Fouad, Nadya A.
  Francisco, Richard P.
  Gloria, Alberta M.
  Kim, Randi I.
  LaFromboise, Teresa
  Lam, Chow S.
  Leong, Frederick T. T.
  Leung, Paul
  Lowe, Susana M.
  Marotta, Sylvia A.
  McNeill, Brian
  McRae, Mary B.
  Morales, Pamilla V.
  Nieto-Cardoso, Ezequiel
  Parks, Fayth M.
  Phelps, Rosemary E.
  Pope-Davis, Donald B.
  Pope, Mark
  Quintana, Stephen M.
  Ribera-Gonzalez, Julio C.
  Ridley, Charles R.
  Rodriguez, Ester R.
  Rojas, Rebecca S.
  Sapp, Marty
  Sodowsky, Gargi R.
  Soriano, Marcel
  Speight, Suzette L.
  Sundararajan, Louise Kuen-Wei
  Sutton, David
  Suzuki, Lisa A.
  Thompson, Chalmer E.
  Valdez, Jesse N.
  Wang, Wen-Hsiu
  Watanabe-Muraoka, Agnes M.
  Wibberly, Kathy H.
  Wong, Martin R.

-Other-

Primary Role
  Daly, Frederica Y.
  Fujimura, Laura E.
  Hargrove, Jr., Jerry E.
  Rivers, Miriam W.

DEVELOPMENTAL PSYCHOLOGY

-Academician-

Primary Role
  Amaro, Hortensia
  Azmitia, Margarita
  Bainum, Charlene K.
  Brookins, Geraldine K.
  Caldera, Yvonne M.
  Campos, Joseph J.
  Chiriboga, David A.
  Cunningham, Michael
  D'Heurle, Adma J.
  DeMeis, Debra K.
  Garcia-Coll, Cynthia
  Garrett, Aline M.
  Gordon, Kimberly A.
  Graham, Sandra
  Grimes, Tresmaine R.
  Grych, Diane S.
  Hestick, Henrietta
  Hossain, Ziarat
  Jones, Elaine F.
  Ko, Hwawei
  Lawrence, Valerie W.
  Mcloyd, Vonnie C.
  Montemayor, Raymond
  Murakami, Sharon
  Nelson-LeGall, Sharon A.
  Nunez, Narina N.
  Oka, Evelyn R.
  Okagaki, Lynn
  Okorodudu, Corahann
  Parks, Carlton
  Richard, Harriette W.
  Roberts, Albert
  Slaughter-Defoe, Diana T.
  Soler, Robin E.
  Somerville, Addison W.
  Ward, Lucretia M.
  Wilson, Shirley B.
  Yang, Raymond K.
  Zayas, Luis H.
  Zepeda, Marlene
  Zhu, Jiajun
Secondary Role
  Balcazar, Fabricio E.
  Beatty, Lula A.
  Blubaugh, Victoria G.
  Burton, Roger V.
  Callahan, Michelle R.
  Delgado-Hachey, Maria
  Kameshima, Shinya
  Reid, Pamela T.
  Scott-Jones, Diane
  Spencer, Margaret B.

-Administrator-

Primary Role
  Beatty, Lula A.
  Coffey, Maryann B.

Harris, Jasper W.
  Horton, Carrell
  Reaves, Juanita Y.
  Reid, Pamela T.
  Toro, Haydee
Secondary Role
  Copeland, Jr., E. Thomas
  Okorodudu, Corahann
  Takanishi, Ruby

-Consultant-

Primary Role
  Baxley, Gladys B.
  Blubaugh, Victoria G.
Secondary Role
  Arriso, Roberta H.
  Bouffard, R. Gerard
  Coffey, Maryann B.
  Figueredo, Migdalia I.
  Grych, Diane S.
  Lee, See-Woo S.
  Lewis, Marva L.
  Montes, Francisco
  Reaves, Juanita Y.
  Richard, Harriette W.
  Rivers, Marie D.
  Romero, Arturo
  Toro, Haydee
  Wong, Dorothy L.

-Practitioner-

Primary Role
  Arboleda, Catalina
  Arriso, Roberta H.
  Bouffard, R. Gerard
  Copeland, Jr., E. Thomas
  Figueredo, Migdalia I.
  Kau, Alice S. M.
  Keefe, Keunho
  Lee, See-Woo S.
  Lewis, Marva L.
  Montes, Francisco
  Pflaum, John H.
  Rivers, Marie D.
  Romero, Arturo
  Williamson, Diane H.
  Wong, Dorothy L.
Secondary Role
  Harris, Jasper W.
  Hestick, Henrietta
  Linares, Lourdes O.
  Somerville, Addison W.

-Researcher-

Primary Role
  Balcazar, Fabricio E.
  Burton, Roger V.
  Callahan, Michelle R.
  Delgado-Hachey, Maria
  Jackson, Jacquelyne F.
  Kameshima, Shinya
  Linares, Lourdes O.

Mink, Iris T.
Mino, Itsuko
Scott-Jones, Diane
Spencer, Margaret B.
Takanishi, Ruby

Secondary Role

Amaro, Hortensia
Azmitia, Margarita
Bainum, Charlene K.
Baxley, Gladys B.
Brookins, Geraldine K
Caldera, Yvonne M.
Campos, Joseph J.
Chiriboga, David A.
Cunningham, Michael
DeMeis, Debra K.
Garcia-Coll, Cynthia
Garrett, Aline M.
Gordon, Kimberly A.
Graham, Sandra
Grimes, Tresmaine R
Hossain, Ziarat
Jones, Elaine F.
Junn, Ellen
Ko, Hwawei
Lawrence, Valerie W.
Mcloyd, Vonnie C.
Montemayor, Raymond
Murakami, Sharon
Nelson-LeGall, Sharon A.
Oka, Evelyn R.
Okagaki, Lynn
Parks, Carlton
Pflaum, John H.
Roberts, Albert
Slaughter-Defoe, Diana T.
Wilson, Shirley B.
Yang, Raymond K.
Zayas, Luis H.
Zepeda, Marlene
Zhu, Jiajun

-Other-

Primary Role
Junn, Ellen

EDUCATIONAL PSYCHOLOGY

-Academician-

Primary Role
Al-tai, Nazar M.
Apenahier, Leonard
Artiles, Alfredo J.
Asamen, Joy K.
Asbury, Charles A.
Baxter, Anthony G.
Brooks, Lewis A.
Carter, Lamore J.
Chen, S. Andrew
Das, Jagannath P.

Duran, Richard P.
Escudero, Micaela
Furukawa, James M.
Garcia, Teresa
Greene, Ruth L.
Herrans, Laura L.
Hong, Eunsook
Hudley, Cynthia
Hutchinson, Kim M.
Jones, Reginald L.
Lequerica, Martha
Lin, Hsin-Tai
Mahy, Yvonne C.
Mendez-Calderon, Luis M.
Miura, Irene T.
Mizokawa, Donald T.
Narvaez, Darcia F.
Price, Linda A.
Sikka, Anjoo
Singg, Sangeeta
Twe, Boikai S.
Velayo, Richard S.
Whang, Patricia A.
Wong, Lily Y.S
Yee, Albert H.

Secondary Role

Chan, Kenyon S.
Kame'enui, Edward J.
Kim, Yang Ja
Okonji, Jacques A.
Rivera-Medina, Eduardo J.
Yan, Bernice
Yu, Howard K.

-Administrator-

Primary Role
Baker, III, Carl E.
Carey, Patricia M.
Chan, Kenyon S.
Henderson Daniel, Jessica
Hill, Anthony L
Johnson, Eugene H.
Mellor, Catherine A.
Spraings, Violet E.

Secondary Role
Carter, Lamore J.
Fields, Amanda H.
Izutsu, Satoru
James, Norman L.
Marrero, Bernie
Roberts, Terrence J.
Thomas, Thomas J.

-Consultant-

Primary Role
Izutsu, Satoru
Moore, Helen B.
Okonji, Jacques A.
Rivera-Medina, Eduardo J.
Thomas, Thomas J.

Secondary Role
Baker, III, Carl E.

Baxter, Anthony G.
Carey, Patricia M.
Coes, Maria R.
de Jesus, Nelson H.
Escudero, Micaela
Gonzalez, John
Lewis, Brenda J.
Meadows-Yancey, Dorothy
Mellor, Catherine A.
Mendez-Calderon, Luis M.
Mendez, Gloria I.
Natalicio, Luiz
O'Brien, B. Marco
Tamayo, Jose M.
Tsui, Ellen C.
Vanderpool, Andrea T.
Yap, Kim O.

-Practitioner-

Primary Role
Adler, Peter J.
Antokoletz, Juana C.
Boggs, Minnie
de Jesus, Nelson H.
Fields, Amanda H.
Fujita, George T.
Gonzalez, John
Hammond, Evelyn S.
James, Norman L.
Kim, Yang Ja
Lewis, Brenda J.
Marrero, Bernie
Mendez, Gloria I.
Natalicio, Luiz
O'Brien, B. Marco
Ramaswami, Sundar
Roberts, Terrence J.
Tamayo, Jose M.
Tsui, Ellen C.
Vanderpool, Andrea T.
Williams, Estelle M.

Secondary Role
Brooks, Lewis A.
Henderson Daniel, Jessica
Herrans, Laura L.
Lequerica, Martha
Moore, Helen B.
Spraings, Violet E.
Twe, Boikai S.

-Researcher-

Primary Role
Coes, Maria R.
Kame'enui, Edward J.
Yan, Bernice
Yap, Kim O.

Secondary Role
Al-tai, Nazar M.
Apenahier, Leonard
Artiles, Alfredo J.
Asamen, Joy K.
Asbury, Charles A.

Chen, S. Andrew
Das, Jagannath P.
Duran, Richard P.
Furukawa, James M.
Garcia, Teresa
Greene, Ruth L.
Hong, Eunsook
Hudley, Cynthia
Hutchinson, Kim M.
Lin, Hsin-Tai
Mahy, Yvonne C.
Miura, Irene T.
Mizokawa, Donald T.
Sikka, Anjoo
Velayo, Richard S.
Wang, Margaret C.
Whang, Patricia A.
Wong, Lily Y.S
Yee, Albert H.

-Other-

Primary Role
Wang, Margaret C.
Yu, Howard K.

ENVIRONMENTAL PSYCHOLOGY

-Academician-

Primary Role
Sinha, Sachchida
Sutton, Sharon E.

-Researcher-

Primary Role
Hilton, William F.
Jennings, Jr., Wilmar A.

EXPERIMENTAL PSYCHOLOGY

-Academician-

Primary Role
Ardila, Ruben
Ashida, Sachio
Cornwell, Henry G.
Edwards, Henry P.
Freeman, James E.
Garcia, Margarita
Gayle, Michael C.
Harleston, Bernard W.
Hom, Harry L.
Izawa, Chizuko
Johnson, Edward E.
Matsumoto, Roy T.
Morgan, Cynthia L.
Mo, Suchoon
Vaid, Jyotsna
Wang, Alvin
Yamaguchi, Harry G.

Zuriff, Gerald E.

Secondary Role
McDonald, Arthur L.
Sakamoto, Katsuyuki
Sax, Kenji W.

-Administrator-

Primary Role
McDonald, Arthur L.
Sakamoto, Katsuyuki

Secondary Role
Garcia, Margarita
Harleston, Bernard W.

-Consultant-

Primary Role
Chinn, Roberta N.

Secondary Role
Barrera, Francisco J.
Cornwell, Henry G.
Edwards, Henry P.
Johnson, Lawrence B.
Tang, Terry
Wong, Jessie

-Practitioner-

Primary Role
Barrera, Francisco J.
Tang, Terry

Secondary Role
Johnson, Edward E.
Zuriff, Gerald E.

-Researcher-

Primary Role
Johnson, Lawrence B.
Sax, Kenji W.
Wong, Jessie

GENERAL PSYCHOLOGY/ METHODS & SYSTEMS

-Academician-

Primary Role
Aradom, Tesfay A
Babb, Harold
Foo, Koong H.
Murray, James L.
Vazquez-Ruiz, Francisco
Williams, Daniel E.

Secondary Role
Jones, Ferdinand
Luna, Donna J.
Teo, Thomas

-Administrator-

Primary Role
Lyles, William B.
Mukherjee, Subhash C.

Secondary Role
Baca, Sandra G.
Sanchez, David M.
Topolski, James M.

-Consultant-

Primary Role
Jones, Ferdinand
Sanchez, David M.

Secondary Role
Blackburn, Winona K.
Diaz-Guerrero, Rogelio
Laosa, Luis M.
Lyles, William B.
Morales, Elias
Vazquez-Ruiz, Francisco

-Practitioner-

Primary Role
Baca, Sandra G.
Hall, Juanita L.
Luna, Donna J.
Morales, Elias

Secondary Role
Aradom, Tesfay A
Williams, Daniel E.

-Researcher-

Primary Role
Blackburn, Winona K.
Diaz-Guerrero, Rogelio
Laosa, Luis M.
Teo, Thomas
Topolski, James M.

GERONTOLOGY

-Administrator-

Primary Role
Mehrotra, Chandra M.N.
Miranda, Manuel R.

-Consultant-

Primary Role
Dos Santos, John F.

Secondary Role
Fuhrmann, Max E.
Gonzales, Linda R.
Johnson, Paul W.

-Practitioner-

Primary Role
Fuhrmann, Max E.
Gonzales, Linda R.
Johnson, Paul W.

-Researcher-

Primary Role
Ai, Amy L.
Yee, Barbara W. K.

HEALTH PSYCHOLOGY

-Academician-

Primary Role
Lim, Patricia J.
Louden, Delroy M.

Secondary Role
Abraido-Lanza, Ana F
Fong, Geoffrey T.
Hong, Barry A.
Thomas, Joseph E.

-Administrator-

Primary Role
Hong, Barry A.
Moore, C. L.

-Practitioner-

Primary Role
Aoki, Melanie F.
Miller, Sarah S.
Pedemonte, Monica
Thomas, Joseph E.

-Researcher-

Primary Role
Abraido-Lanza, Ana F
Fong, Geoffrey T.
Gay, Patricia L.
Wang, Youde

INDUSTRIAL/ ORGANIZATIONAL PSYCHOLOGY

-Academician-

Primary Role
Andujar, Carlos A.
Baba, Vishwanath V.
Chao, Georgia T.
Cooper, Colin
Goltz, Sonia
Johnson, W. Roy
Kanungo, Rabindra
Lee, Jo Ann
Martinez-Lugo, Miguel E.
Reza, Ernesto M.
Shahani-denning, Comila
Tang, Thomas L. P.
Tejeda, Manuel J.
Toro, Carlos A.
Viswesvaran, Chockalingam
Wooten, William

Secondary Role
Caldwell, Barrett S.
Lee, Thomas W.
Mordka, Irwin
Smedley, Joseph W.

-Administrator-

Primary Role
Lin, Thung-Rung
Sanders, Betty M.

Secondary Role
Horsford, Bernard I.
James, Jr., Earnest
Martinez-Lugo, Miguel E.
Pang, Mark G.
Rambo, Lewis M.
Rodriguez, David A.

-Consultant-

Primary Role
Aldrich, John W.
Alfaro-Garcia, Rafael A.
Bosch, Isora
Chan, Paul K. F.
Ching-Yang Hsu, Chris
Garcia, Jose L.
Guzman, Milagros
Horsford, Bernard I.
Hui, Len Dang
Joure, Sylvia A.
Kam, Sherilyn M.
Kop, Tim M.
Majesty, Melvin S.
Mondragon, Nathan J.
Mordka, Irwin
Pereira, Glona M.
Puig, Hector
Rambo, Lewis M.
Rodriguez, David A.
Saner-Yiu, Li-Chia
Smedley, Joseph W.

Secondary Role
Cooper, Colin
Dorr, Bernadette
Henson, Ramon M.
Kramer, Diana R.
Sanchez, Juan
Wellons, Retha V.
Wooten, William

-Practitioner-

Primary Role
Chan, Paul K.
Dorr, Bernadette
Galue, Alberto I.
Graddick, Miriam M.
Henson, Ramon M.
James, Jr., Earnest
Kramer, Diana R.
Lowman, Rodney
Navedo, Christella N.
Pang, Mark G.
Wellons, Retha V.

Secondary Role
Aldrich, John W.
Alfaro-Garcia, Rafael A.
Guzman, Milagros

289

Joure, Sylvia A.
Kam, Sherilyn M.
Mondragon, Nathan J.
Nowatari, Masahiro
Puig, Hector
Sung, Yong H.

-Researcher-

Primary Role
Caldwell, Barrett S.
Lee, Thomas W.
Nowatari, Masahiro
Salas, Eduardo
Sanchez, Juan

Secondary Role
Baba, Vishwanath V.
Chan, Paul K.
Chao, Georgia T.
Garcia, Jose L.
Goltz, Sonia
Hui, Len Dang
Johnson, W. Roy
Kanungo, Rabindra
Kop, Tim M.
Lee, Jo Ann
Lowman, Rodney
Navedo, Christella N.
Reza, Ernesto M.
Saner-Yiu, Li-Chia
Shahani-denning, Comila
Tang, Thomas L P
Tejeda, Manuel J.
Toro, Carlos A.
Viswesvaran, Chockalingam

-Other-

Primary Role
Sung, Yong H.

NEUROSCIENCES

-Academician-

Primary Role
Robertin, Hector
Schmajuk, Nestor
Teng, Evelyn L.

-Administrator-

Primary Role
Winfrey, Angela D.

Secondary Role
Miller, S. Walden

-Practitioner-

Primary Role
Badillo, Diana
Diaz-Machado, Carmen B.
Gasquoine, Philip G.
Hughes-Wheatland, Roxanne
Jay, Milton T.

Nolley, David A.
Shaw, Terry G.

-Researcher-

Primary Role
Banks, Martha E.
Harris, Josette G
Johnson, Fern M.
Miller, S. Walden
Natani, Kirmach

PERSONALITY
PSYCHOLOGY

-Academician-

Primary Role
Benet-Martinez, Veronica
Hyde, Elsie HA
Kannarkat, Joy P.

Secondary Role
Cheng, W. David
Collins, William

-Administrator-

Primary Role
Collins, William
Keita, Gwendolyn P.
Misra, Rajendra K.
Price, Gregory E.
Singleton, Edward G.

-Practitioner-

Primary Role
Cheng, W. David
Ramseur, Howard P.
Roberts, Harrell B.

-Researcher-

Primary Role
Merritt, Marcellus M.

PHYSIOLOGICAL
PSYCHOLOGY

-Academician-

Primary Role
Dalhouse, A. Derick
Del Rio, Augusto B.
Henry, Rolando R.
Hicks, Leslie H.
Hom, Jim
Hoshiko, Michael
Kawahara, Yoshito
Lee, Jerome
Puente, Antonio E.

Secondary Role
Takahashi, Lorey K.

-Administrator-

Primary Role
Diaz, Eduardo I.

Secondary Role
Adams-Esquivel, Henry
de la Pena, Augustin M.
Gladue, Brian A.
Hoshiko, Michael

-Consultant-

Primary Role
Adams-Esquivel, Henry
Baez, Luis
de la Pena, Augustin M.

Secondary Role
Diaz, Eduardo I.
Matsumiya, Yoichi
Pons, Michael B.

-Practitioner-

Primary Role
Artiola, Lydia
Pons, Michael B.

Secondary Role
Del Rio, Augusto B.
Puente, Antonio E.

-Researcher-

Primary Role
Gladue, Brian A.
Matsumiya, Yoichi
Takahashi, Lorey K.

PSYCHOPHARMACOLOGY

-Administrator-

Primary Role
Sharma, Satanand

Secondary Role
Geter-douglas, Beth
Langrod, John
Orabona, Elaine

-Practitioner-

Primary Role
Langrod, John
Orabona, Elaine

-Researcher-

Primary Role
Geter-douglas, Beth

QUAN/MATH &
PSYCHOMETRICS/STAT

-Academician-

Primary Role
Hsu, Louis M.
Johnson, Sylvia T
Kim, Seock-Ho
Liu, An-Yen
Mendoza, Jorge L.
Nihira, Kazuo
Randhawa, Bikkar S.
Urbina, Susana P.

Secondary Role
Hartka, Elizabeth
Insua, Ana Maria
Lee, Howard B.
Li, Xiaoming

-Administrator-

Primary Role
Stone, Lynn J.

-Researcher-

Primary Role
Anthony, Bobbie M.
Boodoo, Gwyneth M.
Hartka, Elizabeth
Insua, Ana Maria
Lee, Howard B.
Li, Xiaoming

SCHOOL
PSYCHOLOGY

-Academician-

Primary Role
Esquivel, Giselle B.
Goh, David S.
Hines, Laura M.
Jackson, John H.
Jew, Cynthia L.
Lopez, Emilia
Mack, Faite R. P.
Palomares, Ronald S.
Patrice, David
Ramirez, Sylvia Z.
Sandoval, Jonathan
Santiago-Negron, Salvador
Santos de Barona, Maryann
Saunders, Janine M.
Taylor, Gary
Walia, Kusum
Worrell, Frank C.
Wyche, Sr., LaMonte G.

Secondary Role
Anderson, Shirley G.
Barona, Andres
Boulon-Diaz, Frances E.

Broadfield, Charles S.
Catarina, Mathilda B.
Chatman, Vera A
Crockett, Deborah P.
Foster, Robert
Hurst, Jurlene
Nuttall, Ena V.

-Administrator-

Primary Role
Anderson, Shirley G.
Bryant, Gerard W.
Catarina, Mathilda B.
Chatman, Vera A
Chin, Jean L
Hammond, W. Rodney
Hurst, Jurlene
McCoy, George F.
Nuttall, Ena V.

Secondary Role
Caraveo, Libardo E.
Gallardo-Cooper, Maria M.
Sandoval, Jonathan
Santiago-Negron, Salvador
Starks-Williams, Mary L.
Wyche, Sr., LaMonte G.

-Consultant-

Primary Role
Boulon-Diaz, Frances E.
Patterson, Drayton R.
Starks-Williams, Mary L.

Secondary Role
Alexander, Allen T.
Alvarez, Maria D.
Aponte, Evelyn I.
Bartholomew, Charles
Congo, Carroll A.
Cruz, Vivian A.
Dawson, Harriett E.
Dozier, Arthur L.
Finkel, Eva
Fleming, Andrea L.
Fong, Donald L.
Hammond, W. Rodney
Hines, Laura M.
Jove-Altman, Jacqueline
Lee, David Y. K.
Loyola, Jaime L.
Martinez, Maria J.
Martorell, Mario F.
Millard, Wilbur A.
Mody, Zarin R.
Patrice, David
Puertas, Lorenzo
Reeves, Alan
Singh, Darshan
Sun, Irene L.

-Practitioner-

Primary Role
Alexander, Allen T.
Alvarez, Maria D.

Aponte, Evelyn I.
Bartholomew, Charles
Broadfield, Charles S.
Caraveo, Libardo E.
Congo, Carroll A.
Cruz, Vivian A.
Dawson, Harriett E.
Dozier, Arthur L.
Finkel, Eva
Fleming, Andrea L.
Fong, Donald L.
Foster, Robert
Gallardo-Cooper, Maria M.
Harte, Lisa M.
Jove-Altman, Jacqueline
Lee, David Y. K.
Loyola, Jaime L.
Martinez, Maria J.
Martorell, Mario F.
Millard, Wilbur A.
Miranda, Jose P.
Modiano, Rachel
Mody, Zarin R.
Puertas, Lorenzo
Reeves, Alan
Rosado, John W.
Singh, Darshan
Sprouse, Agnes A.
Sun, Irene L.

Secondary Role
Chin, Jean L
Jackson, John H.
Mack, Faite R. P.
McCoy, George F.
Palomares, Ronald S.
Patterson, Drayton R.
Saunders, Janine M.
Simms Puig, Jan
Taylor, Gary
Walia, Kusum

-Researcher-

Primary Role
Barona, Andres

Secondary Role
Esquivel, Giselle B.
Goh, David S.
Jew, Cynthia L.
Lopez, Emilia
Ramirez, Sylvia Z.
Santos de Barona, Maryann
Worrell, Frank C.

-Other-

Primary Role
Simms Puig, Jan

SOCIAL PSYCHOLOGY

-Academician-

Primary Role
Adams, Afesa M.
Akimoto, Sharon A
Ambady, Nalina
Asbury, Jo-Ellen
Bailey, Joan W.
Banaji, Mahzarin R.
Beattie, Muriel Y.
Betancourt, Hector
Bhanthumnavin, Duangduen
Borgatta, Edgar F.
Cardalda, Elsa B.
Chang, Weining C.
Clark, Jr., Eddie M.
DeFour, Darlene C.
Edwards, Karen L.
Fairchild, Halford H.
Ferdman, Bernardo M.
Foster, Rachel A.
Fugita, Stephen S.
Gaborit, Mauricio
Gaines, Stanley O.
Garcia, Betty
Genero, Nancy P.
Ginorio, Angela B.
Granberry, Dorothy
Hart, Allen J.
Hu, Li-Tze
Jones, James M.
Kurosawa, Kaoru
Lampkin, Emmett C.
Morishima, James K.
Naidoo, Josephine C.
Niemann, Yolanda F
Olguin, Arthur
Omoto, Allen M.
Ortega, Robert M.
Pope-Tarrence, Jacqueline R.
Pullium, Rita M.
Reaves, Andrew L
Singh, Ramadhar
Stasson, Mark F.
Tanaka, Koji
Thomas, Jr., Charles B.
Trimble, Joseph E.
Willis, Cynthia E.
Wong-Rieger, Durhane
Wong, Frankie Y.
Woo, Tae O.

Secondary Role
Chen, Hongjen
Chia, Rosina
Gonzalez, Alexander
Hall, Christine I.
Jemmott, III, John B.
Le-Xuan-Hy, G. M.
Marin, Gerardo
Matsumoto, David
McCombs, Harriet G.

Salgado de Snyder, V. Nelly S.
Soriano, Fernando I.
Stallworth, Lisa M.

-Administrator-

Primary Role
Allen, Wise E.
Bowen, Peggy C.
Cardoza, Desdemona
Chin, James
Coelho, George V.
Gonzalez, Alexander
Hall, Christine I.
Marin, Gerardo
Maruyama, Geoffrey
McCombs, Harriet G.
Windham, Thomas L.

Secondary Role
Adams, Afesa M.
Derocher, Terry L.
Gaborit, Mauricio
Jones, James M.
Knapp, W. Mace
Lee, Yueh-Ting
Musgrove, Barbara J.
Stasson, Mark F.
Tanaka, Koji
Trimble, Joseph E.

-Consultant-

Primary Role
Burnett, John H.
Hillabrant, Walter J.
Jenkins, Susan M.

Secondary Role
Ariza-Menedez, Maria
Bowen, Peggy C.
Cardoza, Desdemona
Coelho, George V.
Hayles, V. Robert
Jackson, James S.
Jarama, S. Lisbeth
Nagy, Vivian T.
Tiggle, Ronald B.
Windham, Thomas L.
Wong-Rieger, Durhane

-Practitioner-

Primary Role
Derocher, Terry L.
Grant, Swadesh S.
Knapp, W. Mace
Lee, William W.
Musgrove, Barbara J.
Pasamonte, Ana M.

Secondary Role
Allen, Wise E.
Chin, James
Edwards, Karen L.
Ortega, Robert M.

291

-Researcher-

<u>Primary Role</u>

Ariza-Menedez, Maria
Belgrave, Faye Z
Chen, Hongjen
Chia, Rosina
Ebreo, Angela
Guevarra, Josephine S.
Jackson, James S.
Jarama, S. Lisbeth
Jemmott, III, John B.
Le-Xuan-Hy, G. M.
Matsumoto, David
Nagy, Vivian T.
Ng, Pak C.
Nhan, Nguyen
Salgado de Snyder, V. Nelly S.
Soriano, Fernando I.
Stallworth, Lisa M.
Tiggle, Ronald B.

<u>Secondary Role</u>

Akimoto, Sharon A
Ambady, Nalina
Asbury, Jo-Ellen
Banaji, Mahzarin R.
Beattie, Muriel Y.
Betancourt, Hector
Bhanthumnavin, Duangduen
Cardalda, Elsa B.
Chang, Weining C.
Clark, Jr., Eddie M.
DeFour, Darlene C.
Fairchild, Halford H.
Ferdman, Bernardo M.
Foster, Rachel A.
Fugita, Stephen S.
Garcia, Betty
Genero, Nancy P.
Ginorio, Angela B.
Granberry, Dorothy
Hillabrant, Walter J.
Kurosawa, Kaoru
Maruyama, Geoffrey
Morishima, James K.
Naidoo, Josephine C.
Niemann, Yolanda F
Olguin, Arthur
Omoto, Allen M.
Pope-Tarrence, Jacqueline R.
Pullium, Rita M.
Singh, Ramadhar
Thomas, Jr., Charles B.
Willis, Cynthia E.
Wong, Frankie Y.

-Other-

<u>Primary Role</u>

Hayles, V. Robert
Lee, Yueh-Ting

Language
(Non-English)
Listing

The OEMA survey requests respondents to identify whether they have "Non-English language fluency" in one or more of 14 major languages and related dialects. Psychologists of color with non-English language capabilities are listed alphabetically by:

Language Categories (alphabetized)

(and within each of these by:)

State of Residency (alphabetized)

The Language Categories

American Sign Language
Arabic
Chinese (and related dialects)
Filipino (and related dialects)
French
German
Hindi (and related dialects)
Italian
Japanese
Korean
Portuguese
Spanish
Urdu
"Other"

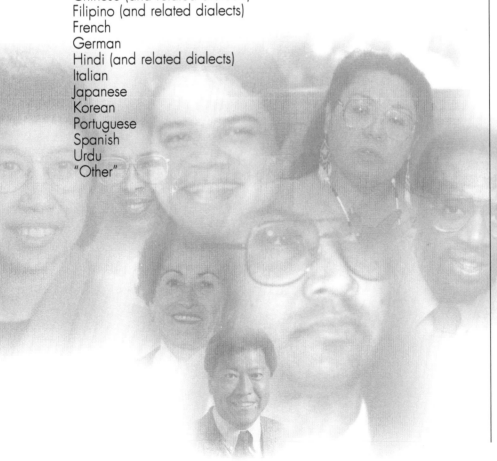

LANGUAGE (Non-English) LISTING

AMERICAN SIGN LANGUAGE

California
Byrd, Robert D.

District of Columbia
Hargrove, Jr., Jerry E.
Peoples, Kathleen

Illinois
Reeves, Alan

Maryland
Gurri Glass, Margarita E.
Thorn, Isabel M.

Texas
De Las Fuentes, Cynthia

ARABIC

District of Columbia
Abudabbeh, Nuha Illinois
Benitez, John C.

Louisiana
Winter, Amal

New York
D'Heurle, Adma J.

CHINESE

California
Chan, Daniel S. (Cantonese, Mandarin)
Chung, Edith C.
Eng, Albert M.
Fong, Donald L.
Gock, Terry S.
Hong, George K.
Ja, Davis Y.
Leung, Alex C. N. (Cantonese, Mandarin)
Lew, Wei M. (Toisanese)
Lin, Thung-Rung (Mandarin)
Liu, Joseph C.
Lu, Elsie G. (Amoy)
Lum, Rodger G.
Ng, James T. (Mandarin, Taiwanese)

Owyang, Walter
Sue, Stanley
Sun, Irene L.
Tang, Terry (Toisanese)
Teng, Evelyn L.
Tung, May
Wong, Hermund (Cantonese, She-Tei)
Wong, Lily Y.S (Mandarin)
Wu, Sheila T. (Mandarin)
Yee, Jane K.
Ying, Yu-Wen
Yu, Howard K. (Mandarin)

Colorado
Lee-Richter, Julie

Florida
Gui, Chui-Liu Serena

Georgia
Chung, Y. Barry (Cantonese)

Hawaii
Ching, June W. J.
Choi, George C.
Lau, Lavay

Illinois
Huang, Wei-Jen William (Mandarin, Taiwanese)
Lam, Chow S.

Indiana
Stephens, Dorothy W. (Mandarin)

Iowa
Chang, Theodore C. H.

Louisiana
Ho, Kay

Maryland
Hsia, Heidi
Kau, Alice S. M.
Li, Xiaoming

Massachusetts
Chan, Connie S.
Chin, Jean L.
Hoshmand, Lisa T.

Lee, Yueh-Ting
Lowe, Susana M.
Wong, Frankie Y.
Wu, Shi-Jiuan

Michigan
Chao, Georgia T.

Minnesota
Lee, Margaret

Mississippi
Liu, An-Yen

Missouri
Duan, Changming

New Jersey
Chin, Lemin
Ho, John E.
Wong, Kit L. (Mandarin, Cantonese)

New York
Chang, Barbara
Chen, Eric C.
Cheng, W. David (Mandarin)
Goh, David S. (Mandarin)
Sundararajan, Louise Kuen-Wei L.
Tana, Joseph
Tsui, Ellen C. (Cantonese)

North Carolina
Chia, Rosina
Pullium, Rita M.

Ohio
Chung, Rita L.
Gee, Carol S.
Leong, Frederick T.
Rigrish, Diana
Shen, John (Mandarin)

Oregon
Yap, Kim O.

Pennsylvania
Chen, Hongjen (Mandarin)
Chen, S. Andrew
Lee, David Y. K.
Wang, Margaret C.

Tennessee
Tang, Thomas L. P.

Texas
Hom, Jim
Hu, Trudy H. C.
Lin, J.C. Gisela G. (Mandarin)
Patterson, Mayin Lau
Tan, Gabriel
Wong, Dorothy L.
Zhu, Jiajun Utah
Loong, James

Virginia
Ching-Yang
Hsu, Chris
Ng, Pak C.
Wang, Youde
Wibberly, Kathy H.

Washington
Ahana, Ellen
Fung, Hellen C. (Cantonese)
Ho, Christine K.
Kuan, Yie-Wen Y.
Lee, Thomas W.
Teng, L. Neal
Tien, Liang
Tsai, Mavis

Wisconsin
Chan, Adrian

FILIPINO

California
Heras, Patricia (Tagalog)
Jurilla-Pastrana, Lina L. (Aklamon, Ilonggo)

Florida
San Luis, Roberto R.

Minnesota
Ascano, Ricardo
Dawis, Rene V.

New Jersey
Henson, Ramon M. (Tagalog)

New York
Laviena, Luis
Sison, Cecile E.
Velayo, Richard S.

Texas
Arana, Olga R.
Quijano, Walter Y.

Virginia
Macaranas, Eduarda A.
(Tagalog)

Wisconsin
Austria, Asuncion M.

FRENCH

Arizona
Artiola, Lydia

California
Adams-Esquivel, Henry
Bainum, Charlene K.
Bersing, Doris S.
Espin, Oliva M.
Fils, David H.
Monteiro, Kenneth P.
Netter, Roberto
Nguyen, Dao Q.
Perez-Arce, Patricia
York, Mary J.

Connecticut
Banks, Karel L.

Delaware
Turner, Alvin L.

District of Columbia
Harper, Mary S.
Myers, Ernest R.
Vontress, Clemmont E.

Florida
Alvarez, Maria D.
Ariza-Menedez, Maria
Herrera-Pino, Jorge A.
Mahy, Yvonne C.
Maldonado, Loretto
Toomer, Jethro W.
Urbina, Susana P.

Hawaii
Robertin, Hector

Illinois
Bennett, Maisha H.
Gallagher, Rosina M.
Gordon, Kimberly A.
Tamayo, Jose M.

Maryland
Cardena, Etzel A.
Coelho, George V.
Gardano, Anna C.
Han, Yu Ling
Nadal-Vazquez, Vilma Y.
Sasscer-Burgos, Julie

Massachusetts
Armengol, Carmen G.
Harleston, Bernard W.
James, Steven E.
Rey-Casserly, Celiane M.
Sedo, Manuel A.
Torres, Mario A.
Whitaker, Arthur L.

Michigan
Chao, Georgia T.

Minnesota
Narvaez, Darcia F.

Nebraska
Sodowsky, Gargi R.

Nevada
Knapp, W. Mace

New Jersey
Finkel, Eva
Gonzalez, Haydee M.
Grant, Wanda F.
Hsu, Louis M.
Laosa, Luis M.
Trotman, Frances K.

New York
Abercombie, Delrita
Altarriba, Jeanette
Araoz, Daniel L.
Arcaya, Jose M.
Burton, Roger V.
Carballo-Dieguez, Alex
Constantine, Madonna G.
Crowder, Virginia B.
D'Heurle, Adma J.
Gular, Enrique
Langrod, John
Sanua, Victor D.

North Carolina
Llorca, Arthur L.
Zayas, Maria A.

Ohio
Banks, Martha E.
Valley, John A.

Pennsylvania
Bryant, Gerard W.
Ellis, Edwin E.
Fried-Cassorla, Martha J.
Nelson-le, Sharon A.
Singh, Silvija S.

Puerto Rico
Ardila, Ruben
Ramirez-Cancel, Carlos M.

Tennessee
Johnson, Johnny

Texas
De Las Fuentes, Cynthia
Galue, Alberto I.
Garnes, Delbert F.
Garrett-Akinsanya, BraVada
Klopner, Michele C.
Lerma, Joe L.
Philp, Frederick W.
Thomas, Thomas J.
Vaid, Jyotsna

Virginia
Anderson, William H.

Wisconsin
Cunha, Maria I.
Sudevan, Padmanbhan

GERMAN

Alabama
Wells, Annie M.

California
Sandoval, Jonathan
Ying, Yu-Wen

District of Columbia
Robinson, John D.
Savage, Jr., James E.

Florida
Urbina, Susana P.

Michigan
Dooley, John A.

Missouri
Acka-Pope, Zeynep K

New Jersey
Coffey, Maryann B.

New York
Araoz, Daniel L.
Cheng, W. David
Laviena, Luis

Ohio
Gladue, Brian A.

Pennsylvania
Baker, III, Carl E.

Texas
Chiu, Loanne
Peniston, Eugene G.
Sacasa, Rafael E.

Virginia
Broadfield, Charles S.
Meadows-Yancey, Dorothy
Richardson, E. Strong-Legs
Williams, Mary Beth

Washington
Teng, L. Neal

HINDI

Alabama
Kothandapani, Virupaksha

Arizona
Mellot, Ramona N.

California
Atwal, Baljit K,
Fanibanda, Darius K.
Kakaiya, Divya
Khorakiwala, Durriyah
Singh, R. K. Janmeha

Colorado
Saleem, Rakhshanda

Connecticut
Banaji, Mahzarin R.

Delaware
Iqbal, S. Mohammed

Florida
Kashikar-Zuck, Susmita M.

Georgia
Asghar, Anila
Campbell, Kamal E.

Illinois
Ahuja, Harmeen
Anand, Shashi (Marath, Gujarti)
Dave, Jagdish P.
Hamid, Mohammad

Iowa
Singh, Darshan Kansas
Jain, Sharat K.

Kentucky
Srinivasan, Sampurna

Maryland
Kupur, Veena

Massachusetts
Ahmed, Mohiuddin
Ambady, Nalina
Garg, Mithlesh
Mukherjee, Subhash C.

Michigan
Vakhariya, Sobha

Minnesota
Mehrotra, Chandra M.N

Nebraska
Sodowsky, Gargi R.

New Jersey
Patel, Sanjiv A.
Saraf, Komal C.
Schroff, Kamal
Sen, Tapas K. Shah,
Vasantkumar B.
Shroff, Kamal

New York
Das, Manju P.
Grant, Swadesh S. (Uttter)
Laviena, Luis
Luthar, Suniya S.
Mehta, Kripal K.
Rajaram, Suparna

Shahani-denning, Comila
Wagner, Aureen Pinto
Walia, Kusum

Ohio
Misra, Rajendra K.

Oregon
Rohila, Pritam K.

Pennsylvania
Sharma, Greesh C.

Tennessee
Khanna, Jaswant L.
Sharma, Vijai P.

Texas
Bhatia, Kiran
Sikka, Anjoo
Singg, Sangeeta
Vaid, Jyotsna

Wisconsin
Sudevan, Padmanbhan

ITALIAN

Arizona
Artiola, Lydia
Bencomo, Armando A.

California
Adams-Esquivel, Henry
Falicov, Celia J.
Hofer, Ricardo
Montesi, Alexandra Saba
Trufant, Carol A.

District of Columbia
Comas-Diaz, Lillian

Florida
Ariza-Menedez, Maria
Urbina, Susana P.

Illinois
Gallagher, Rosina M.

Maryland
Coelho, George V.

Massachusetts
Aradom, Tesfay A.
Sedo, Manuel A.

New Jersey
Lijtmaer, Ruth M.
Perez, Cecilia M.
Puertas, Lorenzo
Trotman, Frances K.

New York
Branche, Leota Susan
Haley, Adriana R.
Sanua, Victor D.

Ohio
Gladue, Brian A.

Pennsylvania
Mitchell, Howard E.

Puerto Rico
Ramirez-Cancel, Carlos M.

Texas
Lerma, Joe L.

Washington
Akutagawa, Donald
Borgatta, Edgar F.

JAPANESE

California
Inoue, Sachi
Ishida, Taeko H.
Kobayashi, Steve K.
Matsumoto, David
Mikamo, Akiko
Miura, Irene T.
Nemoto, Tooru
Nihira, Kazuo
Saito, Gloria C.
True, Reiko Homma
Yamamura, Lorraine M.

Hawaii
Fujinaka, Larry H.
Ishikawa-Fullmer, Janet
Kop, Tim M.
Omizo, Michael M.
Takamine, Sandra

Illinois
Aoki, Melanie F.
Hoshiko, Michael
Koh, Tong-He

Indiana
Yamaguchi, Harry G.

Louisiana
Izawa, Chizuko

Maryland
Furukawa, James M.
McWilliams, Junko O.

Massachusetts
Mino, Itsuko
Michigan Fergus, Esther O.

Minnesota
Akimoto, Sharon A.
Montana Lie, Rudolph T. B.

New York
Ashida, Sachio Tanaka-
Matsumi, Junko

Ohio
Ishiyama, Toaru

Rhode Island
Matsumiya, Yoichi

Texas
Oana, Leilani K. Utah
Higashi, Wilfred H.

Wisconsin
Okazaki, Sumie

KOREAN

California
Keefe, Keunho
Kim, Elizabeth J.
Kim, Randi I.
Kim, Sung C.
Lee, Julie C.
Lee, See-Woo S.
Yi, Kris Y.

Colorado
Mo, Suchoon

Connecticut
Chun, Marvin M.

Georgia
Kim, Seock-Ho

Hawaii
Kop, Tim M.

Illinois
Koh, Tong-He
Rhee, Susan B.
Sung, Yong H.

Michigan
Wilkinson, H. Sook

Nevada
Hong, Eunsook

New Jersey
Kim, Yang Ja

Ohio
Yun, S. B.

Pennsylvania
Woo, Tae O.

Washington
Jun, Heesoon

PORTUGUESE

Arizona
Artiola, Lydia

California
Adams-Esquivel, Henry
Grosso, Federico C.
Hofer, Ricardo
Montesi, Alexandra Saba
Netter, Beatriz E. C.
Netter, Roberto

District of Columbia
Cooper, Donna M.
Nieves-Grafals, Sara

Florida
Dos Santos, John F.
Joffe, Vera
Sanchez-Torrento, Eugenio
Velez-Diaz, Angel

Illinois
Green, Theophilus E.

Indiana
Goltz, Sonia

Maryland
Coelho, George V.
Miranda, David J.

New Jersey
Finkel, Eva
Gonzalez, Haydee M.
Laosa, Luis M.
Perez, Cecilia M.
Trotman, Frances K.

New Mexico
Coes, Maria R.

New York
Beato-Smith, Vera
Branche, Leota Susan
Cleveland, Adriana F.
Langrod, John
Laviena, Luis

North Carolina
Azevedo, Don Fernando

Pennsylvania
Cornwell, Henry G.
Magran, Betty A.
Perez, Carlos A.

Rhode Island
Costa, Armenio S.

Tennessee
Ascencao, Erlete M.

Texas
Natalicio, Luiz

Wisconsin
Cunha, Maria I.

SPANISH

Alabama
Beltran, Joe
Floyd, Bridget J.
Labbe, Elise E.
Suarez-Crowe, Yolanda

Alaska
McNeill, Elizabeth M.
Sanders, Gilbert O. Arizona
Artiola, Lydia
Barona, Andres
Battiest, William V.
Bencomo, Armando A.
Bernal, Martha E.
Bernat, Gloria S.
Caraveo, Libardo E.

de Jesus, Nelson H.
Martinez, Floyd H.
Mordka, Irwin
Rodriguez, Ester R.
Velez, Maria T.

Arkansas
Prado, William M.

California
Adams-Esquivel, Henry
Adler, Peter J.
Alvarez, Paul A.
Alvarez, Vivian
Amezcua, Charlie A.
Arevalo, Luis E.
Artiles, Alfredo J.
Auuilas-Gaxiola, Sergio A.
Aviera, Arlene T.
Azmitia, Margarita
Baca, Sandra G.
Barnes, Charles A.
Bavon, Moises
Beliz, Jr., Efrain A.
Benavides, Jr., Robert
Bersing, Doris S.
Betancourt, Hector
Boulette, Tersea R.
Bruguera, Mark R.
Camarillo, Max
Campos, Joseph J.
Campos, Leonard P.
Cardona, Gilbert
Carr-Casanova, Rosario
Cervantes, Joseph M.
Chatigny, Anita L.
Cherbosque, Jorge
Cordero, Fernando
Cortese, Margaret
Credidio, Vivian F.
Cummings, Joseph D.
De Apodaca, Roberto F.
de Fuentes, Nanette
de la Pena, Augustin M.
de Llano, Carmen
Dehmer-Abalo, Elena M.
Del Rio, Augusto B.
Dosamantes-Beaudry, Irma
Duran, Richard P.
Espin, Oliva M.
Fairchild, Halford H.
Falicov, Celia J.
Fayard, Carlos Ferdman,
Bernardo M.
Fils, David H.
Flaherty, Maria Y.

Flores de Apodaca, Roberto
Flores, Elena
Francisco, Richard P.
Gamez, George L.
Garcia, Betty
Gomez, Jr., Francisco C.
Gonsalves, Carlos J.
Gonzalez, Alexander
Gonzalez, Gerardo M.
Gonzalez, Rocio R.
Gonzalez-Huss, Mary
Grosso, Federico C.
Grunhaus-Belzer, Rosa
Guanipa, Carmen L.
Guerra, Anna Maria
Guerra, Julio J.
Hall, M. Elizabeth L.
Hearn, Kathleen E.
Heller, Beatriz
Heras, Patricia
Hernandez, Maria G.
Hofer, Ricardo
Hyman, Edward J.
Jimenez-Safir, Paula B.
Joshi, Sheila
Lein, H. Beatriz
Lopez, Steven R.
Lowman, Rodney
Lozano, Irma
Mancillas, Paul
Marin, Gerardo
Martin, Laura P.
Martinez, Alejandro M.
Melgoza, Bertha Miccio-
Fonseca, L. C.
Miranda, Manuel R.
Monguio, Ines
Montalvo, Roberto E.
Montesi, Alexandra Saba
Morales, Eduardo S.
Munoz, Marisol
Munoz, Ricardo F.
Murillo, Nathan
Myers, Hector F.
Netter, Roberto
Nogales, Ana Olmedo,
Esteban L. Ortiz, Berta S.
Ortiz, Vilma
Pardo, Ruben C.
Perez, Juan C.
Perez-Arce, Patricia
Pons, Michael B.
Ponton, Marcel O.
Porche-Burke, Lisa M.
Reza, Ernesto M.
Rivera-Lopez, Hector
Rodriguez, Richard A.

Romero, Arturo
Romero, Augusto
Rosales, Israel B.
Ruiz, Fernando
Sanchez, H.G.
Sandoval, Jonathan
Saucedo, Carlos
Saunders, Walter C.
Schenquerman, Berta N.
Shea-Martinez, Herminia E.
Soriano, Fernando I.
Soriano, Marcel
Stewart, Arleen R.
Tabachnik, Samuel
Tazeau, Yvette N.
Tirado, Linda Ann
Valdivia, Lino
Vega, Star
Velasco, Frank E.
Velasquez, Roberto J.
Villela, Leopoldo F.
Zamudio, Anthony
Zavala, Albert
Zepeda, Marlene

Colorado
Aguilar, Martha C.
Chapa, Joel R.
Chavez, Ernest L.
Esparza, Ricardo
Garza, Joe G.
Gomez, Ana L
Irueste-Montes, Ana M.
Montes, Francisco
Rodriguez, Manuel D.
Valdes, Maria
Valdez, Jesse N.
Vega, Jose G.

Connecticut
Badillo, Diana
Guzman, L. Philip
Losada-Paisey, Gloria
Ramos-Grenier, Julia
Rivera, Nelson E.

District of Columbia
Buki, Lydia P.
Carr, Paquita R.
Comas-Diaz, Lillian
Cooper, Donna M.
Hillabrant, Walter J.
Marotta, Sylvia A.
Miranda, M.
Nieves-Grafals, Sara
Robinson, John D.

Florida
Abello, Ana L.
Alonso, Martha R.
Alvarez, Carlos M.
Alvarez, Manuel E.
Alvarez, Maria D.
Anton, William D.
Ariza-Menedez, Maria
Artiles, Laura M.
Azaret, Marisa
Bild-Libbin, Raguel
Bradman, Leo H.
Constanzo, Magda S.
Cornide, Carmen R.
Crane, Rosario S.
Cruz, Vivian A.
Diaz, Eduardo I.
Diaz-Machado, Carmen B.
Dos Santos, John F.
Echavarria, David
Escovar, Luis A.
Faraci, Ana M.
Fernandez, Maria C.
Figueredo, Migdalia I.
Fuentes, Dainery M.
Gallardo-Cooper, Maria M.
Garcia, Hector D.
Garcia, Jose L.
Garcia, Lazaro
Grabau, David
Hernandez, Cibeles
Herrera-Pino, Jorge A.
Hui, Len Dang
Incera, Armando
Labarta, Margarita M.
Leon, Yolanda C.
Lequerica, Martha
Mahy, Yvonne C.
Maldonado, Loretto
Manruque-Reichard, Marta E.
Marina, Dorita
Marrero, Bernie
Montoya, E. Carolina
Mora, Ralph
Morales, Elias
Mussenden, Gerald
Nazario, Jr., Andres
Pacheco, Angel E.
Pedemonte, Monica
Perez, Fred M.
Pico, Daima
Pita, Marcia E.
Porges, Carlos R.
Prado, Haydee
Prieto, Addys
Reyes-Mayer, Erwin
Rivas-Vazquez, Ana A.

Rivera, Enrique
Rodriguez, Lavinia
Ruiz, Sonia I.
Salas, Eduardo
Sanchez, Juan
Sanchez-Torrento, Eugenio
Szapocznik, Jose
Toro, Haydee
Urbina, Susana P.
Velez-Diaz, Angel
Zaldivar, Luis R.
Zayas-Bazan, Carmen

Georgia
Bascuas, Joseph W.
Figueroa, Rolando G.
Gonzalez, Fernando
Lopez, Sarah C.
Mahabee-Harris, Marilyn M.
Perilla, Julia L.

Hawaii
Robertin, Hector

Illinois
Baez, Luis
Balcazar, Fabricio E.
Benitez, John C.
Canovas Welles, Nydia L.
Choca, James
Gallagher, Rosina M.
Green, Theophilus E.
Machabanski, Hector
Manghi, Elina R.
Plazas, Carlos A.
Posner, Carmen A.
Rodriguez, Rogelio E.
Schlesinger, Susana J.
Schmajuk, Nestor
Soto, Tomas A.
Suarez-Balcazar, Yolanda
Tamayo, Jose M.
Vera, Elizabeth M.
Viale-val, Graciela
Whitaker, Sandra V.

Indiana
Hernandez, Vivian O.
Minturn, Robin H.
Prieto, Susan L.
Vargas, Manuel J.

Iowa
Grajales, Elisa M.

Kentucky
Balbona, Manuel

Blair, Deborah G.

Louisiana
Daruna, Jorge H.

Maine
Barry, Martha J.

Maryland
Aguirre-Deandreis, Ana I.
Cardena, Etzel A.
Cruz, Albert R.
Derrickson, Kimberly B.
Gardano, Anna C.
Gurri Glass, Margarita E.
Mastrapa, Selma A.
Miranda, David J.
Nadal-Vazquez, Vilma Y.
Oommen Thomas, Susy
Pinto, Alcides
Ruth, Richard
Sasscer-Burgos, Julie
Thorn, Isabel M.

Massachusetts
Alvarez, Mauricia
Amaro, Hortensia
Arboleda, Catalina
Armengol, Carmen G.
Arredondo, Patricia
Ayoub, Catherine C.
Bacigalupe, Gonzalo M.
Bennasar, Mari C.
Bustamante, Eduardo M.
Cebollero, Ana
Margarita De Louredes
Mattei, Maria
Garrido-Castillo, Pedro
Genero, Nancy P.
Jette, Carmen CB
Lagomasino, Andrew J.
Lawson, Jasper J.
Linares, Lourdes O.
Morales-Barreto, Gisela
Munoz, Leticia S.
Nicks, T. Leon
Nuttall, Ena V.
Rambo, Lewis M.
Rey-Casserly, Celiane M.
Romney, Patricia
Sanchez, William
Sedo, Manuel A.
Torres, Mario A.

Michigan
Arellano-Lopez, Juan

Benet-Martinez, Veronica
Collins, William
Flachier, Roberto
Garcia-Shelton, Linda M.
Gonzalez, Matthew B.
Madrid, Raul P.
Marroquin, Arthur R.
Ortega, Robert M.
Schreier, Raquel L.
Sutton, Sharon E.

Minnesota
Gutterman, Carmen Y.
Moideen, Yasmine
Narvaez, Darcia F.

Missouri
Roehlke, Helen J.
Sancho, Ana M.
Topolski, James M.

Nebraska
Prendes-Lintel, Maria L.

Nevada
Amezaga, Jr., Alfredo M.
Antonuccio, David
Brandenburg, Carlos E.
Knapp, W. Mace

New Jersey
Bosch, Isora
Escudero, Micaela
Esquivel, Giselle B.
Fernandez, Rosemary
Finkel, Eva
Garcia, Margarita
Gonzalez, Haydee M.
Gonzalez, Maria L.
Henson, Ramon M.
Laosa, Luis M.
Latorre, Miriam D.
Lijtmaer, Ruth M
Ludmer, Alba
Martorell, Mario F.
Modiano, Rachel
Pelaez, Carmen
Perez, Cecilia M.
Puertas, Lorenzo
Rodriguez, David A.
Roig, Miguel
Rosado, John W.
Samaniego, Sandra
Trotman, Frances K.

New Mexico
Arroyo, Judith A.

Castillo, Diane T.
Garcia, Melinda A.
Gonzales, Ricardo R.
Marquez, E. Mario
Rivera, Miquela
Roll, Samuel
Sosa, Juan N.
Vargas, Alice M.
Vargas, Luis A.

New York
Abercombie, Delrita
Abraido-Lanza, Ana F.
Altarriba, Jeanette
Anderson, Linda
Aponte, Evelyn I.
Araoz, Daniel L.
Arcaya, Jose M.
Arriso, Roberta H.
Aviles, Alice A.
Balderrama, Sylvia R.
Bastien, IV, Samuel A.
Beato-Smith, Vera
Benamu, Icem
Benzaquen, Isaac
Berrill, Naftali G.
Blandino, Ramon A.
Bracero, William
Branche, Leota Susan
Brooks, Lewis A.
Bursztyn, Alberto M.
Burton, Roger V.
Canedo, Angelo R.
Carballo-Dieguez, Alex
Caro, Yvette
Cleveland, Adriana F.
Correa, Martha L.
Cottingham, Alice L.
Cuesta, George M.
Fleisher, Nancy F.
Foster, RoseMarie P.
Graves, Sherryl B.
Graves-Cooper, Phyllis J.
Gular, Enrique
Haley, Adriana R.
Hooker, Olivia J.
Inclan, Jaime
Javier, Rafael A.
Jove-Altman, Jacqueline
Kahan, Harry
Langrod, John
Lopez, Emilia
Martinez, Maria J.
Martinez-Urrutia, Angel C.
Maynard, Edward S.
Millan, Fred
Mujica, Ernesto

Munoz, John A.
Pasamonte, Ana M.
Peralta, Carmelina
Perez Ebrahimi, Concepcion
Ramos, Arnaldo J.
Rigual-Lynch, Lourdes
Rivera, Carmen J. Rivero,
Estela M.
Rodriguez, Carmen G.
Rogler, Lloyd H.
Romero, Jose
Rosario, Margaret
Sanua, Victor D.
Sobrino, James F.
Soto, Elaine
Suarez, Carlota
Vazquez, Rosa
Wong, Florence C.
Zayas, Luis H.

North Carolina
Llorca, Arthur L.
Puente, Antonio E.
Zayas, Maria A.

Ohio
Bernal, Guillermo A.
Fliman, Vivian P.
Gladue, Brian A.
Lopez-Baez, Sandra I.
Serafica, Felicisima C.
Vicente, Peter J.

Oklahoma
Mendoza, Jorge L.

Oregon
Gonzales, Linda R.
Marmol, Leonardo M.
Morones, Pete A.
Torres-Saenz, Jorge

Pennsylvania
Alonso, Mario
Baker, III, Carl E.
Cornwell, Henry G.
Crespo, Gloria M.
Droz, Elizabeth
Echemendia, Ruben J.
Ellis, Edwin E.
Gutierrez, Manuel J.
Laguna, John N.
Louredes Mattei, Maria De
Loyola, Jaime L.
Lugo, Daisy R.
Magran, Betty A.
Nix-Early, Vivian

Perez, Carlos A.
Poal, Pilar
Ramirez, David E.
Rogers, Melvin L.
Salas, Jesus A.
Salganicoff, Matilde
Tejeda, Manuel J.

Puerto Rico
Alfaro-Garcia, Rafael A.
Alvarez, Rosaligia
Andujar, Carlos A.
Ardila, Ruben
Arsuaga, Enrique N.
Bauermeisten, Jose J.
Belen, Ines I.
Bernal, Guillermo
Berrios, Zaida R.
Boulon-Diaz, Frances E.
Cardalda, Elsa B.
Colon, Ana I.
Cruz-Lopez, Miguel
Fankhanel, Edward H.
Garcia, Pedro I.
Gonzalez, Max A.
Gonzalez-Pabon, Jose F.
Guzman, Milagros
Herrans, Laura L.
Llado, Sarah L.
Llanos, Aracely B.
Margarida, Maria T.
Martinez, Eduardo M.
Martinez-Lugo, Miguel E.
Mendez-Calderon, Luis M.
Montijo, Jorge A.
Navedo, Christella N.
Ocasio-Garcia, Ketty
Olmo, Manuel C.
Ramirez-Cancel, Carlos M.
Ribera-Gonzalez, Julio C.
Rivera, Beatriz D.
Rivera-Medina, Eduardo J.
Rivera-Molina, Elba
Rodriguez, Ramon O.
Roman, Hugo
Romey, Carol M.
Sanchez-Caso, Luis M.
Santini-Hernandez, Ernesto
Serrano-Garcia, Irma
Toro-Alfonso, Jose
Vazquez, Carlos D.
Vazquez, Cesar D.
Vazquez-Ruiz, Francisco

Rhode Island
Costa, Armenio S.

Garcia-Coll, Cynthia
Garrido, Maria C.

Tennessee
Ascencao, Erlete M.
Bueno, Luis F.
Corte, Henry E.
Johnson, Johnny
Masini, Angela

Texas
Ainslie, Ricardo C.
Antokoletz, Juana C.
Arbona, Consuelo
Baron, Augustine
Basco, Monica A.
Caldera, Yvonne M.
Carter, Lamore J.
Cepeda-Benito, Antonio
Contreras, Raquel J.
Cooper, Alan
Cruz, Maria C. de la
Sota, Elizanda M.
De Las Fuentes, Cynthia
DeFerreire, Mary Elizabeth
Delgado-Hachey, Maria
Fernandez, Peter
Galue, Alberto I.
Garcia, Teresa
Garrett-Akinsanya, BraVada
Gonzalez, John
Gonzalez-Sorensen, Anna G.
Hammond, Evelyn S.
Hill, Jr., Sam S. Lerma, Joe L.
Llorente, Antolin M.
Loredo, Carlos M.
Martinez, Raul
Mellor-Crummey, Cynthia A.
Miranda, Jose P.
Morales, Pamilla V.
Natalicio, Luiz
Niemann, Yolanda F.
Otero, Rafael F.
Paniagua, Freddy A.
Paredes, Jr., Frank C.
Pereira, Glona M.
Pettigrew, Dorothy C.
Praderas, Kim
Ramirez, Sylvia Z.
Rosin, Susana A.
Saldana, Delia H.
Silva, Santiago
Somodevilla, S. A.
Sutton, David
Valdes, Thusnelda M.
Vargas, M. Angelica
Vasquez, Melba

Utah
Higashi, Wilfred H.
Mejia, Juan A.
Reyes, Carla J.
Saenz, Javier

Virgin Islands
Garrido, Maria
Mendez, Gloria I.
Moss, Ramona J.

Virginia
Anderson, William H.
Azcarate, Eduardo M.
Fields, Amanda H.
Goebes, Diane D.
Hass, Giselle A.
Hass, Giselle A.
Jarama, S. Lisbeth
Morote, Gloria
Price, Gregory E.
Word, James C.

Washington
Arenas, Jr., Silverio
Borgatta, Edgar F.
Ginorio, Angela B.
Ramirez, John/Juan
Suarez, Alejandra

Wisconsin
Cunha, Maria I.
Mendelberg, Hava E.
O'Brien, B. Marco
Pflaum, John H.
Sapp, Marty Smith, Carol Y.

URDU

Alabama
Kothandapani, Virupaksha

California
Kakaiya, Divya
Khorakiwala, Durriyah
Singh, R. K. Janmeha

Colorado
Saleem, Rakhshanda

Connecticut
Somjee, Lubna

Delaware
Iqbal, S. Mohammed

Georgia
Asghar, Anila

Illinois
Anand, Shashi (Marath)
Hamid, Mohammad

Iowa
Singh, Darshan

Maryland
Kupur, Veena

Massachusetts
Mukherjee, Subhash C.

New Jersey
Saraf, Komal C.

Ohio
Misra, Rajendra K.

Oregon
Rohila, Pritam K.

Pennsylvania
Sharma, Greesh C.

Tennessee
Khanna, Jaswant L.

Texas
Singg, Sangeeta
Stewart, Sunita M.

Virginia
Hamdani-Raab, Asma J.

OTHER

Alabama
Kothandapani, Virupaksha
(Tamil, Telugu)

Arizona
Artiola, Lydia (Catalan)

California
Adler, Peter J. (Hungarian)
Bamgbose, Olujiimi O.
(Yoruba)
Cherbosque, Jorge (Hebrew)
Eskandari, Esfandiar (Farsi)
Grunhaus-Belzer, Rosa
(Hebrew)

Heras, Patricia (Tagalog)
Khorakiwala, Durriyah
(Gujarati)
Lee, Daniel D. (Vietnamese)
Malancharuvil, Joseph M.
(Malayalam)
Nguyen, Dao Q.
(Vietnamese)
Roy, Swati (Bengali)
Sharma, Satanand (Fijian)
Singh, R. K. Janmeha
(Punjabi)
Swan, June A. (Burmese)
Valdivia, Lino (Quechua)
York, Mary J.
(Apache, Penobsot)

District of Columbia
Abudabbeh, Nuha (Turkish)

Florida
Alvarez, Maria D. (Haitian
Creole)
Viswesvaran, Chockalingam
(Tamil)

Georgia
Campbell, Kamal E. (Gujarati)

Hawaii
Kop, Tim M. (Hawaiian)
Robertin, Hector (Thai,
Vietnamese)
Torigoe, Rodney Y.
(Hawaiian)
Roque, Sylvia A. (Hawaiian)

Maryland
Han, Yu Ling
(Dutch, Indonesian)
Kupur, Veena (Punjabi)
Nhan, Nguyen (Vietnamese)
Oommen Thomas, Susy
(Malayalam)

Massachusetts
Ahmed, Mohiuddin (Bengali)
Mukherjee, Subhash C.
(Bengali)
Sedo, Manuel A. (Catalan)

Michigan
Benet-Martinez, Veronica
(Catalan)

Missouri

Acka-Pope, Zeynep K.
(Turkish)

Montana

Lie, Rudolph T.B.
(Dutch, Indonesian)

Nebraska

Sodowsky, Gargi R.
(Bengali, Marathi)

New Jersey

Essandoh, Pius K. (Fante)
Henson, Ramon M.
(Tagalog)
Patel, Sanjiv A. (Gujarati)
Saraf, Komal C.
(Gujarati, Punjabi)
Schroff, Kamal (Marathi)
Sen, Tapas K. (Bengali)

New York

Benamu, Icem (Hebrew)
Benzaquen, Isaac (Hebrew)
Brooks, Lewis A.
(Hungarian)
D'Heurle, Adma J. (Swedish)
Langrod, John (Polish)
Luthar, Suniya S. (Pujai)
Mehta, Kripal K. (Punjabi)
Walia, Kusum (Punjabi)

North Carolina

Ike, Chris A.
(Ibo, Hausa, Yoruba)

Ohio

Fliman, Vivian P. (Hebrew)
Misra, Rajendra K. (Bengali)
Ray, Arun B. (Bengali)
Serafica, Felicisima C.
(Tagalog)
Valley, John A. (Latin)

Pennsylvania

Varki, C. Paily (Malayamam)

Tennessee

Khanna, Jaswant L. (Punjabi)

Texas

Bhatia, Kiran (Punjabi)
Chiu, Loanne
(Dutch, Indonesian)
Gant, Bob L. (Russian)
Klopner, Michele C.

(Haitian Creole)
Singg, Sangeeta (Punjabi)

Virginia

Kannarkat, Joy P.
(Malayalam)
Le-Xuan-Hy, G. M.
(Vietnamese)
Macaranas, Eduarda A.
(Tagalog)

Washington

Ahana, Ellen (Hawaiian)
Suarez, Alejandra
(Esperanto)

Wisconsin

Mendelberg, Hava E.
(Hebrew)
Sudevan, Padmanbhan
(Malayalam, Tamil)

Foreign Countries

Baba, Vishwanath (Tamil)
Sitharthan, Thiagarajan
(Tamil)

Statistical
Profile

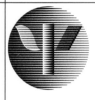

Highlights

*NOTE: Statistical data are based solely on information
on the over 2,400 persons listed in this directory. These persons represent approximately 55% of all of APA's known members of color.
Although this is a most acceptable survey response rate,
caution is warranted in generalizing these data.*

● Of the directory's 2,406 listed psychologists,
33.2% are African American/Black, 32.8% are Hispanic/Latino(a),
27.4% are Asian American/Asian/Pacific Islander,
4.4% are American Indian/Alaska Native, and 2.2% are multiethnic.

● 48.4% of these psychologists are men, 49.0% are women,
and gender was not reported for 2.5%.

● 86.7% of these psychologists hold the PhD,
8.6% hold the EdD or PsyD, 3.0% hold a master's degree,
and 1.7% did not report their degree status.

● 10.9% of these psychologists received their terminal degrees
8 or fewer years ago; 29.8% received their terminal degrees
9 to 15 years ago; 34.7% received their degrees 16 to 25 years ago;
23% received their degrees more than 25 years ago,
and 1.5% did not report this information.

● The geographical areas where these psychologists most frequently reside
are California (20.3%), New York (8.4%), Florida (5.2%), Texas (4.9%),
and Foreign Countries (4.5%). They least frequently reside in Idaho,
North Dakota, South Dakota, Maine, and Wyoming (0.1% or less).

● The most frequently reported major fields were Clinical Psychology
(50.7%), Counseling Psychology (13.5%), Social Psychology (4.9%),
Developmental Psychology (4.4%), and Educational Psychology (4.3%).

● These psychologists are willing to participate in a variety of activities
related to organized psychology. Between 15% and 27% of these
psychologists indicated a willingness to serve on an APA governance
task force, committee, or board related to scientific, educational,
professional, or public interest issues; 21% and 24% respectively
were willing to serve on an editorial board of an APA journal or as an
APA accreditation site visitor.

● The issues of concern most frequently cited by these psychologists were
(1) culturally appropriate research methods; (2) cultural competent
mental health service delivery; and (3) minority recruitment, retention,
and training in psychology.

Table 2

Number and Percent of Psychologists of Color by Ethnic Group

ETHNIC GROUP	NUMBER	PERCENTAGE
African American/Black	798	33.17%
American Indian/Alaska Native	106	4.41%
Asian American/Pacific Islander	659	27.39%
Hispanic/Latino(a)	790	32.83%
Multi-Ethnic	53	2.20%
TOTAL	2406	100.00%

Table 3

Number and Percent of Psychologists of Color by Gender and Ethnic Group

ETHNICITY	GENDER			TOTAL	PERCENTAGE
	Male	Female	Unknown		
African American/Black	358	437	3	798	33.17%
American Indian/Alaska Native	63	41	2	106	4.41%
Asian American/Pacific Islander	303	306	50	659	27.39%
Hispanic/Latino(a)	417	368	5	790	32.83%
Multi-Ethnic	24	29	0	53	2.20%
TOTAL	1165	1181	60	2406	100.00%
PERCENT	48.42%	49.09%	2.49%	100.00%	

Table 4

Number of Psychologists of Color by Major Field and by Ethnic Group

MAJOR FIELD	ETHNIC GROUP						TOTAL	PERCE
	African American/Black	American Indian/ Alaska Native	Asian American/ Pacific Islander	Hispanic/Latino(a)	Multi-Ethnic	Unknown		
Clinical Child Psychology	21	2	19	18	1	0	61	2.54
Clinical Psychology	396	44	296	455	28	0	1219	50.67
Cognitive Psychology	3	0	12	10	0	0	25	1.04
Community Psychology	17	0	4	10	1	0	32	1.33
Comparative Psychology	0	0	1	1	0	0	2	0.08
Counseling Psychology	116	22	78	96	13	0	325	13.51
Developmental Psychology	41	5	31	25	3	0	105	4.36
Educational Psychology	36	6	39	21	1	0	103	4.28
Environmental Psychology	3	0	1	0	0	0	4	0.17
Experimental Psychology	8	1	19	8	1	0	37	1.54
General Psychology/Methods and Systems	6	1	4	8	0	0	19	0.79
Gerontology	0	0	3	5	0	0	8	0.33
Health Psychology	4	1	6	3	0	0	14	0.58
Industrial and Organizational Psychology	15	3	24	26	1	0	69	2.87
Neurosciences	5	2	3	6	1	0	17	0.71
Personality Psychology	9	0	5	1	0	0	15	0.62
Physiological Psychology/Psychobiology	4	1	6	8	0	0	19	0.79
Psychopharmacology	1	0	2	2	0	0	5	0.21
Quantitative//Mathematical Psychometrics/Statistics	3	0	11	3	0	0	17	0.71
School Psychology	40	3	15	26	1	0	85	3.53%
Social Psychology	35	8	44	30	1	0	118	4.90%
Other Major Fields	24	7	34	25	0	0	90	3.74%
No Information[a]							17	0.71%
TOTALS	787	106	657	787	52	0	2406	100.00

a - "No Information" consists of persons who did not indicate a major field of study.

Table 5

Number and Percent of Psychologists of Color by Primary Professional Role and Ethnic Group

PRIMARY ROLE	ETHNIC GROUP						TOTAL	PERCENT
	African American/Black	American Indian/ Alaska Native	Asian American/ Pacific Islander	Hispanic/Latino(a)	Multi-Ethnic	Unknown		
Academician	186	16	158	140	11	0	511	21.24%
Administrator	96	10	49	49	5	0	209	8.69%
Consultant	34	9	17	37	1	0	98	4.07%
Other [a]	8	0	10	5	2	0	25	1.04%
Practitioner	246	40	223	362	25	0	896	37.24%
Researcher	41	4	42	35	3	0	125	5.20%
No Information [b]							542	22.53%
TOTAL	611	79	499	628	47	0	2406	100.00%

- Examples of self-identified "Other" roles are: Test developer, publisher/author, clinical supervisor/manager, human resources staff, psychological examiner, program developer, talk show host, and parent educator

- "No Information" consists of persons who did not indicate a professional role.

Table 6

DIVISIONS	ETHNIC GROUP					TOTAL	PERCENT OF DATABASE
	African	American Indian/	Asian	Hispanic/La	Multi-		

Number of Psychologists of Color in the APA Divisions[a]

DIVISIONS	African	American Indian/	Asian	Hispanic/La	Multi-	TOTAL	PERCENT OF DATABASE
Division 01	15	4	24	23	0	66	2.74%
Division 02	23	2	18	10	2	55	2.29%
Division 03	1	1	9	5	0	16	0.67%
Division 04	No Longer Exists						
Division 05	9	5	22	11	0	47	1.95%
Division 06	0	1	2	5	0	8	0.33%
Division 07	14	0	10	6	1	31	1.29%
Division 08	19	3	24	21	1	68	2.83%
Division 09	55	8	29	30	3	125	5.20%
Division 10	2	0	2	6	1	11	0.46%
Division 11	No Longer Exists						
Division 12	87	11	46	61	7	212	8.81%
Division 13	14	1	11	8	1	35	1.45%
Division 14	9	4	18	24	2	57	2.37%
Division 15	18	3	19	9	3	52	2.16%
Division 16	18	4	4	14	2	42	1.75%
Division 17	49	5	29	35	6	124	5.15%
Division 18	6	4	5	8	0	23	0.96%
Division 19	3	0	1	2	0	6	0.25%
Division 20	6	2	10	22	0	40	1.66%
Division 21	2	1	3	2	0	8	0.33%
Division 22	7	1	10	13	0	31	1.29%
Division 23	1	0	4	6	0	11	0.46%
Division 24	3	1	5	12	0	21	0.87%
Division 25	2	2	3	10	0	17	0.71%
Division 26	5	3	0	5	0	13	0.54%
Division 27	28	1	13	11	0	53	2.20%
Division 28	4	2	2	10	0	18	0.75%
Division 29	45	4	25	33	3	110	4.57%

Table 6 Continued

Number of Psychologists of Color in the APA Divisions[a]

DIVISIONS	ETHNIC GROUP					TOTAL	PERCENT OF DATABASE
	African	American Indian/	Asian	Hispanic/La	Multi-		
ivision 30	10	0	9	9	0	28	1.16%
Division 31	3	0	2	2	0	7	0.29%
Division 32	7	0	6	5	0	18	0.75%
Division 33	6	3	3	7	1	20	0.83%
Division 34	2	0	3	1	0	6	0.25%
Division 35	57	6	25	29	1	118	4.90%
Division 36	4	4	9	5	0	22	0.91%
Division 37	17	1	10	12	1	41	1.70%
Division 38	24	2	27	23	0	76	3.16%
Division 39	17	2	9	28	2	58	2.41%
Division 40	19	9	28	58	2	116	4.82%
Division 41	12	5	14	44	0	75	3.12%
Division 42	67	10	41	64	4	186	7.73%
Division 43	10	4	10	18	1	43	1.79%
Division 44	11	4	10	14	0	39	1.62%
Division 45	176	23	91	139	9	438	18.20%
Division 46	3	0	1	6	0	10	0.42%
Division 47	7	2	8	5	0	22	0.91%
Division 48	4	0	2	6	1	13	0.54%
Division 49	11	3	6	11	2	33	1.37%
Division 50	9	5	7	7	1	29	1.21%
Division 51	7	1	1	7	0	16	0.67%
Division 52	10	1	22	17	0	50	2.08%
Division 53	2	0	5	4	1	12	0.50%
Division 54	4	0	7	10	1	22	0.91%
Division 55	0	1	0	0	0	1	0.04%
No Division Affiliation/No Information						1129	46.92%
TOTALS	944	159	704	933	59	3928	163.26%

[a] – Includes both members and fellows.
[b] – APA Members may affiliate with more than one Division

Table 7

Number of Psychologists of Color Fellows in the APA Divisions

DIVISIONS	ETHNIC GROUP					TOTAL	PERCENT OF RESPONSES
	African American/Black	American Indian/ Alaska Native	Asian American/ Pacific Islander	Hispanic/Latino(a)	Multi-Ethnic		
Division 01	0	1	4	2	0	7	4.24%
Division 02	1	0	1	2	0	4	2.42%
Division 03	1	0	1	0	0	2	1.21%
Division 04	No Longer Exists						
Division 05	0	0	1	0	0	1	0.61%
Division 06	0	0	0	2	0	2	1.21%
Division 07	0	0	1	1	1	3	1.82%
Division 08	0	0	0	1	0	1	0.61%
Division 09	2	1	1	3	0	7	4.24%
Division 10	1	0	0	1	0	2	1.21%
Division 11	No Longer Exists						
Division 12	10	1	4	2	0	17	10.30%
Division 13	2	0	0	0	0	2	1.21%
Division 14	0	0	0	0	0	0	0.00%
Division 15	1	0	2	1	0	4	2.42%
Division 16	3	0	1	1	0	5	3.03%
Division 17	5	1	2	4	0	12	7.27%
Division 18	0	0	0	1	0	1	0.61%
Division 19	0	0	0	0	0	0	0.00%
Division 20	0	0	1	1	0	2	1.21%
Division 21	0	0	0	0	0	0	0.00%
Division 22	0	1	2	0	0	3	1.82%
Division 23	0	0	0	0	0	0	0.00%
Division 24	1	0	0	1	0	2	1.21%
Division 25	1	0	0	0	0	1	0.61%
Division 26	0	0	0	0	0	0	0.00%
Division 27	3	1	2	3	0	9	5.45%
Division 28	0	0	0	1	0	1	0.61%
Division 29	6	1	1	1	0	9	5.45%

Table 7 Continued

Number of Psychologists of Color Fellows in the APA Divisions

DIVISIONS	ETHNIC GROUP					TOTAL	PERCENT OF RESPONSES
	African American/Black	American Indian/ Alaska Native	Asian American/ Pacific Islander	Hispanic/Latino(a)	Multi-Ethnic		
Division 30	0	0	1	0	0	1	0.61%
Division 31	0	0	0	0	0	0	0.00%
Division 32	1	0	0	0	0	1	0.61%
Division 33	2	0	0	0	0	2	1.21%
Division 34	0	0	0	0	0	0	0.00%
Division 35	3	0	3	3	0	9	5.45%
Division 36	0	0	0	0	0	0	0.00%
Division 37	3	1	0	0	0	4	2.42%
Division 38	1	0	1	1	0	3	1.82%
Division 39	0	0	0	0	0	0	0.00%
Division 40	0	1	0	1	0	2	1.21%
Division 41	0	0	0	0	0	0	0.00%
Division 42	0	0	0	0	0	0	0.00%
Division 43	0	0	0	1	0	1	0.61%
Division 44	2	0	1	2	0	5	3.03%
Division 45	16	3	8	9	0	36	21.82%
Division 46	0	0	0	0	0	0	0.00%
Division 47	0	0	1	0	0	1	0.61%
Division 48	0	0	0	0	0	0	0.00%
Division 49	1	0	0	0	0	1	0.61%
Division 50	0	0	0	0	0	0	0.00%
Division 51	1	0	0	0	0	1	0.61%
Division 52	1	0	0	0	0	1	0.61%
Division 53	0	0	0	0	0	0	0.00%
Division 54	0	0	0	0	0	0	0.00%
Division 55	0	0	0	0	0	0	0.00%
TOTALS	68	12	24	45	1	165	100.00%

[a] – APA Members may affiliate with more than one Division

Table 8

Number and Percent of Psychologists of Color by Type of Terminal Degree

Type of Degree	Number	Percent of Total in Directory
PhD	2087	86.74%
EdD	101	4.20%
PsyD	107	4.45%
Masters	71	2.95%
No Information [a]	40	1.66%
TOTAL IN DIRECTORY	2406	100.00%

a – "No Information" consists of persons who did not indicate a degree.

Table 9

Number and Percent of Psychologists of Color by Years Since Terminal Degree and Ethnic Group

ETHNICITY	YEARS SINCE TERMINAL DEGREE					TOTAL	PERCENTAG
	0-8	9-15	16-25	⟩25 Years	No Information		
African American/Black	77	212	313	179		781	32.46%
American Indian/Alaska Native	7	27	38	34		106	4.41%
Asian American/Pacific Islander	81	185	190	·195		651	27.06%
Hispanic/Latino(a)	88	269	284	138		779	32.38%
Multi-Ethnic	9	25	10	8		52	2.16%
TOTAL	262	718	835	554	37	2406	100.00%
PERCENT	10.89%	29.84%	34.70%	23.03%	1.54%		

a – "No Information" consists of persons who did not indicate the year of their terminal degree.

Table 10

Survey Of Involvement In Organized Psychology

INVOLVEMENT ITEMS	ETHNIC GROUP						TOTAL	PERCENT[a]
	African American/Black	American Indian/ Alaska Native	Asian American/ Pacific Islander	Hispanic/Latino(a)	Multi-Ethnic	Unknown		
Member of a national Ethnic Minority Psychological Association (EMPA)	155	9	91	52	9	0	316	18.80%
Served as local or national Officer or Committee Chair of an EMPA	74	4	19	13	5	0	115	6.84%
Member of a State Psychological Association (SPA)	133	13	86	124	17	0	373	22.19%
Served as Officer or Committee Chair of a SPA	38	7	30	42	5	0	122	7.26%
Member of a Regional Psychological Association (RPA)	66	11	46	59	10	0	192	11.42%
Served as Officer or Committee Chair of a RPA	20	8	15	16	1	0	60	3.57%
Served as Asst., Assoc., or Senior Journal Editor	47	11	30	39	3	0	130	7.73%
Served on APA Task Force	52	13	18	39	2	0	124	7.38%
Served on APA Committee	69	14	36	54	5	0	178	10.59%
Served on APA Board	30	6	14	21	0	0	71	4.22%
TOTALS	684	96	385	459	57	0	1681	100.00%

[a]Based on total responses to this item (n=1679).

Table 11

Survey Of Involvement In Organized Psychology

FUTURE[a] INVOLVEMENT ITEMS	ETHNIC GROUP						TOTAL	PERCENT[b]
	African American/Black	American Indian/ Alaska Native	Asian American/ Pacific Islander	Hispanic/Latino(a)	Multi-Ethnic	Unknown		
Willing to serve as APA Accreditation Site Visitor	214	34	121	176	21	0	566	16.31%
Willing to serve on Editorial Board of an APA journal	175	25	126	171	16	0	513	14.78%
Willing to serve on APA Task Force, Committee or Board re: Executive Functions	139	22	97	136	13	0	407	11.73%
Willing to serve on APA Task Force, Committee or Board re: Education Issues	175	26	115	161	17	0	494	14.23%
Willing to serve on APA Task Force, Committee or Board re: Practitioner Issues	169	24	99	160	17	0	469	13.51%
Willing to serve on APA Task Force, Committee or Board re: Public Interest Issues	255	33	138	202	22	0	650	18.73%
Willing to serve on APA Task Force, Committee or Board re: Science Issues	128	22	79	128	15	0	372	10.72%
TOTALS	1255	186	775	1134	121	0	3471	100.00%

a – A respondent often selected more than one of these "future involvement" items.
b - Based on total responses to this item (n=3471)

314

Table 12

Survey Of Involvement In Organized Psychology

ISSUES OF CONCERN	ETHNIC GROUP					TOTAL	PERCENT[a]
	African American/Black	American Indian/ Alaska Native	Asian American/ Pacific Islander	Hispanic/Latino(a)	Multi-Ethnic		
Culturally appropriate research methods	110	17	78	107	13	325	25.55%
Culturally competent MH service delivery	97	12	86	89	6	290	22.80%
Diagnosis/treatment of SMI	3	2	5	4	2	16	1.26%
Families & youth	38	3	28	19	2	90	7.08%
HIV/AIDS	2	2	2	6	0	12	0.94%
Health Care Reform: Effects on Communities of Color	27	4	16	30	1	78	6.13%
Health Care Reform: Effects on Psychologists of Color	5	0	6	2	0	13	1.02%
Minority recruitment, retention & training in psychology	77	2	37	51	7	174	13.68%
Professional advancement/income	19	2	14	18	3	56	4.40%
Public schools/education	26	2	13	19	5	65	5.11%
Research funding	7	1	14	12	0	34	2.67%
Substance abuse	4	3	0	5	0	12	0.94%
Testing & assessment bias	16	3	16	26	1	62	4.87%
Violence prevention	13	1	5	10	2	31	2.44%
Other						14	0.01%
TOTALS	444	54	320	398	42	1272	

a – Based on total responses (n=1272) to this item

Appendices

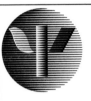

A Chairs of APA's Board/
Committee of Ethnic Minority Affairs
(1980–2000)

B Mission and Goals of APA's
Office of Ethnic Minority Affairs
(OEMA)

C The National Ethnic Minority
Psychological Associations

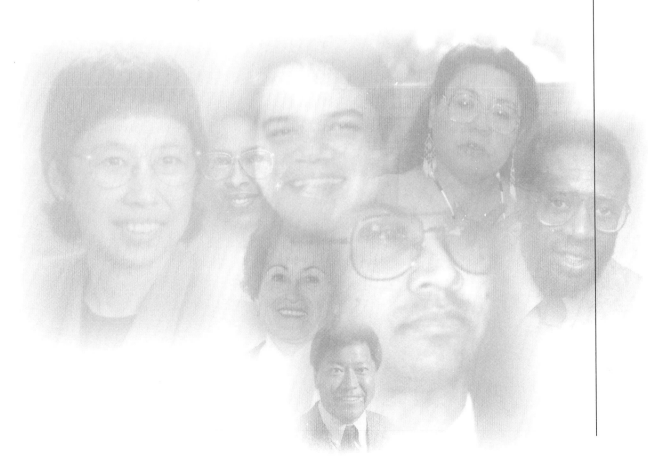

CHAIRS AND MEMBERS OF APA'S BOARD/COMMITTEE OF ETHNIC MINORITY AFFAIRS (1980 - 2000)

Committee on Ethnic Minority Affairs

Chairpersons
Asuncion Miteria Austria, PhD (2000)
Tony L. Strickland, PhD (1999)
Melinda A. Garcia, PhD (1998)
Joseph J. Horvat, Jr., PhD (1997)
Jean L. Chin, EdD (1996)
Fernando I. Soriano, PhD (1995)
Robin A. LaDue, PhD (1994)
Dozier W. Thornton, PhD (1993)
Irma Serrano-Garcia, PhD (1992)
Bertha G. Holliday, PhD (1991)

Membership
Asuncion Miteria Austria, PhD (1998-2000)
Martha E. Banks, PhD (1999-2001)
Sandra K. Bennett Choney, PhD (1996-98)
Alice F. Chang, PhD (1991)
Jean Lau Chin, EdD (!995-98)
Melinda A. Garcia, PhD (1996-98)
Bertha G. Holliday, PhD (1991)
Joseph J. Horvat, Jr., PhD (1995-98)
Adelbert H. Jenkins, PhD (1994-97)
Ernest Johnson, PhD (1993-97)
Robin A. LaDue, PhD (1991-96)
Jeffrey Scott Mio (1998-2000)
Freddy A. Paniagua, PhD (2000-02)
William D. Parham, PhD (2000-02)
W. LaVome Robinson, PhD (1992-96)
Maria P. P. Root, PhD (1992-95)
Irma Serrano-Garcia, PhD (1991-93)
Fernando Soriano, PhD (1994-97)
Tony L. Strickland, PhD (1997-99)
Jeffrey S. Tanaka, PhD (1991-92)
Dozier W. Thornton, PhD (1991-95)
Roberto J. Velasquez, PhD (1997-99)
Diane J. Willis, PhD (1999-2001)

Board of Ethnic Minority Affairs

Chairpersons
G. Rita Dudley Grant, PhD (1990)
Candace M. Fleming, PhD (1989)
Sarah D. Miyahira, PhD (1988)
Joe L. Martinez, PhD (1987)
Teresa D. LaFromboise, PhD (1986)
Maxine L. Rawlings, PhD (1985)
Floyd H. Martinez, PhD (1984)
Richard M. Suinn, PhD (1981-83)

Membership
Martha R. Alonso, PhD (1981-82)
Hortensia Amaro, PhD (1989-90)
Maisha B. H. Bennett, PhD (1985)
Samuel Q. Chan, PhD (1987)
Alice F. Chang, PhD (1989-90)
Catherine A. Cornwell-Jones, PhD (1981-82)
Candace M. Fleming, PhD (1989-90; 1987-88)
Gary A. France, PhD (1981-83)
Pearl Dansby, PhD (1983-85)
G. Rita Dudley-Grant, PhD (1988-90)
Richard P. Duran, PhD (1988-90)
Halford H. Fairchild, PhD (1984-86)
Angela B. Ginorio, PhD (1987-89)
Asa G. Hilliard, PhD (1982-84)
Bertha G. Holliday (1986-87; 1989-90)
Clive D. Kennedy, PhD (1986-88)
Robin A. LaDue, PhD (1990)
Teresa D. LaFromboise, PhD (1984-86)
Gladys Lorenzo, PhD (1983-85)
Dorita R. Marina, PhD (1986-88)
Floyd H. Martinez, PhD (1981-84)
Joe L. Martinez, PhD (1985-87)
Damian A. McShane, PhD (1988-89)
Sarah D. Miyahira, PhD (1986-88)
John Moritsugu, PhD (1988-89)
Charles J. Pine, PhD (1985-87)
Ana M. Ramirez, PhD (1981-83)
Robert A. Ramos, PhD (1984-86)
Maxine L. Rawlings, PhD (1983-85)

Pamela T. Reid, PhD (1989-90)
Diane T. Slaughter, PhD (1986-88)
Irma Serrano-Garcia, PhD (1990)
Guy O. Seymour, PhD (1981-83)
Richard M. Suinn, PhD (1981-83)
Jeffrey S. Tanaka, PhD (1990)
Dalmas A. Taylor, PhD (1987-89)
Dozier W. Thornton, PhD (1990)
Henry Tomes, PhD (1981)
Joseph E. Trimble, PhD (1981-84)
Gail E. Wyatt, PhD (1981-82)
Herbert Z. Wong, PhD (1984-86)
Harry G. Yamaguchi, PhD (1983-85)
Albert H. Yee, PhD (1981-82)

Ad hoc Committee to Establish the Board of Ethnic Minority Affairs - 1980

Chairperson
Henry Tomes, PhD

Membership
Catherine A. Cornwell-Jones, PhD
William A. Hayes, PhD
C. Diane Howell, PhD
Richard E. Lopez, PhD
Jose Szapocznik, PhD
Joseph E. Trimble, PhD
Reiko H. True, PhD
Ana M. Ramirez, PhD
Loye M. Ryan, PhD

MISSION AND GOALS:
APA OFFICE OF ETHNIC MINORITY AFFAIRS

In 1978, APA's Board of Directors and Council of Representatives authorized the establishment of an APA Office of Ethnic Minority Affairs (OEMA) by January, 1979. This action was taken in response to the recommendations of a national conference on "Expanding the roles of culturally diverse people in the profession of psychology". This conference was convened at the Marriott Hotel at Dulles Airport. The "Dulles Conference" was sponsored by the National Institute of Mental Health's Center for Minority Group Mental Health and by APA's Board of Directors and Board of Social and Ethical Responsibility. The Conference's purpose as stated in its agenda was as follows.

> *To bring together ethnic minority psychologists to consider what concerns, needs, and objectives might exist among the different ethnic groups... and to explore how the APA governance structure and function can be altered to improve its relevance, usefulness and representativeness with regard to ethnic minority psychologists and their communities.*

Consistent with the spirit of the Dulles Conference, OEMA is committed to coordinating, advocating, and implementing policies on ethnic minority issues related to education and training, science, and the practice of psychology. OEMA's specific goals and responsibilities are the following.

- Cultivate and advance increased scientific understanding of culture and ethnicity as they relate to psychology.

- Strive to increase the quality and quantity of education and training opportunities in psychology for ethnic minority persons.

- Promote the development of culturally sensitive models for delivery of psychological services.

- Promote the interests of ethnic minority psychologists and their communities by networking and communicating within the APA, its governance structure and divisions, as well as with other organizations, be they public or private, federal or state.

- Increase the number of ethnic minority psychologists within the APA and in the field of psychology.

- Support and facilitate the operations of the APA Committee on Ethnic Minority Affairs and its Task Forces.

<u>Appendix C</u>

THE NATIONAL ETHNIC MINORITY PSYCHOLOGICAL ASSOCIATIONS

The Asian American Psychological Association

The Association of Black Psychologists

The Hispanic Psychological Association

The Society for the Psychological Study of Ethnic Minority Issues
(Division 45 of APA)

The Society of Indian Psychologists

The Presidents of these Associations along with the APA President (or his/her designee) constitute the *Council of National Psychological Associations for the Advancement of Ethnic Minority Interests (CNPAAEMI)*. The goals of the Council are:

- to promote the professional/career development of ethnic/racial minority psychologists;

- to advance multicultural competence of psychologists;

- to promote culturally competent service delivery models of psychological care;

- to increase the recruitment and retention of ethnic/racial minorities in the profession of psychology;

- to liaison and collaborate with other appropriate organizations interested in ethnic/racial minority issues and/or projects;

- to promote research and understanding using alternative cultural paradigms.

The current mailing address, phone number, and roster of officers for the Ethnic Minority Associations can be secured from APA's Office of Ethnic Minority Affairs.